STUDENT WORKBOOK FOR

Medical Assisting: Foundations and Practices

MARGARET SCHELL FRAZIER
CHRISTINE MALONE
KRISTIANA SUE ROUTH

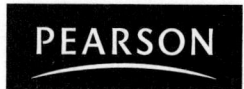

PEARSON

Upper Saddle River, New Jersey 07458

Pearson ® is a registered trademark of Pearson plc

Pearson Education, Ltd., London
Pearson Education Singapore, Pte. Ltd.
Pearson Education Canada, Inc.
Pearson Education—Japan
Pearson Education, Australia PTY, Limited

Pearson Education North Asia, Ltd., Hong Kong
Pearson Education de Mexico, S.A. de C.V.
Pearson Education Malaysia, Pte. Ltd.
Pearson Education, Upper Saddle River, New Jersey

Prentice Hall
is an imprint of

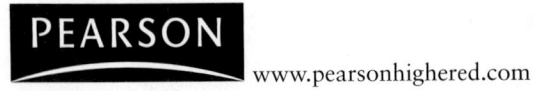

www.pearsonhighered.com

10 9 8 7 6 5 4 3 2 1
ISBN 13: 978-0-13-502363-1
ISBN 10:   0-13-502363-7

Contents

Mastery of Competency Skills

Procedure Number	Procedure Title	Date Mastered	Instructor's Signature
2-1	Adapt to Change		
4-1	Prepare an Informed Consent for Treatment Form		
4-2	Obtain Authorization for the Release of Patient Medical Records		
4-3	Respond to a Request for Copies of a Patient's Medical Record		
5-1	Use Effective Listening Skills in Patient Interviews		
5-2	Communicate with a Hearing-Impaired Patient		
5-3	Communicate with a Sight-Impaired Patient		
5-4	Communicate with a Patient via Interpreter		
5-5	Identify Community Resources		
5-6	Prepare a Patient's Specialist Referral		
6-1	Use the Internet to Find Patient Education Materials		
8-1	Compose a Business Letter		
8-2	Prepare a Document for Photocopying		
8-3	Send a Letter to a Patient About a Missed Appointment		
8-4	Proofread Written Documents		
8-5	Fold Documents for Window Envelopes		
8-6	Open and Sort Mail		
8-7	Annotate Written Correspondence		
9-1	Answer the Telephone in a Professional Manner		
9-2	Take a Telephone Message		
9-3	Call a Pharmacy with Prescription Orders		
10-1	Open the Office		
10-2	Greet and Register Patients		
10-3	Collect Payments at the Front Desk		
10-4	Close the Office		

Procedure Number	Procedure Title	Date Mastered	Instructor's Signature
11-1	Establish an Appointment Matrix		
11-2	Schedule New Patient		
11-3	Schedule an Established Patient Appointment		
11-4	Use Patient Reminder Cards		
11-5	Reschedule a Missed Patient Appointment		
11-6	Manage the Physician's Professional Schedule and Travel		
11-7	Schedule a Hospital Procedure		
11-8	Schedule an Inpatient Admission		
12-1	Prepare and Maintain the Medical Record		
12-2	Chart Patient Telephone Calls		
12-3	File Documents Using the Alphabetic Filing System		
12-4	File Manually Using a Subject Filing System		
12-5	File Documents in Patient Medical Records		
12-6	Use the Numeric System to File Medical Records		
12-7	Correct Errors in the Patient Medical Record		
13-1	Correct an Electronic Medical Record		
14-1	Use Computer Software to Maintain Office Systems		
14-2	Use an Internet Search Engine		
14-3	Verify Preferred Provider Status on an Insurance Company Web Site		
15-1	Take Inventory of Administrative and Clinical Equipment for Maintenance and Other Purposes		
15-2	Perform Routine Maintenance of a Computer Printer		
15-3	Fax a Document		
15-4	Prepare a Purchase Order		
15-5	Receive a Supply Shipment		

Procedure Number	Procedure Title	Date Mastered	Instructor's Signature
16-1	Create an Office Brochure		
16-2	Create a Clinical Procedure for the Procedure Manual		
16-3	Create an Administrative Procedure for the Procedure Manual		
17-1	Calculate Deductible, Coinsurance, and Allowable Amounts		
17-2	Verify a Patient's Insurance Eligibility		
17-3	Obtain a Managed Care Referral		
17-4	Obtain Authorization from an Insurance Company for a Procedure		
17-5	Abstract Data to Complete a Paper CMS-1500 Claim Form		
17-6	Complete a Computerized Insurance Claim Form		
17-7	Handle a Denied Insurance Claim		
18-1	Perform Diagnostic Coding		
19-1	Code for a Procedure		
20-1	Post an Entry on a Day Sheet		
20-2	Prepare an Accounts Receivable Trial Balance		
20-3	Explain Professional Fees to a Patient		
20-4	Calling a Patient Regarding an Overdue Account		
20-5	Send a Patient Billing Statement		
20-6	Post a Nonsufficient Funds Check		
20-7	Post an Adjustment to a Patient Account		
20-8	Post a Collection Agency Payment		
20-9	Process a Patient Refund		
20-10	Process an Insurance Company Overpayment		
21-1	Create a New Employee Record		
21-2	Calculate an Employee's Payroll		
21-3	Write Checks to Pay Bills		

Procedure Number	Procedure Title	Date Mastered	Instructor's Signature
21-4	Pay an Office Supply Invoice		
21-5	Complete a Deposit Slip		
21-6	Account for Petty Cash		
21-7	Reconcile a Bank Statement		
22-1	Direct a Staff Meeting		
22-2	Write a Job Description		
22-3	Conduct an Interview		
22-4	Call Employee References		
22-5	Perform an Employee Evaluation		
22-6	Discipline an Employee		
22-7	Terminate an Employee		
23-1	File a Medical Incident Report		
23-2	Develop an Exposure Control Plan		
24-1	Complete a Patient History Form		
24-2	Document a Clinical Visit and Procedure		
25-1	Perform Correct HandWashing		
25-2	Demonstrate Nonsterile Gloving		
26-1	Demonstrate the Performance of Sanitization		
26-2	Demonstrate Disinfection Procedures		
26-3	Demonstrate How to Wrap Surgical Instruments and Prepare Sterile Trays for Autoclave Sterilization		
26-4	Demonstrate Correct Procedure for Loading and Operating an Autoclave		
26-5	Demonstrate Correct Procedure for Pouring Sterile Solution onto a Sterile Field		
26-6	Demonstrate Correct Procedure for Opening a Sterile Surgical Pack to Create a Sterile Field		
26-7	Demonstrate the Correct Procedure for Using Transfer Forceps		
26-8	Demonstrate a Sterile Scrub (Surgical Hand Washing)		

Procedure Number	Procedure Title	Date Mastered	Instructor's Signature
26-9	Demonstrate How to Glove While Wearing a Sterile Gown		
26-10	Demonstrate Sterile Gloving and Removal		
27-1	Demonstrate Safety Measures to Prepare, Administer, and Document Medication		
27-2	Demonstrate the Preparation of a Prescription for the Physician's Signature		
27-3	Demonstrate Withdrawing Medication from an Ampule		
27-4	Demonstrate Withdrawing Medication from a Vial		
27-5	Demonstrate the Reconstitution of a Powdered Drug for Injection Administration		
27-6	Demonstrate the Administration of Medication during Infusion Therapy		
27-7	Demonstrate the Preparation and Administration of Oral Medication		
27-8	Demonstrate the Administration of a Subcutaneous Injection		
27-9	Demonstrate the Administration of an Intramuscular Injection to Adults and Children		
27-10	Demonstrate the Administration of a Z-Track Injection		
28-1	Obtain an Oral Temperature with an Electronic Digital Thermometer		
28-2	Obtain an Axillary Temperature with an Electronic Digital Thermometer		
28-3	Obtain a Rectal Temperature with an Electronic Digital Thermometer		
28-4	Obtain an Aural Temperature with a Tympanic Thermometer		
28-5	Obtain a Dermal Temperature with a Disposable Thermometer		
28-6	Perform a Radial Pulse Count		
28-7	Perform an Apical Pulse Count		
28-8	Perform a Respiration Count		

Procedure Number	Procedure Title	Date Mastered	Instructor's Signature
28-9	Perform a Blood Pressure Measurement		
28-10	Obtain Weight and Height Measurements		
28-11	Demonstrate Patient Positions Used in a Medical Examination		
28-12	Prepare the Patient for Medical Examination and Assist the Physician		
29-1	Prepare the Skin for Surgical Procedure		
29-2	Set Up a Surgical Tray and Assist the Physician with Minor Surgical Procedures		
29-3	Assist the Physician with Suturing		
29-4	Assist the Physician with Suture or Staple Removal		
29-5	Change a Sterile Dressing		
30-1	Check the Accuracy of Glucometer Results Using Quality Control Methods		
30-2	Screen and Follow up Test Results		
31-1	Demonstrate Correct Use of the Microscope		
31-2	Prepare a Specimen Smear for Microbiological Examination		
31-3	Prepare a Gram Stain		
31-4	Instruct a Patient in the Collection of a Fecal Specimen for Occult Blood or Culture Testing and Develop the Fecal Occult Blood Test		
31-5	Perform a Wound or Throat Culture Collection Using Sterile Swabs		
31-6	Perform Rapid Group A Strep Testing		
32-1	Perform a Butterfly Draw Using a Hand Vein		
32-2	Perform a Venipuncture		
32-3	Demonstrate a Venipuncture Using the Syringe Method		
32-4	Perform a Capillary Puncture		
32-5	Perform a WBC and Platelet Count with a Unopette Vial and Hemacytometer		
32-6	Prepare a Blood Smear for a Differentiated Cell Count		

Procedure Number	Procedure Title	Date Mastered	Instructor's Signature
32-7	Prepare a Smear Stained with Wright's Stain		
32-8	Perform a Microhematocrit by Capillary Tube		
32-9	Perform a Hemoglobin Test Using a Hemoglobulinometer		
32-10	Perform an ESR Using the Wintrobe Method		
32-11	Measure Blood Glucose Using the Accu-Chek™ Glucometer		
32-12	Perform a Blood Cholesterol Measurement Using the ProAct Testing Device		
32-13	Perform a Test for Infectious Mononucleosis		
33-1	Demonstrate Patient Instruction for a Clean-Catch Urine Specimen		
33-2	Demonstrate Patient Instruction for Collection of 24-Hour Urine Specimen		
33-3	Perform Catheterization of a Female Patient		
33-4	Perform Catheterization of a Male Patient		
33-5	Measure Urine Specific Gravity with a Refractometer		
33-6	Perform Urinalysis Using Chemical Test Strips		
33-7	Perform a Multi-Drug Screen Urine Test Using the Instant-View Multi-Drug Screen Test		
33-8	Demonstrate Patient Instruction for Testicular Self-Examination		
34-1	Perform the General Procedure for an X-Ray Examination		
34-2	File and Loan Radiographic Records		
35-1	Perform an Electrocardiogram		
35-2	Demonstrate the Application of a Holter Monitor		
36-1	Demonstrate Performance of Spirometry		
36-2	Demonstrate Performance of Measuring Oxygen Saturation Using a Pulse Oximeter		

Procedure Number	Procedure Title	Date Mastered	Instructor's Signature
36-3	Demonstrate Performance of Peak Flow Testing		
36-4	Demonstrate Performance of the Mantoux Test by Intradermal Injection		
36-5	Demonstrate Patient Instruction in the Use of an Inhaler		
36-6	Demonstrate Patient Assistance in the Use of a Nebulizer		
37-1	Measure Distance Visual Acuity with a Snellen Chart		
37-2	Perform the Ishihara Color Vision Test		
37-3	Perform Eye Irrigation		
37-4	Perform Instillation of Eye Medication		
37-5	Perform Simple Audiometry		
37-6	Perform Ear Irrigation		
37-7	Perform Instillation of Ear Medication		
37-8	Assist with the Nasal Examination and Obtain a Nasopharyngeal Specimen		
41-1	Perform Adult Rescue Breathing and One-Rescuer CPR		
41-2	Use an Automated External Defibrillator (AED)		
41-3	Respond to an Adult with an Obstructed Airway		
41-4	Administer Oxygen		
41-5	Respond to a Patient Who Has Fainted		
41-6	Demonstrate the Application of a Pressure Bandage		
41-7	Demonstrate the Application of Triangular, Figure 8, and Tubular Bandages		
41-8	Demonstrate the Application of a Splint		
41-9	Develop an Environmental Exposure Plan		
42-1	Assist with a Colon Endoscopic/Colonoscopy Exam		
42-2	Assist with a Sigmoidoscopy		

Procedure Number	Procedure Title	Date Mastered	Instructor's Signature
42-3	Insert a Rectal Suppository		
43-1	Assist with Fiberglass Cast Application		
43-2	Assist with Cast Removal		
43-3	Assist the Patient with Cold Application/Cold Compress		
43-4	Assist the Patient with Hot Moist Application/Hot Compress		
43-5	Assisting with Therapeutic Ultrasonography		
43-6	Demonstrate Measuring for Axillary Crutches		
43-7	Assist a Patient with Crutch Walking		
43-8	Assist a Patient Using a Cane		
43-9	Assist a Patient Using a Walker		
43-10	Assist a Patient in a Wheelchair to and from an Exam Table		
44-1	Assist with a Prenatal Exam		
44-2	Instruct the Patient in Breast Self-Examination		
44-3	Assist the Physician in the Performance of a Pelvic Examination and Pap Test		
44-4	Perform a Urine Pregnancy Test		
44-5	Assist with Cryosurgery		
45-1	Perform and Record Measurements of Height or Length, Weight, and Head and Chest Circumference		
45-2	Perform and Record Pediatric Vital Signs and Vision Screening		
45-3	Perform Documentation of Immunizations, Both Stored and Administered		
45-4	Perform Urine Collection with a Pediatric Urine Collection Bag		
46-1	Assisting in a Neurological Exam		
46-2	Assisting with a Lumbar Puncture		
46-3	Prepare a Patient for an Electroencephalogram		

Procedure Number	Procedure Title	Date Mastered	Instructor's Signature
49-1	Role-Play Sensorimotor Changes of the Elderly		
51-1	Write an Effective Resume		
51-2	Compose a Cover Letter		
51-3	Follow Up with an Employer After an Interview		

INTRODUCTION

This student workbook is designed as a study guide and practice tool to accompany the student text, *Medical Assisting: Foundations and Practices*. Read the chapter outlines and use the study guide to reinforce what you have learned. Test your knowledge of medical terminology by completing the variety of activities in the Medical Terminology Review section. Measure whether you have achieved the learning objectives in each chapter by completing the exercises in the Applied Practice and Learning Activities sections of the workbook. Apply your knowledge to real-life situations by answering the Critical Thinking Questions. Use outside resources to complete the research activity at the end of each chapter.

Each chapter of this student workbook includes the following:

Chapter Outline: This is a list of the major content areas in the chapter. Review each of the topics and refer to your textbook for any topics that remain unclear to you.

Student Study Guide: This is of material presented in the chapter. Fill in the blanks, or answer the questions by following PowerPoint presentations in class, or reading through your text.

Applied Practice: Use the knowledge you learned in the chapter to complete these activities.

Learning Activities: These questions/tasks allow you to measure whether or not you have achieved the learning objectives for the chapter.

Medical Terminology Review: This section tests your knowledge of the medical terminology presented in the chapter.

Critical Thinking Questions: These challenging questions allow you to apply your knowledge to real-life situations.

Research Activity: Use outside sources to complete these activities and go beyond the classroom.

Procedure Skill Sheets: These boxed procedures, found in the back of the workbook, correspond to those in the student textbook and allow students to demonstrate the skills needed to become a medical assistant. A space is included for your instructor to document that you have successfully completed the skill. Each step is weighted to better indicate proficiency in the skill.

LIST OF REVIEWERS

Janet R. Sesser, RMA(AMT), CMA(AAMA)
Assistant Vice Provost Academic Administration
High-Tech Institute/The Chubb Institute
Phoenix, AZ

Robyn Gohsman, RMA, CMAS
Former Medical Assisting Program Director
Medical Careers Institute
Newport News, VA

Minda Brown, RMA
Pima Medical Institute
Colorado Springs, CO

CHAPTER 1
The Medical Assistant Profession and the History of Health Care

CHAPTER OUTLINE

General review of the chapter:

    A. Introduction
    B. The Medical Assistant's Role in Health Care
    C. The History of Medicine
    D. Ethics and Patient Rights
    E. Professionalism
    F. The Medical Assistant's Scope of Practice
    G. Job Opportunities
    H. Educational Requirements of Medical Assistants

STUDENT STUDY GUIDE

Use the following guide to assist in your learning of the concepts from the chapter.

  I. The MA's Role in Health Care

    A. MAs fill the need for trained _____ and play a vital role in the health care field.
    B. MAs must:

    _____

    _____

    _____

    _____

    _____

    C. The future provides challenges and unlimited _____ for _____ for MAs.

  II. The History of Medicine and Hand Washing in Health Care

    A. _____ _____ evolved from discovering healing or harmful plants.
    B. Origins of diseases and illnesses were believed to be rooted in the _____.
    C. Medicines
       i. Early medicines were developed from _____ and _____.

    _____

    _____

    _____

_____

_____

   ii. In the world of medicine some plants are still used to treat:

_____

_____

_____

_____

_____

D. Supernatural Causes of Disease
   i. Supernatural, evil spirits or _____ _____ were believed to be the cause of disease.
   ii. Sorcerers and _____ tortured patients to excise spirits or _____ holes in the skull to release _____.
   iii. Less painful methods included dancing, the use of talismans, charms, or _____.

E. Early Egyptian Medicine
   i. Dates back to _____ B.C.:
     (a) Included treating tuberculosis, pneumonia, and even performing surgery
     (b) _____: early Egyptian contributor was thought to have authored information found in the Edwin Smith Papyrus.
     (c) _____ _____ _____: the earliest known medical compilation of cures, examination findings, and prognoses of the time from various authors.

F. Early Chinese Medicine
   i. Believed in living in an interconnected, _____ _____ with the world.
   ii. Classical Chinese practitioners believed in five methods believed to achieve good health:

_____

_____

_____

_____

_____

_____

G. Early Native American Medicine
   i. Dates back _____ years in the United States:
     (a) Concept based on honoring patient's wishes, not forcing treatment
   ii. Suicide was considered the ultimate form of _____:
     (a) The _____ and _____ would often not eat and refuse treatment during times of famine.
   iii. Those who recovered from sickness were believed to have _____ powers.
   iv. Due to lack of written language, early Native American healers passed on medical traditions through oral means.

H. Early Contributors to Medicine
   i. _____: father of medicine
   ii. _____: ideas based on anatomy and physiology
   iii. _____ _____: father of modern anatomy

iv. _____ _____ discovered heart pumped blood
v. _____ founded epidemiology.
vi. _____ _____: first to study bacteria and protozoa with microscope
vii. _____ _____ employed the first anesthesia, ether-based, in 1842.
viii. _____ _____ developed the hypodermic needle in 1853.
ix. _____ _____ discovered X-rays while working with vacuum tubes in 1895.
x. _____ _____ invented the first electrocardiograph (EKG) in the early 1900s.

I. The Hippocratic Oath
   i. Has guided physicians for over _____
   ii. Established as an art of healing, not harming
   iii. Serves as foundation for medical ethics today

J. Hand Washing in Health Care
   i. Ignaz Semmelweiss: In _____ discovered the importance of proper hand hygiene
   ii. He found:

   _____
   _____
   _____
   _____

   iii. Why:

   _____
   _____
   _____
   _____
   _____
   _____
   _____
   _____
   _____

   iv. His study proved death rates _____ _____ when proper hand hygiene was used.

K. Antisepsis in Health Care
   i. _____ _____: in 1867 found that applying antiseptic to wounds would help avoid _____
   ii. He began a study on antisepsis, based on the work of Louis Pasteur.
   iii. Louis Pasteur integrated the use of heat for _____ of surgical instruments.
   iv. Louis Pasteur is considered the father of _____ _____.

III. Important Organizations in Medical History

   A. Over the years, many organizations have formed to advance areas in medicine.
   B. _____ _____ built America's first hospital in 1751.
   C. American Hospital Association (AHA) listed over 5,700 hospitals in the United States in the year 2005.
   D. Hospitals fall into one of four categories:
      i. General or community hospital

   _____
   _____

     ii. Teaching hospitals

_____

_____

_____

    iii. Specialty hospitals

_____

_____

_____

    iv. Research hospitals

_____

_____

_____

  E. The American Medical Association (AMA)
     i. The American Medical Association (AMA) began its contribution to medicine at the University of Pennsylvania in 1847.
    ii. The goals of the AMA include:

_____

_____

_____

_____

  F. American Red Cross
     i. The American Red Cross was founded in _____ by a nurse named _____ _____.
    ii. The American Red Cross is one of the largest_____ organizations in the world.
    iii. Barton, at age _____, also founded the National First Aid Society.

IV. Important Women in Health Care
  A. Women have played a profound role in medical history throughout the years.
  B. _____ _____ is considered one of the first notable women in health care.
     i. She was known for her work with _____.
    ii. In 1903, she became the first woman in France to complete her doctorate.
    iii. She is the only woman, to this day, to win two _____ _____ in two different fields.
  C. _____ _____ is considered the founder of nursing.
     i. She helped advance the care of the poor and improve medical care.
    ii. She founded England Nightingale School of Nursing in _____.
    iii. The Nightingale School of Nursing trains nurses to this day.
  D. _____ _____ was the first degreed female to practice medicine in the United States.

      i. She endured many _____ and _____ in the medical field due to her gender.

      ii. Overcoming these obstacles, she opened her own hospital in _____ in New York.

E. _____ _____, Elizabeth's sister, was the third woman in the United States to earn her medical degree.

      i. She worked at the New York hospital opened by her sister.

      ii. In _____ the Blackwell sisters founded the Women's Medical College in New York.

F. As of 2004, _____ of the physicians in the United States were females.

V. The WHO, Ethics and Patient's Rights

  A. The World Health Organization

      i. Abbreviated WHO

      ii. Founded on April 17, 1948. Today this date is celebrated as World Health Day.

      iii. Goals of WHO include:

_____

_____

_____

_____

_____

_____

_____

_____

  B. AMA's Principles of Medical Ethics

      i. Was developed in 1847

      ii. It covers:

_____

_____

_____

_____

_____

      iii. It was decided that the term ethical refers to _____ _____ or practices and matters of social policy involving issues of morality in practicing medicine.

      iv. Professional conduct not adhering to these standards or policies is considered unethical.

  C. Patient Bill of Rights

      i. Written in _____ by the American Hospital Association

        (a) It focuses on protecting patient rights.

        (b) Rather than physicians telling patients what to do, patients are now more involved in _____ regarding medical care.

      ii. The bill was revised in 1992 and all medical facilities were encouraged to adopt it.

VI. Medical Assistant Professionalism, Job Opportunities, Credentialing and Education

  A. Professional Requirements

      i. Professional requirements include both physical and personal characteristics.

      ii. Physical characteristics include:

_____

_____

_____

_____

_____

_____

_____

_____

B. The MA's Scope of Practice
   i. The MA's Scope of Practice was developed by the American Association of Medical Assistants (AAMA).
      (a) Medical assisting is defined as a/an _____ _____ profession whose practitioners perform _____ and _____ procedures.
      (b) Clinical and administrative duties are performed under a supervising physician's scope of practice that is consistent with the medical assistant's _____.
   ii. Duties will be based on an assigned job description and _____ _____.
   iii. MAs must stay current on laws concerning their scope of practice.
   iv. Medical assistants are not licensed professionals.
      (a) However, their duties may _____ those of licensed health care professionals.
C. Employment Opportunities
   i. Outpatient and inpatient settings:

_____

_____

_____

_____

   ii. Rehabilitation facilities
   iii. Freestanding clinics
   iv. Hospital/physician's office:

_____

_____

_____

_____

D. Job Outlook
   i. Forecast for Medical Assistant careers is promising due to:

_____

_____

_____

   ii. Strength of training in administrative and clinical tasks will allow a greater variety of jobs.
E. Credentialing
   i. AAMA
      (a) Offers the _____ credential
      (b) Eligible candidates must:
         (1) Graduate from a/an _____ or _____ accredited program
         (2) Meet all other AAMA standards
         (3) Submit an application and supporting documentation for consideration

(c) As of _____ _____ testing was made available in a computerized format.

(d) CMAs (AAMA) must recertify every _____ _____ or meet continuing education requirements.

   ii. AMT

     (a) Offers the _____ credential

     (b) Eligible candidates must:

       (1) Graduate from ABHES or CAAHEP accredited school *or*

       (2) Graduate from approved DOE school with _____ hours and externship *or*

       (3) Have formal training in _____ _____ _____ *or* employment for 5 years in field (no more than two years teaching at a post-secondary school)

     (c) Candidates must meet all other AMT standards and submit an application for review.

     (d) Certification Continuation Program requires documentation of activities supporting MA skills every _____ years

F. Educational Requirements

   i. Medical Assistant programs are offered by:

     (a) Vocational and technical training institutes

     (b) Community colleges

   ii. Programs can be accredited by:

_____

_____

_____

_____

_____

   iii. Accredited programs must teach all areas of the AAMA _____ _____ Chart.

   iv. Externship is the _____ phase of medical assisting programs.

   v. In externship, the MA student is working under the supervision of a physician.

   vi. Externship programs can run anywhere between _____ and _____ clock hours.

KEY TERMINOLOGY REVIEW

Complete the sentences below using the correct key terms found at the beginning of the chapter.

1. One of Juan's greatest qualities as a medical assistant was his ability to show _____ to his patients at the oncology clinic where he was employed.

2. Roman was the _____ manager for Sabol Internal Medicine, where he was in charge of scheduling, records management, and billing and coding staff.

3. The _____ _____ _____ often recruits volunteers to help families in emergency crisis, generally after fire, flood, hurricane, and other natural disasters.

4. Malcolm was scheduled to take a Medical Assistant Review class that would prepare him to enter his _____, which was necessary to complete his medical assistant training.

5. Faviola found during her medical assistant training that she favored _____ skills because she loved phlebotomy, injections, and performing EKGs.

6. Often at community colleges, a/an _____ _____ is awarded after 2 years of study.

7. To numb the pain, Dr. Antolik gave his patient a local _____ prior to the removal of an in-grown toenail.

8. Mrs. Krichko took her anatomy and physiology class to the local morgue to view a/an _____ and witness its dissection for pathological study.

9. Michaela received a promising _____ because the cancer was found in its very early stages.

10. Prior to suturing a wound it is important to apply a/an _____ to prevent the growth and reproduction of bacteria.

APPLIED PRACTICE

Match the early contributor of medicine with his or her accomplishment.

a.	Hippocrates	f.	Leeuwenhoek
b.	Galen	g.	Long
c.	Vesalius	h.	Wood
d.	Harvey	i.	Semmelweiss
e.	Sydenham	j.	Lister

_____ 1. Discovered how the heart pumps blood through the circulatory system

_____ 2. First to study bacteria and protozoa using a microscope

_____ 3. His experiment with hand washing reduced the death rate of women who delivered babies in hospitals.

_____ 4. He practiced and taught medicine on the island of Kos, Greece. He is known as the father of medicine.

_____ 5. First to employ modern anesthesia, using an ether-based anesthesia

_____ 6. Through his dissections of the human body, he became known as the father of modern anatomy.

_____ 7. He is known as the English Hippocrates; he founded the science of epidemiology.

_____ 8. He invented the first hypodermic needle in 1853.

_____ 9. He developed the technique for taking a pulse.

_____ 10. Discovered that an antiseptic on wounds helped prevent infection

LEARNING ACTIVITY: TRUE/FALSE

Indicate whether the statement is true (T) or false (F).

_____ 1. The Hippocratic Oath is no longer used, but it has been around for nearly 2,000 years.

_____ 2. The American Medical Association wrote a code of ethics for physicians in 1846.

_____ 3. A medical assistant can only call him- or herself a nurse if certified by either an ABHES- or a CAAHEP-accredited medical assisting program.

_____ 4. Many early and historic plant remedies are still used today for heart conditions, indigestion, bleeding, and urinary tract infections.

_____ 5. The term *trepanning* means to bore a hole in the patient's skull to release evil spirits.

_____ 6. Galen (A.D. 129–199) is known as the Father of Medicine.

_____ 7. Ethics has been a part of medical practice since ancient times.

_____ 8. The medical assistant should understand the _Principles of Medical Ethics_ as explained by the AMA's Council on Ethical and Judicial Affairs.

_____ 9. The AAMA does not have a Code of Ethics for medical assistants.

_____ 10. Medical assistants are licensed, not certified.

CRITICAL THINKING

Answer the following questions to the best of your ability. Use the textbook as a reference.

1. Michelle Manwiller, CMA (AAMA), is working with Harold Chan, a 55-year-old patient. Mr. Chan tells Michelle that he would like to try Chinese medicine treatments instead of taking the medication the physician has prescribed. He asks Michelle if she is familiar with the philosophy behind Chinese medicine. How might Michelle answer?

_____

_____

_____

_____

2. Robert Bautista is taking an administrative medical assisting course as part of his training to earn a certificate in medical assisting. He has been asked to write a paragraph outlining the contributions the Greek physician Galen made to medicine. Robert has been told to include the reasons why Galen's findings were not completely accurate. What could Robert write on this topic?

_____

_____

_____

3. Willie Harrison is creating a presentation for a history class he is enrolled in. Since he is in a medical assisting program, he wants his history paper to revolve around a medical topic. Willie has chosen to write about the history of the use of anesthesia in medicine. How should he start his outline for this presentation?

_____

_____

_____

_____

_____

4. Marian Reiman, CMA (AAMA), is teaching a night class to medical assisting students. Marian wants to lecture on the different types of hospitals that currently exist in the United States. What are the four categories of hospitals she should talk about and how should Marian describe one of these categories?

_____

_____

_____

5. Dayvon Jackson, RMA (AMT), is preparing a presentation for his coworkers on the use of limited-scope radiography by medical assistants. He has decided to include a brief history on the discovery of X-rays. What type of information could he include for his presentation?

_____

_____

_____

_____

_____

RESEARCH ACTIVITY

Use Internet search engines to research the following topics and write a brief description of what is found. It is important to visit reputable Web sites.

1. Using the Internet, choose and research one of the early contributors to medicine and write a 2–3-paragraph summary regarding your findings.

_____

_____

_____

_____

_____

_____

_____

_____

_____

_____

_____

_____

_____

_____

_____

_____

_____

_____

_____

_____

CHAPTER 2

The Medical Assisting Career: Roles and Responsibilities

CHAPTER OUTLINE

General review of the chapter:

    A. The MA's Role in Health Care Today
    B. The History of the Medical Assisting Profession
    C. Qualities of a Good Medical Assistant
    D. Time Management Skills
    E. Other Members of the Health Care Team

STUDENT STUDY GUIDE

Use the following guide to assist in your learning of the concepts from the chapter.

  I. Introduction and the History of Medical Assisting

    A. The MA's Role in Health Care Today
        i. The MA's role in health care is _____.
       ii. Medical assistants are also finding work at _____ companies, hospitals, and _____ _____ facilities.
      iii. MA's role in health care will likely continue to grow as the population ages and more patients enter the health care system.

    B. The History of Medical Assisting
        i. Due to a shortage of nurses in health care, medical assistants began to fill both _____ and _____ needs in physician offices.
       ii. The American Association of Medical Assistants was founded in the

           _____.
          (a) _____ _____ was its first president: There is still a scholarship fund available from the AAMA in her name.
      iii. In the beginning, physicians trained their medical assistants, as there was no formal training available.
      iv. 1978: The U.S. _____ of _____ recognized medical assisting as a profession.
       v. 1991: The AAMA adopted its current definition of medical assisting:

_____

_____

_____

_____

_____

II. Professional Organizations
    A. AMT Professional Certifications

        _____

        _____

        _____

        _____

        _____

        _____

    B. Professional Organizations
        i. American Academy of Professional Coders (AAPC):

        ii. The American Health Information Management Association (AHIMA):

        iii. The Association for Healthcare Documentation Integrity (AHDI):

III. Qualities of a Good Medical Assistant and Time Management
    A. Qualities of a Good MA
        i. Possesses strengths in both the clinical and administrative arenas
        ii. Is the patient's _____
        iii. Has a good understanding of medical _____
        iv. Is aware and proficient in their state's _____ of _____
        v. Strong _____ skills
        vi. Maintains high ethical standards
        vii. Demonstrates _____
        viii. Provides the same level of care to all patients
        ix. Uses proper _____ and avoid _____ terms
        x. MAs should use good personal hygiene:

        xi. Avoid artificial nails and obtrusive jewelry:

xii. Body piercings, except earlobes, and tattoos should not be visible during office hours.

xiii. Avoid scented _____ and _____ that can aggravate patients with allergies.

B. Time Management

   i. Working in a fast paced medical office can be _____.

   ii. A/an _____ _____ work plan is beneficial.

_____

_____

_____

_____

_____

_____

   iii. If other methods fail, create a time-management _____.

   iv. Time-management concerns should be discussed with staff, office management, and physicians.

     (a) Time management can keep staff _____ and patients happy.

IV. Members of the Health Care Team

A. Physicians

   i. The physician's education:

_____

_____

_____

_____

_____

   ii. The physician's role is to provide a/an _____ and direction for patient _____.

   iii. Physicians may also be known as primary care providers (PCPs) or _____.

   iv. In this case the physician is taking on primary responsibility for patient care.

_____

_____

_____

_____

_____

B. Physician's Assistants

   i. Training requirements for the physician's assistant (PA) _____ from _____ to _____.

   ii. The PA provides care to patients under the _____ of a/an _____.

   iii. Duties generally include:

_____

_____

_____

_____

   iv In some states, PAs are permitted to _____ _____.

C. Nurse Practitioner

   i. Nurse practitioners (NPs) have duties similar to _____; however, they have advanced training.

   ii. NPs must obtain the RN degree and then complete a/an _____ nursing program, often in specialized medicine.

iii. After their advanced nursing program, nurses take a state issued licensing exam.

iv. In many states, NPs are allowed to open their own _____ _____ as well as _____ _____.

D. Nurses

i. A licensed practical nurse or vocational nurse (LPN, LVN) requires _____ _____ of training.

ii. A registered nurse (RN):

_____

_____

_____

iii. An RN has more training in _____ and _____ skills, and thus a greater responsibility than an LPN or LVN.

E. Pharmacists

i. Pharmacists _____ drugs prescribed by health care providers.

ii. Pharmacists also educate patients on both _____ and over-the-counter medications.

iii. Information provided by pharmacists includes:

_____

_____

_____

_____

_____

KEY TERMINOLOGY REVIEW

Complete the sentences below using the correct key terms found in the textbook.

(Hint: some terms may be abbreviated and only have one line for the entry of the term)

1. Janice enjoyed learning _____ _____ the most, as the administrative skills seemed not as exciting.

2. All medical assistants must check their state laws regarding the legal _____ of _____ for medical assistants.

3. Because Jonah's school was not _____, he was not able to sit for the CMA (AAMA) examination.

4. Maura scored high on the venipuncture _____, as her skills were exceptional in that area.

5. Maxine Williams was the first president of the _____.

6. Medical assistants must act as a/an _____ on behalf of all of their patients.

7. The _____ offers the certification examinations for medical technologists, medical laboratory technicians, laboratory consultants, and medical administrative specialists.

8. _____ _____ is considered a nonverbal means of communication.

9. After 5 years working in the office triaging calls and scheduling appointments, Mark found that his _____ _____ were stronger than his clinical skills.

10. Blythe's gentle personality and kind spirit enabled her to form a fast and strong _____ with patients.

APPLIED PRACTICE

Give two examples of each positive quality that a medical assistant should possess.

Quality	Example
Loyalty	
Respect	
Dependability	
Courtesy	
Initiative	
Flexibility	
Credibility	
Confidentiality	
Attitude	
Appearance	

LEARNING ACTIVITY: MULTIPLE CHOICE

Circle the correct answer to each of the questions below.

1. The American Health Information Management Association is a national organization of professionals who work in which of the following fields?
   - a. medical records
   - b. coding
   - c. health information management
   - d. all of the above

2. The American Academy of Professional Coders offers a voluntary credentialing program with examinations that confer which of the following?
   - a. CPC
   - b. COLT
   - c. MLT
   - d. CMAS

3. The American Medical Technologists Association offers certification or registration as which of the following?
   - a. RMA
   - b. CPC
   - c. CMA
   - d. all of the above

4. Currently, medical assistants must work under the direction and supervision of which of the following health care professionals?
   - a. physicians
   - b. nurse practitioners
   - c. physician assistants
   - d. all of the above

5. Which of the following is a good tip for success for the medical assistant?

   a. Discuss personal problems only out of the hearing range of patients.

   b. Avoid participating in gossip in the workplace.

   c. Only conduct personal business at the office in between patients.

   d. all of the above

6. Which of the following projects a good image for the medical assistant?

   a. wearing work boots

   b. keeping short artificial nails

   c. having a clean uniform

   d. having a small and tasteful nose ring

7. Which of the following is a reason why the medical assistant should use proper grammar when talking with patients?

   a. Patients who have English as a second language may not understand slang terms or phrases.

   b. Using poor grammar is unprofessional.

   c. Using proper grammar is useful in avoiding miscommunication.

   d. all of the above

8. Who was the first president of the American Association of Medical Assistants?

   a. Florence Nightingale

   b. Wilma Blackford

   c. Maxine Williams

   d. Eleanor McWilliams

9. Performing to the best of one's abilities is an example of

   a. loyalty

   b. dependability

   c. credibility

   d. respect

10. The headquarters of the American Association of Medical Assisting are located in

   a. Philadelphia, PA

   b. Chicago, IL

   c. Baltimore, MD

   d. St. Louis, MO

CRITICAL THINKING

Answer the following questions to the best of your ability. Use the textbook as a reference.

1. Sara Dunn is taking an administrative medical assisting class as part of her training toward earning a medical assisting certificate. She has been assigned the task of writing a paper that outlines the history of medical assisting. Part of the assignment is to include the milestones reached by this profession over the past 50 years. How should Sara outline this paper?

   _____

   _____

   _____

   _____

2. Diane Luder, CMA (AAMA), has been working as an administrative medical assistant in a busy pediatric office for five years. Diane's job has been in the billing and coding department. Helga, a colleague of Diane's in the billing and coding department, tells Diane about the benefits of joining a professional organization of coders. How might Diane benefit from joining such a group?

_____
_____
_____
_____
_____
_____

3. Yelena Rubashka is taking an administrative class as part of her medical assistant training. She has been given an assignment to create a list of the common medical specialties patients will seek care with. What specialties should Yelena include in her list and how should she describe them?

_____
_____
_____
_____
_____

4. James Dugan has nearly completed his training in a medical assisting program. He is considering continuing in his education in order to pursue a nursing degree. What type of education would James have if he pursued a nursing degree?

_____
_____
_____
_____

5. As office manager, Marcia Cody was asked to present information regarding time management to the office staff during the next staff meeting. The physicians had asked Marica to present specific ideas on how the staff can be more effective using their time. What may Marcia include during her presentation?

_____
_____
_____
_____
_____

RESEARCH ACTIVITY

Use Internet search engines to research the following topics and write a brief description of what is found. It is important to visit reputable Web sites.

1. Research your state and local chapters of the American Association of Medical Assistants. What information is available? When and where are meetings located? If a chapter does not exist in your area, what are the requirements for starting a chapter?

_____
_____
_____

CHAPTER 3

Professionalism in the Workplace

CHAPTER OUTLINE

General review of the chapter:

    A. Introduction
    B. The MA's Role in Professionalism
    C. Characteristics of Professional Behavior
    D. Barriers to Professionalism

STUDENT STUDY GUIDE

Use the following guide to assist in your learning of the concepts from the chapter.

  I. Introduction
    A. The MA's Role in Professionalism
       i. Medical assistants have the opportunity to allow a patient to have or a/an _____ or _____ experience with the health care facility.
       ii. A professional-acting medical assistant can be the best _____ for his or her patient.
      iii. Use proper _____ when communicating in the office.
      iv. Avoid making _____ or _____ comments regarding a patient.
    B. Professionalism in the Health Care Setting
       i. Professionalism can be exemplified by a few behaviors:

          _____

          _____

          _____

          _____

       ii. Patients notice both a professional attitude and appearance:
         (a) Especially if the MA _____ _____ in either area
  II. Positive Professional Qualities
    A. _____ MAs should be competent in their knowledge and _____ associated with their profession.
    B. _____—This is important when working with patients and coworkers. This includes only answering questions within the MA's _____ of _____.
    C. _____—Appreciating the pain and fear involved when a patient is enduring a difficult experience and responding in a/an _____ and _____ manner.
    D. _____—MAs should treat each patient as a _____ person and respect his or her differences.
    E. _____—Taking responsibility for his or her own actions, not placing _____ on others, and learning from mistakes made

F. _____—Being loyal to an employer by performing at a person's
_____ _____ and saying positive things regarding the physicians
and the clinic

G. _____ _____—Acting in a thoughtful way by showing respect
for others as well as for oneself

H. _____—The MA's attitude will often set the tone of a patient's visit in the
medical office.

I. _____ tasks and working as a team player also exhibit professionalism:

    i. It is important to assign importance to tasks and complete the most
_____first.

    ii. Helping coworkers when they are running behind or need an extra helping hand

III. Barriers to Professionalism

  A. Bringing personal problems into the workplace:

_____
_____
_____
_____
_____

  B. Taking care of personal business at work:

_____
_____
_____
_____

  C. Inappropriate discussions:

_____
_____
_____
_____
_____

  D. Procrastination of duties:

_____
_____
_____
_____
_____

KEY TERMINOLOGY REVIEW

Place the letter of the key term with its definition below.

    a. compassion   **d.** respect

    b. competence   **e.** responsibility

    c. professionalism

_____ 1. Taking ownership of one's actions

_____ 2. Treating others with dignity

_____ 3. The ability to perform one's job up to standard

_____ 4. Using empathy to sense others' concerns or feelings

_____ 5. Acting in a business-like manner in the workplace

APPLIED PRACTICE

Read the scenario below and answer the questions that follow.

Scenario

John Summers is an office manager at Hillcrest Family Medicine. The physicians at the office have voiced concern to John regarding the lack of professionalism among the office staff. They have asked that John conduct a staff meeting focusing on the importance of professionalism. The physicians have asked that John highlight five qualities of a professional in a health care setting.

1. What five qualities do you think John should choose to discuss during the staff meeting? Explain why.

_____

_____

_____

_____

_____

_____

_____

_____

_____

_____

_____

_____

_____

_____

_____

_____

The physicians have also asked that John decide upon appropriate consequences for unprofessional behavior.

2. How do you think John should handle this request by the physicians? What consequences do you think would be appropriate for unprofessional behavior?

_____

_____

_____

_____

_____

_____

_____

_____

LEARNING ACTIVITY: TRUE/FALSE

Indicate whether the statement is true (T) or false (F).

_____ 1. When prioritizing tasks, it is important always to complete the longest task first.

_____ 2. Discussing a television show is appropriate if the MA and patient share common interests.

_____ 3. Learning from mistakes made is considered a professional characteristic.

_____ 4. It is okay to use slang terms if you know the patient is comfortable with the manner of speaking.

_____ 5. Taking ownership for one's actions is considered acting in a responsible manner.

_____ 6. Patients will take more of notice if a medical staff member is acting in an unprofessional behavior.

_____ 7. Performing to the best of one's ability is an example of being loyal to one's work.

_____ 8. Answering questions outside of one's scope of practice is considered a characteristic of honesty.

_____ 9. It is considered unprofessional to wait until the last minute to complete assigned duties.

_____ 10. When speaking of professionalism, compassion and respect have essentially the same meaning.

CRITICAL THINKING

Answer the following questions to the best of your ability. Use the textbook as a reference.

1. In preparation for his externship, Stefan Marquise has been assigned to write an essay on barriers to professionalism in the health care setting. What information should Stefan include in his essay?

_____

_____

_____

_____

2. A very angry patient asks to talk with the office manager. The patient explains that she overheard two staff members discussing the test results of another patient, who happens to be her sister-in-law. How should the office manager handle this situation?

_____

_____

_____

_____

3. Beth and Grace are both medical assistants working in a busy pediatric office. Beth is upset because Grace is always discussing her marital problems with her and other coworkers. Beth knows that she is not the only person getting irritated by Grace's constant tirades. How should Beth handle this situation?

_____

_____

_____

_____

4. Karen, the office manager, has noticed that the medical assistant, Charles, has been answering his cell phone while at work, as well as checking his e-mail between patients. Today, Charles' wife came to the office to talk with him during the busy hours of the morning. How should Karen address Charles' unprofessional behavior?

_____

_____

_____

_____

5. Bethany, CMA (AAMA), is working with Mrs. Cho in the examination room. Mrs. Cho is there because of a noticeable red patch that has developed on her face, around the eye. Mrs. Cho asks Bethany what is causing the rash. Bethany has seen similar rashes that have been diagnosed as herpes zoster, the shingles virus. How should Bethany respond to Mrs. Cho?

_____

_____

_____

_____

RESEARCH ACTIVITY

Use Internet search engines to research the following topics and write a brief description of what is found. It is important to visit reputable Web sites.

1. Type the word "professionalism" into an Internet search engine. What are some of the most interesting and helpful results that are returned with your search?

_____

_____

_____

_____

_____

_____

_____

CHAPTER 6
Patient-Centered Care and Education

CHAPTER OUTLINE

General review of the chapter:

    A. Introduction
    B. The MA's Role in Patient Centered Care
    C. Wellness
    D. A Holistic Approach to Health Care
    E. Pain
       i. Types
       ii. Assessment
       iii. Management
    F. Educating the Patient

STUDENT STUDY GUIDE

Use the following guide to assist in your learning of the concepts from the chapter.

I. Introduction

    A. The MA's Role in Patient-Centered Care

    _____
    _____
    _____
    _____
    _____

II. Wellness

    A. Wellness
       i. Wellness = practicing a/an _____ _____ on a regular _____.
       ii. Wellness is:

    _____
    _____
    _____

    B. Risk Factors
       i. Affect a person's _____
       ii. Can be _____
       iii. Risk factors are also determined by _____ _____.

C. Life Span
    i. The average lifespan in the U.S. is _____ years.
    ii. Ignoring risk factors can cause _____ _____ and illness.
D. Influences
    i. A person's lifestyle may be influenced by

_____

_____

_____

    ii. Aside from genetics, _____ and _____ risk factors can be changed.
E. Healthy Habits
    i. Positive _____, being active, _____, and avoiding addictive substances are examples of healthy habits.
F. Holistic Health
    i. Focuses on the person's surroundings, including:

_____

_____

_____

_____

_____

G. Holistic Medicine
    i. Facilitates _____ and _____ wellness
    ii. Connects the mind and body
    iii. Includes the patient in decisions, _____, and _____ of health
H. Stress
    i. Large contributor to illness
    ii. _____ _____ help to control stress.
    iii. Teaching these to patients is a good example of holistic health.
I. Mind-Body Connection
    i. Human spirit and _____ are a part of healing.
    ii. Emotions of joy, happiness, and love cause release of _____, which boost _____ to disease.
    iii. Negative emotions cause elevated body responses that are unhealthy.
    iv. Be aware of your patient's _____ and _____ state when dealing with their health.

III. Pain

A. Tolerance levels of pain vary among individuals.
B. Past _____ and _____ can affect pain
C. The pain experience can be heightened by _____ or _____.
D. Acute vs. Chronic Pain
    i. Acute =

_____

_____

_____

    ii. Chronic =

_____

_____

_____

E. Long-term Effects of Pain
    i.   Long-term pain can affect a person's mental state.
    ii. Including:

    _____

    _____

    _____

    _____

    _____

    _____

    _____

    _____

F. Physical pain
    i.   Physical pain = body's sign of _____ or _____ and serves
         as a protective mechanism
    ii. Physical pain can be _____ or on the body's surface, or deep within the
         bones, muscles, or tendons.
    iii. _____: pertaining to internal organs
    iv. Visceral pain is usually _____ _____.
G. Psychological Pain
    i.   Psychological pain = acute or chronic
    ii. Described as:

    _____

    _____

    _____

    _____

    _____

    iii. Common diagnoses include

    _____

    _____

    _____

    _____

    _____

H. Phantom Pain
    i.   Phantom pain occurs after the _____ of a body part. Nerve endings feel as
         if they are still getting _____.
    ii. Can be painful but will _____ and _____ over time
I. Pain Assessment
    i.   It is vital that a Medical Assistant can assess a patient's pain level.
    ii. Use _____ questions.
    iii. Use the _____ _____, _____
         _____, or full body picture.
J. Options for Pain Management

    _____

    _____

    _____

    _____

    _____

K. Pain Medications
  i. Some medications, such as _____ _____, may be prescribed.
  ii. Educate patient on _____, _____, use, and importance of keeping followup appointments.
  iii. Some patients choose not to use controlled substances because of their side effects and the possibility of drug dependence.
L. Alternative Therapies for Pain Management
  i. Relaxation
  ii. _____ remedies
  iii. _____ therapy
  iv. Biofeedback, acupuncture, _____
  v. Chiropractic

IV. Patient Education

A. All patient education must be performed under the _____ of the physician.
B. Patient information should be gathered:

_____

_____

_____

_____

_____

C. Plan what _____ will best be used when educating the patient.
D. This could include:
  i. Pamphlets or other preprinted information
  ii. Equipment that will be used for demonstration purposes.
E. Implementing the instruction is the actual _____ _____.
  i. The MA may need to demonstrate a new skill to a patient.
  ii. The patient should then demonstrate the skill to the MA, verifying that he or she understands.
F. _____ is vital to patient education.
  i. After the education is completed:
    (a) The MA should document in the patient's medical record the _____ _____ in the teaching process.
    (b) The level of patient _____
    (c) Any _____ the MA may have regarding the patient's _____.
G. Evaluation is the final step in patient education.
  i. This may be done by a patient _____ the office with a progress report.
  ii. It is important to ensure that the patient is complying with instructions.
  iii. _____ should be made aware of noncompliance, and documentation of the noncompliance should be charted in the patient's _____.
H. The Proper Learning Environment
  i. When educating patients, the teaching environment must be conducive to learning.
  ii. Consider the following list of items when determining a learning environment:
    (a) The area should be quiet and free from _____.
    (b) The area should be well _____.
    (c) Avoid hallways and the _____ area.
    (d) The space should encourage the patients to feel relaxed, comfortable, and able to _____ _____.
    (e) MA's should have a strong knowledge of the _____ they are teaching.

     (f) If an MA is not sure of an answer to a question the patient asks, the MA should be honest.

     (g) The MA should let the patient know that he or she will find the answer and get back to them.

I. Preventing Medication Errors

    i. It is important to educate patients on the _____ of medication errors.

    ii. Often errors are _____; however, they happen far too often.

    iii. It is important to review with the patient their medications, including:

_____

_____

_____

_____

J. Dieting and Weight Loss

    i. It is a good idea to provide patients with a copy of the new food guide.

     (a) It is called _____.

    ii. Also provide patients with information regarding how to read _____ _____.

    iii. This can help patients make _____ _____ in their diet.

K. Exercise

    i. MAs will often discuss with patients the benefits of exercise.

     (a) Pamphlets may be given outlining the benefits of exercise.

    ii. It is important to teach patients to _____ into an exercise program.

     (a) Also, how _____ and proper _____-up will help avoid injury.

    iii. *Always* remember that the physician must authorize any information given to a patient.

L. Reducing Stress

    i. High levels of stress can impede health.

    ii. Information pertaining to stress reduction can be very useful for patients.

    iii. This information may include:

_____

_____

_____

_____

M. Smoking and Substance Abuse Cessation

    i. Medical assistants may be asked to educate patients on the cessation of smoking or substance abuse.

    ii. Information and resources should be provided both for _____ and _____ services.

    iii. The American Cancer Society's Web site has valuable information regarding _____ _____.

    iv. The National Institute on Drug Abuse maintains a Web site with information pertaining to drug _____ and _____.

N. Teaching Resources
    i. Teaching resources may include:

    _____

    _____

    ii. The _____ provides another forum for patient education.
    iii. Only use information from reputable Web sites:

    _____

    _____

    _____

    _____

    iv. The physician should approve any material before it's given to a patient.

KEY TERMINOLOGY REVIEW

Place the letter of the key term with its definition below.

a.	afferent nerves	h.	efferent nerves
b.	analgesic	i.	endorphins
c.	assess	j.	evaluation
d.	cerebral	k.	implementing
e.	chronic	l.	planning
f.	controlled substances	m.	referred pain
g.	documenting	n.	risk factor

_____ 1. To evaluate

_____ 2. Determining how to begin the task of teaching the patient

_____ 3. Motor nerves that carry impulses from the central nervous system to the peripheral nervous system

_____ 4. Narcotics, stimulants, and certain sedatives

_____ 5. Pain that is felt in a different area from the injured or diseased part of the body

_____ 6. Pertaining to the cerebrum, the forepart of the brain

_____ 7. Factor that makes a person particularly vulnerable to certain diseases or disorders

_____ 8. Checking to see how well the patient has understood what has been taught

_____ 9. Sensory nerves that carry impulses to the central nervous system

_____ 10. The actual teaching phase

_____ 11. Pain reducing

_____ 12. Recording the education process in the patient's medical record

_____ 13. Proteins in the brain that have analgesic properties

_____ 14. Of long duration, often with slow progression

APPLIED PRACTICE

Read the scenario below and answer the questions that follow.

Scenario

Ethan is a RMA (AMT) working at a pain management clinic. He often conducts patient education seminars on proper medication administration and methods of pain management. Today Ethan is working with Mr. Baker, a patient who had a below-the-knee right leg amputation. The following conversation occurs between Ethan and Mr. Baker:

Ethan: "How have you been feeling since your surgery last month, Mr. Baker?"

Mr. Baker: "I have been okay for the most part. It is difficult getting adjusted to a wheelchair and I have been experiencing odd sensations."

Ethan: "Can you explain the sensations to me?"

Mr. Baker: "It sounds weird, but I have been feeling an intense pain in my right calf area, as if it were still there."

1. What type of pain is Mr. Baker experiencing? Explain your answer.

   _____

   _____

   _____

   _____

2. What are some questions that Ethan should ask next?

   _____

   _____

   _____

   _____

3. Of the three methods discussed in the textbook that can be used to assess pain, which would be the logical method Ethan should use to assess Mr. Baker's pain? Why?

   _____

   _____

   _____

   _____

LEARNING ACTIVITY: MULTIPLE CHOICE

Circle the correct answer to each of the questions below.

1. Which of the following is an open-ended question?
   a. Do you feel nauseated?
   b. Does the pain feel severe and sharp?
   c. Where is the pain located?
   d. Did the pain start yesterday?

2. An amputation often causes
   a. phantom pain
   b. emotional pain
   c. psychological pain
   d. physical pain

3. In the list of common words that can be used to describe pain, *intermittent* means
   a. deep inside
   b. the very worst pain imaginable
   c. comes and goes
   d. pain in children

4. Which of the following is *not* a treatment goal for patients with pain?
   a. lessen the pain
   b. reduce stress that makes pain worse
   c. keep the pain tolerable
   d. promote physical functioning

5. Which of the following is *not* one of the three types of physical pain?
   a. superficial
   b. deep
   c. visceral
   d. organic

6. Which of the following is conducive to a proper learning environment?
   a. the reception area
   b. a private examination room
   c. the hallway
   d. the front desk

7. Which of the following is *not* an appropriate teaching resource?
   a. audiocassette
   b. videos
   c. pamphlets
   d. personal Web sites

8. An acceptable form of stress-reducing therapy is:
   a. social smoking
   b. sex
   c. overeating
   d. destructive therapy

9. When educating patients regarding diet and weight loss, what information should *not* be included?
   a. successful fad diets
   b. information regarding how to read food labels
   c. copies of MyPyramid
   d. all of the above should be given

10. Which of the following is *not* a phase of patient education?
    a. implementing
    b. documenting
    c. producing
    d. planning

CRITICAL THINKING

Answer the following questions to the best of your ability. Use the textbook as a reference.

1. In the case study at the beginning of this chapter, Marina is smoking outside of the clinic. How might this make a patient feel about Marina? About the practice?

    _____

    _____

    _____

    _____

2. What would you recommend that Marina say to the patient after noticing his reaction? If the patient tells the physician, what do you feel the physician should do or say about the incident with Marina?

    _____

    _____

    _____

    _____

3. a. Consider that you are a family member of a patient with chronic pain going with him or her to a clinic visit. You know that the patient is truly in pain and is not a drug seeker. What do you think you would say or do if the MA or any staff gave the impression, through body language only, of not believing the patient had as much pain as the patient indicated?

    _____

    _____

    _____

    _____

    b. What do you think you would say or do if the MA did not make eye contact, was not warm and caring, and didn't chat at all except to ask the required questions then hurried out when the patient started to ask a question?

    _____

    _____

    _____

    _____

    c. What do you think you would say or do if the MA would not talk over the medication treatment with you, only the patient, stating that the patient needs to be able to handle their medications themselves?

    _____

    _____

_____

_____

_____

4. You are a new medical assistant and the physician has asked you to go into the exam room and give patient teaching to Mrs. McCarty about her rheumatoid arthritis pain management plan. The physician has written in the chart what the plan is but you are not very familiar with rheumatoid arthritis. Would you (a) try to do the best you can? (b) ask another MA to tell you what to do or how to do it? (c) ask the patient to wait while you research by office policy manuals and the Internet to figure it out? Choose one of the options and then explain your reasoning.

_____

_____

_____

_____

5. You are a medical assistant at OB/GYN. The physician has recently put you in charge of creating a list of resources and materials to be used in a patient education library. What patient education topics would you include in an OB/GYN resource library? List at least three topics and explain why you chose them.

_____

_____

_____

_____

RESEARCH ACTIVITY

Use Internet search engines to research the following topics and write a brief description of what is found. It is important to visit reputable Web sites.

1. Choose a topic for patient education and search the Internet for reputable information. List at least five reputable Web sites that could be used for patient education. Also, list at least five items of special interest that you learned.

_____

_____

_____

_____

_____

_____

_____

_____

CHAPTER 7

Considerations of Extended Life

CHAPTER OUTLINE

General review of the chapter:

    A. The Medical Assistant's Role in Extended Life Care
    B. Organ and Tissue Harvesting
        i. Organ and tissue harvesting
       ii. Donation issues and concerns
      iii. Transplant costs
      iv. Organ and tissue donation rules and regulations
       v. Uniform Anatomical Gift Act
    C. Advance Medical Directives
    D. Life-Prolonging Declarations
    E. Hospice

STUDENT STUDY GUIDE

Use the following guide to assist in your learning of the concepts from the chapter.

  I. The Medical Assistant's Role in Extended Life Care

    A. Medical advances in _____ and _____ transplants has extended life.
    B. Medical Assistants need to know rules regarding organ and tissue donations and transplants.
    C. Medical Assistants should be knowledgeable regarding:

      _____

      _____

      _____

      _____

      _____

      _____

       i. Offer the patient sources of information to research such topics including:

        _____

        _____

        _____

        _____

       ii. Document the patient's _____ and _____ in his or her chart.

 II. The Gift of Life

    A. The gift of life may be given through organ and tissue donation.
    B. Body _____ available to donate include skin, heart valves, cornea, and more.

C. Body _____ available to donate include hearts, lungs, kidneys, and more.
D. The Removal of Organs and Tissue
   i. Based on three factors:

      _____

      _____

      _____

      _____

   ii. In order to reduce rejection, _____ must be determined first.
   iii. _____ is crucial regarding the harvesting of tissues and organs.
   iv. Warm ischemic time cannot exceed _____ after circulation and respiration has ceased.
   v. Cold ischemic time cannot exceed _____ after circulation and respiration has ceased.
E. Organ/Tissue Donors
   i. The heart, lungs, kidneys, liver, pancreas, stomach, and intestines must be harvested _____ the patient has been pronounced dead.
     (a) The donor must have sustained _____ _____ in which respiration and circulation can be supported _____ by ventilators and machines.
   ii. Certain tissues, bone marrow, stem cells, cord blood, kidneys, or a portion of the liver may be given by _____ _____ .
F. Refusal of Organ Donation
   i. Usually stems from

      _____

      _____

      _____

      _____

G. Legality of Organ Donation
   i. Illegal to _____ organs in the United States.
   ii. The United Network for Organ Sharing (UNOS) oversees organ/tissue harvesting and transplants.
   iii. Organ procurement organizations handle the _____ of _____ organs.
H. Donor Cards
   i. Common to see organ donor status on a/an _____ _____
   ii. In some cases, exact tissues and organs can be specified.
   iii. A signed _____ _____ card is considered a legal document in some states.
I. Family Involvement
   i. Some institutions still ask a family's permission before procuring organs.
   ii. If the decision is overridden, a final decision is usually given by order of priority:

      _____

      _____

      _____

      _____

   iii. A person who states they do not wish to donate organs prior to death will have their decision honored.
J. The Uniform Anatomical Gift Act
   i. Uniform Anatomical Gift Act was passed in _____ to regulated state variances.

    ii. The act was updated in 1987 to make people aware of the need for donations.

    iii. Basic rules include:

_____

_____

_____

_____

_____

K. The Social Security Act for Organ Donation

    i. _____ amendment requires Medicaid/Medicare hospitals to make families of potential donors aware they can _____ organ donation

    ii. Upon admission, patients are asked their preference regarding organ donation.

    iii. If permission is granted to donate, the patient must provide _____ _____.

    iv. This is documented in the _____ _____ and only valid upon death.

L. OPTN

    i. *The Organ Procurement and Transplant Network* established rules that hospitals must follow to be _____ for _____/_____ services regarding transplants.

    ii. The OPTN set goals:

_____

_____

_____

_____

M. UNOS

    i. *United Network for Organ Sharing* created a national data base for patients requiring transplants.

    ii. Information in the data base includes the following patient information:

_____

_____

_____

_____

III. Legalities, Life-Prolonging Procedures, and Hospice

  A. Advance Medical Directives

    i. Documents that show patient wishes in a/an _____ state

    ii. Life prolonging procedure laws will vary by _____.

    iii. It is helpful to discuss such decisions with a family, a/an _____, _____, _____, or health providers.

  B. Durable Power of Attorney

    i. This person is appointed to make medical decisions when the patient is mentally incompetent.

    ii. Guidelines for appointing a DPA include:

      (a) _____ competent witnesses over the age of 18, not related to the patient.

      (b) Must be notarized

      (c) The appointment becomes effective when the patient's physician certifies in writing the patient is no longer able to consent.

      (d) The appointment can be _____ by _____ the appointment document.

C. The Living Will
    i. Legal document that states a personal wish to die _____ rather than be kept _____ when death is _____.
    ii. Identifies medical procedures that should/shouldn't be done in extenuating circumstances.
    iii. It also allows for procedures or medications to provide _____ measures, and/or the desire to receive artificial nutrition and hydration.
    iv. In order for the Living Will to take effect, a physician must certify:

_____

_____

_____

_____

_____

_____

D. Life Prolonging Procedures
    i. Document declaring that a person _____ life-prolonging medical treatments

_____

_____

    ii. Should be discussed with family, an attorney, and a physician
    iii. Must be made in good health, before hospitalization and not under stress:

_____

_____

_____

_____

E. Hospice
    i. Originated in _____ and came to the U.S. in _____
    ii. Hospice is a facility that cares for _____ ill patients.
    iii. Quality of life is improved with palliative care versus life-extending procedures.
    iv. A team-oriented approach is taken to provide _____, _____, and _____ support for both patients and their families.

KEY TERMINOLOGY REVIEW

A. Define the key terms listed below.

1. Cadaver:

_____

2. Hospice:

_____

3. Ischemic:

_____

4. Organ:

_____

5. Palliative:

_____

6. Tissue:

_____

B. Use each word above to correctly complete the sentences below.

1. Lung _____ is composed of cells that work together during the pulmonary process.

2. When Austin realized his cancer was incurable, he opted for _____ care to aid in his pain and discomfort.

3. Jill worked as a CMA (AAMA) in the office of a/an _____ facility for the terminally ill.

4. After a myocardial infarction, cardiac muscle may display _____ qualities due to the lack of blood supply to a portion of the heart.

5. Dr. Sayid, the St. Louis Medical Examiner, had the _____ on the autopsy table ready for examination.

6. The appendix is considered an accessory _____ located within the gastrointestinal tract.

APPLIED PRACTICE

Follow the directions as instructed with each question below.

1. Practice filling out a *Power of Attorney for Health Care* form from the scenario listed below. Pay careful attention to each section that is required to be filled out.

Scenario 1

Today, you are working with patient Timothy Goldblum. Timothy resides at 3215 Sprucetree Drive, Springfield, NY, 11234. Mr. Goldblum is 65 years old, born October 17, 1943. He is choosing his son, Adam Goldblum, as his agent for health care decisions. Adam lives at 155 North Winchester Blvd., Springfield, NY, 11234. His home phone number is 555-122-3343, and his work phone number is 555-877-3393.

Timothy Goldblum's alternate agent is his niece, Josie Westerfield. She lives at 2992 Apple Orchard Dr., Westport, NY, 11283. Her home phone number is 555-124-6436.

Timothy Goldblum chooses not to receive prolonging life measures. He also would like only to donate his heart, kidneys, and pancreas, for transplant only.

Alternate Scenario

Fill out either your own *Power of Attorney for Health Care,* or that of a family member using Figure 7-1 (page 62).

LEARNING ACTIVITY: FILL IN THE BLANK

Using words from the list below, fill in the blanks to complete the following statements.

competent	in a short time	physician
death	inconsistencies	procurement fees
decedent	interest	refusal
decisions	in writing	removal
designated recipient	live	the patient and family
donation	living will	members
driver's license	local/regional	tissue
durable power	national	Uniform Anatomical Gift Act
family	naturally	waiting
honor that decision	need	
hospital stay	organ donor card	

1. The removal of organs or tissues is based on three factors: the source of the _____, the _____ period, and the _____ order.

2. A/an _____ for health care tells the _____ and the _____ that if the patient is no longer mentally _____, the appointed person with that power of attorney can make _____ for the patient's best _____.

3. When an organ or _____ is donated from a/an _____ donor, it may be given to a/an _____.

4. If a/an _____ prior to death has indicated a/an _____ to make an organ donation, the institution or health care provider must _____.

5. Medical costs for transplants can include _____, lost wages for _____, and the _____ and surgical procedures.

6. The National Conference on Uniform State Laws, approved by the _____ in 1968, addresses the _____ among states.

7. When a patient agrees to donate, a request is made to see and document the _____, the _____, and any other documentation of the intent to donate.

8. Organ and tissue distribution was expanded from a/an _____ system to a/an _____ system based on _____.

9. A/an _____ advises the physician of a person's wish to die _____.

10. A living will must have _____ by the attending physician that, for one thing, the patient's _____ will occur _____.

CRITICAL THINKING

Answer the following questions to the best of your ability. Use the textbook as a reference.

1. What do you feel are some of the benefits of hospice?

   _____
   _____
   _____
   _____
   _____

2. Living donors can donate certain tissues. What are some of the concerns you would have if you were considering being a live donor?

   _____
   _____
   _____
   _____
   _____

3. Review the case study at the beginning of the chapter. Can Ori's mother keep him from being an organ donor on his driver's license? How do you feel about a parent denying an 18-year-old's request to donate?

   _____
   _____
   _____

POWER OF ATTORNEY FOR HEALTH CARE

(1) **DESIGNATION OF AGENT:** I designate the following individual as my agent to make health care decisions for me: _____

_____
(Name of individual you choose as agent)

_____
(address) (city) (state) (zip code)

_____
(home phone) (work phone)

OPTIONAL: If I revoke my agent's authority or if my agent is not willing, able, or reasonably available to make a health-care decision for me, I designate as my first alternate agent:

_____
(Name of individual you choose as first alternate agent)

_____
(address) (city) (state) (zip code)

_____
(home phone) (work phone)

OPTIONAL: If I revoke the authority of my agent and first alternate agent or if neither is willing, able, or reasonably available to make a health care decision for me, I designate as my second alternate agent:

_____
(Name of individual you choose as second alternate agent)

_____
(address) (city) (state) (zip code)

_____
(home phone) (work phone)

(2) **AGENT'S AUTHORITY:** My agent is authorized to make all health care decisions for me, including decisions to provide, withhold, or withdraw artificial nutrition and hydration, and all other forms of health care to keep me alive, **except** as I state here:

(3) **WHEN AGENT'S AUTHORITY BECOMES EFFECTIVE:** My agent's authority becomes effective when my primary physician determines that I am unable to make my own health care decisions unless I mark the following box. If I mark this box [ ], my agent's authority to make health care decisions for me takes effect immediately.

(4) **AGENT'S OBLIGATION:** My agent shall make health care decisions for me in accordance with this power of attorney for health care, any instructions I give below, and my other wishes to the extent known to my agent. To the extent my wishes are unknown, my agent shall make health care decisions for me in accordance with what my agent determines to be in my best interest. In determining my best interest, my agent shall consider my personal values to the extent known to my agent.

(5) **AGENT'S POSTDEATH AUTHORITY:** My agent is authorized to make anatomical gifts, authorize an autopsy, and direct disposition of my remains, except as I state here or elsewhere in this form:

INSTRUCTIONS FOR HEALTH CARE
Strike any wording you do not want.

(6) **END-OF-LIFE DECISIONS:** I direct that my health care providers and others involved in my care provide, withhold, or withdraw treatment in accordance with the choice I have marked below: **(Initial only one box)**
[ ] (a) **Choice NOT To Prolong Life**
I do not want my life to be prolonged if (1) I have an incurable and irreversible condition that will result in my death within a relatively short time, (2) I become unconscious and, to a reasonable degree of medical certainty, I will not regain consciousness, or (3) the likely risks and burdens of treatment would outweigh the expected benefits, **OR**
[ ] (b) **Choice To Prolong Life**
I want my life to be prolonged as long as possible within the limits of generally accepted health care standards.

(7) **RELIEF FROM PAIN:** Except as I state in the following space, I direct that treatment for alleviation of pain or discomfort should be provided at all times even if it hastens my death:

DONATION OF ORGANS AT DEATH
(8) Upon my death: (mark applicable box)
[ ] (a) I give any needed organs, tissues, or parts,
OR
[ ] (b) I give the following organs, tissues, or parts only: _____
[ ] (c) My gift is for the following purposes:
(strike any of the following you do not want)
(1) Transplant
(2) Therapy
(3) Research
(4) Education

(9) **EFFECT OF COPY:** A copy of this form has the same effect as the original.

(10) **SIGNATURE:** Sign and date the form here:

_____	_____
(date)	(sign your name)
_____	_____
(address)	(print your name)
_____	_____
(city)	(state)

(11) **WITNESSES:** This advance health care directive will not be valid for making health care decisions unless it is either: (1) signed by two (2) qualified adult witnesses who are personally known to you and who are present when you sign or acknowledge your signature; or (2) acknowledged before a notary public.

FIGURE 7-1 Sample of power of attorney for health care

Source: Ramont, Roberta Pavy, Niedrighaus, Dee Maldonado,Towle, Mary Ann, Comprehensive Nursing Care, © 2006, pp. 845, 900. Reprinted by permission of Pearson Education, Upper Saddle River, NJ.

4. Referring to the same case study, how do you feel about the mother's belief that CPR would not be performed on people who were known organ donors because it is less expensive to let the patient die and then harvest the organs?

_____

_____

_____

_____

5. Read the Uniform Anatomical Gift Act and the rules. List any rules that you feel are wrong or unfair, and explain why you think so.

_____

_____

_____

_____

RESEARCH ACTIVITY

Use Internet search engines to research the following topics and write a brief description of what is found. It is important to visit reputable Web sites.

1. Research your state laws regarding extended life rules and regulations.

   What are your state's laws regarding living wills?
   What are some statistics regarding organ donation within your state of residence?
   How can one become an organ donor in your state of residence?

_____

_____

_____

_____

_____

_____

_____

_____

_____

_____

_____

_____

CHAPTER 8
Written Communication

CHAPTER OUTLINE

General review of the chapter:

    A. Introduction
    B. The Medical Assistant's Role in Written Communication and Professional Correspondence
    C. Components of a Business Letter
    D. Using Fonts in Typed Communication
    E. Sending Letters to Patients
    F. Proofreading
    G. Creating Memos
    H. Mailing Written Communication
    I. Using E-Mail to Communicate
    J. Managing Mail and Correspondence

STUDENT STUDY GUIDE

Use the following guide to assist in your learning of the concepts from the chapter.

  I. The MA's Role in Written Communication and Professional Communication
    A. The MA's Role in Written Communication

    _____

    _____

    _____

    _____

    _____

    B. Professional Communication
      i. Writing letters is a responsibility of an administrative MA.
     ii. Correct _____, _____, and _____ are essential to maintaining a professional image.
    iii. Letters should be accurate, _____, and to the point.
    iv. Paragraphs in letters:

    _____

    _____

    _____

     v. Many computers have spell-check software.

    _____

    _____

    _____

    _____

_____

_____

    vi. Always check letters for grammatical errors:

_____

_____

    vii. If making corrections, be sure to keep the original _____ of _____ of the letter.

    viii. Punctuation can also be _____.

II. Components of a Business Letter

    A. All letters from the medical office should appear on _____.

    B. A nonabbreviated date is typed _____ lines below the letterhead—the day the letter was _____, not _____.

    C. The inside address, which is the _____address, is typed _____ to _____lines below date.

    D. The _____typically appears _____ lines below the inside address. The salutations of formal letters should include the recipients' proper names and courtesy titles.

    E. The _____ line describes the letter's purpose and is two lines below the salutation. RE: is used to indicate the subject of a business letter.

    F. The body of the letter begins _____ lines after the subject line, and contains the main information of the letter.

    G. The _____ of the letter is written _____ lines below the final paragraph of the body of the letter.

    H. _____ to _____ spaces should be included before typing the sender's name—space allows for a/an _____ signature.

    I. Reference initials are typed four to five _____ below the closing.

        i. Reference initials include the all-capital initials of the _____who wrote the letter, followed by the all-lowercase initials of the _____ who _____ the letter.

    J. Enclosures are additional documents that accompany a letter.

        i. If enclosures are present, _____ _____ is typically written two lines below the reference initials.

        ii. The number of enclosures is written in _____.

    K. The notation c: follows two lines below the enclosure if another person is receiving a copy of the letter.

    L. Subsequent pages begin with the _____ of the letter, followed by the _____ line.

    M. These pages do not require letterhead; however, they should appear on paper that matches the _____ and _____ of the letterhead.

III. Styles, Fonts, Proofreading, and Abbreviations

    A. Various styles of business letters include*:

_____

_____

_____

_____

    B. Font

        i. Font style is another consideration:

        (a) Lettering size should be _____.

*The physician's preference will dictate which style is used.

    ii. Professional font should be used,

_____

_____

  C. Proofreading
    i. Proofreading is the process of checking written information for _____ or
      other errors.
    ii. MAs should proofread all documents at least _____ before printing.
    iii. Documents need to be _____, _____, and logically
      organized.
    iv. After printing, the document should be read one last time for formatting, spelling,
      punctuation, and grammatical errors.
    v. The MA should use proofreader _____ if changes are needed to the
      document before reprinting.
  D. Abbreviations
    i. Abbreviations for medical terms are often used.
    ii. _____ has named some abbreviations that should no longer be used.

_____

_____

    iii. If the MA is unsure of an abbreviation, they should _____ the word.

IV. Memos, Mail, and Correspondence
  A. Memos

_____

_____

_____

_____

_____

_____

  B. Sending Mail
    i. $8 \frac{1}{2}'' \times 11''$ paper and _____ envelopes are standard.
    ii. A business letter to be mailed in a size 10 envelope should be folded into

    _____.
    iii. The sender's address should appear in the _____ _____
      corner of an envelope.
    iv. The recipient's name and address is in the _____ of the envelope.
    v. Personal or Confidential should appear if the contents of the envelope are personal in
      nature.
    vi. Window envelopes are commonly used for billing:

_____

_____

  C. Postage Meters
    i. Determine the weight and the proper postage for letters being sent.
    ii. Meters are generally user friendly and reduce _____ within the office.
    iii. Meters are _____ from mailing companies.
    iv. To use the meter, the MA will contact the leasing company's customer service department
      and provide necessary information.
  D. United States Postal Service Mailing Services
    i. A first-class stamp from the USPS will mail a letter that weighs less than

    _____.

    ii. Priority mail is used for mail weighing more than 13 ounces and no more than 70 pounds:

_____

_____

_____

  iii. Express mail guarantees next-day delivery seven days a week.
  iv. Media mail is an economic choice for printed and bound materials such as:

_____

_____

_____

_____

    v. For an additional charge, the USPS offers:

_____

_____

_____

_____

_____

_____

  vi. _____ mail is preferred when sending important documents.
 vii. Is available for first-class and priority mail
viii. Insurance can be purchased for any item shipped via the USPS.
  ix. The cost of the insurance rises with the _____ of the item.

E. E-mail

_____

_____

_____

_____

_____

F. Incoming Mail and Correspondence
    i. Administrative medical assistants are responsible for _____ incoming mail.
   ii. Sorting mail is a time-sensitive task that needs to be completed on a daily basis.
  iii. The MA usually opens each item of mail and _____ it.
  iv. _____ items are only to be opened by the intended receiver.
   v. Offices have sorting systems to determine who gets what mail.
  vi. A physician may receive _____, whereas an office manager may receive _____.

G. Annotation
    i. Administrative MAs may annotate mail for the physician:

_____

_____

_____

_____

_____

_____

_____

KEY TERMINOLOGY REVIEW

Write a sentence using the selected key terms in the correct context.

1. Annotation:

_____

_____

2. Closing:

_____

_____

3. Font:

_____

_____

4. Memo:

_____

_____

5. Proofreading:

_____

_____

6. Reference initials:

_____

_____

7. Salutation:

_____

_____

8. Thesaurus:

_____

_____

APPLIED PRACTICE

Follow the directions as instructed with each question below.

1. Proofread the following body of a business letter and make changes as necessary, using proofreader's marks. (Refer to Figure 8-11 in your textbook.)

    Mr. SUSAN Rowe (8-12-1877 was seen in my office today. She presents with complaints of

    uper right quadrant pain times too weeks. Mrs. rowe states that alon g with the pain, she

    is experiencing nausea and vomitting. Upon palpation the abdomen appears bloted and is

    sensitive to the touch

2. Using word processing software, create an interoffice memo. Andrew Edwards, CMA (AAMA) is the sender of the memo and all clinical staff members are intended to be the recipients. The purpose of the memo is to inform the clinical staff that a pharmaceutical sales representative will be presenting information on a new cardiac drug that Dr. Sheila Tyrone is considering using for patient therapy. The presentation will occur on Friday during the lunch hour.

LEARNING ACTIVITY: MULTIPLE CHOICE

Circle the correct answer to each of the questions below.

1. Which of the following types of mail would be appropriate for use with a window envelope?
    a. insurance claim forms
    b. patient laboratory slips
    c. patient operative reports
    d. all of the above

2. Which of the following is the size of a standard business envelope?
    a. $3 \frac{1}{2}'' \times 8 \frac{1}{2}''$
    b. $4 \ 1/8'' \times 9 \frac{1}{2}''$
    c. $4 \frac{1}{4}'' \times 9 \frac{1}{4}''$
    d. none of the above

3. How much postage is required to mail an interoffice memo?
    a. \$.31
    b. \$.23
    c. \$.20
    d. none of the above

4. If the medical assistant is unsure whether a certain medical abbreviation is correct, how should he proceed?
    a. make his best guess
    b. skip the abbreviation and write the term out in full
    c. ask a coworker
    d. any of the above

5. In order to catch all errors in a written document, how many times should the medical assistant read a letter before sending it out?
    a. once
    b. twice
    c. three times
    d. four times

6. Martin F. Susman, MD has dictated a letter to a patient. The medical assistant who types the letter is Kendra M. Oncler, CMA (AAMA). Which of the following is the correct way to use the reference initials on the letter?

  a. MS/KO
  b. MFS/KMO
  c. ms/ko
  d. MFS/kmo

7. The _____ of a professional letter typically appears two lines down from the ending portion of the body.

  a. closing
  b. subject line
  c. salutation
  d. letterhead

8. Which of the following pieces of information are typically included in the office letterhead?

  a. the office name
  b. the office address
  c. the office e-mail address
  d. all of the above

9. Which of the following statements is written correctly?

  a. The patient is taking five milligrams of the medication every hour.
  b. The patient is taking 5 milligrams of the medication every hour.
  c. The patient is taking five (5) milligrams of the medication every hour.
  d. All of the above are correct.

10. Which of the following words is misspelled?

  a. Foriegn
  b. Occurrance
  c. Liason
  d. All of the above are misspelled.

CRITICAL THINKING

Answer the following questions to the best of your ability. Use the textbook as a reference.

1. Missie Hurst, RMA (AMT), is working as an administrative medical assistant with a gastroenterology practice. Dr. Brown has asked Missie to annotate the laboratory reports that come back from the lab. What is he asking Missie to do?

  _____

  _____

  _____

  _____

2. Henry Connelly, CMA (AAMA), has just been hired to work at the front desk in a family practice clinic. Part of his job is to open and sort the mail. There is no written office policy about this task currently on file in the office so Henry decides to create one. How should Henry proceed and what might his policy look like?

  _____

  _____

  _____

3. Willie Rachenko, RMA (AMT), has been working with Dr. Stuart for several years. Dr. Stuart asks Willie to contact Mr. Brocheer with his lab results from earlier this week. Willie looks into Mr. Brocheer's chart and sees that the patient has listed his work e-mail address. Willie isn't able to reach Mr. Brocheer by telephone and instead of leaving a voice-mail message asking the patient to return his call, Willie decides to e-mail the patient with his lab results. Later that day, Mr. Brocheer calls the office very upset. He tells Willie that his boss intercepted the e-mail and now knows that his employee was screened for a sexually transmitted disease. What did Willie do wrong?

4. Mallory Valdez is taking an administrative medical assisting class. She has been given the assignment of writing a short paper that outlines the various mailing services offered by the U.S. Postal Service. What should Mallory include in her paper?

5. Ronna Howard, RMA (AMT), is working for Dr. Jameelah Brown. Dr. Brown is considering purchasing a postage meter for the clinic and has asked Ronna to find out the pros of having such a piece of equipment. What should Ronna include in her evaluation?

RESEARCH ACTIVITY

Use Internet search engines to research the following topics and write a brief description of what is found. It is important to visit reputable Web sites.

1. Visit www.usps.com and research information regarding certified mail, rates, and extra services available. When could some of the extra services be useful when dealing with written correspondence between the medical office and patients?

CHAPTER 9

Telephone Procedures

CHAPTER OUTLINE

General review of the chapter:

    A. Introduction
    B. The MA's Role in Telephone Procedures
    C. Telephone System Features
    D. Answering the Telephone
    E. Messages and Prescription Refills
    F. Calling Patients
    G. Telephone Directories

STUDENT STUDY GUIDE

Use the following guide to assist in your learning of the concepts from the chapter.

I. Telephone Procedures
    A. The MA's Role in Telephone Procedure
        i. MAs must be able to handle a variety of calls.
            (a) Medical office calls could range from _____ _____ to _____.
        ii. MAs should always remain calm, regardless of the _____of the caller.
    B. The Telephone
        i. The first _____ of _____ between the medical office and a patient is a/an _____ _____.
        ii. To ensure a good first impression:
            (a) Always be _____ and _____.
            (b) Answer the telephone by the _____ _____.
            (c) Select a proper greeting for the medical office:

            _____
            _____
            _____

            (d) An example might be:

            _____
            _____
            _____

II. Telephone Features
    A. Multifunction telephone systems require _____ _____.
    B. Hands-free devices are gaining popularity:

    _____
    _____
    _____
    _____

C. _____ _____ phones store up to 100 programmed numbers which are easily accessed with the touch of a single button.

D. _____ dials the last number called, also with the touch of a single button.

E. _____ _____ allows more than two parties to speak on the same phone line at the same time.

   i. *Example:* A conference call among a physician, his or her patient, and a physical therapist.

F. _____ _____ allows more than one person in the same location to participate in a telephone call.

_____

_____

_____

G. _____ _____ routes incoming phone calls to another telephone number.

_____

_____

_____

H. _____ _____ _____ eliminate hold times because they allow the caller to be routed directly to the desired party.

   i. Medical offices must have multiple phone lines.

I. _____ _____ _____: Patients call a main number then choose an extension to dial to reach their desired party.

   i. Drawbacks to this system may include:

_____

_____

_____

_____

J. The hold feature:

_____

_____

_____

_____

_____

_____

_____

K. Larger offices may choose to purchase additional telephone features:

   i. Automatic calls to patients with _____ _____ reminding the patient of an appointment

   ii. Automatic reverse redial:

_____

_____

_____

L. Answering Services

   i. Answering services are used when the medical office is _____: *before and after hours and lunchtime.*

   ii. They forward patient messages to the _____ _____.

    iii. Medical offices should only use answering services with _____ _____ _____.

    iv. Physician _____ _____ must be left with the answering service should they have to contact him or her with a patient emergency after office hours.

    v. When the office reopens, the office staff will contact the answering service to obtain messages.

_____

_____

III. Triage and Emergency Calls

  A. Telephone Triage

    i. Triage is a duty of the administrative medical assistant.

    ii. Telephone triaging involves _____ _____ _____ based on the _____ of the need.

    iii. Life-threatening emergencies that require urgent care:

_____

_____

_____

_____

_____

_____

_____

_____

    iv. Often triage _____ are used.

_____

_____

_____

    v. _____ are usually involved in constructing these notebooks.

    vi. Usually a/an _____ _____ that categorizes emergency situations presented in phone calls to the office

  B. Emergency Calls

    i. Handling emergency calls while a physician is in the office:

      (a) MA should obtain the patient's _____, _____, and _____

      (b) Immediately inform the _____ of the emergency call: Physicians will often take emergency phone calls.

  C. Emergency Calls Without a Physician in the Office:

_____

_____

_____

_____

_____

  D. Emergencies in the Office

    i. A physician may request that _____ _____ be called to the office.

ii. Obtain the patient's _____, _____ _____,
description of the problem, and requested emergency service.

iii. Office _____ and _____ should be listed near the
phone—provide floor, suite, or office numbers when appropriate.

iv. Obtain an estimated _____ of _____.

E. Patient with Speech Impediments

_____

_____

_____

_____

F. Angry Callers
   i. Angry callers must be dealt with _____ and _____.
   ii. An understanding voice and a/an _____ can usually _____
   an angry caller.
   iii. Do not stand for _____ _____.
   iv. _____ _____ must be documented in the patient's chart.
   v. Physicians must be made aware of _____ _____ regarding
   angry patients.

G. Emotional/Grieving Patients
   i. Grieving or emotional patients require more time.
   ii. These calls are _____ in nature and must be _____ in the
   patient's chart.
   iii. If an accident has occurred:

   _____

   _____

   iv. It may be appropriate to have the physician call the patient.

H. Charting Calls

_____

_____

_____

_____

IV. Telephone Messages
   A. Telephone message pads are available at most offices.
   B. Specific information must be obtained when taking a telephone message.
      i. Always include:

      _____

      _____

      _____

      _____

      _____

   C. Let patients know when they can _____ to _____ a return call.
   D. Give messages to the intended parties in a timely manner.
   E. Prescription Refill Messages
      i. Refill policies vary by office—however, _____ is generally required
      for processing.

    ii. Transfer refill requests to a/an _____ _____
          _____: A call may come from a patient or pharmacist.
    iii. Physicians may want to see the patient prior to issuing a refill.

  F. Messages Regarding Prescription Refills:
     i. If a physician is not in the office when a request comes in:

_____

_____

_____

_____

  G. Calling a Patient
     i. Have necessary information and the patient's chart prior to calling.
    ii. _____ _____ phone calls must be charted in the
         patient's chart.
    iii. Maintain HIPAA standards and maintain patient confidentiality when leaving a message.
    iv. State who the message is for:

_____

_____

     v. State your name:

_____

_____

    vi. The name and number of the doctor's office you are calling from:

_____

_____

  H. Telephone Directories
     i. Telephone books:

_____

_____

_____

_____

_____

    ii. Online directories:

_____

_____

_____

_____

    iii. Commonly called numbers should be kept in a/an _____ card system or
         _____.

V. The Telephone and Patient Confidentiality
  A. Patient information must never be discussed within the _____
     _____ of _____ _____.
     i. Doing so violates HIPAA and _____ may be _____.
  B. Maintaining patient confidentially reinforces a professional image.

C. Patient identity cannot be verified over the phone:

_____

_____

_____

_____

KEY TERMINOLOGY REVIEW

Use the key terms found at the beginning of the chapter to finish the sentences below. Key terms may be more than one word in length.

1. Maria liked using the _____ when triaging calls; it allowed her to move about freely throughout the office because she wasn't using the telephone receiver.

2. Dr. Adamson's pager was programmed as number 2 on the _____ because he was called most often from the medical office.

3. Shelly was often _____ patient calls because she was skilled at prioritizing patient needs.

4. The physician placed Dr. Michaels on _____ in order for all the physicians to hear the consulting physician's remarks.

5. _____ is a feature allowing incoming calls to go directly to another number.

6. "Good afternoon and thank you for calling. The office is now closed and will reopen at 9:00 A.M." This is an example of a/an _____.

7. Shelly will often refer to the _____ to handle calls from patients with potentially life-threatening conditions.

8. "Thank you for calling Springfield Family Medicine. For the receptionist, press 1; for prescription refills, press 2; for our billing department, press 3." This telephone feature is an example of _____.

9. This is similar to an automatic dialer, _____.

10. Anthony needed to schedule a/an _____ for Dr. Hagenson in Miami, FL, as well as Dr. Hin in Los Angeles, CA, and Dr. Pennybrook in Seattle, WA. The physicians need to discuss a new procedure involving rhinoplasty.

11. A receptionist will generally _____ incoming telephone calls to their correct departments.

12. While Mikayla was on the phone with Mr. Martinez, she had to utilize the _____ because another phone line was ringing that she needed to answer.

13. _____ allow callers direct access to a particular person without having to be routed through a receptionist.

14. The _____ will call the last number dialed from that phone.

15. Because Marco Antolik was seen last week, he is now considered a/an _____.

APPLIED PRACTICE

Using your textbook, answer the questions that follow each scenario below.

1. Using the box, create a message pad template that could be used in a medical office to take telephone messages.*

[ ]

2. Manuel Vinnzio is an administrative medical assistant. He receives a phone call from a woman requesting a refill for one of her prescription medications. How should Manuel handle this call? What information must Manuel obtain from the patient? What should he do with the message after the call has ended?

_____

_____

_____

_____

_____

LEARNING ACTIVITY: MULTIPLE CHOICE

Circle the correct answer to each of the questions below.

1. Which of the following would be appropriate to play for callers who are on hold?
   a. a local radio station
   b. prerecorded music
   c. a message about seasonal allergies
   d. all of the above

*Consider the important items to be obtained from callers when they call the office.

2. Which of the following might be offensive or irritating for callers to listen to while they are on hold?

   a. religious music
   b. prerecorded music

   c. a message about seasonal allergies
   d. a local radio station

3. How long is an acceptable period of time to leave a caller on hold?

   a. less than 10 seconds
   b. 20–30 seconds

   c. 45–60 seconds
   d. 1–2 minutes

4. What items should the medical assistant have available before answering the office telephone?

   a. pen or pencil
   b. paper

   c. telephone message pad
   d. all of the above

5. The medical office telephone should be answered within how many rings?

   a. on the first ring
   b. between 2–3 rings

   c. between 3–4 rings
   d. no more than 5 rings

6. Which of the following pieces of information should the medical assistant be able to give callers?

   a. directions to the office
   b. parking fees

   c. the insurance plans the physician is participating with
   d. all of the above

7. Which of the following telephone calls should be taken care of first?

   a. a patient who says she needs to schedule her yearly mammogram
   b. an angry patient who is calling about her bill

   c. a patient who says he is having chest pains
   d. a patient who is calling to find out his laboratory results

8. What information would you expect to find in a telephone triage notebook?

   a. driving directions to the medical office
   b. the hours the clinic is open

   c. the questions to ask a patient who complains of chest pain
   d. all of the above

9. In the event of a medical emergency in the office, what information should the medical assistant have available before calling for emergency services?

   a. the patient's name
   b. the patient's age

   c. the patient's gender
   d. all of the above

10. Which of the following emergency telephone numbers should the medical assistant have readily available at the front desk?

   a. poison control
   b. the local police department

   c. the local fire department
   d. all of the above

CRITICAL THINKING

Answer the following questions to the best of your ability. Use the textbook as a reference.

1. Rosie Sanchez, CMA (AAMA), has been working as an administrative medical assistant in an internal medicine clinic for the past year. A large part of her day is spent answering the office telephone and scheduling appointments. She would like the office to provide her with a hands-free headset for the telephone system. The clinic director has asked Rosie to create a list that outlines the benefits of having a hands-free headset over a conventional telephone headset. What should Rosie list?

_____

_____

_____

_____

2. Mackenzie Quinn, RMA (AMT), has just been hired to work as an administrative medical assistant in a family practice clinic. The telephone system Mackenzie will use has an automatic dialing feature, which allows the user to program up to 100 commonly dialed telephone numbers. What type of telephone numbers should Mackenzie include in her telephone?

_____

_____

_____

_____

3. Ron Douglas is a student in an administrative medical assisting class. He has been given an assignment to create an office policy that discusses how the speaker telephone function of the front desk telephone system can be used without violating patient confidentiality. What should Ron write?

_____

_____

_____

_____

4. Yelena Sheytovski, CMA (AAMA), is working with Dr. Francis. The office has just purchased a new telephone system that allows the user to record telephone calls. Dr. Francis has asked Yelena to create a recorded message to alert callers that their call may be recorded. What should Yelena's message include?

_____

_____

_____

_____

5. Martin Taylor, RMA (AMT), is working in an audiology clinic. The clinic is researching the possibility of purchasing a new telephone system that will include an automatic routing unit where callers can dial an extension to reach their desired party. Martin has been asked to create a list of pros and cons for this type of system. What should Martin include on his list?

_____

_____

_____

_____

_____

RESEARCH ACTIVITY

Use Internet search engines to research the following topics and write a brief description of what is found. It is important to visit reputable Web sites.

1. Search the Internet for on-call answering services that are provided for medical offices after hours. What types of services are offered by these companies? What is the general cost for on-call answering services?

_____

_____

_____

_____

_____

_____

_____

_____

_____

_____

_____

_____

_____

_____

_____

_____

_____

_____

_____

_____

CHAPTER 10

Front Desk Reception

CHAPTER OUTLINE

General review of the chapter:

A. Introduction
B. The MA's Role in Front Desk Reception
C. Opening the Office
D. Preparing Patient Files
E. Greeting and Registering Patients
F. Managing Difficult Patients
G. Closing the Office

STUDENT STUDY GUIDE

Use the following guide to assist in your learning of the concepts from the chapter.

I. Duties of the Front Desk Receptionist

A. The MA's Role in Front Desk Reception
   i. The duties of the front desk receptionist include:

   _____

   _____

   _____

   _____

   _____

B. Opening and Closing the Office
   i. Opening and closing procedures vary office to office.
   ii. Generally these are the responsibility of the _____ _____

   _____.
   iii. A/an _____ outlines the steps for each procedure.
      (a) Also assists in properly _____ _____ staff members.
   iv. Opening staff should arrive at least _____ prior to the first scheduled patient.
C. Opening the Office

   _____

   _____

   _____

   _____

   _____

D. Closing the Office

_____

_____

_____

_____

_____

E. Preparing Patient Files
  i. Patient files are prepared at the _____ of a business day, in preparation for the _____.
  ii. Files must be created for new patients.
  iii. The number and types of _____ vary from office to office.
  iv. All offices include in their patient charts:

  _____

  _____

  v. Administrative staff must verify reports are accounted for and filed:

  _____

  _____

  vi. Patient files must be kept in a/an _____ location to ensure

  _____.

II. Reception Duties
  A. Greeting Patients
    i. The receptionist should:
      (a) _____ greet all who enter the office.
      (b) Acknowledge all patients, even if he or she is busy with another task.
    ii. Medical offices used to have windows to separate the office from the reception area.

  _____

  _____

    iii. A new patient should be shown the locations of the _____,
    _____, and the coat rack.
    iv. When greeting an established patient, verify all information on file is correct and make necessary changes.
    v. If insurance has changed, copy _____ _____ of the new insurance card.
  B. Patient Confidentiality
    i. Confidential discussions with patients must be conducted out of the _____
    _____ of other _____.
    ii. Patient sign-in sheets must be _____ compliant:

  _____

  _____

  _____

  _____

  C. Obtaining Patient Information
    i. Sometimes patients are _____ to provide personal information.
    ii. Inform the patient that information can only be given out:

  _____

  _____

_____

_____

    iii. Make a note in the patient's file and inform the physician if the patient still
_____ to _____ information.

D. Delays in the Medical Office Schedule

    i. _____ and _____ _____ concerns can absorb the physician's time.

    ii. Notify patients when a physician's schedule is delayed _____ or more.

    iii. Attempt to reach patients _____ to their arrival at the office, or _____ _____ their arrival.

    iv. Informing the patient and providing a rescheduling option lets a patient know that the medical office realizes that his or her time is _____.

_____

_____

E. Disruptive Patients

    i. Administrative medical assistants will likely encounter disruptive patients.

    ii. Remove the patient from the _____ _____.

    iii. This will relieve the _____ of the other patients.

    iv. This doesn't provide for a/an _____ that the disruptive patient may be seeking.

    v. Attempt to _____ the patient's concern—or find another staff member who can help.

F. Sick Patients

    i. Patients with certain _____ or _____ should not be expected to wait in a reception area.

    ii. Patients who should be moved to an exam room upon check-in include:

_____

_____

_____

_____

_____

G. The Reception Room

    i. The reception room should be kept _____ and free of _____ _____.

    ii. The MA should circulate the reception room throughout the day to throw away _____ and collect items _____ _____ by patients.

    iii. If necessary, the MA should ask children to remain quiet.

    iv. Patients should be instructed that food should not enter the medical office.

    v. There should be enough seating for _____ worth of patients and their companions _____ _____.

    vi. Office furniture should be sturdy and comfortable, as well as easy to _____ and _____.

    vii. Office décor should be tasteful and reflect the office's patient base.

H. Reading Material

    i. Reading material should be consistent with the medical office's specialty.

    ii. Material should be _____, _____, and in good condition.

I. Children in the Reception Area
    i. Medical offices have areas designated for children:

_____

_____

_____

    ii. The toys and furniture should be cleaned and checked regularly for _____ and _____.

    iii. State guidelines may dictate cleaning requirements for toys in _____ _____.

    iv. Children should never be left unattended in a reception room.

    v. If a child is unattended, and the MA does not speak out against it, the MA is providing _____ _____ to care for the child.

    vi. Parents should be made aware of the office's policy regarding children in the reception area.

KEY TERMINOLOGY REVIEW

Match the key terms to their definitions below.

a. Americans with Disabilities Act	**g.** office policy
b. checklist	**h.** reception area
c. copayment	**i.** receptionist
d. front desk	**j.** service animal
e. hazard	**k.** sign-in sheet
f. HIPAA compliant	

_____ 1. In line with federal patient confidentiality laws.

_____ 2. List of activities or steps to take to perform a task.

_____ 3. Place in a medical office where the receptionist welcomes patients as they enter.

_____ 4. Medical staff member who greets patients, answers the telephone and directs office flow.

_____ 5. Paper or electronic document on which patients sign their names upon entering the office.

_____ 6. Agreed-upon standard for handling a situation or procedure in the office.

_____ 7. Animal that has been trained to assist a person with a handicap.

_____ 8. A predetermined amount of money a patient must pay for each physician's visit.

_____ 9. Federal law that outlines appropriate treatment or accommodations for patients or employees with disabilities.

_____ 10. Waiting area for patients in the medical office.

_____ 11. Something that is dangerous or possibly dangerous.

APPLIED PRACTICE

Using your textbook, answer the questions or complete the activities that follow.

1. Aubrey Cody is a CMA (AAMA) who has been hired as a medical office for a new pediatric practice that is being built. The physicians within the practice have asked her to design and decorate the reception area. In the practice there are three physicians who can see up to four patients each hour. How could Aubrey design the medical office reception area? What is the minimum amount of seating that should be in the reception area? What theme, toys, and reading materials may be appropriate for the reception area? Explain your answer after you have designed the reception area.

_____

_____

_____

_____

_____

_____

_____

_____

LEARNING ACTIVITY: MULTIPLE CHOICE

Circle the correct answer to each of the questions below.

1. If the medical assistant is on the telephone when a patient arrives at the office, what should she do to let the patient know she is aware of their presence?

   a. continue looking down at the desk so the patient realizes she is on the telephone and won't be able to help right away

   b. make eye contact with the patient, smile and hold up an index finger to indicate she'll be with them in just a moment

   c. turn her back to the patient in order to keep the telephone conversation more private

   d. any of the above

2. If the patient needs to share private information with the front desk receptionist, what should the receptionist do?

   a. lower his voice so other patients cannot hear the conversation

   b. ask the patient to come into a more private area of the medical office to continue the conversation

   c. ask the patient to write down their comment so other patients won't overhear

   d. any of the above

3. When established patients check in at the front desk, what information should the receptionist confirm with the patient?

   a. patient's marital status has not changed since their last visit

   b. the type of medications the patient is taking

   c. patient's address has not changed since their last visit

   d. all of the above

4. Which of the following sign-in sheet methods would be HIPAA compliant?

   a. an electronic sign-in sheet where signatures are not viewable to the patient

   b. a paper sign-in sheet where the receptionist covers up the names of other patients

   c. a paper sign-in sheet where the receptionist blackens out the names of other patients with a marker pen

   d. any of the above

5. Patient information forms should contain which of the following pieces of information?

   a. the patient's home address
   b. the patient's insurance information

   c. the patient's contact telephone numbers

   d. all of the above

6. Many offices use _____ to track fees charged to patients.

   a. a checklist
   b. superbills or encounter forms

   c. a patient booklet
   d. any of the above

7. How should the receptionist respond when confronted with an angry patient?

    a. move the patient out of the front desk area

    b. ask the patient to sit down in the reception room until they have calmed down

    c. walk away from the front desk until the patient calms down

    d. any of the above

8. Which of the following patients should be moved out of the reception room as soon as possible?

    a. a patient with HIV

    b. a patient with conjunctivitis

    c. a patient with a fever

    d. a patient with a headache

9. How should the receptionist handle a patient who brings in food to eat while in the reception room?

    a. The receptionist should ignore it unless the patient is making a mess.

    b. The receptionist should ask the patient to share the food with the other patients in the reception room.

    c. The receptionist should ask the patient to take the food outside to finish eating it.

    d. The receptionist should ask the physician to come out and speak with the patient.

10. How much seating should the reception room have for patients?

    a. enough to accommodate 15 minutes' worth of patients per physician, as well as the patient's friends and relatives

    b. enough to accommodate 30 minutes' worth of patients per physician, as well as the patient's friends and relatives

    c. enough to accommodate 1 hour's worth of patients per physician, as well as the patient's friends and relatives

    d. enough to accommodate 2 hours' worth of patients per physician, as well as the patient's friends and relatives

CRITICAL THINKING

Answer the following questions to the best of your ability. Use the textbook as a reference.

1. Marcus Winston, RMA (AMT), has been hired to work as an administrative medical assistant at the front desk in a small, one-physician medical office. Dr. Quan has been using a paper sign-in sheet for his patients for many years. Marcus has recently completed his medical assisting education and remembers learning that sign-in sheets must be HIPAA compliant. What can Marcus tell Dr. Quan about the paper sign-in system he is currently using?

_____

_____

_____

_____

_____

2. Sara Womack, CMA (AAMA), is the medical office manager in a women's clinic. She has two employees who share the job of front desk receptionist. Aaron Shelley, CMA (AAMA), doesn't like to work at the front desk. He is often short with the patients, some of whom have complained to the physician. Michael Sulley, RMA (AMT), is the other front desk receptionist. Michael has a sunny personality and thoroughly enjoys the fast pace at the front desk. Would Sara be better serving the patients of the women's clinic if she moved Aaron out of that position and had Michael work there full time? Why or why not? What sort of ramifications might occur if Sara leaves Aaron in the front desk position?

_____

_____

_____

_____

3. Marjorie Sorensen, CMA (AAMA), has just been hired to work as the office manager for Dr. Rodriguez. The doctor tells Marjorie that she has noticed that many tasks are being skipped by the front desk staff when opening the office in the morning. Dr. Rodriguez believes the front desk staff is forgetting these tasks and has asked Marjorie to come up a solution to this problem. What might Marjorie suggest?

_____

_____

_____

_____

4. Isaiah Chung is taking an administrative medical assisting course as part of his training to become a medical assistant. His instructor has assigned the task of creating an office policy for opening the medical office. How might Isaiah's policy read?

_____

_____

_____

_____

5. Wally Harrison, RMA (AMT), has just come back from an administrative medical assisting continuing education workshop. He has learned that many medical offices are sending new patient paperwork to patients in the mail prior to their appointment. How can Wally explain the benefits of doing this to his coworkers and the physicians where he works?

_____

_____

_____

_____

RESEARCH ACTIVITY

Use Internet search engines to research the following topics and write a brief description of what is found. It is important to visit reputable Web sites.

1. Using the information and décor theme of the reception area that you designed in the applied practice activity, research the Internet and obtain figures and estimates regarding the cost of decorating a reception area. Take into consideration paint, accessories, seating, tables, etc. Be sure to cite the Web sites you use to find your materials.

CHAPTER 11

Patient Scheduling

CHAPTER OUTLINE

General review of the chapter:

    A. Scheduling Patient Appointments
    B. Methods of Appointment Scheduling
        i. Appointment types
       ii. Buffer time
      iii. Patient reminders
      iv. Correcting the appointment schedule
    C. Managing the Physician's Professional Schedule
    D. Arranging for Interpreters
    E. Arranging for Transportation

STUDENT STUDY GUIDE

Use the following guide to assist in your learning of the concepts from the chapter.

   I. Patient Scheduling
     A. The MA's Role in Patient Scheduling
        i. The MA will schedule a variety of appointments:
           (a) Office appointments for new and established patients
           (b) _____ and _____ appointments at outside medical facilities
     B. Scheduling Guidelines
        i. First determine if a patient is _____ or _____.
       ii. Anyone seen within the past _____ is considered established.
          (a) This is a guideline set by many _____ _____ for billing purposes.
      iii. Scheduling a new patient for an appointment over the phone generally involves the use of a new patient information checklist.
      iv. New information checklist includes:

_____

_____

_____

_____

_____

_____

_____

_____

_____

_____

_____

v. Office policies vary concerning appointment _____.

vi. New patients generally have _____ appointment times.

vii. Some offices may also only perform certain _____ on certain _____.

viii. Documenting scheduling policies is important so that everyone is aware of the physician's scheduling preferences.

ix. An appointment _____ identifies _____ and _____ available for scheduling patient appointments.

    (a) Holidays, _____ _____, and the _____ _____ _____ must be _____ so that appointments cannot be scheduled during those times.

x. Abbreviations used during matrix annotations must be standard for the office.

xi. Patient or staffing needs must be recognized when scheduling appointments:

_____

_____

_____

_____

_____

_____

_____

C. Scheduling Systems

   i. Electronic scheduling systems are becoming the norm.

    (a) This allows _____ _____ to schedule appointments at the same time.

  ii. Appointment books are still used.

    (a) Books must support all _____ in the practice.

    (b) Multipractice offices may utilize _____ _____ appointment books.

D. Appointment Types

   i. Cluster scheduling:

_____

_____

_____

_____

  ii. Double booking:

_____

_____

_____

_____

  iii. Fixed appointment:

_____

_____

_____

_____

  iv. Open hours:

_____

_____

_____

   v. Wave scheduling:

_____

_____

_____

_____

   vi. Modified wave scheduling:

_____

_____

_____

_____

   vii. _____ time: 15-20 minutes at the end of the morning, afternoon, and
         evening.
         (a) Allows the physician time to catch up on _____
         (b) Allows appointment times for patients who need _____ -
              _____ appointments
E. Reminder Cards
    i. Reminder cards are often given to patients when an appointment is _____.
    ii. Reminder cards or _____ may be sent to patients via the postal system.
         (a) Usually for patients who have scheduled appointments more than a/an
              _____ in advance.
         (b) If sending postcards, patient _____ must be considered.
F. Changes to the Appointment Book
    i. "_____-_____" patients fail to arrive, cancel, or
        reschedule an appointment.
    ii. If a change to the appointment book needs to be made, a/an _____ line
         should be drawn through the appointment with a/an _____ regarding the
         _____ for the change.
    iii. _____ _____, _____ and
          _____ are not permitted in the appointment book.
G. Following Up Missed Appointments
    i. The MA should call the patient _____ minutes after the missed
        appointment.
    ii. A message may be left requesting the patient to call the office.
    iii. If unable to reach a patient, a/an _____ can be _____ ask-
          ing the patient to call and reschedule the appointment.
    iv. _____ is vital for all missed appointments.
    v. Missed appointments and attempts made to reach the patient must be
        _____ in the _____ _____.
    vi. If a patient encounters adverse reactions or outcomes due to not appearing for his or her
         appointment, _____ _____ backs up the medical office
         during _____.

II. Other Scheduling Duties
    A. The Physician's Travel Schedule
        i. The physician's travel schedule is usually maintained by the _____.
        ii. This includes blocking appointment times when the physician is away from the office.
       iii. All information must be clearly documented:

_____

_____

_____

_____

       iv. A copy of the physician's _____ should be kept at the
          _____ as reference for the staff.
        v. _____ _____ _____ the physician earns
          during his travels is recorded by the MA.
    B. Hospital Admission Procedures
        i. Hospital services or admission should be scheduled while the patient is in the office.
        ii. Many insurance companies require _____ prior to testing or a/an
          _____.
       iii. Obtain preapproval authorization prior to scheduling an appointment.
       iv. Various procedures that are performed in the hospital setting should have established
         guidelines.
        v. Guidelines should include:

_____

_____

_____

_____

_____

    C. Interpreter Services
        i. Patients who require language translation often bring a friend or family member to his or
         her doctor visit.
        ii. The medical office must _____ _____
          _____ if the patient is unable.
       iii. _____ _____ of translators that are used by the office
         should be kept at the front desk.
       iv. Many states offer translation services for their _____ covered programs.

KEY TERMINOLOGY REVIEW

Match the correct medical term with the definition listed below.

    a. buffer time   **h.** new patient
    b. cluster scheduling   **i.** office brochure
    c. double booking   **j.** open hours
    d. established patient   **k.** pre-approvals
    e. fixed-appointment   **l.** slack time
    f. matrix   **m.** wave scheduling
    g. modified wave scheduling

_____ 1. Calling an insurance carrier for authorization prior to scheduling a test in a hospital.

_____ 2. Scheduling more than one patient for the same appointment time.

_____ 3. A time of the day left open for same-day appointments or time for the physician to catch up on charting.

_____ 4. A patient whom the provider has not seen in more than 3 years.

_____ 5. Scheduling method where patients are not given appointment times.

_____ 6. Also known as slack time.

_____ 7. A pamphlet outlining an office's staff and services.

_____ 8. A patient whom has been seen by a practitioner within the past 3 years.

_____ 9. Process of blocking out times in the appointment schedule when the provider is unavailable or out of the office.

_____ 10. Patients are only scheduled during the first half of an hour and are served on a first-come, first-served basis.

_____ 11. Patients, with similar appointment types, are scheduled around the same block of time.

_____ 12. The most common form of appointment scheduling.

_____ 13. Two or three patients are scheduled at the beginning of each hour, followed by single patient appointments every 10 to 20 minutes for the rest of that hour.

APPLIED PRACTICE

Follow the directions as instructed with each question below.

1. Using the information below and the manual schedule on the following pages, create a matrix for the medical office. (Remember to use a pencil.)

   a. The medical office opens at 8:30 A.M. every day.
   b. The last appointment for the day is scheduled no later than 3:30 P.M.
   c. The office is closed for appointments for lunch starting at 12:00 P.M. and reopening at 1:15 P.M.
   d. Dr. Cho has hospital rounds every Wednesday from 7:30 A.M. to 10:00 A.M.
   e. Dr. Jackson has hospital rounds every Thursday from 7:45 A.M. to 10:15 A.M.
   f. On February 3, Dr. Cho has a meeting at Alliance Assisted Living that starts at 3:30 P.M.
   g. On February 2, Dr. Jackson has a meeting with a pharmaceutical representative that is scheduled from 12:45 to 1:30 P.M.

2. Schedule the following patients on the appointment schedule.

   a. LaToya Atwater is a new patient to see Dr. Cho. Wednesdays work best for LaToya.
   b. Sujin Dalywhal wants to see Dr. Jackson Thursday afternoon for an abdominal suture removal.
   c. José Alvarez calls on Wednesday morning because he has had a terrible headache for the past two days.
   d. Anna Maria DeCamillo is a diabetic patient who wants to see Dr. Jackson for her 3-month diabetic check-up on Wednesday afternoon.
   e. Mark Tomlinson wants to see Dr. Cho for his annual check-up on Thursday.
   f. Aiden Taylor needs to be seen on Thursday morning for his 3-year well-child visit with Dr. Jackson.
   g. Dr. Cho requests that an appointment be made on Wednesday morning with her patient, Lydia Pazmino, regarding her blood test results.

WEDNESDAY, FEBRUARY 2, 20XX

	Dr. S. Cho	Dr. A. Jackson
7:30		
7:45		
8:00		
8:15		
8:30		
8:45		
9:00		
9:15		
9:30		
9:45		
10:00		
10:15		
10:30		
10:45		
11:00		
11:15		
11:30		
11:45		
12:00		
12:15		
12:30		
12:45		
1:00		
1:15		
1:30		
1:45		
2:00		
2:15		
2:30		
2:45		
3:00		
3:15		
3:30		
3:45		
4:00		

THURSDAY, FEBRUARY 3, 20XX

	Dr. S. Cho	Dr. A. Jackson
7:30		
7:45		
8:00		
8:15		
8:30		
8:45		
9:00		
9:15		
9:30		
9:45		
10:00		
10:15		
10:30		
10:45		
11:00		
11:15		
11:30		
11:45		
12:00		
12:15		
12:30		
12:45		
1:00		
1:15		
1:30		
1:45		
2:00		
2:15		
2:30		
2:45		
3:00		
3:15		
3:30		
3:45		
4:00		

LEARNING ACTIVITY: MULTIPLE CHOICE

Circle the correct answer to each of the questions below

1. How much time should the medical assistant wait before calling a patient who has missed his appointment?

   a. 5–10 minutes
   b. 10–15 minutes

   c. 15–30 minutes
   d. 60 minutes

2. Which of the following is an acceptable way to note a missed appointment in a paper appointment book?

   a. Use white correction fluid to cover the patient's name.
   b. Use a black marker to obliterate the patient's name.

   c. Use an eraser to remove the patient's name.
   d. Draw a single line through the patient's name.

3. What is one way to remind patients of their upcoming appointment in the medical office?

   a. Send out a reminder card to the patient just prior to the appointment.
   b. Call the patient to remind them of their appointment.

   c. Send an email to the patient to remind them of their appointment.
   d. any of the above

4. Which of the following messages would be appropriate to leave on a patient's voice-mail?

   a. "This is Martha calling from Dr. Brown's office to remind John of his appointment tomorrow at 9 A.M."
   b. "This is Martha calling from Dr. Brown's office to remind John of his appointment for a culture and sensitivity test tomorrow at 9 A.M."

   c. "This is Martha calling from Dr. Brown's office to remind John of his appointment tomorrow at 9 A.M. He will need to fast for 12 hours prior to this appointment."
   d. any of the above

5. A typical reminder card for patient appointments contains which of the following pieces of information?

   a. the date of the upcoming appointment
   b. the time of the upcoming appointment

   c. the name of the medical facility
   d. all of the above

6. Which of the following correctly defines "buffer" or "slack" time in the appointment schedule?

   a. times in the appointment book that are left open to accommodate patients who call for same-day appointments
   b. times in the appointment book that are left open to accommodate emergency patients

   c. times in the appointment book that are left open for physicians to catch up on charting
   d. all of the above

7. The _____ method of scheduling is where two or three patients are scheduled at the beginning of each hour, followed by single patient appointments every 10 to 20 minutes for the rest of that hour.

   a. wave scheduling
   b. modified wave scheduling

   c. open hours scheduling
   d. fixed appointment scheduling

8. The _____ method of scheduling is where patients are scheduled only for the first half of each hour. The first patient to arrive is seen first.

   a. wave scheduling
   b. modified wave scheduling

   c. open hours scheduling
   d. fixed appointment scheduling

9. The _____ method of scheduling is most commonly used in walk-in clinics, laboratories, and X-ray facilities where patients are typically seen on a first-come, first-served basis.

   a. wave scheduling
   b. modified wave scheduling

   c. open hours scheduling
   d. fixed appointment scheduling

10. The _____ method of scheduling is one where each patient is given a specific appointment time.

    a. wave scheduling
    b. modified wave scheduling

    c. open hours scheduling
    d. fixed appointment scheduling

CRITICAL THINKING

Answer the following questions to the best of your ability. Use the textbook as a reference.

1. Dylan Reilly, CMA (AAMA), is working in a busy family practice office. The physicians and staff all agree that the appointment scheduling system is not working and patients are frequently waiting long periods of time for appointments. How should Dylan go about creating a new scheduling procedure for this office?

   _____

   _____

   _____

   _____

2. Mallory Shannon, RMA (AMT), has been asked by the clinic director to create a written policy for how to arrange for language interpreters for patients who need them. What sort of policy might Mallory create?

   _____

   _____

   _____

   _____

   _____

3. Armando Alonso is taking an administrative medical assisting course as part of his medical assisting training. He has been given an assignment to create a list of the information patients should be given in order to help prepare the patient for medical procedures when scheduling the patient. What sort of information should Armando list?

_____

_____

_____

_____

_____

4. Anna Simonenko, CMA (AAMA), is working at the front desk in a family practice clinic. Anna has been asked to schedule Roger Edetsberger for a procedure to be performed in the hospital. Anna tells Roger that she will need to call his insurance company before she can schedule the procedure. Roger says, "Why do you need to do that? Can't you just schedule the procedure now and call the insurance company some other time?" What can Anna say to Roger?

_____

_____

_____

_____

_____

5. Ronna DeLancer, RMA (AMT), is working as an administrative medical assistant for Dr. Angela Chien. Dr. Chien is traveling out of town for a continuing education seminar and has asked Ronna to make all of the arrangements. What sort of arrangements will Ronna likely make for Dr. Chien?

_____

_____

_____

_____

_____

RESEARCH ACTIVITY

Use Internet search engines to research the following topics and write a brief description of what is found. It is important to visit reputable Web sites.

1. Research various appointment scheduling software programs for medical offices.

   What products are available?
   What must be considered prior to purchasing medical office software?
   What type of technical support is available?

_____

_____

_____

_____

_____

CHAPTER 12
Medical Records Management

CHAPTER OUTLINE

General review of the chapter:

- A. Key Terminology
- B. Information in the Medical Record
- C. Forms of Charting
- D. Charting Patient Communication
- E. File Storage Systems
- F. Retaining, Correcting, and Adding to Medical Records

STUDENT STUDY GUIDE

Use the following guide to assist in your learning of the concepts from the chapter.

I. The MA's Role and Medical Record Information
   A. The MA's Role in Medical Record Management
      i. MAs work with medical records on a/an _____ _____.
      ii. MAs must understand how to handle patient records.
      iii. Offices may be subject to _____ if patient privacy is _____.
   B. Information Contained in the Medical Record
      i. The medical record contains _____, _____, _____, and _____ information for each patient.
      ii. Personal information includes:

      _____

      _____

      _____

      iii. Financial information includes:

      _____

      _____

      _____

      iv. Medical information includes:

      _____

      _____

      _____

      _____

v. Social information includes:

_____

_____

_____

_____

II. Charting Styles and Cross Referencing
   A. Narrative Charting
      i. _____ form of medical charting
     ii. A/an _____ account
    iii. Often physicians have their narrative notes _____ after dictation.
    iv. The _____ notes are placed in the patient's chart.
   B. SOAP Charting
      i. "S" reflects _____ findings: patient statements and information about chief complaints.
     ii. "O" includes _____ clinical findings: vital signs and examination findings.
    iii. "A" represents the _____ found by the physician which is a diagnosis or possible diagnosis.
    iv. "P" represents the _____ that the physician will take to treat the patient: prescriptions, tests, referrals, etc.
   C. Problem-Oriented Medical Records (POMR)
      i. A/an _____ is assigned to every patient's problem.
     ii. That number is referred to when the patient seeks help for that specific problem.
   D. Patient Communication
      i. Medically relevant communication must be charted in a patient's medical record.
     ii. This includes communication with patients _____ of office visits.

_____

_____

    iii. Information including _____ or _____ appointments and _____ refill requests
    iv. Every office should have policies regarding what information must be charted.
   E. Cross-Referencing
      i. Alphabetical filing can become complicated when the patient's last name is _____.
     ii. With cross-referencing, both the _____ patient chart and a _____ patient chart is filed.
    iii. The blank patient file is filed under the _____ last name.
   F. Cross-Referencing Example

_____

_____

_____

_____

   G. Missing Medical Records
      i. A patient medical file may be _____ from its correct _____.
     ii. This is often due to _____.
    iii. First check to see if the chart was filed under the patient's _____ _____.
    iv. If the chart is still missing, check the following locations:

_____

_____

_____

_____

III. Filing Systems, File Storage, and File Status

    A. Color-Coded File Systems

        i. Color-coded filing is often used along with _____ filing.

        ii. Color-coded alphabetic _____ are used.

        iii. The first _____ _____ of a patient's last name is used for alphabetic color-coding.

            (a) Various _____/_____ combinations may be used.

        iv. Color-coded stickers are affixed to the outside of the patient's chart.

        v. Alphabetic filing causes the same colored stickers to be _____ together.

        vi. This easily identifies _____ charts.

    B. Numeric Filing

        i. Medical office may choose to use numeric filing instead of alphabetical filing

        ii. Often used if patient information is highly _____:

_____

_____

_____

_____

        iii. This system makes it more difficult to retrieve medical files.

        iv. Staff members must be aware of codes pertaining to numerical filing.

        v. Patient names and their corresponding file number should be kept in a/an

_____ _____.

    C. File Storage Systems

        i. File storage systems are usually _____.

        ii. Metal towers with pull-out drawers are a/an _____ filing system.

        iii. _____ filing systems having drawers that reveal the sides of the files are commonly used.

        iv. Larger offices may use file storage cabinets that can be moved in their entirety.

            (a) This system allows for additional filing space, _____ _____, and _____.

    D. Status of Patient Files

        i. Paper files take up a lot of valuable space.

        ii. Offices will commonly _____ patient files that are closed or inactive.

        iii. Purged files may either be stored at a secured off-site location, or be transferred to a digital file.

        iv. Active patients have recently seen a practitioner within the practice.

        v. Inactive patient may not have seen a physician within _____ years.

_____

_____

        vi. Removing inactive charts takes up less space and makes it easier to locate active charts.

        vii. Closed files include:

_____

_____

_____

_____

    E. Paper and Electronic Medical Records

        i. Paper records may be converted to electronic records for _____ storage.

        ii. Once the paper file has been completely transferred, it must be _____.

  iii. This is done by _____ the paper files.
  iv. All medical offices should have paper shredders to shred confidential information.
    (a) Shredding companies can be hired to complete large projects.
 F. Storing Inactive Files
  i. Inactive medical files should be stored so that they take up as little room as possible:
    (a) Records can be scanned and kept on _____, _____,
    _____, or any other safe electronic format.
  ii. Medical records must be stored in a secure environment:
    (a) Safe from _____ or _____ damage
    (b) Easily accessible by the health care team as needed
 G. Destroying Patient Files
  i. There may be times when it is determined appropriate to destroy a medical record.
  ii. HIPAA dictates that the record must be shredded _____
  _____.
  iii. It cannot be in a condition such that it can be put back together to reveal personal patient information.
 H. Correcting a Medical Record
  i. To correct an error that is made in the medical record:

_____

_____

_____

  ii. Errors in the medical record should never be obliterated, scribbled out, or covered with
  _____ _____.

 I. Patient-Directed Changes to the Medical Record
  i. The physical documents that compose a medical record belong to the

_____

_____

  ii. The patient owns the

_____

_____

  iii. If a patient believes that an error exists in the medical record, he or she may request that a change be made.
  iv. If a patient wishes to change information in the record:

_____

_____

_____

_____

_____

_____

_____

KEY TERMINOLOGY REVIEW

Match the correct medical term with the definition listed below.

a. active patient files
b. chief complaint
c. closed patient files
d. flow charts
e. inactive patient charts

f. indecipherable
g. narrative
h. obliterate
i. POMR
j. progress note

k. purge
l. shingling
m. SOAP
n. statute of limitations
o. subpoena

_____ 1. Files for patients who have not seen the physician for extended periods.

_____ 2. To remove closed or inactive patient medical records from the medical office.

_____ 3. Type of medical record charting that focuses on patient's health care problems and addresses those problems at each health care visit.

_____ 4. Files for patients who have seen a physician recently.

_____ 5. Type of charting that considers the patient's subjective and objective findings and the provider's assessment, and the prescribed plan of action for treatment.

_____ 6. Unreadable.

_____ 7. Notes in patients' medical charts outlining those patients' progress or complaints.

_____ 8. Main reason a patient seeks care.

_____ 9. Process of attaching small pieces of paper to standard-size sheets of paper so the small items are easy to locate in patient charts.

_____ 10. Type of medical charting in which the health care provider writes a narrative version of patient contact.

_____ 11. Court order demanding that a party appear in court or copies of the medical record be sent to a third party.

_____ 12. Graphs in patient medical records that track such things as weight gain or newborn growth.

_____ 13. Period within which a patient must file a lawsuit after an injury.

_____ 14. To make unreadable or unrecognizable.

_____ 15. Files for patients that will not be returning to the clinic.

APPLIED PRACTICE

Follow the directions as instructed with each question below.

1. Indicate if the following patients would be considered active, inactive, or closed patient files.

   a. Lori Hughes, a patient who has moved out of the state
      Patient file status: _____

   b. Quin Tao, a patient who has not been seen in the office for five years
      Patient file status: _____

c. Gloria Sanchez, a patient who was in the office for care last week

Patient file status: _____

d. Sara Womack, a patient who died last year

Patient file status: _____

2. Using the progress note, accurately place the statements below into SOAP format. Mario Reynolds, born August 12, 1990 presents to the office.

- T: 100.3°
- Positive Rapid Strep-Test
- My throat is sore.
- Pharyngitis and strep throat
- Throat appears red, and white spots present on tonsils.
- Penicillin V 250mg bid × 10 days
- BP: 118/86
- Wt: 192#
- Patient has been sick with a fever for 3 days.

Progress Note

Patient:_____ DOB:_____

	S	O	A	P

LEARNING ACTIVITY: MULTIPLE CHOICE

Circle the correct answer to each of the questions below.

1. Which of the following techniques is the appropriate way to correct an error in the patient's medical record?

   a. Use white correction fluid to obliterate the error.
   b. Use a black marker to obliterate the error.
   c. Draw a single line through the error, initial and date the correction.
   d. any of the above

2. Under which of the following circumstances can the patient's medical record be copied and released?

   a. when the patient's spouse comes to the office to request a copy
   b. when the patient's employer calls the office to request a copy
   c. when the office receives a subpoena signed by a judge requesting a copy
   d. when the patient's brother sends in a letter asking for a copy

3. Medicare guidelines dictate that patient medical records must be kept in the office for at least _____ years from the patient's last date of service.

   a. 5

   b. 10

   c. 15

   d. 20

4. Once an office is out of room for storing patient medical records, which of the following is an appropriate way to store records?

   a. scan the record and record it onto a CD

   b. scan the record and record it onto a DVD

   c. scan the record and record it onto microfilm

   d. any of the above

5. Which of the following is true about retaining patient medical records?

   a. The record should be kept for 3 years from the date of the last service.

   b. The length of time the record is kept is determined by the statute of limitations in any particular state.

   c. The record should be kept until the patient reaches age 18.

   d. All of the above are true.

6. _____ patient files are the files of patients who have moved and will not be continuing to treat with the physician or facility.

   a. Open

   b. Closed

   c. Inactive

   d. none of the above

7. _____ patient files are the files of patients who have not been in to see the physician for a period of between 2 to 5 years, depending upon the type of practice.

   a. Open

   b. Closed

   c. Inactive

   d. none of the above

8. _____ patient files are the files of patients who have been in to see the physician recently.

   a. Open

   b. Closed

   c. Inactive

   d. none of the above

9. Which of the following is a situation where the medical office might use a flow chart to track patient care?

   a. to track an infant's weight and length

   b. to chart appropriate patient telephone calls

   c. to chart needed patient medical procedures

   d. any of the above

10. _____ is a type of medical charting that tracks a patient's problems throughout medical care by assigning a number to each of the patient's medical problems.

   a. Narrative notes

   b. SOAP notes

   c. POMR notes

   d. none of the above

CRITICAL THINKING

Answer the following questions to the best of your ability. Use the textbook as a reference.

1. Lily Foote, CMA (AAMA), is working with Dr. Marla Tiffany. Dr. Tiffany has asked Lily to create a policy for how medical records will be handled for patients who are involved in the medical research programs that Dr. Tiffany participates in. How should Lily proceed?

_____

_____

_____

_____

_____

2. Susan Haufe, RMA (AMT), is working with a small, one-doctor internal medicine clinic. The physician, Dr. Chentow, is retiring and will not be transferring his files to another physician. How should Susan proceed with working with the patient files that are in the office?

_____

_____

_____

_____

_____

3. Rodney Jarvis is in an administrative medical assisting class. He has been given an assignment to create a policy for documenting prescription refill requests in the medical office. What might Rodney create?

_____

_____

_____

_____

_____

4. Michael Manson, RMA (AMT), has just been hired to work in a family practice clinic. On his first day in the office, he notices that many patient charts have words such as "problem" and "talker" listed on them. He asks the MA who is training him about these words and is told it is the office's way of noting those patients who are difficult to work with or who talk excessively during their visit. What kinds of problems might this facility encounter when using these notations?

_____

_____

_____

_____

5. Chris Nichols, CMA (AAMA), has been given the task of deciding which patient files to purge from the clinic in order to create more storage room. How should Chris proceed with this project?

_____

_____

_____

RESEARCH ACTIVITY

Use Internet search engines to research the following topics and write a brief description of what is found. It is important to visit reputable Web sites.

1. Using the Internet as a research source, research the types of filing systems that may be found in a medical setting. Describe the pros and cons of each system.

CHAPTER 13
Electronic Medical Records

CHAPTER OUTLINE

General review of the chapter:

    A. Introduction
    B. The MA's Role in Medical Assisting
    C. Paper Charting vs. Electronic Charting
    D. Making the Conversion
    E. EMR and HIPAA Compliance
    F. Using PDAs with EMRs
    G. Benefits of EMRs

STUDENT STUDY GUIDE

Use the following guide to assist in your learning of the concepts from the chapter.

  I. The Electronic Medical Record

    A. The MA's Role in Electronic Medical Records
       i. The EMR is a part of the _____ of health care.
      ii. MAs must be comfortable with computers:
         (a) They must be able to navigate an EMR.
      iii. _____ used varies from office to office; however, the premise for each system is similar.

    B. Paper vs. Electronic Records
       i. Electronic medical records:
         (a) Allow for easy _____ of patient information between health care providers
         (b) Should reduce medical _____ _____
         (c) Offers an overall _____ in health care
         (d) Most Americans will have electronic medical records by _____.
         (e) Many offices now have _____ _____ in each examination room
      ii. Some physicians and medical assistants use electronic _____ to enter patient data into a computer system.
      iii. With paper files, patient records are only available to one _____ _____ at a time.
      iv. With electronic files, patient records are accessible by _____ staff members at the same time.
      v. When using paper records:
         (a) Patient information must be _____. It is sometimes difficult to read.
         (b) Staff members have to _____ insurance information.
         (c) Charts for new patients must be _____ and _____.

(d) All information obtained during the patient's visit is written into the paper record:

_____

_____

_____

(e) Patient education material must be _____ and _____ according to topic.

C. Converting Paper Medical Records

   i. Converting paper medical records to electronic medical records is _____ _____.

   ii. However, the _____-_____utilizing the electronic medical record can save a great deal of time.

   iii. Offices must determine which type of _____will be used according to the preferences of the staff.

   iv. Offices may choose to _____documents into a computer system.

   v. Offices may also choose to _____ _____information from the paper chart to the electronic chart.

D. Using the EMR

   i. An electronic medical record can be started when a new patient _____ _____the office to schedule an appointment.

   ii. When using electronic records:

_____

_____

_____

_____

_____

_____

_____

_____

_____

_____

_____

E. Correcting the EMR

   i. Charting errors may still occur while using the electronic medical record.

   ii. The error must be corrected _____after it has been recognized.

   iii. Software programs vary regarding how to make changes to the EMR.

   iv. Generally, a/an _____ _____is _____through the entry, and corrected information is entered.

   v. The _____ _____is still viewable, though it might be on a separate screen or shown with a line drawn through it.

F. Destroying the Paper Record

   i. If an office has converted to EMRs, the _____ _____record must be dealt with accordingly.

   ii. Offices may choose to _____ the records.

   (a) To do this properly, all documents within the record must be _____.

   iii. Office may choose not to _____ the _____.

   (a) Files would be stored at a/an _____ _____.

G. HIPAA Compliance

   i. EMRs must be _____compliant.

   ii. This is accomplished by:

   (a) All computers must be _____protected.

   (b) Each staff member must have his or her own _____ and _____ to access patient files.

(1) This tracks who made _____, _____, and deletions to the EMR.

(c) Computer stations must be _____ _____ when a person is away from the desk.

(d) Computer screens with patient information can not be visible to other patients.

(e) Offices must safeguard the EMR by _____ _____ the computer systems:

_____

_____

H. Personal Digital Assistants

_____

_____

_____

_____

_____

_____

I. Benefits of the EMR

   i. The ability to use an electronic signature as opposed to a/an _____ _____ signature

     (a) A/an _____ _____ of the _____ must be kept on file in the office.

  ii. Forms and _____ can be completed in an electronic format:

_____

_____

  iii. EMRs save time:

_____

_____

_____

_____

_____

_____

  iv. Results from tests performed in the medical office can be sent _____ to the patient's EMR.

   v. The EMR can serve as _____ between staff members.

  vi. The EMR is useful during marketing purposes.

 vii. The EMR can assist in making patient records available _____.

KEY TERMINOLOGY REVIEW

Create sentences using the key terminology within the correct context.

1. Electronic medical record:

_____

_____

2. Electronic signature:

_____

_____

3. Indecipherable:

_____

_____

APPLIED PRACTICE

Read the scenario and then answer the questions that follow.

Scenario

Jeffery Cody, RMA (AMT), is the office manager for Foothills Family Medicine. The office has slowly been transferring from paper medical records to electronic medical records.

1. In the final stages, how will the medical office include written reports and consultations from other facilities?

_____

_____

2. Jeffery is writing a memo to the office staff regarding making corrections to the medical record. What information should he include in his memo?

_____

_____

_____

_____

LEARNING ACTIVITY: TRUE/FALSE

Indicate whether the statement is true (T) or false (F).

_____ 1. Electronic medical records offer enhanced ease, efficiency, and accessibility.

_____ 2. Using electronic medical records, a medical office can send reminder post cards to patients more easily than performing this task using paper medical records.

_____ 3. Using electronic medical records a medical office is able to perform many tests in the office and have the results show immediately within the electronic medical record.

_____ 4. It is much more difficult to remain HIPAA compliant with patient medical records if the office is using electronic medical records instead of paper medical records.

_____ 5. Once the medical office has converted from paper to electronic medical records, the paper medical record should still be stored in the medical office.

_____ 6. Most electronic medical records programs have drop-down menus that allow the user to choose information from a list.

_____ 7. As a result of a study released in 1999, the Institute of Medicine suggested that some medical errors are caused by indecipherable handwriting.

_____ 8. Using electronic medical records, health care providers may be alerted to possible medication errors.

_____ 9. In medical offices where electronic signatures are used, an original version of the user's signature must be kept on file in the office.

_____ 10. All medical facilities use the same software for electronic medical records.

CRITICAL THINKING

Answer the following questions to the best of your ability. Use the textbook as a reference.

1. Rosa Valdez, CMA (AAMA), is working in the billing office in a urology practice. The office uses electronic medical records for patient charting. Rosa frequently finds that she needs to alert other staff members to her need to speak with a patient about their account. How might Rosa devise a way to alert her coworkers to the need to see patients when the patient comes into the office?

_____

_____

_____

_____

2. Chris Hernandez, RMA (AMT), is the office manager of a busy family practice clinic. Chris has been asked by the physicians to come up with some ideas for using the electronic medical record software to create a marketing program. What kinds of ideas could Chris suggest for this project?

_____

_____

_____

_____

3. Mickey Cape is taking a course on electronic medical records. Mickey has been given an assignment to write a policy on how to dispose of paper medical records once the record has been converted to electronic form. What might Mickey come up with?

_____

_____

_____

_____

4. Barret Risenhour, RMA (AMT), is the office manager in a women's clinic. The physicians in the clinic are considering moving to electronic medical records from the paper records they have been using for years. Barret has been asked to create a list of pros and cons to using paper records as opposed to using electronic medical records. What might Barret's list contain?

_____

_____

_____

5. Dr. Shawn Hagen has been using paper medical records in his practice for over 20 years. He is reluctant to change to electronic medical records because he feels his computer skills are poor. What sort of information can his office manager give to him about the ease of converting from paper to electronic medical records?

_____

_____

_____

_____

_____

RESEARCH ACTIVITY

Use Internet search engines to research the following topics and write a brief description of what is found. It is important to visit reputable Web sites.

1. Using the Internet as a research source, locate three companies that sell electronic medical records software. Create a list of the pros and cons of each system.

_____

_____

_____

_____

_____

_____

_____

_____

_____

_____

_____

_____

CHAPTER 14
Computers in the Medical Office

CHAPTER OUTLINE

General review of the chapter:

A. Introduction
B. The MA's Role in Computers in the Medical Office
C. Components of the Computer System
D. Computer Peripherals
E. Maintaining Computer Equipment
F. Computer Software
G. Personal Computer Use in the Office
H. Computer Ergonomics

STUDENT STUDY GUIDE

Use the following guide to assist in your learning of the concepts from the chapter.

I. The MA's Role and Computers in the Medical Office

  A. The MA's Role Using Computers in the Medical Office
    i. The MA will use the computer to:
      (a) Enter _____ _____
      (b) Charge and _____ for billing services
      (c) _____ appointments
      (d) Various other tasks as needed

  B. Computers in the Medical Office
    i. Computers have many uses in the medical office:

    _____

    _____

    _____

    _____

    _____

  C. Technology has advanced the use of computers:
    i. Scanners
    ii. Digital cameras
    iii. Electronic sign-in sheets
    iv. Barcode readers are also becoming common in medical offices.
    v. They can be used for:

    _____

    _____

_____

_____

II. Computer Purchasing, Types, Components, Maintenance, and Security

   A. Purchasing a Computer

      i. _____ is highly recommended before purchasing a computer for the office.

     ii. Things to consider:

        (a) _____ _____ _____: the brain of the computer. The faster the CPU runs, the more _____ the computer.

        (b) Memory: the _____ memory, the higher the cost.

        (c) Software: Consumes memory. Various software applications are available. See Table 14-3 for commonly used software in the medical field.

        (d) Computer monitor: Monitor resolution is measured in dots per _____ _____ or DSI. The _____ the DSI, the higher the price.

        (e) Flat panel monitor: More costly than the traditional computer monitor; however, it saves valuable _____ _____.

   B. Types of Computers

      i. _____ _____: fastest processing capacity; introduced in the 1960s

     ii. _____ computer: used for large volume applications, such as government statistics

    iii. _____: a multiuser computer, and falls in size between the mainframe and the microcomputer

    iv. _____: most commonly used in health care; _____ and _____ are examples.

   C. Components of a Computer

      i. Hardware:

_____

_____

     ii. Software:

_____

_____

_____

_____

_____

    iii. Peripherals:

_____

_____

   D. Computer Maintenance

      i. Maintenance should be performed to ensure that computers are running efficiently.

     ii. Avoid _____ and _____ near the computer.

    iii. Keep computer systems and any discs:

_____

_____

_____

_____

    iv. Handle any discs carefully and _____ them appropriately.

     v. Dust _____ and _____ regularly.

    vi. Performance or maintenance issues should be handled by _____ _____.

E. Computer Security
   i. Medical office computers must be secured because they store _____ _____.
   ii. All staff should have personal _____ passwords to access computers.
   iii. Never share or leave passwords in plain view.
   iv. _____ _____ after using the computer.
   v. HIPAA requires:
      (a) Patient health information (PHI) must be _____ _____ periodically.
      (b) A/an _____ _____ must exist for backed-up data that leaves the medical facility.
      (c) Access to backed-up data must be _____ to _____ parties.
      (d) A backup plan and _____ _____ plan must be in place.
      (e) Data must be a retrievable, exact copy.
      (f) All computers must be password protected.

III. Internet, Personal Use, PDAs and Ergonomics

   A. Internet Research
      i. Contemporary physicians and medical offices utilize the Internet to conduct research.
      ii. Only _____ _____ _____ should be used when conducting a search.
      iii. Pharmaceutical and insurance companies often maintain comprehensive Web sites that contain valuable information:

      _____

      _____

      _____

      _____

      _____

   B. Personal Computer Use
      i. Every office will develop its own _____ regarding personal computer use in the office.
      ii. Some offices _____ any form of personal computer use.
      iii. Other offices may allow personal computer use during _____, _____, or before and after shifts.
      iv. Each office's policies should be written out and strictly followed by all employees.
   C. PDAs
      i. Physicians use PDAs to:

      _____

      _____

      _____

      _____

   D. Computer Ergonomics
      i. Ergonomics help prevent _____ associated with _____ - _____ computer use.
      ii. _____ _____ and carpal tunnel syndrome may result from repeated improper computer use:
         (a) Antiglare screens, ergonomic keyboards, and keyboard wrist rests are useful.
      iii. _____ and _____ are crucial to computer ergonomics.

iv. Chairs should have lower _____ _____ and armrests, which should not be used while typing.
v. Elbows should be positioned at _____ _____ and close enough to the keyboard so the user doesn't have to _____ _____.
vi. Monitors should be at _____ _____ and legs should be uncrossed with feet positioned flat on the floor.

KEY TERMINOLOGY REVIEW

Match the vocabulary term to the correct definition below.

a. bar-code scanners
b. battery backup systems
c. computer peripherals
d. computer viruses
e. electronic sign-in sheet
f. ergonomic
g. flash drives

h. health-related calculators
i. Internet search engines
j. malware
k. medical management software
l. personal digital assistants
m. scanners
n. thumb drives

_____ 1. Programs written to disrupt computer function.
_____ 2. Web sites that search the Internet for information based on set criteria.
_____ 3. Software medical offices use to perform day-to-day functions.
_____ 4. Designed for proper body posture.
_____ 5. Systems that protect computers in the event of power surges or power outages.
_____ 6. Computer programs that can destroy a computer's programs.
_____ 7. Devices that copy documents or pictures for transfer to computer systems.
_____ 8. Devices that connect to computers to add function or use.
_____ 9. Small external computer storage devices.
_____ 10. Small portable devices that store and transmit data.
_____ 11. Devices that scan or view barcodes for transfer to attached computers.
_____ 12. Computer programs that quantify health-related conditions.
_____ 13. Similar to a flash drives.
_____ 14. Computer programs that display the names of those that sign in.

APPLIED PRACTICE

Read the scenario and answer the questions that follow.

Scenario

Shane Eiler, RMA (AMT), is an office manager for Inner Harbor Sports Medicine. His office computer has had a recent attack from a malware program. This attack has left his computer unusable.

1. Shane has been asked to research the price of purchasing a new computer for the medical office. Create a list of the steps he should take to determine the type of system best for the office.

   _____

   _____

   _____

   _____

2. The physicians have also asked Shane to create a list of suggestions for securing the office computers from unauthorized access. What suggestions may Shane state?

   _____

   _____

   _____

   _____

LEARNING ACTIVITY: MULTIPLE CHOICE

Circle the correct answer to each of the questions below.

1. _____ are devices that allow documents to be copied and transferred into the computer system.

   a. Thumb drives
   b. Personal digital assistants

   c. Printers
   d. Scanners

2. DPI stands for:

   a. data per information
   b. dots per square inch

   c. data performance institution
   d. data performance information

3. _____ is the computer equipment.

   a. The hardware
   b. The software

   c. The peripheral
   d. The USB

4. _____ were introduced in the 1960s and have the fastest processing capacity of today's computers.

   a. Mainframe computers
   b. Supercomputers

   c. Minicomputers
   d. Microcomputers

5. _____ are used for large-volume applications such as government statistics.

   a. Supercomputers
   b. Mainframe computers

   c. Minicomputers
   d. Microcomputers

6. _____ are generally small computers, ranging from desktop models to handheld versions.

   a. Supercomputers
   b. Mainframe computers

   c. Minicomputers
   d. Microcomputers

7. The computer's CPU is considered the computer's _____.

   a. brain

   b. memory

   c. keyboard

   d. mouse

8. An ergonomic keyboard is used to:

   a. connect to the computer via a wireless connection.

   b. reduce typing stress by supporting the hands and wrists comfortably.

   c. type faster than using a conventional keyboard.

   d. maintain patient privacy when using the keyboard.

9. A flat screen computer monitor may be appropriate in which of the following situations?

   a. an office that has staff with limited computer skills

   b. an office that has a limited amount of money to spend on computer parts

   c. an office with limited desk space

   d. an office that needs to back up data frequently

10. As computer technology advances, _____ are becoming obsolete.

   a. floppy disk drives

   b. CD drives

   c. DVD drives

   d. thumb drives

CRITICAL THINKING

Answer the following questions to the best of your ability. Use the textbook as a reference

1. Marcia Dukat is taking a computer applications class in the medical assisting program she is attending. She has been given an assignment to create a list of steps medical office staff can take in order to protect the office computers from viruses. What should Marcia's list include?

_____

_____

_____

_____

2. Rolf Von Trapp, RMA (AMT), is discussing the need for a new computer system with the physician. Dr. Nyrse has asked Rolf to describe the difference between the hardware, the software, and the peripherals that go with various computer systems. How might Rolf define these three components?

_____

_____

_____

_____

_____

3. Wanda Vallone is writing an essay on the main types of computer systems for a class she is taking. What are the computer types Wanda should include in her essay, and how would she define them?

_____

_____

_____

_____

4. George El Fashir, CMA (AAMA), has been asked to describe the various computer drives that might be used to store information from the computer systems in his office. What information should George prepare?

_____

_____

_____

_____

5. Riley Gaddum is taking a computer class as part of his medical assisting training. He has been given an assignment to describe the difference between ROM and RAM. What might Riley write for this assignment?

_____

_____

_____

_____

_____

RESEARCH ACTIVITY

Use Internet search engines to research the following topics and write a brief description of what is found. It is important to visit reputable Web sites.

1. Use the Internet to research medical office software programs. You may choose to use the Web sites found in Figure 14-7 as a guide. What software program do you seem to like the most? What features does it have? Why would you recommend its use?

_____

_____

_____

_____

_____

_____

CHAPTER 15
Equipment, Maintenance, and Supply Inventory

CHAPTER OUTLINE

General review of the chapter:

    A. Introduction
    B. The MA's Role: Components of the Computer System
    C. Working with Medical Office Equipment
    D. Medical Transcription
    E. Logging Medical Office Supplies
    F. Handling Drug Samples
    G. Stocking Clerical Supplies
    H. Tracking Supplies with Computer Software

STUDENT STUDY GUIDE

Use the following guide to assist in your learning of the concepts from the chapter.

  I. Equipment and Maintenance
    A. The MA's Role

      _____

      _____

      _____

      _____

    B. Equipment Manuals
       i. Equipment manuals are invaluable resources:
         (a) Provide _____ and _____ regarding the proper use of equipment.
         (b) Every piece of equipment has an individual _____ in the manual that outlines its proper use.
         (c) Employees will sign off and date the manual page after _____ is _____.
    C. Maintenance Logs
       i. Maintenance logs are kept for _____.
       ii. Anyone who performs maintenance on equipment should _____ the log.
      iii. Logs provide _____ of proper upkeep of the equipment.
         (a) Useful for issues regarding _____ and manufacturing concerns
    D. Researching Equipment
       i. Research tools include:

      _____

      _____

_____

_____

_____

_____

   E. Leasing Equipment
      i. Leasing or purchasing will depend on the office needs and _____ _____.
     ii. When equipment is leased:
        (a) No down _____ is needed.
        (b) If the equipment breaks or malfunctions, it is usually _____ or _____.
        (c) The medical office has no ownership of the equipment.
   F. Purchasing Equipment
      i. When equipment is purchased:

_____

_____

_____

_____

II. Office Equipment

   A. Faxing
      i. Fax machines should be used only if absolutely necessary.
     ii. Some offices choose to use a/an _____ _____ when patient information is highly _____.
    iii. The fax machine should be placed in an area that is inaccessible to patients and away from the _____ _____.
    iv. A HIPAA-compliant fax coversheet must accompany the document.

_____

_____

_____

_____

   B. The Photocopier
      i. Medical offices should have _____ _____ photocopiers.
     ii. They should be maintained and serviced often.
    iii. Copies of _____ _____, insurance cards, and other billing information are made daily.
    iv. A malfunctioning photocopier can _____ the daily functioning of the medical office.
     v. Machines are placed behind the _____ _____ and near the billing area for easy _____.
   C. The Adding Machine
      i. Ten-key adding machines are usually _____ and have a roll of paper for printing numbers.
     ii. They are often used to tally columns of numbers found on _____ _____ day sheets or patient ledgers.
    iii. The clinical staff generally uses handheld calculators.

D. The Transcription Machine
   i. A transcription machine is used to _____ out the _____ words of a physician.
   ii. A physician will dictate notes into a handheld tape recorder and an administrative MA would obtain the tape.
   iii. The machine:
      (a) _____ are used to listen to the tape.
      (b) _____ _____ to control the speed and volume of the tape
   iv. The physician reviews the document for _____.
E. Outside Transcription Services
   i. Most offices utilize _____ medical transcription services.
   ii. Research transcription companies.
   iii. Find out the company's patient _____ policies, costs, and turnaround time.
   iv. Obtain _____ from others in the medical community.
   v. Some transcription services are located outside of the United States.
   vi. Work with a company that will adhere to HIPAA's patient _____ laws.

III. Inventory

A. Inventory Control Manual
   i. Efficient medical offices have enough supplies to sustain the functioning of the office, but not an excessive amount.
   ii. All _____ supplies should be listed in an inventory manual or list.
   iii. Clinical and administrative areas should be compiled on separate inventory lists.
   iv. The inventory list should include:

_____

_____

_____

_____

_____

B. Drug Supplies
   i. Medical offices receive samples of new drugs from _____

      _____ _____.

   ii. Some states allow the medical assistant to sign for the medications that the representative is giving to the office.
   iii. Most states require the _____ to sign for the medication.
   iv. Medicines should be:

_____

_____

_____

_____

   v. Group and store samples according to the drug's _____.
   vi. Drugs with an early expiration date should be stored in _____ of those with later dates.
   vii. Expired drugs must be _____, as it is illegal to use expired drugs or supplies.
   viii. Drug supplies should also be tracked.
   ix. In some states tracking supplies is _____.
   x. Tracking supplies supports proper _____ and _____.

C. Stocking Clerical Supplies
    i. Clerical supplies are _____ to stock than clinical supplies.
    ii. Clerical supplies do not _____.
    iii. They are available at local supply stores.
    iv. Suppliers may provide a discount for _____ purchasing.
      (a) This may be problematic if space is limited.
D. Barcode Scanners
    i. Inventory supply_____is available that utilizes barcode scanners.
    ii. The process includes:
      (a) As items _____, their bar codes are scanned.
      (b) Items are then _____
      (c) As staff members remove items, they are to scan the item that is being _____from stock.
      (d) When stock becomes low, the person in charge of inventory will receive a notice to reorder supplies.
    iii. This scanning process helps track inventory, but it only works if staff members are compliant with the process.

KEY TERMINOLOGY REVIEW

Use the key terms found at the beginning of the chapter to complete the sentences below.

1. The copy machine had been well _____ throughout the 8 years of its use, due to proper usage and routine cleanings.

2. Dr. Sabol chose to purchase an extended _____ that would cover repair and maintenance for an additional 7 years.

3. Michayla used the _____ to transfer the image of the patient's insurance card into the computer.

4. Always check the _____ of clinical supplies prior to any patient use or consumption.

5. Austin was proficient on the _____ because he was proficient in spelling medical terminology and was a very fast typist, making very few errors.

6. Maxine was asked to create a/an _____ for instruction and proper use of the fax machine.

7. Dr. Linn asked his clinical manager to create a/an _____ of all the supplies located in the supply closet.

8. After Antoinette received the shipment of supplies, she immediately checked the items received against the _____.

9. One of Maura's favorite administrative tasks was to _____ the physician's dictated patient notes from the tape recorder.

APPLIED PRACTICE

Read the scenario and answer the questions that follow.

Scenario

Javier Gomez, CMA (AAMA), is working in the front office of a busy family practice. His manager, Chris, has asked him to create a detailed inventory list of all supplies needed for his station at the patient check-out desk. Below is a list that Javier has started.

Item Name	Company	Amount on Hand
Pens	Office Supplies R Us	14
Message pad	Office Supplies R Us	2 tablets
Ink pad	Office Supplies R Us	2 pads

1. Based on the inventory list, what additional important information is Javier to include before submitting his list to Chris?

   _____

   _____

   _____

2. Considering that Javier is working at a patient check-out desk, where patients pay copayments and schedule follow-up appointments as needed, what additional items would Javier be likely to add to his inventory list? Name at least five.

   _____

   _____

   _____

   _____

   _____

LEARNING ACTIVITY: MULTIPLE CHOICE

Circle the correct answer to each of the questions below.

1. When researching new office equipment, which of the following is an appropriate avenue for the medical assistant in determining the best equipment for the office to purchase?

   a. Ask the vendor to bring the equipment to the office for a demonstration.

   b. Call other medical offices that are using the equipment.

   c. Go to stores where the equipment is being sold to look at the equipment.

   d. all of the above

2. Which of the following is an advantage of leasing over buying a piece of equipment?

   a. Little or no money is required at the time of acquiring the equipment.

   b. The medical office owns the equipment.

   c. The equipment repair is not covered by the manufacturer.

   d. all of the above

3. Which of the following is an appropriate place for the fax machine to be located in the medical office?

   a. in the reception room
   b. in a treatment room

   c. in the billing office
   d. all of the above

4. When the medical office needs to send confidential patient information to another medical facility, which of the following is the most secure way to do so?

   a. send the documents via fax
   b. send the document via courier

   c. send the document via the postal service
   d. send the document attached to an e-mail

5. When faxing a document from the medical office, which of the following pieces of information should be included on the fax cover sheet?

   a. the name of the clinic sending the document
   b. the name of the clinic receiving the document

   c. the number of pages included in the fax
   d. all of the above

6. Which of the following considerations should be made when researching possible copy machines to purchase for the medical office?

   a. the cost of supplies for the copier
   b. the price of the copier

   c. the warranty associated with the copier
   d. all of the above

7. When researching outside transcription services, what is the most important consideration the medical office must make?

   a. the cost of the transcription service
   b. the speed with which the service will return transcribed documents

   c. whether the transcription company is HIPAA compliant
   d. the availability of the transcription company to come to the medical office in person

8. In order effectively to keep track of medical office supplies, which of the following should be included in the list of inventory?

   a. the shipping company
   b. the order or part number

   c. item dimensions
   d. all of the above

9. In order to manage office inventory effectively, how often should the medical office perform inventory?

   a. daily
   b. weekly

   c. monthly
   d. This will vary; it depends upon the needs of the office.

10. What information should be included on the packing slip that comes with a shipment of supplies?

a. a list of the supplies included in the shipment

b. a list of supplies that may be ordered in the future

c. a list of upcoming sales or promotions the supplier is advertising

d. all of the above

CRITICAL THINKING

Answer the following questions to the best of your ability. Use the textbook as a reference.

1. Corey Steinberg, CMA (AAMA), has recently been hired to work as an administrative medical assistant in a busy cardiology practice. Corey has been given the task of creating a manual that outlines the warranty information as well as maintenance schedule for each piece of medical office equipment. How should Corey go about beginning this task?

_____

_____

_____

_____

_____

2. Monte Beaton, RMA (AMT), is the office manager in a gastroenterology practice. Monte has recently hired three new medical assistants and wants to be sure they are properly trained to use each piece of equipment in the medical office. How can Monte be sure the training is done properly?

_____

_____

_____

_____

_____

3. Krystle Shawger is taking an administrative class as part of her medical assisting training. She has been given an assignment to write an essay describing how an equipment maintenance log would be useful in the medical office. What might Krystle include in her paper?

_____

_____

_____

_____

4. Marian Harrison, RMA (AMT), is the administrative office manager in a family practice clinic. She is writing an office policy for inventory of administrative office equipment. What might her policy include?

_____

_____

_____

_____

_____

5. Joann Felmer, CMA (AAMA), works in a walk-in clinic. At the weekly office staff meeting, the office manager mentioned the need for purchasing a new EKG machine. The office manager has asked Joann to research the various options available. How should Joann handle this task?

_____

_____

_____

_____

_____

RESEARCH ACTIVITY

Use Internet search engines to research the following topics and write a brief description of what is found. It is important to visit reputable Web sites.

1. Create an Internet search for office and medical supply companies. Which companies supply products at a competitive price? What is the cost of shipping charges? Which company seems to have the best variety of products? How could this information be useful for medical offices?

_____

_____

_____

_____

_____

_____

_____

_____

_____

_____

_____

_____

_____

_____

_____

_____

_____

_____

_____

_____

CHAPTER 16

Office Policies and Procedures

CHAPTER OUTLINE

General review of the chapter:

    A. Introduction
    B. The Medical Assistant's Role in Policies and Procedures
    C. Creating Patient Information Pamphlets
    D. Creating Policies and Procedures for the Medical Office

STUDENT STUDY GUIDE

Use the following guide to assist in your learning of the concepts from the chapter.

I. The MA's Role in Policies and Procedures

    A. Upon being hired at a new job, the MA should be provided a/an _____ and _____ for review.
    B. Procedures may need to be _____ that pertain to new aspects or considerations of the MA's job.
    C. Policy and procedure manuals are valuable tools.
        i. They aid in avoiding _____.

II. Information Pamphlet

    A. _____ _____ is the responsibility of the entire health care team.
    B. Pamphlets assist in patient education:
       _____
       _____
       _____
       _____

III. Manuals

    A. Personnel
        i. Personnel manuals are also known as _____ _____.
        ii. Developed by office _____ and _____
        iii. Manuals list rules and regulations for all staff members.
        iv. Manuals must adhere to _____ and _____ laws.
    B. Policy and Procedure Manuals
        i. Policy and procedure manuals will vary from office to office.

ii. Most manuals will contain:
  (a) _____ _____: a concise statement that outlines the mission, or goal of the medical office. Many times the mission statement is also displayed where patients are able to read it, such as in the reception area.
  (b) _____ _____: This is a chart that lists the hierarchy of the medical office, from physicians to entry-level staff members. By having an organizational chart, everyone in the office will understand who their supervisor is, as well as the chain of command in the office.
  (c) _____ _____: Information could include policies regarding relationships between office staff, relationships between staff and patients, and termination policies.
  (d) _____ _____: Clinical procedures will vary from office to office, depending on medical specialty. All clinical procedures should include steps to complete the procedure, patient education, documentation, and infection control.
  (e) _____ _____: Documented administrative procedures will also vary from office to office.
    (1) Some of the most common administrative procedures include :

    _____

    _____

    _____

    _____

  (f) A/an _____ of _____ is found at the beginning of the manual for easy reference.
  (g) Separate infection control and risk management manuals must be kept.
    (1) This complies with _____ and _____ guidelines.

KEY TERMINOLOGY REVIEW

Write a sentence using each key term below in its correct context.

1. Brochure:

  _____

  _____

2. Compulsory:

  _____

  _____

3. Mission statement:

  _____

  _____

4. Organizational chart:

  _____

  _____

5. Personnel manual:

_____

_____

6. Policy:

_____

_____

7. Procedure:

_____

_____

APPLIED PRACTICE

Read the scenario below and answer the questions that follow.

Scenario

Ivan Opleski, MA works for a busy pediatric office. He has been asked by the office manager to organize an office risk-management team and conduct an office meeting during the lunch hour next Friday.

1. How would Ivan explain the purpose of a risk management as he attempts to recruit his fellow coworkers?

_____

_____

_____

_____

_____

2. List five procedures that Ivan and his team may choose to implement:

_____

_____

_____

_____

_____

3. Using one of the topics listed in the previous questions, create a policy regarding that topic using the form on page 138.

Policy Title:
Policy
Created By
Date Created or Revised

LEARNING ACTIVITY: MULTIPLE CHOICE

Circle the correct answer to each of the questions below.

1. Which of the following is an example of an administrative office procedure?
   a. how to handle an accidental needle stick
   b. the steps to handling a missed patient appointment
   c. how to properly fill out a laboratory requisition form
   d. steps to calculating a medication dosage

2. Which of the following is an example of a clinical office policy?

   a. the steps to cleaning the exam room tables

   b. the steps to printing the daily appointment list

   c. how to handle an accidental needle stick

   d. the steps for cleaning the reception room

3. Which of the following is an example of a risk management office policy?

   a. how to handle life-threatening patient events in the office

   b. steps to opening and sorting mail

   c. steps to taking a telephone message

   d. how to deal with overdue patient accounts

4. Which of the following may be found in a personnel manual?

   a. how to answer the office telephone

   b. validating patient parking

   c. a complete patient list

   d. sexual harassment

5. Which of the following is an example of a quality improvement policy?

   a. decreasing patient wait times for appointments

   b. appropriate reception room reading materials

   c. planning the physician's travel itinerary

   d. all of the above

6. How often should the office policy and procedure manual be updated?

   a. yearly

   b. semiannually

   c. as needed

   d. It is not necessary to update the policy and procedure manual.

7. According to _____, quality improvement and risk management procedures must be kept in a separate notebook that is clearly marked and updated regularly.

   a. CLIAA

   b. HIPAA

   c. CMS

   d. all of the above

8. According to _____, infection control procedures must be kept separate from other procedures manuals in the office.

   a. CLIAA

   b. OSHA

   c. HIPAA

   d. CMS

9. Which of the following is an example of an infection control procedure?

   a. cleaning children's toys in the reception room

   b. how to schedule sick patient appointments

   c. steps to sorting the mail

   d. employee needlestick injuries

10. A policy regarding releasing medical information to a patient is an example of what kind of policy?

   a. administrative

   b. clinical

   c. risk management

   d. infection control

CRITICAL THINKING

Answer the following questions to the best of your ability. Use the textbook as a reference.

1. Macey Goldsmith is taking an administrative medical assisting class. She has been asked to design and create an informational pamphlet that could be given to a patient in a health care setting. What should Macy consider before starting this project? What should she include?

   _____

   _____

   _____

   _____

2. Hiro Yoshi, CMA (AAMA), has recently been hired to work in a busy walk-in clinic. Hiro wants to find out what the office policy is regarding taking time off after the birth of a new child. He doesn't want to ask his coworkers or the office manager because he doesn't want his new employer to know he and his wife are trying to have a baby. How can Hiro find this information without having to discuss the issue with his coworkers?

   _____

   _____

   _____

   _____

3. Larry Anderson, RMA (AMT), has been working for Dr. Bacon for 7 years. Last year he asked to take time off over the July 4th holiday. At that time, Larry was told the office did not allow time off over holidays. The office personnel policy manual confirms this as the office policy. Sara Hastings, CMA (AAMA), has just been hired by Dr. Bacon. Larry overhears Sara ask for time off over the upcoming Memorial Day weekend. The office manager grants Sara her request. What can Larry do about this seemingly unfair application of the office policy regarding time off over holidays?

   _____

   _____

   _____

   _____

4. Julie Ryan, CMA (AAMA), is the office manager in a busy urology practice. The clinic has an office policy manual but it has not been updated in over 10 years. As Julie looks through the manual, she sees several policies that are outdated and no longer apply to the office. How should Julie go about the process of updating her clinic policy manual?

   _____

   _____

   _____

   _____

5. Beth Watanabe, RMA (AMT), is the office manager in a pediatric clinic. Joe Jensen, CMA (AAMA), was hired to work in this clinic one month ago. Though Joe wore appropriate attire, including clean scrubs and shoes at the beginning of his employment, he has been gradually moving away from the office dress code policy and has recently been wearing street clothes and open-toed shoes to work. Beth has asked Joe to wear the appropriate attire but Joe says he doesn't see why he should have to dress so blandly. What can Beth do to address this situation?

_____

_____

_____

_____

_____

RESEARCH ACTIVITY

Use Internet search engines to research the following topics and write a brief description of what is found. It is important to visit reputable Web sites.

1. Search the Internet to find information that is available for risk-management and quality management committees. What type of information is available and how can it be useful in a medical office?

_____

_____

_____

_____

_____

_____

_____

_____

_____

_____

_____

_____

CHAPTER 17
Insurance Billing and Authorization

CHAPTER OUTLINE

General review of the chapter:

A. The Medical Assistant's Role in Insurance Billing and Authorizations
B. The History of Health Insurance
C. Health Insurance Today
D. Private Health Insurance
E. Types of Plans
F. Types of Coverage
G. Government Insurance
H. Reimbursement Methods
I. Processing Claims
J. Health Insurance Claim Forms
K. Working with Fee Schedules
L. Posting Payments
M. Tracing Claims
N. The Office of the Insurance Commissioner
O. Projecting Health Insurance Costs in the Future

STUDENT STUDY GUIDE

Use the following guide to assist in your learning of the concepts from the chapter.

I. Introduction
   A. The MA's Role in Insurance and Authorization
      i. Processing claims correctly requires:
         (a) A strong knowledge in _____ _____
         (b) A strong knowledge in basic _____ _____ terminology
      ii. Medical assistants will:
         (a) _____ insurance coverage.
         (b) Determine if it is necessary to obtain _____ for procedures.
         (c) Explain how _____ health care works.
         (d) Accurately process insurance claim forms.
         (e) Follow up on _____ _____ claims.
         (f) Pursue account _____.
      iii. The MA's involvement in insurance billing will depend on the _____ of the physician's practice.
      iv. MAs may have more _____ in smaller offices.
      v. In larger offices, there may be an entire _____ devoted to insurance billing.

B. History of Health Insurance
  i. Mid-1800s:
    _____

    _____

  ii. 1847:
    _____

    _____

  iii. 1890:
    _____

    _____

  iv. 1929:
    _____

    (a) Started after a group of _____ school teachers formed a contract with
        a local hospital guaranteeing _____ days of hospital care for a pre-
        mium of _____ per year.
  v. During World War II:
    _____

    _____

  vi. 1954:
    _____

    _____

  vii. 1965:
    _____

    _____

  viii. 1980s and 1990s:
    _____

    _____

  ix. This caused many employers to move _____ _____ plans.
  x. Managed care plans were _____ expensive.
C. Health Insurance Today
  i. Half of insured Americans have health insurance through _____ or
     _____ _____ companies.
  ii. Employers may choose to sponsor group health insurance policies
  iii. Some employers choose to self-insure:
     (a) Paying directly for their employees' _____ _____
  iv. Americans without private insurance may qualify for government programs:
    _____

    _____

    _____

    _____

    _____

  v. _____-_____ million Americans have no health insurance coverage.
  vi. For these patients, offices may establish a/an _____ _____
     scale.

Insurance Billing and Authorization   **143**

vii. Some cities have free or low-cost clinics.

_____

_____

II. Health Insurance Terminology

   A. The person who owns the insurance policy may be known as the _____,

     _____, _____, or policyholder.

   B. The term _____ is used for those covered by government policies.

   C. Family members, covered under the member's policy, are known as _____:

     i. Including

_____

_____

   D. Premiums are paid by the _____ to obtain the health insurance policy:

     i. Usually paid in _____ installments for the next _____ coverage.

     ii. With group coverage, the _____ will pay the majority of the premium.

     iii. Employees will generally authorize the remainder of the premium to be _____ from _____.

   E. A fee schedule is a list of charges providers charge for each service they provide:

     i. Generally organized by type of _____ and _____ code

   F. A/an _____ _____ is what an insurer averages for the same specialty within the same geographic area for the same charge.

     i. This is also termed the _____ or _____ amount.

   G. If a provider's usual charge is lower than the allowed charge, he or she will be paid the

     _____ _____.

   H. If a provider's actual charge is higher than the allowed charge, he or she will be paid the

     _____ _____.

   I. A/an _____ is an out-of-pocket expense paid by the patient.

     i. This must be paid before an insurance plan will pay for benefits.

   J. Deductibles can range from _____ to _____.

   K. Some plans require that both individual _____ and _____ deductibles be paid.

   L. After the required deductible has been paid, the _____ _____ will begin to pick up the cost of medical services.

   M. A/an _____ is a set dollar amount that a patient pays at the time of a service.

   N. _____ is a set percentage that a patient must pay.

     i. An 80/20 coinsurance plan means that the insurance company pays _____ of approved charges, and the patient pays _____.

   O. Preferred or participating providers _____ with an insurance company, agreeing to accept the insurance's _____ amount as full payment.

     i. Providers cannot bill the patient for the difference between the actual charge and the allowed amount.

   P. _____ _____ occurs when a patient sees a provider that is not participating or contracted:

     i. The provider will accept the allowed amount from the insurance company and in turn bill the patient for the _____ _____.

   Q. Insurance policies often carry a stop loss and lifetime maximum benefits clauses.

   R. Stop loss is the _____ amount that a/an _____ must pay for out-of-pocket expenses.

   S. After the stop loss is paid, the insurance company will cover any remaining expenses at _____ for the remaining _____ year.

T. Lifetime maximum benefit is the maximum that the _____ _____ will pay for individual members over the course of the _____ _____.

    i. Often this amount is $1 million; however, it could be as low as $100,000.

U. A waiting period is a set time that must pass before the insured's _____ condition is covered.

    i. Including anything the patient was diagnosed with or treated for, including receiving _____ _____, before beginning coverage with a new insurance plan.

III. Health Insurance

A. Sources of Coverage

    i. Private health insurance coverage can include:

_____

_____

_____

B. Group Health Insurance

    i. Offers coverage where the risk or _____ of _____ is spread over a group of people

    ii. Everyone pays the same _____ for protection.

    iii. Employer-sponsored group insurance is most widely used.

    iv. Various health insurance packages are available for selection.

    v. Employers determine how much money their _____ will pay for _____.

C. Self-Insurance

    i. Self-insurance is often utilized through _____ _____.

    ii. With self-insurance, a large set of money is set aside to _____ employees for their _____ _____ expenses.

    (a) A policy is not purchased from a/an _____ carrier.

D. COBRA

    i. COBRA offers the opportunity to continue _____ _____ after an employee leaves his or her place of employment.

    ii. This is done at the _____ expense.

    (a) They are responsible for paying their portion of the premium in addition to that which the employer had been paying.

    iii. COBRA allows employees to keep insurance in force until new _____ is obtained.

E. Individual Insurance

    i. Individuals purchase their own policies from _____ carriers.

    ii. Generally, benefits are not as good as _____ _____ _____.

    iii. They result in _____ deductibles and other out-of-pocket expenses.

    iv. _____ govern minimum level benefit coverage for individual insurance policies.

    (a) As a result of the restrictions, only a few companies may offer the option to purchase individual policies.

F. Managed Care Plans

    i. These plans work to control health care _____.

    ii. Managed care _____ (MCOs) contract with health care providers to provide care to certain patients.

    iii. Contracted providers are known as _____ providers.

    iv. Contracts stipulate _____ rates and _____ guidelines.

G. Types of Managed Care Plans

_____

_____

H. Types of HMOs

_____

_____

_____

_____

I. Consumer-Directed Health Care Plans
   i. Allow consumers to delegate how their health care _____ are
    _____.
  ii. Generally there is a three-tiered structure of payment:
    (a) A/an _____-_____ health savings account
    (b) A/an _____-_____ health insurance policy
    (c) A gap between the two, for which individuals pay health care expenses out of pocket

J. Blue Cross/Blue Shield
   i. Nearly _____ of Americans are covered by some type of Blue Cross or Blue
    Shield (BCBS) plan.
  ii. Each BCBS plan is separate, with unique benefit terms.
  iii. BCBS includes:
    (a) _____coverage and managed care plans
    (b) A _____ employee program (FEP)
    (c) Medicare _____plans
    (d) Health care _____plans
  iv. The member _____ _____indicates the individual's form of
    coverage.
  v. Each BCBS processes its own claims.
    (a) It is important to verify the correct filing address upon _____ patients.

K. Third Party Liability
   i. Covers medical bills arising from _____-_____–related
    accidents.
  ii. Business, home, and vehicle owners carry liability insurance.
    (a) This covers injuries that occur on their _____.

IV. Insurance Coverage

A. Coverage refers to the specific services that are covered under health insurance plans.
B. Plans are tailored to offer benefits most desired and affordable for each group or individual.
   i. Hospital coverage:

_____

_____

_____

_____

_____

  ii. Medical coverage:

_____

_____

_____

_____

   iii. Surgical coverage:

_____

_____

_____

   iv. Outpatient coverage:

_____

_____

_____

   v. Major medical:

_____

_____

_____

   vi. Home health care:

_____

_____

_____

   vii. Catastrophic health insurance:

_____

_____

_____

   viii. Long term care insurance:

_____

_____

_____

   ix. Ancillary coverage:

_____

_____

_____

_____

V. Government Insurance

   A. Government-sponsored health insurance is made available for:

_____

_____

_____

_____

B. Eligibility requirements and benefits vary with each program.
C. Medicare
    i. Administered by the Centers for Medicare and Medicaid Services
    ii. Medicare Administrative Contractors (MAC):

_____

_____

    iii. MedLearn:
      (a) Found on the _____ Web site
      (b) Provides free online training for _____ on many Medicare topics
    iv. All claims should be processed within _____ days of service.
    v. Medicare has four major components:
      (a) Part A _____
      (b) Part B _____
      (c) Part C _____
      (d) Part D _____
    vi. National Provider Identification
      (a) A/an _____-digit number assigned to health care providers by the

      _____

      (b) Each number is unique to the provider.
      (c) All health care providers are required to use NPIs on patient _____

      _____.

      (d) Specialists who receive referrals from other physicians must place the referring physician's NPI and their own NPI on billing forms.
    vii. Medicare Part A
      (a) Covers hospital insurance for up to _____ days
      (b) No _____ is required.
      (c) It also covers:

_____

_____

_____

_____

_____

    viii. Medicare Part B
      (a) Covers:

_____

_____

_____

_____

      (b) Participation is voluntary and members are required to pay:
        (1) An annual _____
        (2) Monthly _____ based on the recipient's _____
        (3) 20 percent _____ on services
    ix. Medicare Part C
      (a) This is known as Medicare _____ plans.
        (1) These plans are offered by _____ _____ companies to replace Parts A, B, and D.
      (b) Part C plans may provide more _____ care.
      (c) However, the choice of _____ is limited.

x. Medicare Part D
    (a) This is Medicare's _____ _____ plan.
    (b) It's optional for Medicare members.
    (c) Part D covers both _____ and _____
        _____ prescription drugs.
    (d) Plans are provided by private carriers:
        (1) Plans carry a/an _____ deductible.
        (2) _____ or coinsurance is required.
        (3) There is a maximum benefit level.
xi. Advanced Beneficiary Notice
    (a) This is a form signed by _____ before receiving recommended services
        that may be _____ by Medicare.
    (b) The patient has the ability to _____ or _____ a service.
        (1) While knowing that he or she will be obligated to pay if Medicare denies coverage
    (c) MAs must review the ABN with patients and obtain a signature _____
        service is provided.
D. Medicaid
    i. Medicaid is a federal program for _____ _____ patients.
    ii. It is run by CMS, though each _____ dictates the amount and types of
        services Medicaid covers.
    iii. _____ rates for services are low.
        (a) Many providers have chosen to stop treating Medicaid patients.
    iv. Providers who treat Medicaid patients must become _____ by their state.
    v. Medicaid qualifications:

        _____

        _____

        _____

        _____

        _____

    vi. Medicaid and other insurance
        (a) Low-income elderly patients may have both _____ and
            _____.
            (1) Medicare is always the _____ insurance.
            (2) Medicaid is always considered the "_____ of last
                _____."
            (3) If a patient has other insurance coverage, Medicaid is always the last to be billed.
E. TRICARE
    i. Tricare provides health care benefits to families of _____ and
        _____ military personnel.
    ii. The three benefit types offered by Tricare include:

        _____

        _____

        _____

    iii. Enrollees are automatically enrolled in Tricare Standard and Tricare Extra.
F. CHAMPVA
    i. CHAMPVA covers health care expenses of families of _____ with total,
        permanent, _____ _____ disabilities.
    ii. CHAMPVA also covers _____ and _____ of veterans who
        died in the line of duty.
    iii. CHAMPVA allows the use of any civilian health care provider.
        (a) _____ are not required.

G. Worker's Compensation
    i. Covers employees injured in the _____ or suffering from work-related
    _____.
    ii. MAs must be aware of their _____ _____ for workman's
    compensation coverage.
      (a) Detailed _____ are crucial to these cases.
    iii. Worker's compensations cases should have newly created files.
    iv. These should be kept separate from other patients' medical records.
    v. State labor departments usually provide:

    vi. Benefits to injured workers include:

    vii. Benefits to injured workers include (continued):
      (a) Death benefits to _____ when the accident is a cause of the worker's
      death
      (b) _____ to allow workers to return to work
      (c) _____ if a different line of work is necessary

H. Disability Insurance
    i. Covers a patient's lost wages due to a/an _____-
    _____–related disability
    ii. This must prevent the individual from working.
    iii. Generally this is _____ of the person's wages.
    iv. Disability benefits are not _____ _____
    v. Social Security Disability Insurance (SSDI) is for workers who are _____
    disabled.

I. Other Government Insurance
    i. Supplemental Security Income:

    ii. Veteran's Disability Compensation:

    iii. Veteran's Disability Pension Benefits:

    iv. Civil Service and Federal Employees Retirement System:

VI. Reimbursement Methods and Processing Claims

A. Reimbursement Methods
    i. Usual, customary, and reasonable (UCR) method: Insurers establish a "customary" fee.
      (a) This is based on what similar _____ of the same
      _____ within the same _____ charge.
    ii. Insurers will pay providers the customary fee or the provider's usual fee, whichever is the
    _____ of the two.
    iii. Negotiated fee schedule method: The MCO develops a list of fees for providers that are
    then _____ upon and _____.

iv. Capitation method: The insurer pays providers a/an _____ _____ per member per month regardless of the services used by the patient.
  (a) This is the _____ _____ reimbursement method.
v. Per diem method: means "_____ _____" and is used for inpatient care.
  (a) Facilities receive a/an _____ _____per day the patient remains in the facility, regardless of what services are provided.
vi. Per case method: Payment is also used for hospitals.
  (a) Hospital receives a pre-established amount per patient per day which is based on the patient's _____.
  (b) This form of payment is used by _____: called diagnosis _____ _____ (DRG)
B. Processing Claims: Patient Registration
  i. New patients should fill out a patient registration form that contains important information
  ii. This information should be _____.
    (a) Keep in mind that this information is considered highly protected.
  iii. It is vital to have _____ and _____ information.
C. Processing Claims: Insurance Verification
  i. Insurance information may be obtained over the _____ or in person with the patient.
  ii. MAs should verify the _____ with the insurance company.
  iii. Each patient is given a member identification number.
    (a) Usually _____ or _____
  iv. Insurance company phone numbers are usually on the back of the member's insurance card.
  v. Utilizing online means of verification generally quicker and easier
D. Processing Claims: Coordination of Benefits
  i. Coordination of benefits (COB) occurs when patients have _____ than _____insurance carrier.
  ii. COB determines which insurance is considered the _____ and which is considered _____ insurance.
  iii. If spouses or partners are covered by each other's policy:
    (a) The patient's own policy is always their _____ insurance.
    (b) Their spouse's insurance is considered their secondary insurance.
E. Processing Claims: The Birthday Rule
  i. When both parents carry coverage for their children:
    (a) The parent with the birthday _____ in the year will use his or her insurance as _____ for their children.
    (b) The parent's birthday that falls _____ in the year carries _____ coverage for their children.
F. Processing Claims: Referrals, Authorizations, and Precertifications
  i. Referrals, authorizations, and precertifications may be necessary for _____, _____ procedures.
  ii. MAs should call insurance carriers to:
    (a) Verify patient eligibility for the desired services
    (b) Obtain any needed preauthorizations
  iii. A referral from the patient's primary care provider (PCP) may be necessary prior to obtaining a/an _____.
  iv. MAs who work for the PCP will coordinate the referral.
  v. Authorization numbers for specialist visits or tests should immediately be recorded in the _____ _____.
  vi. Also document the authorization number on the _____ form at the time of billing.

G. Processing Claims: Documenting Insurance Company Calls
  i. MAs with questions about a patient's insurance coverage should contact the insurance provider's customer service number.
    (a) This is done if online information is not available.
  ii. MAs should document all calls made to an insurance carrier, including:

  _____

  _____

  _____

VII. Health Insurance Claim Forms and Fee Schedules
  A. Claim Forms
    i. The _____ is used by physicians and professional health care providers.
    ii. It is accepted by _____ health insurance carriers.
    iii. The boxes on the CMS-1500 form are referred to as _____
       _____ (FL).
    iv. The form is divided in to two major sections:
      (a) _____ and _____ information: found in FL 1-13
      (b) _____ and _____ information: found in FL 14-33
    v. Government insurance carriers as well as workman's compensation have specific _____ for form completion.
    vi. MAs should be aware of various guidelines.
    vii. MAs should also know whom to contact should questions arise.
      (a) MAs must _____ data and use various sources to find the required information to complete the form.
    viii. Accuracy when completing the form is vital.
      (a) A single error or _____ could cause the claim to be rejected.
    ix. The CMS form is printed in _____ ink.
    x. This allows it to be recognized by _____ _____ recognition scanners.
    xi. These scanners are used to process claims because of their speed and _____.
    xii. When using these forms:
      (a) Use _____ approved forms.
      (b) Use _____ letters.
      (c) Use a standard monospaced serif font, such as Courier.
      (d) Do not use any _____ marks.
      (e) Keep all text within the _____ of the red box for each FL.
      (f) Use _____ digit dates for _____; other dates can be six or eight digits.
      (g) If a mistake is made, _____ _____: Never erase, strike out, overtype, or white out.
      (h) Do not use _____ or pen to make any extra markings.
      (i) Do not tape or _____ anything to the form.
  B. Fee Schedules
    i. Two common methods are used to determine fee structure:
      (a) Charge-based fee schedule

  _____

  _____

  _____

  _____

  _____

(b) Resource-based fee schedule

_____
_____
_____
_____
_____

   ii. Medicare Fee Determination
     (a) Payments are based on the _____-_____relative value scale (RBVS).
     (b) This consists of three parts:
       (1) The _____ _____value (RVU): based on the cost of the physician's work, overhead and malpractice cost
       (2) The _____ _____factor (GAF): considers the areas of the country in which a physician practices, adjusting higher or lower based on that area's cost of living
       (3) _____ _____conversion factor: used to determine the dollar amount for payment amounts for services

VIII. Processed Claims, the EOB, and Tracing Payments
  A. After claims are processed, the insurance carrier sends a/an _____to the provider.
    i. An explanation of _____ (EOB) is also sent to the physician.
    ii. The EOB will list:

_____
_____
_____
_____

    iii. The EOB has three sections that explain how a claim was processed:
     (a) Service Information:

_____
_____

     (b) Coverage Determination:

_____
_____

     (c) Benefit Payment Information:

_____
_____

    iv. Patients with _____should pay at the time of service.
    v. Those with _____should be billed after information and notification from the insurance carrier has been received.
    vi. Payments are posted to specific _____ and _____.
    vii. Positive or negative changes to a patient's account balance will result in an adjustment.
     (a) This could be due to _____, changes, or write-offs to a patient's account.
     (b) It is necessary to note if there is a/an _____ _____ from a patient, or if a refund is due to the patient or the insurance carrier.
  B. Tracing Claims
    i. It may be necessary to trace a claim if payment hasn't been received:
     (a) More than _____ days after submission of a paper claim
     (b) More than _____ days after submission of an electronic claim
    ii. This may vary by state.

    iii. Each state has a/an _____ indicating when an insurance carrier must pay or deny a claim.

    iv. MAs will telephone the insurance carrier for followup of the claim.

    v. If a claim is not on file, the MA may request a/an _____
_____ to send the claim.

        (a) Usually it is sent directly to the customer service representative for processing.

    vi. Payment might not have been made due to a/an _____ on file.

        (a) MAs may be asked to verbally fix the claim over the phone.

    vii. It may be necessary to _____ the claim.

    viii. Document the telephone call indicating:

_____

_____

_____

  C. Rejections and Denials

    i. Claims may be rejected due to mistakes made by the medical office.

    ii. Common mistakes for a claim rejection include:

_____

_____

_____

_____

_____

    iii. Claims are denied because of benefits or coverage issues.

        (a) The reason for a denial is often listed in the _____.

    iv. Appeals can be made to _____ the claim.

        (a) This process is very time consuming and requires extra _____.

    v. MAs must be aware of the payer's appeal process before beginning.

    vi. Generally an appeal will include:

        (a) _____ a/an _____ that clearly states why the provider believes the denial was not justified.

        (b) A copy of the _____

        (c) Supporting _____

IX. Office of the Insurance Commissioner and Future Costs of Insurance

  A. Office of the Insurance Commissioner

    i. Each _____ has an Office of the Insurance Commissioner.

    ii. Written complaints to the commissioner are made when claims were incorrectly _____ and appeal attempts are _____.

    iii. Patient involvement is crucial.

        (a) The commissioner is in charge of protecting the _____, which is the patient.

    iv. Patients are often unfamiliar with the process.

        (a) MAs may want to write a letter on behalf of the _____ to the Commissioner.

        (b) The _____ will sign the letter.

    v. The simple threat of a letter to the Insurance Commissioner may inspire insurance carriers to review a claim.

B. Future Costs of Health Insurance Coverage
   i. Health care costs continue to rise in America.
   ii. The U.S. health care system will likely be _____ _____ in the future.
      (a) Employers may start to offer employees _____ for health care coverage to be used to purchase health care plans that suit their needs.
      (b) Americans could also be offered _____ _____ or rebates for purchasing health insurance coverage.
   iii. Medical assistants must stay current on the _____ that affects health care and health insurance coverage.

KEY TERMINOLOGY REVIEW

Match the selected key terms to their definitions below.

a.	allowed amount	p.	long-term disability insurance
b.	ancillary coverage	q.	Medicaid
c.	allowed amount	r.	Medicare
d.	beneficiary	s.	member
e.	catastrophic	t.	physician services
f.	CHAMPVA	u.	policyholder
g.	covered	v.	preauthorization
h.	dependents	w.	premium
i.	end-stage renal disease	x.	self-insurance
j.	fee schedule	y.	sliding fee scale
k.	group health insurance	z.	stop loss
l.	hospital services	aa.	TRICARE
m.	individual health insurance	bb.	unbundling
n.	insured	cc.	usual, customary, and reasonable
o.	liability insurance	dd.	Worker's Compensation

_____ 1. Covers dependents of veterans who have total and permanent service-connected disabilities.

_____ 2. A standard set of fees the provider charges to all insurers.

_____ 3. The dollar amount that an insurance company considers acceptable and uses to determine benefit payments.

_____ 4. A commercial insurance policy with rates based on individual health criteria.

_____ 5. Insurance that covers lost wages and certain other benefits due to a disability that prevents the individual from working, usually for more than one year.

_____ 6. Person who owns or holds an insurance policy.

_____ 7. When an employer sets aside a large reserve fund to directly reimburse employees for medical expenses rather than purchase commercial insurance.

_____ 8. Person who is eligible to receive services under an insurance policy.

_____ 9. Patient care provided by a licensed acute care hospital.

_____ 10. Covers active duty military personnel, retired service personnel, and their eligible dependents.

_____ 11. Also known as a beneficiary.

_____ 12. Fees for a service that are based on the patient's financial ability to pay.

_____ 13. Total or nearly complete failure of the kidneys.

_____ 14. Usually a monthly amount that is paid to an insurance company to keep coverage in force.

_____ 15. Joint federal and state program that helps with medical costs for those with low income and limited resources.

_____ 16. Services potentially eligible for reimbursement.

_____ 17. Fee determined by third-party payers to reimburse providers based on the provider's normal fee, the range of fees charged by those of the same specialty in the same geographic area, and other factors.

_____ 18. Dollar amount for a service that an insurance company considers acceptable and uses to determine benefit payments.

_____ 19. Insurance that covers injuries that occur on, in, or because of the insured's property.

_____ 20. Large and usually unforeseen.

_____ 21. Approval for treatment or service obtained from an insurance company before the care is provided.

_____ 22. Billing multiple services with separate CPT codes and separate charges that should be combined under a single CPT code and one charge.

_____ 23. The maximum amount the patient must pay out of pocket for copayments and coinsurance.

_____ 24. A commercial insurance policy with rates based on a group of people, usually offered by an employer.

_____ 25. Also known as the member or policyholder.

_____ 26. A family member or other individual who qualifies for coverage on the insured's policy.

_____ 27. A federal program that covers medical expenses for those aged 65 and over.

_____ 28. Insurance for services such as dental, vision, or chiropractic care.

_____ 29. Insurance coverage for job-related illness or injury provided by employers.

_____ 30. Patient care provided by a licensed physician.

APPLIED PRACTICE

Complete the CMS-1500 form (Figure 17-1) using the patient registration form, the encounter form, and the fee schedule that is provided.

Note: _This activity has been adapted from Vines,_ Comprehensive Health Insurance: Billing, Coding, and Reimbursement _Student CD. © 2008 Pearson Education, Inc. Upper Saddle River, NJ 07458._

HEALTH INSURANCE CLAIM FORM

APPROVED BY NATIONAL UNIFORM CLAIM COMMITTEE 08/05

| | PICA | | | | | | | PICA | |

1. MEDICARE □ (Medicare #) MEDICAID □ (Medicaid #) TRICARE CHAMPUS □ (Sponsor's SSN) CHAMPVA □ (Member ID#) GROUP HEALTH PLAN □ (SSN or ID) FECA BLK LUNG □ (SSN) OTHER □ (ID)

1a. INSURED'S I.D. NUMBER _(For Program in Item 1)_

2. PATIENT'S NAME (Last Name, First Name, Middle Initial)

3. PATIENT'S BIRTH DATE MM DD YY SEX M □ F □

4. INSURED'S NAME (Last Name, First Name, Middle Initial)

5. PATIENT'S ADDRESS (No., Street)

6. PATIENT RELATIONSHIP TO INSURED Self □ Spouse □ Child □ Other □

7. INSURED'S ADDRESS (No., Street)

CITY STATE

8. PATIENT STATUS Single □ Married □ Other □

Employed □ Full-Time Student □ Part-Time Student □

CITY STATE

ZIP CODE TELEPHONE (Include Area Code) ( )

ZIP CODE TELEPHONE (Include Area Code) ( )

9. OTHER INSURED'S NAME (Last Name, First Name, Middle Initial)

10. IS PATIENT'S CONDITION RELATED TO:

11. INSURED'S POLICY GROUP OR FECA NUMBER

a. OTHER INSURED'S POLICY OR GROUP NUMBER

a. EMPLOYMENT? (Current or Previous) YES □ NO □

a. INSURED'S DATE OF BIRTH MM DD YY SEX M □ F □

b. OTHER INSURED'S DATE OF BIRTH MM DD YY SEX M □ F □

b. AUTO ACCIDENT? PLACE (State) YES □ NO □

b. EMPLOYER'S NAME OR SCHOOL NAME

c. EMPLOYER'S NAME OR SCHOOL NAME

c. OTHER ACCIDENT? YES □ NO □

c. INSURANCE PLAN NAME OR PROGRAM NAME

d. INSURANCE PLAN NAME OR PROGRAM NAME

10d. RESERVED FOR LOCAL USE

d. IS THERE ANOTHER HEALTH BENEFIT PLAN? YES □ NO □ _If yes_, return to and complete item 9 a-d.

READ BACK OF FORM BEFORE COMPLETING & SIGNING THIS FORM.
12. PATIENT'S OR AUTHORIZED PERSON'S SIGNATURE I authorize the release of any medical or other information necessary to process this claim. I also request payment of government benefits either to myself or to the party who accepts assignment below.

SIGNED _____ DATE _____

13. INSURED'S OR AUTHORIZED PERSON'S SIGNATURE I authorize payment of medical benefits to the undersigned physician or supplier for services described below.

SIGNED _____

14. DATE OF CURRENT: MM DD YY ◄ ILLNESS (First symptom) OR INJURY (Accident) OR PREGNANCY(LMP)

15. IF PATIENT HAS HAD SAME OR SIMILAR ILLNESS. GIVE FIRST DATE MM DD YY

16. DATES PATIENT UNABLE TO WORK IN CURRENT OCCUPATION MM DD YY MM DD YY FROM TO

17. NAME OF REFERRING PROVIDER OR OTHER SOURCE

17a.
17b. NPI

18. HOSPITALIZATION DATES RELATED TO CURRENT SERVICES MM DD YY MM DD YY FROM TO

19. RESERVED FOR LOCAL USE

20. OUTSIDE LAB? $ CHARGES YES □ NO □

21. DIAGNOSIS OR NATURE OF ILLNESS OR INJURY (Relate Items 1, 2, 3 or 4 to Item 24E by Line)

1. |___.___
2. |___.___
3. |___.___
4. |___.___

22. MEDICAID RESUBMISSION CODE ORIGINAL REF. NO.

23. PRIOR AUTHORIZATION NUMBER

24. A. DATE(S) OF SERVICE		B. PLACE OF SERVICE	C. EMG	D. PROCEDURES, SERVICES, OR SUPPLIES (Explain Unusual Circumstances)		E. DIAGNOSIS POINTER	F. $ CHARGES	G. DAYS OR UNITS	H. EPSDT Family Plan	I. ID. QUAL	J. RENDERING PROVIDER ID. #
From MM DD YY	To MM DD YY			CPT/HCPCS	MODIFIER						
1										NPI	
2										NPI	
3										NPI	
4										NPI	
5										NPI	
6										NPI	

25. FEDERAL TAX I.D. NUMBER SSN □ EIN □

26. PATIENT'S ACCOUNT NO.

27. ACCEPT ASSIGNMENT? (For govt. claims, see back) YES □ NO □

28. TOTAL CHARGE $

29. AMOUNT PAID $

30. BALANCE DUE $

31. SIGNATURE OF PHYSICIAN OR SUPPLIER INCLUDING DEGREES OR CREDENTIALS (I certify that the statements on the reverse apply to this bill and are made a part thereof.)

SIGNED _____ DATE _____

32. SERVICE FACILITY LOCATION INFORMATION

a. NPI b.

33. BILLING PROVIDER INFO & PH # ( )

a. NPI b.

790-0129 (08-05) (OCR) 1 PT.

NUCC Instruction Manual available at: www.nucc.org

APPROVED OMB-0938-0999 FORM CMS-1500 (08-05)

Figure 17-1

Capital City Medical—123 Unknown Boulevard, Capital City, NY 12345-2222 (555)555-1234 Phil Wells, MD, Mannie Mends, MD, Bette R. Soone, MD	Patient Information Form Tax ID: 75-0246810 Group NPI: 1513171216

Patient Information:

Name: (Last, First) Colich, Guy   ☒ Male   ❑ Female   Birth Date: 04/23/1958

Address: 872 Hickory Pl, Capital City, NY 12345   Phone: (555) 555-9069

Social Security Number: 142-86-2078   Full-Time Student: ❑ Yes   ☒ No

Marital Status: ❑ Single   ☒ Married   ❑ Divorced   ❑ Other

Employment:

Employer: None   Phone: ( )

Address:

Condition Related to: ❑ Auto Accident   ❑ Employment   ❑ Other Accident

Date of Accident: _____ State _____

Emergency Contact: _____ **Phone: ( )** _____

Primary Insurance: Aetna   Phone: ( )

Address: 1625 Healthcare Bldg, Capital City, NY 12345

Insurance Policyholder's Name: Same   ❑ M ❑ F DOB: _____

Address:

Phone: _____ Relationship to Insured: ☒ Self ❑ Spouse ❑ Child ❑ Other

Employer: _____ Phone: _____

Employer's Address:

Policy/ID No: 9567305   Group No: 511669 Percent Covered: ____%, Copay Amt: $ 35.00

Secondary Insurance: _____ Phone: ( )

Address:

Insurance Policyholder's Name: _____ ❑ M ❑ F DOB: _____

Address:

Phone: _____ Relationship to Insured: ❑ Self ❑ Spouse ❑ Child ❑ Other

Employer: _____ Phone: ( )

Employer's Address:

Policy/ID No: _____ Group No: _____ Percent Covered: ____%, Copay Amt: $_____

Reason for Visit: I am here for a recheck on my manic depression

Known Allergies:

Were you referred here? If so, by whom?:

Patient Name *Guy Colich*

Capital City Medical
123 Unknown Boulevard, Capital City, NY 12345-2222

Date of Service
10-07-20XX

New Patient			Arthrocentesis/Aspiration/Injection			Laboratory	
Problem Focused	99201		Small Joint		20600	Amylase	82150
Expanded Problem, Focused	99202		Interm Joint		20605	B12	82607
Detailed	99203		Major Joint		20610	CBC & Diff	85025
Comprehensive	99204		**Other Invasive/Noninvasive**			Comp Metabolic Panel	80053
Comprehensive/High Complex	99205		Audiometry		92552	Chlamydia Screen	87110
Well Exam Infant (up to 12 mos.)	99381		Cast Application			Cholesterol	82465
Well Exam 1–4 yrs.	99382		Location Long Short			Digoxin	80162
Well Exam 5–11 yrs.	99383		Catheterization		51701	Electrolytes	80051
Well Exam 12–17 yrs.	99384		Circumcision		54150	Ferritin	82728
Well Exam 18–39 yrs.	99385		Colposcopy		57452	Folate	82746
Well Exam 40–64 yrs.	99386		Colposcopy w/Biopsy		57454	GC Screen	87070
			Cryosurgery Premalignant Lesion			Glucose	82947
			Location (s):			Glucose 1 HR	82950
						Glycosylated HGB A1C	83036
Established Patient			Cryosurgery Warts			HCT	85014
Post-Op Follow Up Visit	99024		Location (s):			HDL	83718
Minimum	99211		Curettement Lesion			Hep BSAG	87340
Problem Focused	99212		Single		11055	Hepatitis panel, acute	80074
Expanded Problem Focused	99213	X	2–4		11056	HGB	85018
Detailed	99214		>4		11057	HIV	86703
Comprehensive/High Complex	99215		Diaphragm Fitting		57170	Iron & TIBC	83550
Well Exam Infant (up to 12 mos.)	99391		Ear Irrigation		69210	Kidney Profile	80069
Well exam 1–4 yrs.	99392		ECG		93000	Lead	83655
Well Exam 5–11 yrs.	99393		Endometrial Biopsy		58100	Liver Profile	80076
Well Exam 12–17 yrs.	99394		Exc. Lesion Malignant			Mono Test	86308
Well Exam 18–39 yrs.	99395		Benign			Pap Smear	88155
Well Exam 40–64 yrs.	99396		Location			Pregnancy Test	84703
Obstetrics			Exc. Skin Tags (1–15)		11200	Obstetric Panel	80055
Total OB Care	59400		Each Additional 10		11201	Pro Time	85610
Injections			Fracture Treatment			PSA	84153
Administration Sub. / IM	90772		Loc			RPR	86592
Drug			w/Reduc		w/o Reduc	Sed. Rate	85651
Dosage			I & D Abscess Single/Simple		10060	Stool Culture	87045
Allergy	95115		Multiple or Comp		10061	Stool O & P	87177
Cocci Skin Test	86490		I & D Pilonidal Cyst Simple		10080	Strep Screen	87880
DPT	90701		Pilonidal Cyst Complex		10081	Theophylline	80198
Hemophilus	90646		IV Therapy—To One Hour		90760	Thyroid Uptake	84479
Influenza	90658		Each Additional Hour		90761	TSH	84443
MMR	90707		Laceration Repair			Urinalysis	81000
OPV	90712		Location Size Simp/Comp			Urine Culture	87088
Pneumovax	90732		Laryngoscopy		31505	Drawing Fee	36415
TB Skin Test	86580		Oximetry		94760	Specimen Collection	99000
TD	90718		Punch Biopsy			**Other:**	
Unlisted Immun	90749		Rhythm Strip		93040		
Tetanus Toxoid	90703		Treadmill		93015		
Vaccine/Toxoid Admin <8 Yr Old w/ Counseling	90465		Trigger Point or Tendon Sheath Inj.		20550		
Vaccine/Toxoid Administration for Adult	90471		Tympanometry		92567		

Diagnosis/ICD-9:**296.80**

I acknowledge receipt of medical services and authorize the release of any medical information necessary to process this claim for healthcare payment only. I do authorize payment to the provider.

Patient Signature *Guy Colich*

Total Estimated Charges:_____

Payment Amount:_____

Next Appointment:_____

New Patient Examinations		
Office Visit, Level 1	99201	$ 55.00
Office Visit, Level 2	99202	$110.00
Office Visit, Level 3	99203	$154.00
Office Visit, Level 4	99204	$226.00
Office Visit, Level 5	99205	$299.00
Established Patient Examinations		
Office Visit, Level 1	99211	$ 45.00
Office Visit, Level 2	99212	$ 60.00
Office Visit, Level 3	99213	$ 80.00
Office Visit, Level 4	99214	$123.00
Office Visit, Level 5	99215	$199.00

Fee schedule.

LEARNING ACTIVITY: TRUE/FALSE

Indicate whether the statement is true (T) or false (F).

_____ 1. Insurance plans always cover the children of the insured member.

_____ 2. Two patients with the same insurance carrier may have varying coverage, even under the same employer.

_____ 3. Under COBRA coverage, the employee pays the entire insurance premium.

_____ 4. Most patients are well aware of what their insurance covers.

_____ 5. Under consumer directed health care plans, the patient is more aware of the cost of the health care they are receiving.

_____ 6. From the medical provider's point of view, consumer-directed health care plans work much the same as traditional health insurance plans.

_____ 7. Managed care plans control the costs associated with plan purchase by controlling the amounts they reimburse health care providers.

_____ 8. Patients do not have copays under capitated insurance plans.

_____ 9. Managed care fee schedules vary greatly between plans.

_____ 10. Most insurance plans have lifetime maximum benefits.

CRITICAL THINKING

Answer the following questions to the best of your ability. Use the textbook as a reference.

1. Josie Svien, CMA (AAMA), is working in the billing office of a family practice clinic. Josie is having trouble reading the hand-written chart notes of one of the clinic physicians. How should Josie proceed with billing for the services in this patient's chart?

   _____

   _____

   _____

   _____

   _____

2. Sean Quinn, RMA (AMT), has been hired to work in the billing office of a large general surgery practice. Sean has been asked to go through several outstanding insurance claims and determine why they have not been paid. As Sean looks through the files, he discovers that many of the claims have never been billed to the insurance carrier. Some of the claims are over a year old and Sean realizes those may be considered past timely filing limits. What can Sean do in this situation?

   _____

   _____

   _____

   _____

   _____

3. Monica Swinger is taking an administrative medical assisting course. She has been given the assignment to write an essay describing how health insurance began in the United States. What information should Monica include?

   _____

   _____

   _____

   _____

   _____

4. Erica Owsley, CMA (AAMA), is working with Charles Wong, a patient in the clinic where Erica works. Charles tells Erica he has the option of buying into the group insurance plan his employer offers or he can buy an individual policy on his own. He isn't sure which option to choose and asks Erica if she can tell him the difference between individual and group insurance plans. What can Erica tell Charles?

_____

_____

_____

_____

_____

5. Abrama Tesfe is a patient of Dr. Roland's. Abrama has recently gotten married and his wife has two children from a previous marriage. Abrama tells Dr. Roland's medical assistant that both he and his new wife have insurance coverage and he wants to know how to determine which insurance plan will be primary and which will be secondary for Abrama's step-children. What can the medical assistant tell Abrama?

_____

_____

_____

_____

_____

RESEARCH ACTIVITY

Use Internet search engines to research the following topics and write a brief description of what is found. It is important to visit reputable Web sites.

1. Using the Internet as a research source, find your state's Medicaid Web site and research the criteria for being covered under Medicaid in your state. Write an essay describing the persons who may be covered under Medicaid in your state.

_____

_____

_____

_____

_____

_____

_____

CHAPTER 18

ICD-9-CM Coding

CHAPTER OUTLINE

General review of the chapter:

    A. The Medical Assistant's Role in Diagnostic Coding
    B. The History of Diagnostic Coding
    C. Coding with the ICD-9-CM Book
    D. The Volumes of ICD-9-CM
    E. Determining the Correct Diagnosis Code
    F. Coding for Special Situations
    G. Pursuing Professional Certification

STUDENT STUDY GUIDE

Use the following guide to assist in your learning of the concepts from the chapter.

I. Introduction
    A. The MA Role in Diagnostic Coding
        i. MAs assign a code to the diagnosis that a/an _____ provides.
        ii. Attention to detail is vital for accurate coding.
        iii. Inaccurate coding will result in _____ or _____-_____ for services.
        iv. MAs maintain _____ _____ so that they can be utilized by coders.
    B. History of Diagnostic Coding
        i. 1893:

        ii. 1898:

        iii. 1901:

        iv. 1979:

(a) Up to this point, volumes had been updated about every _____ _____.

    v. Today, the ICD-9-CM is still used in the United States.
      (a) Most major countries are utilizing the _____.
      (b) No implementation date has been set for the United States for the ICD-10.

II. Function and Layout of the ICD-9-CM
  A. There are over _____ diagnosis codes that are organized and arranged in three volumes.
  B. The coding manual is updated every _____.
  C. The volumes appear in the following order:
    i. Volume _____, Volume _____, Volume _____
  D. Physician offices generally use volumes _____ and _____ and hospitals utilize all three volumes.
  E. Volume II
    i. Has two sections:
    ii. Section 1: _____ _____ to _____: Conditions and diseases are listed alphabetically by main term and subterms.
    iii. After selecting a diagnosis code, _____ it by referring to Volume _____.
    iv. Section 2: Alphabetic Index to External Causes of _____ _____ of Drugs and Other _____ Substances, _____, and Poisonings: supplemental codes to describe a condition caused by an accident or poisoning
  F. Volume I
    i. Volume I is used as a/an _____ reference.
    ii. Codes are arranged _____ and divided into _____ chapters based on etiology.
    iii. Each disease has a/an _____ _____ code combination.
    iv. Fourth and fifth digits of a code supply more _____ _____ of the disorder.
    v. A/an _____-digit code confers the highest level of definition.
  G. Volume I Appendices
    i. Appendix A:

      _____

      _____

    ii. Appendix B:

      _____

      _____

    iii. Appendix C:

      _____

      _____

    iv. Appendix D:

      _____

      _____

    v. Appendix E:

      _____

      _____

H. Volume I: V & E Codes
   i. V Codes classify the reason for care, other than the _____

     _____.
     (a) V Codes range from _____ to _____.
   ii. E codes are the second supplementary classification found within Volume II.
     (a) These codes classify causes of _____ and _____.
     (b) E codes range from _____ to _____.

I. Volume III
   i. Volume III is used for _____ _____ coding.
   ii. MAs will only use this if they work in _____ settings.
   iii. The majority of hospitals hire professional certified coders to code inpatient charts.

III. Steps to Diagnostic Coding
A. Step 1:

B. Step 2:

C. Step 3:

D. Step 4:

E. Step 5:

F. Step 6:

_____

_____

_____

_____

_____

_____

G. Step 7:

_____

_____

_____

_____

_____

_____

H. Step 8:

_____

_____

_____

_____

_____

_____

I. Steps 9–11:

_____

_____

_____

_____

_____

_____

IV. Coding for Special Circumstances
   A. Signs and symptoms codes—assigned when a/an _____ _____ is not yet available.
   B. Coding for neoplasms:
      i. Volume II provides the index to the _____ and _____ _____ of neoplasms.
      ii. _____ possible codes are available for each site depending on neoplasm behavior.
   C. V Codes: mainly for annual checkups, physical exams, and _____
      i. These encounters do not pertain to a/an _____ or injury.
   D. E Codes: never used alone and are never the _____-_____ diagnosis

    i. These are a supplementary classification that describes the external cause of an illness or injury.

E. Coding for drugs or chemicals that have caused poisoning or adverse reactions:
    i. MAs will need to know:

_____

_____

_____

_____

    ii. E codes are mandatory.

F. Coding for fractures
    i. The MA will need to know:

_____

_____

_____

_____

G. Coding for burns
    i. MAs will need to know:

_____

_____

_____

    ii. First, code the _____ and _____ of the burn:
        (a) The most severe is coded first.
    iii. Second, code the percentage of total body surface area (based on the _____ of _____).
    iv. Finally, use a/an _____ to describe the cause of the burn.

H. Late effects: arise from old injuries or conditions that have been resolved
    i. This is dependent on the physician's judgment.
    ii. Key words indicating a late effect include:

_____

_____

I. Coding for Obstetrics
    i. Obstetrics is a complex area of coding.
    ii. Codes must be considered for:

_____

_____

_____

_____

_____

    iii. Multiple births, caesarean sections, and complicated deliveries require _____ codes.

J. Coding for Diabetes Mellitus
    i. The diabetes mellitus (DM) is a category often used.
    ii. DM is always coded to the _____ _____.
        (a) It often requires _____ and multiple coding.

iii. It is important to know:

_____

_____

_____

_____

K. Inpatient services: provided by the physician in the inpatient setting
   i. Patients are assigned a/an _____ _____.
   ii. A principal diagnosis is assigned after all tests, studies, and results are completed.
   iii. The _____ _____ must be assigned prior to final billing.

V. Pursuing Professional Certifications
   A. The most widely recognized coding certifications include:
      i. Certified Professional Coder (CPC):

_____

_____

_____

      ii. Certified Coding Specialist-Physician (CCS-P):

_____

_____

_____

   B. Passing the examination requires an in-depth knowledge of:

_____

_____

_____

_____

KEY TERMINOLOGY REVIEW

Match the selected key terms to their definitions below.

a. category

b. chapter

c. combination code

d. conventions

e. E codes

f. first-listed

g. late effect

h. main term

i. M codes

j. nonessential modifier

k. not-elsewhere classified

l. not otherwise specified

m. sequelae

n. subcategory

o. subclassification

p. tabular list

q. V codes

_____ 1. A single code that describes two or more conditions that frequently occur together.

_____ 2. Current condition that results from a previous resolved condition.

_____ 3. A four digit code in the ICD-9-CM tabular list.

_____ 4. Words in parentheses after a main term in the ICD-9-CM, clarifying the main term, but need not be present in the medical record.

_____ 5. A three digit code in ICD-9-CM tabular list.

_____ 6. Volume I of ICD-9-CM which lists all diagnostic codes in numerical order.

_____ 7. The diagnosis that is chiefly responsible for the outpatient services provided; formally called primary diagnosis.

_____ 8. A general code used when details are not available in the medical record.

_____ 9. A three digit code in ICD-9-CM tabular list.

_____ 10. Words by which conditions and diseases are alphabetized in ICD-9-CM Volume II; may be the name of condition, eponym, acronym, or synonym, but not an anatomical site.

_____ 11. ICD-9-CM coding rules, abbreviations, symbols or formatting intended to ensure consistency in coding.

_____ 12. Code that cannot be found elsewhere in the coding book.

_____ 13. An abnormal condition resulting from previous injury, condition, or disease.

_____ 14. Codes for visits' reasons, other than disease or illness.

_____ 15. A five digit code in ICD-9-CM tabular list.

_____ 16. Identify neoplasm type and tumor behavior, used by tumor registries.

_____ 17. Codes that indicate the external cause of an illness or condition.

APPLIED PRACTICE

Using Volume II and Volume I of the ICD-9-CM, identify the diagnostic code for each of the following diagnoses.

1. Diabetes with ketoacidosis: _____

2. Acute idiopathic pericarditis: _____

3. Acute lymphadenitis: _____

4. Pneumococcal meningitis: _____

5. Acute pharyngitis: _____

6. Hirsutism: _____

7. Chest pains, unspecified: _____

8. Special screening for diabetes mellitus: _____

9. Cushing's syndrome: _____

10. Glycosuria: _____

LEARNING ACTIVITY: MULTIPLE CHOICE

Circle the correct answer to each of the questions below.

1. Diagnostic coding has existed since what year?

    a. 1793
    b. 1893
    c. 1993
    d. 2003

2. The first Internal Classification of Diseases (ICD) book was published in what year?

    a. 1810
    b. 1710
    c. 2001
    d. 1910

3. The ICD-10 book contains which of the following new chapters?

    a. mental disorders
    b. eye doctors
    c. urinary disorders
    d. cardiac disorders

4. Which volume of the ICD-9-CM contains a tabular list of diseases?

    a. Volume I
    b. Volume II
    c. Volume III
    d. Volume IV

5. Which volume of the ICD-9-CM contains an alphabetic index of diseases?

    a. Volume I
    b. Volume II
    c. Volume III
    d. Volume IV

6. Which volume of the ICD-9-CM contains a list of diagnosis codes used for hospital billing?

    a. Volume I
    b. Volume II
    c. Volume III
    d. Volume IV

7. Volume I of the ICD-9-CM coding book has _____ chapters.

    a. 15
    b. 16
    c. 17
    d. 18

8. Volume I of the ICD-9-CM coding book has _____ appendices.

    a. 4
    b. 5
    c. 6
    d. 7

9. Appendix _____ contains a list of the morphology of neoplasms.

    a. A
    b. B
    c. C
    d. D

10. Appendix _____ contains a glossary of mental disorders.

    a. A
    b. B
    c. C
    d. D

CRITICAL THINKING

Answer the following questions to the best of your ability. Use the textbook as a reference.

1. Teresa Clymer is taking a course in medical insurance billing as part of her medical assistant training. She has been asked to write a paper describing how proper diagnosis coding is linked to proper reimbursement from insurance carriers. What information should Teresa include in her paper?

   _____

   _____

   _____

   _____

   _____

2. Mavis Raschenko, RMA (AMT), has been asked by her office manager to explain the difference between Volumes I and II of the ICD-9-CM coding book. How might Mavis explain the differences?

   _____

   _____

   _____

   _____

   _____

3. Benjamin Tho is taking a billing and coding course as part of his medical assistant training. He has been asked to prepare a list of the appendices of the ICD-9-CM coding book, including the information contained within. What should Benjamin include?

   _____

   _____

   _____

   _____

   _____

4. Marc Alaimo, RMA (AMT), has been newly hired to work in the billing office in a family practice clinic. Marc has been asked to explain to the physicians how V codes are to be used. What should Marc include in his explanation?

   _____

   _____

   _____

   _____

5. Sonya Kraski, CMA (AAMA), is working as the billing office manager in a urology practice. She has been asked to explain to the physicians how E codes are to be used. What should Sonya include in her explanation?

   _____

   _____

_____

_____

_____

RESEARCH ACTIVITY

Use Internet search engines to research the following topics and write a brief description of what is found. It is important to visit reputable Web sites.

1. Using the Internet as a research source, find three to five Web sites that would be beneficial for those working with diagnostic coding on a day-to-day basis. Explain how these sites would be helpful.

_____

_____

_____

_____

_____

_____

_____

_____

_____

_____

_____

_____

CHAPTER 19

Procedural Coding

CHAPTER OUTLINE

General review of the chapter:

A. Key Terminology
B. The MA's Role in Procedural Coding
C. The History of Procedural Coding
D. Coding with the CPT-4 Manual
E. Organization of the CPT Manual
F. Using CPT Modifiers
G. Coding for Evaluation and Management Services
H. Using Code Modifiers Appropriately
I. Coding for Special Situations
J. The Health Care Common Procedure Coding System (HCPCS)

STUDENT STUDY GUIDE

Use the following guide to assist in your learning of the concepts from the chapter.

I. Introduction
    A. The MA's Role in Procedural Coding
        i. MAs assign procedural codes that reflect _____ that are performed by providers.
        ii. This involves _____ data from the medical record to determine the proper code.
        iii. MAs may need to clarify information with a physician.
        iv. MAs also may discuss with _____ _____ the reason that a code was assigned to a patient.
    B. The History of Procedural Coding
        i. The _____, _____, and _____ system was used before procedural coding.
            (a) It was developed by insurance companies to determine reasonable fees for services provided within a/an _____area.
        ii. Before the mid-1960s, the UCR system was used without any standardized medical billing forms or _____ _____.
        iii. In _____, the first Current Procedural Terminology was published.
        iv. The last major revision of the CPT occurred in _____.
        v. In _____, the U.S. Congress devised the relative value unit (RVU) to increase the accuracy of coding.
        vi. Today, the CPT covers all procedures allowed by the _____ and _____ _____.

II. The CPT-4® Manual
   A. Purpose of the CPT-4® Manual
      i. The Current Procedural Terminology, Fourth Edition
         (a) Published by the _____ _____ _____
      ii. Lists procedures and services performed by physicians
      iii. Provides a uniform language to describe medical, _____, and
           _____ services
   B. Fraudulent Practices in Billing and Coding
      i. Though procedural coding may be challenging, MAs should avoid _____
         or _____.
      ii. This could result in _____ or _____ of the billing system.
      iii. It is best to consult with the physician, a colleague, or a professional organization if coding
           issues arise.
      iv. Fraudulent coding practices may result in loss of the provider's _____,
          practice, and reputation.
      v. Those who commit this offense may be _____ and charged with crimes.
      vi. Examples of fraudulent coding and billing practices include:

      _____

      _____

      _____

III. Organization of the CPT-4® Manual
   A. Over _____ procedural codes are listed in the manual.
   B. The CPT Manual is organized as follows:
      i. The inside covers offer a list of commonly used _____,
         _____ and place of service codes.
      ii. The back cover lists commonly used medical _____.
      iii. The tabular index provides a numerical listing of all CPT codes.
         (a) The tabular index is divided into three categories:
            (1) Category I:

            _____

            _____

            _____

            (2) Category II:

            _____

            _____

            _____

            (3) Category III:

            _____

            _____

            _____

      iv. Appendices:
         (a) Appendix A:

            _____

            _____

            _____

(b) Appendix B:

_____

_____

(c) Appendix C:

_____

_____

(d) Appendix D:

_____

_____

(e) Appendix E:

_____

_____

(f) Appendix F:

_____

_____

(g) Appendix G:

_____

_____

(h) Appendix H:

_____

_____

(i) Appendix I:

_____

_____

(j) Appendix J:

_____

_____

(k) Appendix K:

_____

_____

       (l) Appendix L:

_____

_____

_____

       (m) Appendix M:

_____

_____

_____

   v. The Alphabetical Index lists all procedures and services in the CPT manual.
      (a) These are listed alphabetically by the _____ _____ and
         _____ terms.
      (b) This aids in locating the most appropriate code or range of codes for procedures and services.

IV. Steps to Procedural Coding

A. Step 1:

_____

_____

_____

_____

B. Step 2:

_____

_____

_____

_____

C. Step 3:

_____

_____

_____

_____

D. Step 4:

_____

_____

_____

_____

E. Step 5:

_____

_____

_____

_____

F. Step 6:

_____

_____

G. Step 7:

_____

_____

_____

_____

H. Step 8:

_____

_____

I. Step 9:

_____

_____

J. Step 10:

_____

_____

_____

_____

K. Step 11: Assign the code.

V. Modifiers

A. Modifiers are _____-digit suffixes used with CPT codes.

B. Proper use of modifiers can speed up claims processing and _____ reimbursement.

C. Misusing modifiers could cause billing _____ and possibly claim _____.

D. Modifers are used:
   i. To report only the _____ _____ of a procedure or service
   ii. To report a service mandated by a/an _____-_____ payer
   iii. To indicate that a procedure was performed _____
   iv. To report _____ _____ performed at the same session by the same provider
   v. To report a portion of a service or procedure that was _____ or eliminated at the physician's discretion.

E. Commonly Used Modifiers
   i. 22 *Unusual Procedural Service:*

   _____

   _____

   ii. 47 *Anesthesia by Surgeon:*

   _____

   _____

   iii. 50 *Bilateral Procedure:*

   _____

   _____

   iv. 51 *Multiple Procedures:* Specifically has four applications to identify—

   _____

   _____

v. *53 Discontinued Procedure:*

_____

_____

vi. *54 Surgical Care Only:*

_____

_____

vii. *55 Postoperative Management Only:*

_____

_____

viii. *56 Preoperative Management Only:*

_____

_____

ix. *58 Staged or Related Procedure by the Same Physician During the Postoperative Period:*
If a procedure was performed during the postoperative period, the physician may need to indicate if the procedure was:
(a) Planned _____ at the time of the original procedure
(b) More _____ than the original procedure
(c) For therapy following a/an _____ _____ procedure

x. *59 Distinct Procedural Service:*

_____

_____

xi. *62 Two Surgeons:*

_____

_____

xii. *78 Return to the Operating Room for a Related Procedure During the Postoperative Period:*

_____

_____

xiii. *79 Unrelated Procedure or Service by the Same Physician During the Postoperative Period:*

_____

_____

xiv. *80 Assistant Surgeon:*

_____

_____

VI. Evaluation and Management Coding, Coding for Special Situations, HCPCS
   A. E&M codes describe patient _____ with a physician.
   B. Codes are usually marked on the encounter form.
   C. _____ in the medical record should be consistent with the codes that are checked off.
   D. Steps for E&M Coding
      i. Step 1: Identify the category of service.

_____

_____

_____

ii. Step 2: Identify the subcategory of service.

_____

_____

iii. Step 3: Review the reporting instructions for the selected category or subcategory.

_____

_____

iv. Step 4: Determine the key components.

_____

_____

v. Step 5: Identify the contributing factors.

_____

_____

vi. Step 6: Verify and assign the code.
vii. Step 7: Identify bundled and separately billable services.

_____

_____

_____

_____

viii. Step 8: Identify modifiers.
ix. Common Modifiers Used in E&M Coding
   (a) _____ Prolonged Evaluation and Management Service
   (b) _____ Unrelated Evaluation and Management Service by the Same Physician During a Postoperative Period
   (c) _____ Significant, Separately Identifiable Evaluation and Management Service by the Same Physician on the Same Day of the Procedure or Other Service
   (d) _____ Mandated Services
   (e) _____ Reduced Services
   (f) _____ Decision for Surgery
x. Step 9: Identify the place of service for the CMS-1500.
   (a) The place of service (POS) code is required for block _____ on the _____ form.
E. Coding for Anesthesia
  i. Anesthesia codes are used for _____ and _____ anesthesia
   (a) Also supplementation of local anesthesia
  ii. Codes are determined using the B＊T＊M formula:

_____

_____

_____

_____

F. Coding for Surgery
    i. The Surgery section is the _____ in the CPT.
    ii. Surgical codes are divided into _____ based on the systems of the body.
    iii. They are further divided into _____ arrangements of each subsection.
    iv. Surgical codes are bundled into a package that includes:

_____

_____

_____

_____

_____

_____

    v. Services not included in the surgical package codes include:

_____

_____

_____

_____

_____

G. Coding for Radiology
    i. Radiological codes have two parts:
      (a) The _____ component, which deals with components associated with the procedure
      (b) The _____ component, which deals with the physician's skill, time, and expertise used for reading and interpreting the radiological examination
    ii. Contrast material may be given for image _____.
    iii. It can be coded "_____ _____," as long as the contrast material was not administered orally and/or rectally.

H. Coding for Pathology and Laboratory
    i. A complete pathology or laboratory service completed or supervised by a physician includes:

_____

_____

    ii. A panel is a group of tests ordered together.
      (a) A panel will detect particular _____ or malfunctioning _____.
    iii. When coding a panel, all tests must have been performed without any substitution.
    iv. _____ the code may be necessary if fewer tests are performed than the entire panel.
      (a) Individual tests would then be coded.

I. Coding for Medicine
    i. Codes that pertain to medicine vary by reporting, and procedures and services.
    ii. These codes may be often used by physical therapists, occupational therapists, and audiologists.
    iii. Two codes must be provided for immunizations:

_____

_____

_____

J. Unlisted Codes
  i. Used if a physician performs a procedure that is not listed in the coding book.
  ii. A copy of the _____ _____ must be submitted with the claim.
     (a) Failure to send the procedure report could result in _____ of the claims.
K. The Health Care Common Procedure Coding System (HCPCS)
  i. Used for reporting:

  _____

  _____

  _____

  ii. Level I Codes—CPT codes for professional services
  iii. Level II Codes—Codes beginning with a letter followed by _____ numbers
     (a) These codes cover supplies, DME, drugs, nonphysician providers, and certain physician services for Medicare and Medicaid.
     (b) Always use the _____ code if a CPT code is available for the same service.
     (c) Level II codes are updated _____.
     (d) Updates are available on the CMS Web site at www.cms.gov.
  iv. Level III codes are being phased out.
     (a) This is due to HIPAA's _____ _____ provision and the need for uniform code sets.
     (b) Originally, Level III codes were developed by_____ Medicare carriers.
L. Documentation and Reimbursement
  i. Accurate and complete medical records are the _____ of medical billing.
  ii. MAs may be faced with incomplete service or procedure documentation.
     (a) MA must send the chart back to the proper health care professional for
        _____.
     (b) This is a much quicker and easier solution than providing an insurance company with an incomplete or inaccurate insurance claim.
  iii. Only correct and complete documentation will ensure _____ at the _____ level.

KEY TERMINOLOGY REVIEW

Match the selected key terms to their definitions below.

a. abuse
b. add-on code
c. alphabetic index
d. audit
e. bundling
f. category
g. common descriptor
h. downcode
i. Evaluation and Management (E&M)

j. examination
k. fraud
l. guidelines
m. history
n. key component
o. main term
p. medical decisionmaking
q. modifier
r. physical status modifier

s. section
t. special instruction
u. standalone code
v. subcategory
w. subsection
x. tabular index
y. unbundling
z. upcode

_____ 1. To bill intentionally for services that were never given.

_____ 2. A review process that verifies every detail of a CPT code is clearly documented in the medical record.

_____ 3. One of six major divisions of the CPT manual.

_____ 4. To assign a code for a lower level of service that was actually performed.

_____ 5. Directions within each section describing specific rules and definitions for use of codes within a particular category or subcategory.

_____ 6. Improper behavior and billing practices that result in financial gain but are not fraudulent.

_____ 7. Words by which procedures and services are alphabetized in the CPT index.

_____ 8. To code and bill for a higher level of service than was actually provided.

_____ 9. CPT codes used for billing physician services to evaluate and manage patient care, such as office visits.

_____ 10. A division of a category within the tabular index.

_____ 11. Billing multiple services with separate CPT codes and separate charges that should be combined under a single CPT code and one charge.

_____ 12. Three primary determining criteria in selecting an E&M code; include history, examination, and medical decisionmaking.

_____ 13. A CPT code designated by the (+) that cannot be used alone and must be used with another CPT code.

_____ 14. Specific instructions at the beginning of each section of the CPT manual that define terms and describe specific information about how to use codes in that section.

_____ 15. A key component of E&M coding that describes the complexity establishing a diagnosis and/or selecting a management option.

_____ 16. A CPT code that contains a full description and is not dependent on another code for complete meaning.

_____ 17. The portion of a standalone code before the semicolon that is shared with the indented codes that follow.

_____ 18. Subdivisions within a CPT section of the tabular index.

_____ 19. Two-digit alphanumeric codes appended to CPT or Level II codes to further describe circumstances.

_____ 20. The numerical listing of all CPT codes, accompanied by guidelines and notes.

_____ 21. Two-digit alphanumeric codes (P1 to P6) appended to anesthesia codes, which indicate the health status of the patient at the beginning of the procedure.

_____ 22. Alphabetical listing of CPT codes by procedure name, condition, eponym, and acronym.

_____ 23. A key component of E&M coding that describes the background, onset, and progression of the patient's current condition.

_____ 24. A division of a subheading within the tabular index.

_____ 25. Combining multiple services under a single, all-inclusive CPT code and one charge.

_____ 26. A key component of E&M coding that describes the complexity of the physical assessment of the patient.

APPLIED PRACTICE

Follow the directions that apply to each section.

A. Provide the correct modifier for each of the following descriptions.

1. Bilateral procedure _____

2. Discontinued procedure _____

3. Unusual procedural service _____

4. Preoperative management only _____

5. General anesthesia provided by the surgeon _____

B. Code the following using the CPT code book:

1. Debridement of 10 nails by any method _____

2. Chemical peel, facial; dermal _____

3. Mastectomy, subcutaneous _____

4. Incision and draining (I&D) of hematoma, soft tissue of neck _____

5. Manipulation, elbow, under anesthesia _____

6. Endoscopy, surgical; operative tissue ablation and reconstruction of atria, without cardiopulmonary bypass _____

7. Laparoscopy, surgical, appendectomy _____

8. Vaginal delivery only, including postpartum care _____

9. Mammography, bilateral _____

10. Spirometry, including graphic record, total and timed vital capacity, expiratory flow rate measurement with or without maximal voluntary ventilation _____

Note: This activity has been adapted from Vines, Comprehensive Health Insurance: Billing, Coding, and Reimbursement. *© 2008 Pearson Education, Inc. Upper Saddle River, NJ 07458.*

LEARNING ACTIVITY: MULTIPLE CHOICE

Circle the correct answer to each of the questions below.

1. Procedure codes have been standardized since _____.
   a. 1946
   b. 1956
   c. 1966
   d. 1976

2. The United States Congress developed the relative value unit system in _____.
   a. 1972
   b. 1982
   c. 1992
   d. 2002

3. The CPT book has _____ major sections.
   a. 3
   b. 4
   c. 5
   d. 6

4. The last major revision to the CPT coding book was made in _____.
   a. 1967
   b. 1977
   c. 1987
   d. 1997

5. All CPT codes are _____ digits long.
   a. 4
   b. 5
   c. 6
   d. all of the above

6. Within the CPT book, _____ means this is a new code.
   a. a black circle
   b. a triangle
   c. two triangles
   d. a circle with inner dot

7. Within the CPT book, _____ means this is a revised code.
   a. a black circle
   b. a triangle
   c. two triangles
   d. a circle with inner dot

8. Within the CPT book, _____ means a new or revised description.
   a. a black circle
   b. a triangle
   c. two triangles
   d. a circle with inner dot

9. Within the CPT book, _____ means this code includes conscious sedation.
   a. a black circle
   b. a triangle
   c. two triangles
   d. a circle with inner dot

10. When physicians perform procedures that are not listed in the CPT coding book, what must the medical assistant do?
    a. choose a code for the closest procedure to what was done
    b. not bill for the service
    c. ask the physician to choose an appropriate code
    d. use an unlisted procedure code and submit copies of the procedure report with the claim

CRITICAL THINKING

Answer the following questions to the best of your ability. Use the textbook as a reference.

1. Henry Bagualin is taking an administrative medical assisting course. He has been given an assignment to explain how to code for a procedure that is not listed in the CPT coding book. What can Henry do for this assignment?

_____

_____

_____

_____

_____

2. Kira Stansfield, CMA (AAMA), is working with Dr. Ramey in an internal medicine clinic. Dr. Ramey is unsure which evaluation and management code to choose for certain patients she has seen. How can Kira advise Dr. Ramey in choosing the appropriate code?

_____

_____

_____

_____

3. Joyce Shawger is taking an administrative medical assisting course. She has been given the assignment of explaining how E&M codes are used in determining the level of physical examination done by the physician. What should Joyce include in her assignment?

_____

_____

_____

_____

4. Gloria Heritage, RMA (AMT), is working in the billing office of a pediatric practice. One of the physicians in the practice frequently chooses a high level E&M code when billing for his patients. When Gloria consults the patient's charts, she finds there is not sufficient information to use the higher billing codes and determines a lower code would be more appropriate. What can Gloria do in this situation?

_____

_____

_____

_____

5. James Douglas, CMA (AAMA), is working for Dr. Boyan. James notices that Dr. Boyan frequently forgets to chart every detail about his patients' visits. Often, Dr. Boyan circles a procedure code for something he hasn't completely charted in the patient's chart. James is concerned that Dr. Boyan will be accused of fraudulent billing practices in the event an insurance company requests copies of a patient's medical chart. How can James address this situation?

_____

_____

_____

_____

RESEARCH ACTIVITY

Use Internet search engines to research the following topics and write a brief description of what is found. It is important to visit reputable Web sites.

1. Using the Internet as a research source, go to your state's Web site for the Department of Health. Research the laws that apply to billing for medical services in your state. Create a list of the laws you find relating to fraudulent practices in billing and coding.

    _____

    _____

    _____

    _____

    _____

    _____

    _____

    _____

    _____

    _____

    _____

    _____

CHAPTER 20

Billing, Collections, and Credit

CHAPTER OUTLINE

General review of the chapter:

    A. Introduction
    B. The MA's Role in Billing, Collections, and Credit
    C. Billing
        i. Fee schedules, participating provider agreements
    D. Credit and Collections
        i. Patient identification, accounts receivable, collection in managed care
        ii. Nonpaying patients, uncollectible accounts, small claims court

STUDENT STUDY GUIDE

Use the following guide to assist in your learning of the concepts from the chapter.

  I. Introduction to Billing, Collections, and Credit
    A. The MA's Role
        i. The medical assistant will be responsible for _____ fees for services to patients.
          (a) This should be done _____ _____ are _____.
          (b) An explanation of fees will help avoid _____ and misunderstandings over patient accounts.
        ii. The medical assistant will also be responsible for _____ payments from patients.
    B. Methods of Payment
        i. Cash: Keep a copy of the _____ of the cash received.
          (a) This discourages _____ among office staff.
        ii. Personal checks: Verify that the check amount is correctly written, _____, and _____.
          (a) If "Payment in Full" appears on the check, verify that the check is for the full amount owed in order to avoid _____ at a later _____.
        iii. Credit/debit cards _____ are issued with this form of payment and generally are _____ to _____ percent of the charges.
    C. Manual Billing Systems
        i. The manual billing system is commonly referred to as the _____ _____.
        ii. This system utilizes day sheets.
          (a) Day sheets are placed on a pegboard at the _____ of each day.
        iii. Patient _____ cards are placed on the day sheets under the superbills.
          (a) Ledger cards contain patient information and _____ _____.

    iv. The day sheet lists charges for services and _____ received throughout the day.

    v. At the end of each day sheet or business day, whichever occurs first, all charges and collections are tallied.

    vi. The collection total must match the _____ _____ _____.

D. Computerized Billing Systems

    i. Manual billing systems are becoming outdated as computerized billing becomes the norm.

    ii. With computerized billing:

_____

_____

_____

_____

_____

_____

    iii. _____ _____ document the money owed to the medical office and how long the account has been _____.

E. Features of Computerized Billing

    i. Computerized medical billing systems come equipped with multiple features.
    (a) The ability to run multiple _____ is a common feature.

    ii. High-level features often _____ the price of the software package system.

    iii. Some high-level features include:

_____

_____

_____

_____

_____

_____

    iv. Extensive _____ should be completed prior to purchasing a software package.
    (a) This will ensure that the medical office is receiving the best software package, at an affordable price, that will meet its needs.

II. Posting Payments, Fee Schedules, and Managed Care Contracts

A. Posting Payments Manually

    i. Place the patient's _____ _____ on the day sheet.

    ii. Enter the type of _____ on the ledger card.

    iii. _____ adjustments as appropriate.

    iv. Calculate the new balance.

    v. Enter the new balance on the _____ _____.

B. Posting Payments with Computerized Billing

_____

_____

_____

_____

C. Fee Schedules

    i. Fee schedules set maximum amounts for services using the resource-based relative value scale (RBRVS).

   ii. This was designed to reduce _____ _____ and establish a
        national standard for physician payment.
  iii. Medicare bases fee schedules on:

_____

_____

_____

_____

_____

   iv. Physician's fees are adjusted using the _____ _____ cost
        index (GPCI).
    v. The Centers for Medicare and Medicaid Services established the relative value unit (RVU).
   vi. The RVU combines the _____ and the GPCI.
  vii. Most health insurance plans base their fees on the _____ fee schedule.
      (a) This fee schedule generally sets the maximum charge allowed for any given service or
           procedure.
  viii. Yearly, Medicare assigns a/an _____ _____
        _____.
   ix. The national conversion factor is multiplied by the physician's _____ to
        determine the allowed fee for that service.

  D. Managed Care Contracts
     i. Managed care contracts are required to be signed _____ to becoming
        preferred provider by a managed care company.
    ii. Contracts can be very lengthy.
      (a) It is strongly suggested that the entire contract be reviewed prior to signing.
   iii. Medical assistants may help physicians with _____ the contract.
   iv. The MA will often use a highlighter to reference points of conflict or interest.
      (a) _____ _____ and provider _____
          restrictions should certainly be highlighted.
    v. All highlighted areas should be reviewed with the physician.
   vi. When a contract is signed, the physician is _____ to see patients for the
        agreed-upon fees.

III. Accounts Receivable and Collections

  A. Accounts Receivable
     i. Accounts receivable includes all monies owed to the practice.
    ii. This includes money owed from:

_____

_____

_____

_____

   iii. Accounts receivable is a very important task that requires regular monitoring and paying
        close attention to detail.
   iv. Information obtained and checked during accounts receivable include:

_____

_____

_____

_____

_____

    v. If a patient's account is past due, it is best to talk with patients when they are in the office.
   vi. Contacting the patient via the telephone is the next best option.
  vii. When calling the patient:

_____

_____

_____

_____

_____

_____

B. Collection Policies
    i. Specific information should be covered when creating a collection policy.
   ii. Information should include:

_____

_____

_____

_____

_____

_____

_____

_____

_____

C. Collection Issues in Managed Care

_____

_____

_____

_____

_____

_____

_____

_____

_____

D. Collection Agencies
    i. A medical office may choose to enlist the services of a collection agency.
    (a) This is after _____ _____ by the office via phone and mail to collect an outstanding balanced owed by the patient.
   ii. It is best to get _____ from other offices who have utilized collection agencies.
  iii. Collection agencies must:
    (a) Abide by the _____ _____ _____ Act
    (b) Actively pursue patient accounts while not _____ or offending patients

(c) Utilizing a collection agency will increase the chance of recouping a payment.

    iv. Collection agencies will charge a percentage of the amount owed by the patient.

    v. The percentage fee is often _____ of the patient's balance.

    vi. Some companies charge a/an _____ for their services.

       (a) This can prove to be cost effective for offices with large outstanding account balances.

E. Small Claims Court

    i. Small claims court is another method of collecting _____

    _____.

    ii. _____ vary from state to state regarding filing:

       (a) You may file a claim online, via the postal service, or you may have to file a claim in person at the local courthouse.

    iii. The medical office must prove that the patient _____

    _____ and _____ the charges for the service.

       (a) The patient chart as well as _____ _____ by the patient regarding payment of outstanding bills can verify this.

    iv. Providers often win these sorts of cases; however, there is cost associated with filing a claim.

    v. The provider must weigh the benefit of receiving payment against the costs associated with filing.

KEY TERMINOLOGY REVIEW

Match the selected key terms with their appropriate definitions.

a.	accounts receivable	j.	patient billing statements
b.	aging report	k.	pegboard accounting system
c.	collection agency	l.	posting
d.	day sheet	m.	professional courtesy
e.	fee schedule	n.	RVU
f.	GPCI	o.	superbill
g.	hardship agreement	p.	tickler file
h.	ledger card	q.	uncollectible
i.	national standard	r.	write off

_____ 1. Document used to track services rendered that is used with manual pegboard systems.

_____ 2. Used with manual pegboard system to document and track the charges and payments within the medical office.

_____ 3. To give a patient a discount due to the fact that the patient is a health care professional.

_____ 4. Money owed to the medical office.

_____ 5. Tool for tracking future events, such as patient appointments.

_____ 6. Process of adding charges or payments to a patient's accounts.

_____ 7. Medicare system for adjusting fees based on the area in which the health care provider practices.

_____ 8. Monthly statements sent to patients who have an outstanding balance.

_____ 9. Point of reference for developing charges for health care services used throughout the United States.

_____ 10. List of services and their fees.

_____ 11. To remove a balance from a patient account.

_____ 12. Numeric value assigned by Medicare to formulate schedules for health care providers.

_____ 13. Account believed never to be paid.

_____ 14. Documentation of the money owed the medical office and how long accounts have been outstanding.

_____ 15. Document that indicates the services performed with a patient on a given visit.

_____ 16. Agreement a patient signs to indicate an inability to pay full health care costs due to financial hardship.

_____ 17. Manual bookkeeping system.

_____ 18. Company that pursues overdue accounts for a fee.

APPLIED PRACTICE

Complete the activities and answer the questions that follow.

1. Call a local medical office in your area and ask to speak to someone in the billing office. Interview this person about their job function. Ask them the following questions:

   a. What type of system does this office use for billing (manual or computerized)?

   _____

   _____

   b. If the office uses a computer system for billing, what is the name of the software used?

   _____

   _____

   c. What functions does the computer system have that helps the billing office staff better perform their jobs?

   _____

   _____

2. Read the scenario below and answer the questions that follow.

Scenario

Kaley McManus, RMA (AMT), works for Havensburg Audiology. The payment policy for the audiology practice states that all copayments are expected at the time of service. Arturo is responsible for paying 20 percent of all services and his insurance company, Healthy Care, will reimburse the physician the remaining 80 percent.

Arturo Alamos was seen today by Dr. Lynst. Two procedures were performed, a comprehensive audio and a tympanography. Below is the fee schedule for the office.

AUDIOLOGY SERVICES		
Screening audio air only	92551	$ 38.00
Pure tone air	92552	$ 37.00
Pure tone air and bone	92553	$ 50.00
Comprehensive audio	92557	$101.00
Loudness balance test	92562	$ 38.00
Tone decay	92563	$ 41.00
Tympanography	92567	$ 40.00
Acoustic reflex	92568	$ 42.00
Reflex decay	92569	$ 43.00
Visual reinforced audio	92579	$ 78.00
Brain stem audiogram	92585	$327.00

Sample fee schedule.

a. How much will Kaley collect from Mr. Alamos today?

b. How much will Healthy Care be billed for the services rendered by Mr. Alamos?

c. As Mr. Alamos gets ready to pay for his office visit, he realizes he only has a $20 bill. What should Kaley do?

LEARNING ACTIVITY: MULTIPLE CHOICE

Circle the correct answer to each of the questions below.

1. _____ are documents that detail the money owed to the medical practice and how long the account has been outstanding.
   a. Accounts payable
   b. Aging reports
   c. Superbills
   d. none of the above

2. Medical billing software programs can print reports such as:
   a. patients' birthdays
   b. female patients over the age of 40 who have not had a mammogram in the past year
   c. male patients over the age of 50 who have not had a colonoscopy in the past year
   d. all of the above

3. Computerized billing systems can typically perform which of the following?
   a. send electronic insurance bills
   b. appointment book systems
   c. post insurance payments electronically
   d. all of the above

4. The Omnibus Budget Reconciliation Act was passed in _____.
   a. 1993
   b. 1973
   c. 1983
   d. 2003

5. The resource-based relative value scale was designed to:
   a. reduce fraudulent billing
   b. reduce Medicare costs
   c. create a fee schedule that can never be raised
   d. none of the above

6. Medicare service fees are calculated based on which of the following factors?
   a. service intensity
   b. time needed for the service
   c. the practice's malpractice premiums
   d. all of the above

7. The geographical practice cost index adjusts physicians' fees according to what criteria?
   a. the type of specialty the physician practices
   b. the amount of the physician's overhead
   c. where the practice is located within the United States
   d. the number of employees the physician has

8. The relative value unit was devised by _____ as a way for physicians to create a fee schedule for the services they render.
   a. OSHA
   b. COBRA
   c. CMS
   d. JCAHO

9. Managed care participating provider agreements are _____ pages in length.
   a. 10–20
   b. 20–30
   c. 30–40
   d. It depends upon the managed care plan.

10. When should fees be discussed with patients?
   a. before care is rendered
   b. while care is being rendered
   c. after care is rendered
   d. never

CRITICAL THINKING

Answer the following questions to the best of your ability. Use the textbook as a reference.

1. Marissa Duchenne, CMA (AAMA), has been newly hired as the office manager in a multispecialty clinic. When she goes over the clinic's fee schedule, Marissa finds that the clinic has several different fee levels associated with the same procedure codes. When Marissa questions the office staff, she finds that patients who have no insurance coverage are charged nearly 40 percent less for the same services as patients who have insurance coverage. What can Marissa say to the physicians about this practice?

   _____

   _____

   _____

   _____

2. Susan Doerr, RMA (AMT), is working in the billing office in a small family practice clinic. The physicians are considering the pros and cons of taking credit card payments in the clinic and have asked Susan to research the options available and give a report of her findings to the physicians at the weekly staff meeting. What can Susan tell the physicians about taking credit card payments?

   _____

   _____

   _____

   _____

3. Christopher Hernandez, CMA (AAMA), is working at the front desk of a gastroenterology practice. The office has been having difficulty with patients' personal checks being returned from the bank for nonsufficient funds. What might Christopher suggest to the office manager to help alleviate this problem?

   _____

   _____

   _____

4. Dr. Roger Dominguez operates a single-physician practice. Dr. Dominguez employs one medical assistant, Garrick Sinclair, CMA (AAMA). The clinic has been using a manual accounting system for many years and Dr. Dominguez has asked Garrick to research the pros and cons of moving to a computerized system as opposed to keeping the manual system. What might Garrick list as pros and cons for using a manual system vs. a computerized system?

_____

_____

_____

_____

5. Margaret Larson, RMA (AMT), is working in the billing office in a family practice clinic. The clinic uses a superbill for physicians to indicate the charges assigned to each patient on each patient visit. The superbill used by this clinic was designed nearly 5 years ago and contains several codes that are no longer used by the clinic. Also, there are several codes the physicians use that are not on the printed superbill, causing the physicians to handwrite these codes when used. What might Margaret suggest the facility do to solve this problem and make the superbill more accurate for use in this office?

_____

_____

_____

_____

RESEARCH ACTIVITY

Use Internet search engines to research the following topics and write a brief description of what is found. It is important to visit reputable Web sites.

1. Using the Internet as a research source, look up three collection agencies that offer their services in your area. List the pros and cons of using these three companies.

_____

_____

_____

_____

_____

CHAPTER 21

Payroll, Accounts Payable, and Banking Procedures

CHAPTER OUTLINE

General review of the chapter:

    A. Introduction
    B. The MA's Role
    C. Processing Payroll
    D. Accounts Payable
    E. Accessing Bank Accounts via the Internet
    F. Petty Cash
    G. Reconciling Bank Statements

STUDENT STUDY GUIDE

Use the following guide to assist in your learning of the concepts from the chapter.

I. Introduction

    A. The MA's Role

    _____

    _____

    _____

    _____

    _____

    _____

II. Payroll

    A. Legality
        i. Payroll is strictly regulated by various laws.
        ii. Laws regulate the calculating of an employee's _____ and the amount of _____ to be withheld from an employee's _____ pay.

    B. Responsibilities
        i. Staying current with _____ and _____ laws for payroll taxes
        ii. Keeping _____ records of employees' hours and wages
        iii. Computing the taxes and other _____ to be taken from employees' paychecks
        iv. Documenting the wages, deductions, and _____ _____ for each employee
        v. Preparing and distributing _____ to employees
        vi. Calculating office payroll taxes and depositing the funds
        vii. Preparing quarterly payroll reports

      viii. Maintaining and updating employee _____ as necessary.

      ix. Each employee, upon hiring, must fill out a/an _____ form indicating any withholding taken from the employee's earnings each payroll cycle.

      x. Employees are generally responsible for keeping track of their hours worked.

C. Calculating Payroll

    i. To calculate an hourly employee's wages:

      (a) The total number of hours worked is _____ by the employee's

           _____ _____.

      (b) Any overtime hours are paid at _____ times the regular hourly rate.

    ii. The gross earnings of a/an _____ employee do not change within a 40 hour a week pay period.

      (a) Any hours worked over 40 hours per week are generally paid _____.

D. Manual Payroll Processing

    i. The _____ is an IRS publication used to manually process payroll.

    ii. The _____ is updated annually and states the amount of federal tax that is to be withheld from each employee's earnings.

    iii. To process payroll manually, the medical assistant must have:

_____

_____

_____

_____

_____

_____

    iv. Processing payroll manually requires close attention to detail.

E. Computerized Payroll Processing

    i. Computerized payroll systems run much smoother.

    ii. Computerized payroll requires the office to set up each new employee.

    iii. It is much easier to enter employee hours and calculate employee withholding.

    iv. Payroll _____ _____ can also print checks for employees and run scheduled reports.

III. Accounts Payable

A. Overview

    i. Accounts payable is responsible for paying the _____ required to operate the medical office.

    ii. Examples of bills paid by accounts payable include:

_____

_____

_____

_____

    iii. Review bills for _____ prior to making a payment.

    iv. Keep adequate records of all checks being sent out.

B. Writing a Check

    i. It is necessary to use a checkbook _____ to keep accurate account of all checks written.

    ii. Checkbook registers can be kept _____ or be _____.

    iii. The register should include columns that indicate the type of expenditure.

      (a) This will help offices keep track of payments.

iv. To write a payroll check, complete the following steps.

_____

_____

_____

_____

_____

C. Expenses
  i. Expenses are paid in either _____ or _____ installments.
  ii. Single installment accounts could include supplies that are paid after receiving an invoice.
    (a) Often suppliers will offer a/an _____ if invoices are paid in full within a certain date of receiving the invoice.
  iii. Accounts that are paid monthly could include:

_____

_____

IV. Banking Procedures

A. Deposit Slips
  i. Deposit slips are created at the end of each day in the medical office.
  ii. Monies included in the deposit slip include:

_____

_____

_____

_____

  iii. Payments for deposit are made in the form of cash, check, or _____ _____.
  iv. All daily collections indicated from the pegboard or computer must match the day's deposit amount.
    (a) This must be done prior to completing the deposit slip.
  v. If these numbers do not match, it is necessary to find and correct the error.
B. Petty Cash
  i. Petty cash is a small amount of cash that is kept on hand in the medical office used to purchase spur of the moment items.
    (a) Example: Replacing out-of-stock office supplies and buying postage
  ii. When petty cash is used, the _____ should be placed in the envelope replacing the money taken out.
C. Reconciling a Bank Statement
  i. When reconciling a bank statement, the deposits and _____ _____ appearing on the statement must correlate to the checkbook register.
  ii. Any _____ _____ must be added to the end-of-the month balance listed on the register.
  iii. Outstanding checks should be _____ from this amount.
  iv. The adjusted reconciled bank statement amount should then match the final balance found in the _____ _____.

KEY TERMINOLOGY REVIEW

Match the selected key terms with their appropriate definitions.

a. auditors

b. Circular E

c. deductions

d. endorsement stamp

e. Fair Labor Standards Act (FLSA)

f. Federal Insurance Contributions Act (FICA)

g. Federal Unemployment Tax Act (FUTA)

h. garnish

i. gross pay

j. net pay

k. outsource

l. payroll

m. Social Security Act

n. W-2 form

o. W-4 form

_____ 1. Number of allowances to be withheld from wages.

_____ 2. Law passed by U.S. Congress in 1938 to address employment issues like federal minimum wage.

_____ 3. Amount earned before taxes or deductions are subtracted.

_____ 4. Law passed by the U.S. Congress in 1935 to provide workers and their families financial security post-retirement.

_____ 5. Those who review personal or corporate bank or tax records on behalf of an agency such as the Internal Revenue Service (IRS).

_____ 6. Law that addresses Social Security withholding taxes.

_____ 7. Amount remaining after deductions and taxes are subtracted.

_____ 8. Law that addresses federal unemployment tax withholding.

_____ 9. U.S. federal form that annually documents the wages employees drew the previous year.

_____ 10. Rubber tool that imprints a receiving agency's banking information.

_____ 11. Yearly booklet published by the IRS that outlines the federal tax deductions to be taken from individuals' wages depending on marital status and number of exemptions.

_____ 12. To send to another business for completion.

_____ 13. Process of calculating the amounts employees receive for their work.

_____ 14. To withhold wages from an employee's paycheck due to a court order.

_____ 15. U.S. federal form that indicates employees' marital status and federal tax exemptions.

APPLIED PRACTICE

Complete the activities and answer the questions that follow.

Scenario

Daniel Evans, CMA (AAMA), works as the administrative medical assistant for Happy Valley Medical Center. Handling payroll, accounts payable, and banking procedures are part of his work responsibilities. It is Thursday, and he must perform these duties.

1. Daniel must calculate the gross earnings for the two clinical medical assistants who work in the back office. The office pays its employees every week, for the previous week's work. For every hour over 40 hours worked, employees get paid time and a half. Last week, Shelby Coleman worked 43.5 hours. She earns $13.00 per hour. Chantal Jefferson worked 45 hours last week. Chantal earns $13.75 per hour.

   a. What are Shelby's gross earnings?

   _____

   b. What are Chantal's gross earnings?

   _____

2. Daniel has received an invoice from a vendor that supplied the physician with new business cards. The invoice reads:

SELECT STATIONERY UNLIMITED			
Bill to: Happy Valley Medical Center 1129 Felicity Road Springfield, PA 00010 Account #: 288901HVMC		Remit Payment to: Select Stationery Unlimited PO Box 588 New York, NY 11110	
Item Number	Description	Price	Total
0123	250 Business Cards	32.99	32.99
		Tax (0.05%)	1.65
		Shipping and Handling	4.95
		Total	$39.59

   a. Complete the check (Figure 21-1) below according to how Daniel should pay this bill.

Happy Valley Medical Center	13003
1129 Felicity Road	Date_____ 20____
Springfield, PA 00010	

   Pay to the order of: _____ [   ]

   _____

   _____ dollars

   MEMO: _____   _____

   Figure 21-1

LEARNING ACTIVITY: MULTIPLE CHOICE

Circle the correct answer to each of the questions below.

1. Which of the following would be considered deductions on an employee's payroll?

   a. federal tax withholding
   b. vacation pay
   c. overtime pay
   d. all of the above

2. Quarterly tax reports are computed how often?

   a. once per month
   b. every 3 months
   c. every 6 months
   d. once per year

3. Which of the following items might be found in an employee's personnel file?

   a. a copy of the employee's driver's license
   b. a copy of the employee's employment application
   c. a copy of the employee's resume
   d. all of the above

4. How often should an employee's personnel file be updated?

   a. monthly
   b. yearly
   c. as necessary when information changes
   d. at each employee evaluation

5. Which pieces of information from the employee's personnel file must be kept confidential?

   a. the employee's Social Security number
   b. the employee's home phone number
   c. the employee's rate of pay
   d. all of the above

6. Which IRS form is used to indicate the employee's withholding allowance?

   a. the W-4 form
   b. the W-2 form
   c. the W-3 form
   d. the quarterly form

7. How often should employees update their W-4 form?

   a. yearly
   b. every 5 years
   c. every 10 years
   d. whenever withholding information changes

8. How much is typically paid to employees for overtime wages?

   a. twice the employee's normal rate of pay
   b. 1.5 times the employee's normal rate of pay
   c. three times the employee's normal rate of pay
   d. none of the above

9. The _____ IRS form is used to calculate the correct amount of federal withholding tax for an employee.

a. quarterly report

b. W-2 form

c. Circular E

d. none of the above

10. FICA withholding is _____ percent of the employee's gross wage.

a. 7

b. 6.2

c. 7.2

d. 6

CRITICAL THINKING

Answer the following questions to the best of your ability. Use the textbook as a reference.

1. Ronnie Nguyen, CMA (AAMA), is the office manager for Dr. Hyun Kim. Ronnie has been handling the office payroll with a manual system for several years. Dr. Kim has asked Ronnie to research the possibility of buying software for the payroll function. Dr. Kim wants Ronnie to provide her with a list of pros and cons for manual and computerized systems for the payroll function. What should Ronnie include?

_____

_____

_____

_____

2. As part of an assignment for an administrative medical assisting course, Jordyn Hughes has been asked to write an essay describing the history of payroll in the United States. What should Jordyn include in her essay?

_____

_____

_____

_____

3. Francie Crook, RMA (AMT), has been newly hired to work in a busy family practice clinic. When Francie looks at her first paycheck, she notices tax has been taken out for something called FICA. She asks her office manager to explain what this tax is. How might the office manager explain this tax to Francie?

_____

_____

_____

_____

_____

4. Linnea Wagner is taking an administrative course as part of her medical assistant training. She has been asked to write an essay explaining how an injured worker's medical bills would be taken care of. What might Linnea include in her paper?

_____

_____

_____

_____

5. Mark Jameelah is taking a course in payroll processing. He has been asked to write a short essay explaining the difference between gross pay and net pay. What might Mark write?

_____

_____

_____

_____

RESEARCH ACTIVITY

Use Internet search engines to research the following topics and write a brief description of what is found. It is important to visit reputable Web sites.

1. Using the Internet as a research source, look up three different software programs that can perform the payroll function. Create a list of the pros and cons of these three programs as well as manual vs. computerized payroll systems.

_____

_____

_____

_____

_____

_____

_____

_____

_____

CHAPTER 22
Managing the Medical Office

CHAPTER OUTLINE

General review of the chapter:

    A. The MA's Role in Managing the Medical Office
    B. Characteristics of the Medical Office Manager
    C. Leadership Styles
    D. Conducting Effective Staff Meetings
    E. Staffing the Medical Office
    F. Sexual Harassment in the Medical Office
    G. Employment Resources
    H. Providing Employee References
    I. Improving Quality and Managing Risk in the Medical Office

STUDENT STUDY GUIDE

Use the following guide to assist in your learning of the concepts from the chapter.

I. The Medical Office Manager

    A. The Medical Assistant's Responsibilities
        i. Medical assistants may become medical office managers.
        ii. Managers must possess excellent _____ skills.
        iii. Those from either a/an _____ or _____ background may be eligible to be an office manager.

    B. An Effective Office Manager
        i. A successful medical office relies on the _____ and _____ of a strong office manager(s).
        ii. Office managers oversee and facilitate all office activities.
        iii. Effective office managers lead by _____ and encourage others to work at their highest _____.
        iv. Office managers should be able to _____ and display _____.

        v. Additional traits for an effective office manager include:

        _____

        _____

        _____

        _____

        _____

        _____

C. Management Styles
   i. Office managers tailor management styles to meet the needs of the medical office as well as their own personal traits.
   ii. _____ _____ leader makes all decisions without seeking input; best for emergencies when orders must be given quickly and followed exactly.
   iii. _____ _____ leader tends to ask for opinions and/or advice before making decisions, may seek consensus or retail sole decisionmaking authority.
   iv. _____ - _____ _____ leader tends to allow others to make their own decisions, becoming involved only when _____ needed.

II. Duties of a Medical Office Manager

  A. Staff Meetings
   i. Staff meetings keep the lines of communication open between _____ and _____.
   ii. Staff meetings should be held_____ of regular business hours.
   iii. All employees should be _____ for additional time during attendance of a meeting.
   iv. The staff meeting is generally led by a/an _____ _____ or a physician.
   v. To conduct a staff meeting:
    (a) Start the meeting _____ _____.
    (b) Note staff in _____ and staff who are absent.
    (c) Discuss the agenda items one at a time, being mindful of the time.
    (d) When nonagenda items arise, determine if they should be included in this meeting or moved to the next.
    (e) Address any _____ or _____ that arise.
    (f) End the meeting at the _____ time.
   vi. Agendas for staff meetings
    (a) Staff should receive an agenda of the meeting _____ to the start of the meeting.
    (b) The agenda will _____ topics of _____.
    (c) Meeting start and end times should be listed on the agenda.

  B. Job Descriptions
   i. A job description should be written for every staff member of the medical office with outlined _____ and _____.
   ii. The following information should be included in a job description:

_____

_____

_____

_____

_____

_____

_____

_____

_____

_____

_____

C. Job Advertisement
  i. Job placement ads
    (a) Effective job placement ads should include:

    _____

    _____

    _____

    _____

  ii. Medical offices may choose to advertise for staff at:

    _____

    _____

    _____

    _____

D. Interviews
  i. Effective interviews
    (a) A/an _____ list of questions should be used for _____
        candidate.
    (b) Additional questions can be tailored to fit prospective candidates.
    (c) Notes on each candidate should be taken during the interview including:

    _____

    _____

    _____

    _____

  ii. Interview questions

    _____

    _____

    _____

    _____

    _____

    _____

    _____

    _____

E. Employment References
  i. The office manager should obtain _____ to obtain reference information.
  ii. Previous employment information is usually provided on a/an _____ or an
      application.
  iii. _____ from a prospective employee to provide such information may be a
      signal of potential _____.
  iv. A prospective employee may not want a reference call made to his or her current employer.

    _____

    _____

  v. When reference calls are made, it is beneficial to use _____ -
      _____ questions.
  vi. Descriptions of the person's work _____ are commonly discussed.

F. Effective Office Management
    i. Office managers must determine the best supervisory approach to each area of the office.
    ii. Office managers must also ensure that all new staff members have been trained according to office policy.
    iii. _____ staff members usually assist in the training of new staff.
    iv. Office managers must make sure that the new employee is aware of his or her expectations.

G. Scheduling
    i. Adequately staffed schedules ensure that _____ and _____ needs are being met.
    ii. Managers should follow a fair _____ policy.
    iii. A time-off request should be submitted in _____ to the office manager at least _____ _____ prior to the requested dates off.

III. Evaluations, Policies and Patient Safety

A. Employee Evaluations
    i. Employee evaluations:

_____

_____

_____

_____

_____

    ii. Employees should be given a/an _____ _____ form prior to the evaluation.
    iii. The office manager should provide a/an _____ copy of his or her evaluation to the employee.
    iv. Both the office manager and the employee should sign the evaluation.
    v. Evaluations usually include:

_____

_____

_____

_____

_____

    vi. Target dates for improvement in specific categories may be made to overcome issues.
    vii. Employee evaluations should be conducted in _____ settings away from other _____ _____.

B. Office Policies
    i. Office employment policies are generally listed in a/an _____ _____ which is generally given to an employee on the _____ day of work.
    ii. Some policies listed in the handbook are related to employee _____ and _____.

     iii. _____ and poor job performance are examples of issues that may be grounds for discipline.

     iv. Policies vary from office to office.

     v. Most offices will provide _____ and _____ warnings prior to suspensions or termination.

     vi. Serious implications such as breach of _____ _____ may be handled in a more aggressive manner.

     vii. The use of _____ _____ may be grounds for immediate termination.

C. Sexual Harassment

     i. Sexual harassment is _____ in all workplaces.

     ii. If an employee feels that he or she is being sexually harassed, he or she must bring the situation to the attention of the _____.

     iii. Office managers presented with a sexual harassment allegation against a staff member must immediately _____ the claim.

     iv. If the office manager fails to do so, the employee may sue the medical office for allowing a/an _____ work _____ to continue.

     v. The conduct that is considered harassment must be clearly unwelcome by the accuser.

     vi. It may include:

_____

_____

_____

_____

_____

_____

_____

_____

_____

_____

_____

D. Employee Assistance Programs

     i. Common in large _____ _____ and _____

     ii. These programs assist employees going through personal _____.

     iii. Available resources should be outlined in office _____.

     iv. _____ _____ should have this list readily available as an added reference.

     v. Employee referrals for assistance programs appear in personnel files and must be kept _____.

E. Employee References

     i. Strict and consistent policies must be followed when providing references for _____ _____.

     ii. Office managers must provide references for all previous employees.

     iii. Only _____ relating to their employment should be discussed.

     iv. Opinions or _____ are not acceptable.

     v. Information provided during an employee reference includes:

_____

_____

_____

_____

    vi. _____ positive or negative employee references could be grounds for legal action.

  F. Teamwork and Patient Safety

    i. Working as a team is important when working with patients in the medical office.

    ii. With teamwork, issues are resolved more easily and quickly.

  G. Quality Improvement

    i. Quality improvement programs increase the _____ and _____ well-being of patients.

    ii. The office manager should be made aware of issues of concern regarding the patient's safety or satisfaction.

    iii. Often these issues are the basis for quality improvement programs.

    iv. Examples of these issues include:

_____

_____

_____

_____

_____

_____

  H. Improving Patient Safety

    i. If a medical assistant notices a potential _____ _____ to a patient, he or she should address the issue with the appropriate person.

    ii. Medical assistants must voice their _____ when patient safety issues arise.

    iii. Patient safety is the responsibility of _____ _____ of the health care team.

    iv. Patients who trust their health care providers can be a tremendous asset.

    v. Medical assistants should always:

      (a) Pay close attention to the patient's body language

      (b) Listen closely to their questions

      (c) Talk with the patient's family when communication is misunderstood or foreign language is a barrier

KEY TERMINOLOGY REVIEW

Write a sentence using the chosen key terms within their correct context.

1. Adverse outcome:

_____

_____

2. Agenda:

_____

_____

3. Delegate:

_____

_____

4. Employment assistance programs:

_____

_____

5. Sentinel event:

_____

_____

APPLIED PRACTICE

Read the scenario below and answer the questions that follow.

Scenario

Pretend that you are a medical office manager for a busy ob/gyn office and need to hire an administrative medical assistant to perform patient scheduling, answer telephones, patient check-out, light filing, and billing procedures.

1. Write an effective job advertisement for this position.

_____

_____

_____

_____

_____

_____

2. List three places within your city where you could place this advertisement.

_____

_____

_____

3. Make a list of five questions you would ask during the interview.

_____

_____

_____

_____

_____

LEARNING ACTIVITY: TRUE/FALSE

Indicate whether the statement is true (T) or false (F).

_____ 1. The medical office manager should be able to adopt different leadership styles depending upon the situation.

_____ 2. Staff meetings should always be lead by the physician.

_____ 3. The job description may be used to evaluate current employees' performance.

_____ 4. Job descriptions will vary from one office to another.

_____ 5. Medical offices may recruit employees by posting openings with medical assisting programs local to their area.

_____ 6. Resumes with poor grammar or typographical errors may be discarded by office managers.

_____ 7. When interviewing potential employees the office manager should change the interview questions to best suit the needs of the candidate.

_____ 8. The office manager should take notes when interviewing potential employees.

_____ 9. The Equal Employment Opportunity Commission enforces the laws against discriminating in hiring practices.

_____ 10. When an employer calls the office for a reference on a former employee, the office manager can decide what information to release on a case by case basis.

CRITICAL THINKING

Answer the following questions to the best of your ability. Use the textbook as a reference.

1. Shannon Nelson, RMA (AMT), is working as the office manager in a walk-in clinic. Shannon is alerted to a patient in the reception room who is angry about the wait time he has experienced during his visit today. How should Shannon handle this situation?

_____

_____

_____

_____

2. Walter Nichols is taking an administrative medical assisting class. He has been given an assignment to create a list of skills an effective office manager should have. What might Walter include in his list?

_____

_____

_____

_____

3. Gina Hagen, CMA (AAMA), has been asked to create an office policy for how the weekly staff meetings should be conducted. What might Gina include?

_____

_____

_____

_____

_____

4. Bobbie Kilpatrick, RMA (AMT), has been newly hired to work in a small general practice office. On her first day, Bobbie finds out that the office holds staff meetings twice weekly during the lunch hour. Bobbie's coworkers tell her that lunch is not provided and the time spent at the staff meetings is not compensated. The general feeling from the office staff is one of dislike of these meetings. How might this office change the employees' attitude toward the staff meetings?

_____

_____

_____

_____

_____

5. At the weekly staff meeting, several items that were not on the agenda have been brought up. Julie, the office manager, wants to end the meeting on time. What can she do about the unexpected items that are brought up?

_____

_____

_____

_____

_____

RESEARCH ACTIVITY

Use Internet search engines to research the following topics and write a brief description of what is found. It is important to visit reputable Web sites.

1. Using the Internet and local newspaper as a resource, look for the current job listings for medical assistants in your area. Create a list of these jobs, including any required qualifications.

_____

_____

_____

_____

_____

CHAPTER 23

The Clinical Environment and Safety in the Medical Office

CHAPTER OUTLINE

General review of the chapter:

    A. The Medical Assistant's Role in Office Safety
    B. Personal Safety Measures
    C. General Office Safety
    D. Emergency Plans
    E. OSHA Bloodborne Pathogen Standards
    F. Exposure Control Plan
        i. Standard precautions
        ii. Control practices
        iii. PPE
        iv. Hepatitis B vaccinations
        v. Training and record keeping
        vi. Exposure, post-exposure evaluation, and followup

STUDENT STUDY GUIDE

Use the following guide to assist in your learning of the concepts from the chapter.

  I. The MA Role in Office Safety

    A. Medical assistants must have knowledge regarding medical office safety procedures.
    B. _____ conditions must be reported _____ and safety measures followed.
    C. Personal safety requires:
        i. Avoiding loose or baggy clothing
        ii. _____
        iii. _____
        iv. Wearing long hair back in a tie
        v. _____

  II. Safety in the Office

    A. Body Mechanics and Lifting:
        i. Check for the _____ of an object before lifting.
        ii. Make sure the floor is _____ and dry where you're going to lift boxes.
        iii. Move feet apart to _____ _____ and put one foot slightly forward.
        iv. Tighten stomach muscles and keep back straight.
        v. Lift the objects with your _____ versus _____ muscles.

B. Patient and Employee Safety in the Medical Office:

_____

_____

_____

_____

_____

_____

_____

_____

_____

_____

C. Examination Room Safety:
   i. Keeping all medications locked in cabinets
   ii. Disposing of expired medications by flushing them or returning to manufacturer
   iii. _____
   iv. Securing equipment at the proper wall height
   v. _____
   vi. _____
   vii. _____

D. Emergency Plans:
   i. Fire safety:

_____

_____

_____

_____

   ii. Electrical safety:

_____

_____

_____

_____

   iii. Natural disasters:

_____

_____

_____

_____

   iv. Violence:

_____

_____

_____

_____

v. Workplace security:

_____

_____

_____

_____

_____

E. _____ reports are filed when there is a/an _____ in the office.

    i. Examples include:

_____

_____

_____

III. Bloodborne Pathogen Standards

  A. Every medical office must adhere to standards:

_____

_____

_____

_____

_____

_____

_____

_____

_____

  B. Medical offices must have written exposure control plans that cover:

    i. _____

    ii. _____

    iii. Decontamination

    iv. _____

    v. Post-exposure evaluation and followup

  C. HBV and HIV:

_____

_____

_____

_____

  D. The CDC:

    i. Recommend that employees be tested for _____

    ii. The _____ _____ test is most common for screening.

    iii. The CDC also recommends health care facilities have a TB exposure plan in place.

    iv. Guidelines will vary from state to state regarding _____ _____ _____ and guidelines.

E. Exposure Control Plans:

_____

_____

_____

_____

_____

F. Employees are categorized according to likelihood of exposure.

IV. Standard Precautions
    A. Standard precautions include:
        i. Infection control guidelines developed by the _____.
          (a) All _____ _____ and body fluids are considered
          _____.
    B. PPE includes:
        i. _____
        ii. _____
        iii. _____
        iv. _____
        v. Employers must provide this at no cost to the employee.
    C. _____ and _____ staff must have _____
    training.
        i. Entitled to same vaccination protection, PPE, and standards of the facility
    D. Hepatitis B vaccinations
        i. Must be offered within _____ days of _____ employment.
        ii. Vaccine must be _____ to the employee.
        iii. Employees can accept or decline.
    E. Hazardous Waste:

_____

_____

_____

_____

_____

V. Exposure Training
    A. Employers must provide training on risk of exposure within _____ days of hire and annually.
    B. Records must be kept for _____ years.
        i. Confidential records for at-risk medical office employees are kept for _____ years after employment.
    C. Procedures must exist for exposure incidents and post-exposure treatments.
    D. Post-exposure evaluation should include:
        i. _____
        ii. _____
        iii. _____

VI. Engineering Controls
    A. Engineering controls are devices that isolate or remove health hazards.
    B. President Clinton signed the _____ _____ and Prevention Act in _____.

C. Includes the use of:

_____

_____

_____

D. Equipment contaminated with _____ and _____ fluids must be _____ before it is cleaned.

KEY TERMINOLOGY REVIEW

Write a sentence using the vocabulary term in the correct context.

1. Decontamination:

_____

_____

2. Pathogen:

_____

_____

APPLIED PRACTICE

Follow the directions as instructed with each question below.

1. Categorize each medical office employee based on the level of occupational exposure to blood and other potentially infectious materials.

        a. Ongoing occupational risk
        b. Accidental or potential risk
        c. No exposure risk

_____ 1. Medical Records Technician
_____ 2. Physician
_____ 3. Janitor
_____ 4. Medical office accountant
_____ 5. Clinical medical assistant
_____ 6. Laundry service technician
_____ 7. Phlebotomist

LEARNING ACTIVITY: FILL IN THE BLANK

Using words from the list below, fill in the blanks to complete the following statements.

accidents	classifications	evaluation and treatment
all patients	DEA	filed
banned	employees	fire departments
chance of exposure	evacuation	hand washing

HIV or HBV   Ongoing Occupational Exposure   review committee
incident   Risk   safety
law enforcement   physician   spread
meeting place   prescription pad   telephone
mercury thermometers   reduce   unusual occurrences
no charge   relay services

1. Frequent _____ is one of the best ways to _____ the _____ of infection.

2. Post-exposure medical _____ is/are provided by the employer. There is _____ to the employee.

3. Incident reports are used to document _____ or _____ in the medical office.

4. Telecommunications _____ service to the general public must also provide_____, such as TTY.

5. Many facilities are removing _____ from use and some communities have _____ them completely.

6. An employee with _____ should not perform patient care until given advice from a _____ and a medical _____.

7. If a/an _____ is required of the office and/or building, assist _____ to your assigned _____.

8. Local _____ generally train _____ regarding fire_____ in the office.

9. If a/an _____ is missing, a/an _____ report should be _____, and _____ and/or the _____ should be notified.

10. In the exposure control plan, there are _____ for employees relating to their _____ to blood or OPIM. A medical assistant or other clinical/lab person is at the classification of _____.

CRITICAL THINKING

Answer the following questions to the best of your ability. Use the textbook as a reference.

1. What is the main premise of Standard and Universal Precautions and Body Substance Isolation? What impact on patient discrimination do you think this has had?

_____

_____

_____

_____

2. If you were confronted in the office with an angry patient who is threatening you, you should try to alert another staff member to call the police. What would you do if you were not able to alert someone or if you were alone?

_____

_____

_____

_____

3. Imagine you are working in the lab doing weekly cleaning tasks at the end of the day. When you reach under the sink to get bleach to mix a 10:1 cleaning solution, the lid to the bottle is loose and some of the bleach splashes in your face and eyes. What would you do *first* according to OSHA's guidelines?

_____

_____

_____

_____

4. You have a reaction to the powdered gloves at your new job, and your hands are quite itchy from the powder. You ask the office manager to purchase a few boxes of powder-free gloves because of your sensitivity, and the manager says, "No, the doctors want powder and we always buy all of the same kind. If you need a special kind, you will need to purchase them yourself and bring them in to work."

   a. Is it right for your employer to refuse the PPE that you need?

_____

_____

_____

_____

   b. What would you do or say to support your right by OSHA to have PPE provided at no cost to you?

_____

_____

_____

_____

5. In your clinic, one of the laundry receptacles has a biohazard label and another is for regular laundry without visible blood or body fluids. Your manager tells you that the laundry services will be a day late due to snow, and asks you to take home the regular laundry to do and bring back tomorrow. Would you do this? Explain why or why not.

_____

_____

_____

_____

RESEARCH ACTIVITY

Use Internet search engines to research the following topics and write a brief description of what is found. It is important to visit reputable Web sites.

1. Research the Web site for the Occupational Safety and Health Administration, www.osha.gov.

    What information can be found for health care facilities?
    List some facts found within the Web site:

    _____

    _____

    _____

    _____

    _____

    _____

    _____

    _____

    _____

    _____

    _____

    _____

    _____

    _____

    _____

    _____

    _____

    _____

    _____

    _____

    _____

    _____

    _____

    _____

    _____

    _____

CHAPTER 24

The Clinical Visit: Office Preparation and the Patient Encounter

CHAPTER OUTLINE

General review of the chapter:

A. Introduction
B. The MA's Role in the Clinical Visit
C. The Standard Medical Office
D. Preparing and Maintaining the Examination and Treatment Areas
E. Triage
    a. Critically Ill or Severely Injured Patients
F. Consent
G. Charting Medical History and the Clinical Visit
    a. Completing a Patient History
    b. Charting a Clinical Visit
    c. Charting Procedures

STUDENT STUDY GUIDE

Use the following guide to assist in your learning of the concepts from the chapter.

I. Introduction
    A. The MA's Role in the Clinical Visit
        i. The MA must ensure that examination and treatment areas are _____ and _____.

        ii. Administrative duties relating to the clinical visit include:

_____

_____

_____

_____

        iii. Clinical duties relating to the clinical visit include:

_____

_____

_____

_____

B. Examination Room Items
   i. Equipped with standard setup

   _____

   _____

   _____

   _____

   ii. Stocked with standard medical equipment

   _____

   _____

   _____

   _____

   iii. MAs should make sure equipment is in good _____ _____.
C. Maintaining the Exam Room
   i. The MA is responsible for:
      (a) Cleaning and setting up the _____ _____.
      (b) Checking and stocking _____.
      (c) Clean room according to office protocol:
         (1) After _____ _____, the exam room should be cleaned and the examination table paper changed.
      (d) _____ and _____ disposing of all waste.

II. Triage

A. Triage in the Medical Office
   i. Triaging determines the _____ for the treatment for patients on the _____ and in the _____.
   ii. Review medical offices policy and procedure on triage.
   iii. Call EMS if a patient has _____ _____ or difficulty _____.

B. Emergencies Requiring Immediate Assessment or Intervention

   _____

   _____

   _____

   _____

   _____

   _____

   _____

   _____

   _____

   _____

   _____

C. Common Sense
   i. Use common sense when triaging patients
   ii. Put patients in an exam room when:

   _____

   _____

   _____

   _____

III. Consent
    A. Implied Consent
        i. Medical offices rely on implied consent for _____ _____
           and treatment.
          (a) Implied consent for examination and treatment is given when the
              _____ _____ to the office for a routine visit.
    B. The Physician-Patient Contract
        i. Includes:

_____

_____

_____

_____

        ii. Patients have the right to:

_____

_____

_____

_____

    C. Signed Consent
        i. Signed consent forms are _____ _____ documents.
          (a) They state a patient is giving permission for certain procedures to be performed.
        ii. A signed consent form must include:

_____

_____

_____

_____

    D. Consent to Release Information
        i. This form must be signed by a patient before the provider can apply for
          _____ - _____ _____.
        ii. These forms should contain:

_____

_____

_____

_____

IV. The Clinical Visit
    A. Initial Assessment
        i. The medical assistant will review the patient's health history, including information
          based on:
          (a) Personal history

_____

_____

_____

_____

_____

_____

(b) Previous medical history

_____

_____

_____

_____

_____

(c) Family medical history

_____

_____

_____

_____

_____

(d) Chief complaint (CC)

_____

_____

_____

_____

_____

(e) Present illness

_____

_____

_____

_____

_____

B. Guidelines for Charting the Clinical Visit
    i.   After selecting the correct patient chart, verify the patient's _____ and
         _____ of _____.
    ii. Using _____ or _____ ink, write or print legibly.
         _____ ink is used for marking patient allergies.
    iii. Make sure the patient's name appears on each page.
    iv. _____ and _____ each entry, writing brief but
         complete notes.
    v.   Use only accepted medical abbreviations and make sure all medical terms are spelled
         correctly.
    vi. _____ erase or white out mistakes.
    vii. Document phone conversations and _____ _____.
C. Charting Methods
    i.   Common charting methods include:
         (a) _____ charting entries

(b) Problem-oriented medical records, also termed POMR.
    (1) When using the POMR method, entries are made using the _____, _____, _____, and _____ format (SOAP).

D. Charting a Clinical Procedure
  i. Medical assistants will chart many procedures performed on the patient.
    (a) A physician may _____ _____ or operative procedures.
  ii. Legally speaking:
    (a) A procedure that was not _____ in the medical chart was not completed.
    (b) Charting prior to a procedure is _____.
  iii. When documenting a procedure include:
    (a) The patient's vital signs:

    _____

    _____

    (b) _____ assessment
    (c) _____ administration
    (d) Specimen collection and laboratory tests
    (e) _____ and _____ testing

KEY TERMINOLOGY REVIEW

Match the selected key terms to their definitions below.

a.	charting	**g.**	sign
b.	diagnosis	**h.**	sphygmomanometer
c.	informed consent	**i.**	stethoscope
d.	ophthalmoscope	**j.**	symptom
e.	otoscope	**k.**	thermometer
f.	prognosis	**l.**	triage

_____ 1. Instrument used to examine the eyes.

_____ 2. Documentation of all the events of a patient's visit.

_____ 3. That which can be seen, heard, measured, or felt by the examiner.

_____ 4. A perceptible change in the body related by the patient.

_____ 5. Prioritizing patient needs by assessing symptoms, situations, and external factors and arranging patients according to most immediate need.

_____ 6. Instrument used to examine the eyes.

_____ 7. Instrument used to measure blood pressure.

_____ 8. Instrument used to measure body temperature.

_____ 9. Conclusion made about the patient's condition by interpretation of data.

_____ 10. Instrument used to listen to sounds within the body.

_____ 11. An outcome prediction for the course of a disease and patient recovery.

_____ 12. Consent given by a patient after all potential treatments and outcomes have been discussed for a specific medical condition, including risks and possible negative outcomes.

APPLIED PRACTICE

Answer the questions that follow each scenario.

Scenario

Medical assistant, Diego Ramirez is working with a new patient. Below is a list of statements made by the patient while Diego reviewed the patient history form.

Using the following abbreviations, identify the section in which each statement would be applicable on the patient history form.

SH	Social History
OH	Occupational History
PH	Personal History
PMH	Previous Medical History
FMH	Family Medical History
CC	Chief Complaint
PI	Present Illness

_____ 1. My father died of a massive heart attack at age 63.

_____ 2. I have been in a monogamous relationship for the past 5 years.

_____ 3. I served in the armed forces for 6 years.

_____ 4. I have been having headaches that seem to be getting worse every day.

_____ 5. I had my appendix removed when I was 21 years old.

_____ 6. I live alone in my apartment.

_____ 7. I exercise about four times a week.

_____ 8. I am allergic to codeine.

_____ 9. My sister has high blood pressure.

_____ 10. My mother's dad died of an aortic aneurysm when he was 59.

_____ 11. I do not always wear my seat belt.

_____ 12. I am a history teacher.

_____ 13. I had whooping cough and chicken pox when I was a child.

_____ 14. I have been having the headaches for the past 2 weeks and my vision seems to be blurry.

_____ 15. I drink about seven alcoholic drinks a month.

LEARNING ACTIVITY: FILL IN THE BLANK

Using words from the list below, fill in the blanks to complete the following statements. Note: Some words may be used in more than one statement.

all personnel
assume
before
best decisions
care or treatment
common sense
complications
condition or disease
cyanosis
diagnosis
diagnostic
electrocardiogram
epistaxis
eructation

imaging
incomplete possible
incontinence
informed
jaundice
label
laryngitis
legal
liability
medical record
otoscope
outcomes
patient teaching
phone calls

policies
predict
prognosis
pull-out
respiratory
risks
severe
sphygmomanometer
staff member
stethoscope
stirrups
syncope
that is to be done
thermometer

1. The conclusion about a patient's condition is a/an _____, which the physician determines after an exam, diagnostics, reports and the patient's history. The physician can anticipate or _____ the outcome of a/an _____ and the patient's recovery, which is called the _____.

2. Occasionally, equipment may malfunction in the office. It is vital that the MA or any _____ should not forget, ignore, or _____ someone else will take care of the problem. In a court of law, the _____ would be more _____ if it is found that staff knew about it and did not take steps to _____ or get it repaired.

3. A/an _____ is used to measure the patient's temperature. A/an _____ is used to listen to internal body sounds. An exam table with _____ and a/an _____ footrest is best. A/an _____ is an instrument to examine ears. To measure blood pressure, a/an _____ is used.

4. Diagnostic reports that would be filed in the medical record include a/an _____ and other cardiology reports, _____ therapy reports, _____ reports and other radiology reports, and any additional _____ procedure reports.

5. If a procedure is not charted in the _____, it would be considered _____ by the _____ system.

6. In your textbook, Table 24-3: Common Signs and Symptoms Related by and Observed in Patients, provides medical terms to use for brief statements of the signs and symptoms. Provide the medical term for the definitions that follow:

   belching _____

   yellow color to skin and white parts of the eyes _____

   bluish tint to the skin _____

   inability to hold urine _____

   fainting _____

   nosebleed _____

   loss of voice, hoarseness with little volume _____

7. In the _____ all employees should chart information when providing
_____, _____ or _____, among other
interactions with the patient.

8. In triage, a good guideline in general is _____. Of course, the policy of the individual workplace is to be followed and _____ _____ must be familiar
with these _____ whether they have direct patient care or not.

9. _____ consent must contain four items of information that must be conveyed to
the patient so he or she can make the _____ based on all aspects of the treatment,
surgery, or procedure _____ giving their consent to it. Those four items are the
procedure _____, the expected _____, the _____ and
_____ involved.

CRITICAL THINKING

Answer the following questions to the best of your ability. Use the textbook as a reference.

1. If a patient does not speak English very well, how will you ensure that the medical information you
collect for the patient history form is accurate?

_____

_____

_____

_____

2. A patient walks into the clinic and is having life-threatening symptoms; however, the doctor is not
present in the clinic. The office manager and the RN clinical manager are out to lunch for another
20 minutes, and you are alone covering the phones during this time period. What should you do?
List three or four tasks that would be vital.

_____

_____

_____

_____

3. A patient is in the exam room and you are taking vital signs prior to the physician's examination. As
you are taking the blood pressure, you look up at the patient and notice that she is trying to say
something but appears to be unable to speak normally and that one side of her face seems to be
drooping where it wasn't prior to the start of the vital signs. What is your first thought on what the
problem could be? What actions would you take?

_____

_____

_____

_____

_____

4. Consider that the occupational history of the patient is one of the parts of a patient history. Although not stated in detail in the book, why do you think a patient's past occupation(s) would be important in a medical history? List two examples of occupations that do have an effect on a person's medical state.

_____

_____

_____

_____

5. You are a new graduate on your first job as a medical assistant. You are in with the physician, a patient, and his wife. The patient was seen for upper abdominal pain, and the physician has diagnosed gallstones. The doctor proposes the removal of the gallbladder. The doctor explains the procedure, why it is needed, and then explains the risks of the surgery. The patient and his wife look at each other and say nothing, but then whisper to each other a little. The patient shakes his head yes and signs the informed consent form. The doctor signs and asks you to sign as a witness. You feel that the patient was not given all the required information for informed consent but are not confident about how to handle this: Should you tell the physician in front of the patient? Sign the form and then tell the doctor later that you did not feel comfortable signing it and why? Ask another staff member for advice on how to handle it? Refuse to sign it? There are many options. Consider all options you can think of and choose what you feel is best; write an explanation of how you would handle this.

_____

_____

_____

_____

_____

RESEARCH ACTIVITY

Use Internet search engines to research the following topics and write a brief description of what is found. It is important to visit reputable Web sites.

1. Search the Internet for medical malpractice issues regarding a lack of informed consent. Choose one of the issues found and write a two-paragraph summary of the malpractice case. Be sure to include the Web site information where the topic was found.

_____

_____

_____

_____

_____

_____

_____

_____

_____

CHAPTER 25
Medical Asepsis

CHAPTER OUTLINE

General review of the chapter:

    A. The Medical Assistant's Role in Medical Asepsis
    B. The Cycle of Infection
    C. Natural Defenses Against Infection
        i. The Integumentary System
       ii. The Immune System
      iii. Other Natural Defenses
    D. Asepsis and Infection Control
        i. Occupational Safety and Health Administration (OSHA)
       ii. Centers for Disease Control and Prevention (CDC)
    E. Infection Control Precautions
    F. Infectious Diseases
    G. Hand Washing, Nonsterile Gloving
        i. Latex Allergy

STUDENT STUDY GUIDE

Use the following guide to assist in your learning of the concepts from the chapter.

  I. The MA's Role in Medical Asepsis
    A. Medical settings harbor infectious microorganisms:

_____

_____

_____

_____

    B. _____ for infection prevention established by _____ agencies:
        i. The CDC
       ii. OSHA
    C. The MA must learn and practice Universal Precautions:

_____

_____

_____

_____

_____

  II. Microorganisms and Cycle of Infection
    A. Microorganisms:

_____

_____

B. Pathogens:

_____

_____

_____

C. _____ are _____ microorganisms.

D. _____ circulate in the blood stream.

E. The Infection Cycle:

    i. _____

    ii. _____

    iii. _____

    iv. _____

    v. _____

F. The body's natural defense against infection:

_____

_____

_____

_____

_____

G. Layers of the skin:

    i. _____: outer protective layer made up of five stratified layers of epithelial cells

    ii. _____: middle layer containing hair follicles, nerve endings, connective tissues, sweat and oil glands

    iii. _____: deepest layer containing fat, blood, lymph vessels and other connective tissue

III. Types of Immunity

A. Two Types of Immunity:

    i. Cell-mediated:

_____

_____

    ii. Humoral:

_____

_____

B. Active Immunity:

_____

_____

C. Passive Immunity:

_____

_____

D. Healthy Lifestyle Aids Immune System:

_____

_____

_____

_____

_____

_____

_____

_____

E. Natural Defense Mechanisms:

_____

_____

_____

_____

_____

_____

_____

_____

_____

_____

_____

_____

_____

IV. Asepsis

A. _____ or _____ controlled environment

B. Medical asepsis (_____) reduces number of pathogens.

C. Universal Precautions are practiced.

D. _____ _____is most important prevention

E. OSHA:

_____

_____

_____

_____

_____

_____

F. The CDC:

_____

_____

_____

_____

_____

G. Universal Precautions:

_____

_____

_____

_____

_____

_____

_____
_____
_____
_____
_____
_____
_____
_____

H. Body substance isolation was developed in _____.
   i. More extensive and inclusive than _____

I. Nosocomial infection:
_____
_____
_____

J. Personal Protective Equipment Examples:
_____
_____
_____
_____
_____
_____

V. Infectious Diseases
  A. Hepatitis:
     i. Caused by _____ of the _____
    ii. Type and state of health will determine a patient's severity of symptoms
  B. Types of hepatitis include:
     i. Hep A (HAV): _____ and _____ routes
    ii. _____: percutaneous and permucosal contact, blood, IV drug use, sexual contact
   iii. Hep C (HCV): percutaneous and permucosal contact, blood, IV drug use
    iv. _____: percutaneous and permucosal contact, blood, IV drug use
     v. Hep E (HEV): _____ and _____ routes
  C. HIV/AIDS:
_____
_____
_____
_____
_____
_____
_____
_____
_____

D. HIV/AIDS Diagnosis and Treatment:

_____

_____

_____

_____

_____

_____

_____

_____

_____

E. Caring for the HIV/AIDS patient:

_____

_____

_____

_____

_____

_____

_____

_____

_____

_____

_____

_____

_____

_____

VI. Hand Washing and Gloving
   A. Hand Washing:

   _____

   _____

   _____

   _____

   B. Key Points to Hand Washing:
      i. Use warm_____.
      ii. Keep _____ _____.
      iii. _____
      iv. Lotion should be used to prevent drying and cracking.
      v. Avoid _____ _____ unless it can be rinsed and placed on a
         _____ tray.

C. When to Wash Your Hands:

_____

_____

_____

_____

_____

_____

_____

_____

_____

_____

D. Nonsterile Gloves:
   i.   Barrier device that prevents the _____ of disease
   ii. Hands sweat, providing a perfect environment for _____ growth.
   iii. Wash hands _____ and _____ using gloves.
   iv. Never use gloves more than once.
E. Latex Glove Allergies

_____

_____

_____

_____

_____

_____

_____

_____

_____

_____

KEY TERMINOLOGY REVIEW

Use terminology words throughout the chapter to correctly complete the sentences below.

1. The hair _____ is located in middle layer of the skin.

2. In normal circumstances, urine is _____ or free from microorganisms.

3. Some microorganisms are _____ and thrive without oxygen.

4. The _____ system is the first line of defense against infection.

5. Markus had a scratchy throat three-days before developing a fever. The three-day period is considered _____.

6. _____ _____ is also known as the clean technique.

7. While hospitalized, Howard developed a staph infection after his open-heart surgery. This infection is known as _____.

8. When the body is in a state of optimal functioning, it is considered to be in a state of _____.

9. A person who is able to carry and transmit a specific disease is known as a/an _____.

10. Harmless microorganisms are also called _____.

11. In 1992, _____ _____ _____ was developed and regards all body substances as infectious materials.

12. The CDC developed this in 1985 _____ _____.

13. A/an _____ develops after a pathogenic microorganism invades the body.

14. _____ occurs when leukocytes surround and destroy pathogens.

15. Acidic pH serves as a/an _____ agent, killing bacteria within the gastrointestinal track.

APPLIED PRACTICE

Follow the directions as instructed with each question below.

1. Identify the links of the cycle of infection, as well as the incubation and prodromal periods.

Scenario

Shandra Grahm, CMA (AAMA), did not know that she was infected with the flu virus when she went to work at Peachtree Medical Center. She forgot to wash her hands after she had coughed just prior to rooming her patient, Adam Kenney. While she was checking Mr. Kenney's blood pressure, Shandra sneezed and, unfortunately, was unable to cover her mouth.

Two days later, Mr. Kenney developed some muscle aches which he had attributed to his exercise regimen. By day five, post his office visit, Mr. Kenney had a high fever, chills, and intense muscular aches.

a. Who, in this scenario, represents the reservoir host within the cycle of infection?

_____

b. What is the means of exit of the infectious pathogen?

_____

c. What is the means of transmission of the pathogen?

_____

d. Who is the susceptible host?

_____

e. What is the incubation period for the reservoir host?

_____

f. What is the prodromal period for the person who became infected?

_____

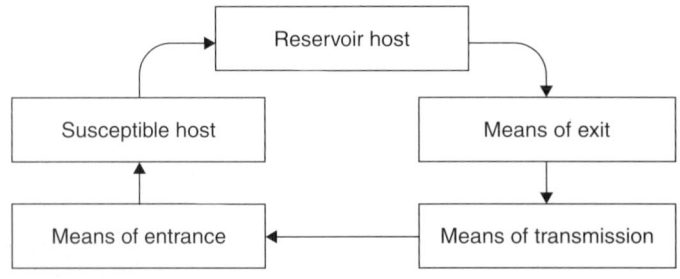

FIGURE 25-1 Five links in the cycle of infection

LEARNING ACTIVITY: MULTIPLE CHOICE

Circle the correct answer to each of the questions below.

1. Since _____, the United States has been screening all blood transfusions for HIV antibodies.

   a. 1980
   b. 1990
   c. 1978
   d. 1985

2. The primary stage of HIV infection may last a few weeks and cause _____ symptoms.

   a. opportunistic
   b. flulike
   c. Kaposi's sarcoma
   d. no symptoms in primary stage

3. The greatest number of microorganisms on the hands are found (circle all that apply):

   a. under the nails
   b. around the nails
   c. in the creases of the palms
   d. in rings

4. The deepest layer of the skin is the

   a. epidermis
   b. subcutaneous
   c. stratum corneum
   d. statum granulosum

5. The purpose of medical asepsis is to (circle all that apply):

   a. protect the healthcare worker from infections
   b. maintain a clean environment
   c. teach only handwashing
   d. prevent the transmission of disease

6. The CDC (circle all that apply):

   a. works to protect the public health and safety
   b. is a state agency of the United States Department of Health and Human Services
   c. provides immunization services and health information
   d. had the original name of Communicable Disease Center

7. A 10:1 solution is one part of 10% sodium hypochlorite mixed with nine parts of water. The sodium hypochlorite is actually

   a. alcohol
   b. salt with chloride
   c. household bleach
   d. none of the above

8. The personal protective equipment you will wear for various tasks is determined by

   a. actual or anticipated exposure to microorganisms
   b. actual or anticipated exposure to blood and body fluids and OPIM
   c. actual or anticipated exposure to nosocomial infections
   d. actual or anticipated exposure to hepatitis B or HIV/AIDS

9. Some states are now requiring _____ to have the series of three HBV immunizations before _____.

   a. men and women, getting married
   b. women, getting pregnant
   c. all healthcare workers, doing direct patient care
   d. children, kindergarden

10. HIV can be passed from the infected patient only by contact with their blood or body fluids. It is only when their infected blood or body fluids _____ of someone else that the recipient is infected.

    a. get into the mucous membranes of the genitals

    b. get into the bloodstream

    c. get under the skin where they can be absorbed and get into the blood

    d. get absorbed into tissue and eventually the whole system

CRITICAL THINKING

Answer the following questions to the best of your ability. Use the textbook as a reference.

1. Although not specifically stated in this chapter, explain why hands cannot be sterilized even though we wash them with soap and water. If sterilization is not something you have learned yet, consider what you already know or think about surgery (from TV or personal experience) and offer your best idea.

   _____

   _____

   _____

   _____

2. In the case study at the beginning of this chapter, list each thing in the last paragraph that Gloria did wrong (that could spread infection).

   _____

   _____

   _____

   _____

3. Since OSHA monitors and regulates workplaces for safety and health of the workers, many businesses see OSHA as an unfair regulatory agency. Some labor groups feel that OSHA doesn't do enough. What is your opinion on this? Is the role of OSHA good, bad, could be improved, not necessary, too regulating? Recall the things that you have already learned that OSHA requires. Consider the amount of work and money that many of the requirements would involve for an employer, both big and small. Explain your opinion.

   _____

   _____

   _____

   _____

4. A new couple has unprotected sex and then wonders if one of them could have contracted HIV from the other. They go together to a clinic to be tested and both get negative results. However, they still cannot be sure that the initial test proves that they are HIV free. Explain why one HIV test cannot definitely tell the presence of HIV.

   _____

   _____

5. After reading the section Caring for the HIV/AIDS Patient in this chapter, carefully reread the longest paragraph, which deals with instructing the significant other or family on the more personal aspects of care. There are many more nonmedical things the patient must deal with that a caregiver can help with, such as lack of money because he or she can't work, bills that may be unpaid, driving to appointments and the store, etc. Choose three aspects of the personal effects on the patient and offer at least two things each that a caregiver could help with.

RESEARCH ACTIVITY

Use Internet search engines to research the following topics and write a brief description of what is found. It is important to visit reputable Web sites.

1. Research the Web site for the Centers for Disease Control and Prevention, www.cdc.gov/niosh.

   What does NIOSH stand for?

   List some topics discussed within the NIOSH Web site specifically for health care workers:

CHAPTER 26
Surgical Asepsis

CHAPTER OUTLINE

General review of the chapter:

    A. The Medical Assistant's Role in Surgical Asepsis
    B. Surgical Asepsis
    C. Sanitization, Disinfection, and Sterilization
    D. Wrapping Instruments and Preparing Sterile Trays
    E. Preparing the Surgical Field

STUDENT STUDY GUIDE

Use the following guide to assist in your learning of the concepts from the chapter.

I. The MA's Role in Surgical Asepsis

    A. The MA must know what areas are to remain _____ as well as _____ areas during ambulatory surgery or an invasive procedure.
    B. The MA remains in a/an _____, able to:
        i. Obtain supplies
        ii. Open sterile packages while maintaining a sterile field
        iii. Place sterile contents onto a sterile field by dropping or using sterile transfer forceps
        iv. Prepare specimens for laboratory testing.
    C. What is surgical asepsis?

    _____

    _____

    _____

    _____

    _____

    _____

    _____

    _____

II. Sanitization, Disinfection, and Sterilization

    A. Decontamination consists of three processes:
        i. _____ bacterial growth or inactivates pathogens: does not _____
        ii. Disinfection _____ or inhibits pathogenic microorganisms:

           _____

        iii. _____ destroys all living forms of microorganisms, including _____.
    B. Sanitization
        i. Treatment rooms and equipment must be disinfected and sanitized.

ii. This can be done in one of two ways:

_____

_____

_____

_____

_____

iii. Manual sanitization

_____

_____

_____

_____

_____

_____

C. Ultrasonic Sanitization
   i. Considered _____ because instruments are _____

     _____.

   ii. Certain _____ may not be _____ in the same load.

  iii. Instruments are not allowed to _____.

  iv. This may cause this form of sanitization to take longer.

   v. Make sure all _____are covered in _____

     _____.

D. Disinfection
   i. _____

   ii. _____

  iii. _____

  iv. Levels and types of disinfectants:

_____

_____

_____

_____

_____

_____

_____

_____

_____

_____

E. Disinfectant Procedure

_____

_____

_____

_____

_____

_____

F. Sterilization

   i. Forms of sterilization

_____

_____

_____

_____

_____

_____

   ii. The autoclave

_____

_____

_____

_____

_____

_____

_____

_____

_____

_____

G. Other Methods of Sterilization

   i. _____

   ii. _____

   iii. _____

   iv. _____

H. Autoclaving Procedures

_____

_____

_____

_____

_____

_____

_____

_____

I. Wrapping Instruments
    i. Instruments can be wrapped in a variety of items.
      (a) _____
    ii. Sterilization _____ are placed in the _____.
    iii. Specific _____ is necessary to maintain _____after _____ is complete.

III. The Surgical Field
  A. The Surgical Field

_____

_____

_____

_____

_____

_____

  B. Guidelines for a Sterile Field
    i. Never _____ over a sterile field.
    ii. Sterile areas should be set up away from areas with potential _____.
    iii. Never _____ over a sterile field.
    iv. _____ areas on the sterile field lead to _____.
    v. Movement around the sterile field should be _____ and _____.
    vi. Place all items toward the _____ of the sterile field.
  C. Alcohol-Based Hand Rub
    i. CDC issued _____ for use of alcohol-based hand rubs in lieu of _____ _____ are as follows:
      (a) Remove _____, _____, and bracelets prior to beginning a surgical scrub.
      (b) Remove debris from underneath_____.
      (c) Prewash hands and forearms with a/an _____-_____ soap and dry completely.
      (d) Apply alcohol-based product in the palm of one hand and rub hands together, covering all _____.

KEY TERMINOLOGY REVIEW

Match the correct medical term with the definition listed below.

    a. autoclave
    b. debris
    c. emesis
    d. endoscope
    e. Mayo stand

    f. noncritical
    g. spore
    h. sterile field
    i. sterilization indicator
    j. ultrasonic cleaning

_____ 1. An instrument used to view the internal aspect of the GI tract.

_____ 2. A protective shell formed by some bacteria.

_____ 3. Considered to be safer than manual sanitization.

_____ 4. Extraneous material that interferes with proper functioning or cleaning of supplies or equipment.

_____ 5. Items that do not touch the patient or only intact skin.

_____ 6. This provides verification of an autoclave's effectiveness.

_____ 7. A two-compartment device that utilizes steam and pressure to sterilize items.

_____ 8. A microorganism-free environment used during procedures.

_____ 9. A moveable table used for the placement of supplies and instruments.

_____ 10. Vomit.

APPLIED PRACTICE

Follow the directions as instructed with each question below.

1. Arrange the following steps in order to reflect the process of sanitization, disinfection, and sterilization of instruments. Read through all the steps carefully. When you find what you think is the first step, write its corresponding letter in the space provided for Step 1. Continue this process until you have the final step assigned.

   a. Completely immerse instruments in a container of disinfectant, cover, and let soak for the recommended length of time.
   b. With hinges open, allow instruments to air dry on a cotton towel.
   c. Remove instruments from disinfectant, rinse thoroughly, and dry with paper towels.
   d. Place contaminated instruments in an empty basin, cover the basin, and transport to the cleaning area.
   e. Load the autoclave.
   f. Read MSDS for disinfectant and check expiration date.
   g. Place disinfected instruments in center of dry wrapping paper.
   h. Fold wrapping paper as directed and apply sterilization indicator tape.
   i. Place instruments in a neutral low-suds detergent.
   j. Remove instruments to a clean container using sterile transfer forceps.
   k. Check distilled water level in autoclave reservoir, add distilled water as necessary.
   l. Use a soft brush on all serrated and smooth edges, grooves, and open hinges, cleaning one instrument at a time.
   m. Turn on the autoclave.
   n. Apply disposable gloves and then utility gloves before handling disinfectant.

   Step 1: _____
   Step 2: _____
   Step 3: _____
   Step 4: _____
   Step 5: _____
   Step 6: _____
   Step 7: _____

Step 8: _____
Step 9: _____
Step 10: _____
Step 11: _____
Step 12: _____
Step 13: _____
Step 14: _____

LEARNING ACTIVITY: FILL IN THE BLANK

Using words from the list below, fill in the blanks to complete the following statements. **Note:** *Some terms may be used in more than one statement.*

alcohol prep	invasive	steam
aseptic	local anesthetic	sterilant
bracelets	one-inch	sterile
chamber	penetrate	sterilization
contaminated	required	surgical
disinfection	rings	time tips
distilled water	sanitization	touching
fingernails	skin	upside down
forceps	spores	watches

1. When loading packs into an autoclave correctly, steam must _____ all surfaces for the _____ and at the _____ temperature to kill all microorganisms and their_____.

2. Three ways to clean items of microorganisms are _____, _____, and _____.

3. The autoclave reservoir is filled with _____ to produce _____ for sterilization.

4. There is a/an _____ perimeter of the sterile field that is considered _____.

5. Prior to assisting with a minor surgical procedure, _____, _____, and _____ should be removed before the _____ hand scrub, and debris should be removed from underneath the _____.

6. To help reduce errors when donning or removing sterile gloves, remembering this simple saying will help: _____ to _____, _____ to _____.

7. Sterile or _____ technique is used at all times during _____ procedures and when _____ integrity is or will be broken.

8. When loading an autoclave, ask yourself some questions, one of which is: Are any of the packs _____ the inside of the autoclave _____?

9. During a surgical procedure, the doctor needs to withdraw _____ from a vial, so the MA uses a/an _____ to clean the vial top, then holds the vial _____ outside of the sterile field and with the label facing the doctor.

10. Transfer _____, when not in use to prepare a/an _____ tray, must have the _____ not the handles kept in a chemical _____.

CRITICAL THINKING

Answer the following questions to the best of your ability. Use the textbook as a reference.

1. Picture yourself in an aseptic environment wearing a surgical gown, gloves, and mask. You are assisting with a minor surgical procedure. In the middle of the procedure, you let your hands go below your waist. What should you do?

   _____

   _____

   _____

   _____

2. In the same scenario as above, you have opened a sterile package of instruments and placed them on the tray prior to the procedure, added a small cup of a solution, and draped the tray until the doctor comes in. When you remove the drape so the doctor may begin, you spill the solution on the sterile field. Since the field is sterile and the instruments are sterile, is it all right to proceed? Explain the reasoning behind your answer.

   _____

   _____

   _____

   _____

3. In the same scenario as above, following the procedure, you are cleaning up the sterile field. Two of the instruments on the tray were not used and did not touch any blood or body fluids. Do you have to sanitize and disinfect them prior to sterilizing or can you simply wrap them again? Explain your answer.

   _____

   _____

   _____

   _____

4. Read Tips for Success: Which Decontamination Steps Should You Perform? It lists certain items that vary in the way they are decontaminated. Consider the same process for these items: the exam table, a scalpel (nondisposable) to be used for the next incision and drainage procedure, a tourniquet used when drawing blood. Explain how to decontaminate each item below.

   Exam table:

   _____

   Scalpel for surgery:

   _____

   Tourniquet:

   _____

5. You are working on preparing the sterile field and go to the autoclave for the paper-wrapped packs of instruments you ran earlier that day. The tape on the outside of the packs has the darkened stripes so you know that the outside of the pack has been sterilized. The physician is behind schedule and irritated about that. There are no extra instruments for this particular procedure, which is why you planned ahead and autoclaved them beforehand. You open all the packs and transfer the contents to the sterile tray and put the sterile cover over it. As you clean up the empty paper and packages, you notice that the sterilization indicator from the inside of the packs had not changed color. What would you do—say nothing and assume that the tape on outside indicated that the entire package had been sterilized? Tell the doctor that it will take another 40 minutes to reautoclave the items and get them ready for the procedure? Say nothing because you fear the physician's anger or even losing your job?

_____

_____

_____

_____

_____

RESEARCH ACTIVITY

Use Internet search engines to research the following topics and write a brief description of what is found. It is important to visit reputable Web sites.

1. Use Internet search engines to find the prices for various disinfection and sterilization items. Include the Web site address where you find your information.

   What is the price range for autoclaves?

   What is the price range for autoclave indicator tapes or sterility check strips?

   What are the pros and cons of purchasing high-priced items, such as an autoclave, from a Web site such as www.ebay.com?

_____

_____

_____

_____

_____

_____

_____

_____

_____

_____

_____

_____

CHAPTER 27
Pharmacology and Medication Administration

CHAPTER OUTLINE

General review of the chapter:

   I. The MA's Role in Administering and Dispensing Drugs
  II. Basic Pharmacology
 III. Medication Measurement and Conversion
 IV. Safety Guidelines and the Prescription
  V. Forms and Routes of Administration

STUDENT STUDY GUIDE

Use the following guide to assist in your learning of the concepts from the chapter.

I. The MA's Role in Pharmacology and Drug Administration and Basic Pharmacology

  A. The MA's Role in Pharmacology and Drug Administration. An MA must understand:
     i. _____ legal guidelines
     ii. How to read medication orders or prescriptions
     iii. How to _____ medications under physician's order
     iv. Know and recognize side effects
     v. _____ patients about their medication
     vi. Search _____ for additional information

  B. Drug Processing
     i. Absorption

_____

_____

_____

_____

_____

_____

     ii. Distribution
       (a) Involves the _____ of the drug in the body
       (b) Cardiovascular/circulatory diseases could cause _____ changes in patients.
     iii. Metabolism and _____
       (a) Occurs in the _____
       (b) Separating unusable and useable substances from the drug
       (c) Unusable substances are excreted via _____, _____, etc.
       (d) Useable substances are circulated to obtain chemical and _____ effects.

C. Effects of Drugs on the Body
   i. _____ effect: desired effect of a drug
   ii. _____ effect: adverse reactions to medications
   iii. _____ effects: overdose, allergic reaction, interactions with other drugs
   iv. _____ effect: cannot be explained or predicted
   v. Contraindications: reasons _____ prescribing or administering a drug

D. Basic Functions of Drugs
   i. **Therapeutic:**

_____

_____

   ii. **Diagnostic:**

_____

_____

   iii. **Curative:**

_____

_____

   iv. **Replacement:**

_____

_____

   v. **Preventive or prophylactic:**

_____

_____

E. Forms of Drug Classifications
   i. Prescription medication:

_____

_____

   ii. Over-the-counter (OTC):

_____

_____

F. Drug Safety
   i. The _____ _____ regulates quality and safety of drugs.
   ii. Read all labels when taking OTC medications.
   iii. Some OTC drugs can have serious _____ with other medications.

II. Drug Nomenclature, Reference Sources, and Dosage Calculations

A. Drug Nomenclature
   i. Drugs are given three names:

_____

_____

_____

_____

_____

_____

B. Drug Reference Sources
   i. Two common sources for drug information:
     (a) *U.S.* _____ *and National* _____ (**USP-NF**)
       (1) Lists and describes all accepted therapeutic drugs and chemical name

(b) *Physician's Desk Reference*

_____
_____
_____
_____
_____

C. Drug Classifications: In the left-hand column write the drug name, and in the right-hand column write the action that it has on the body:

Drug	Action on the Body

D. The Controlled Substance Act
    i. This is enforced by the _____.
   ii. Controlled substances are also called scheduled drugs:
      (a) They include drugs with potential abuse such as narcotics, depressants, stimulants or hallucinogenics.
  iii. Records concerning the _____ and _____ of controlled substances must be kept away from patient charts.
   iv. Records must be kept for _____ _____ and always available for the DEA.
    v. Schedule drugs must be stored in a/an _____ _____ box that is securely fastened to the wall.
   vi. All scheduled drugs must be accounted for at all times.
  vii. Those drugs administered to patients must be recorded in a log:

_____

_____

E. Drug Measurement Systems and Dosages
    i. Apothecary:

_____

_____

_____

_____

   ii. Metric:

_____

_____

_____

_____

  iii. Medication-specific:
      (a) _____ for electrolytes (e.g., potassium)
      (b) Units (e.g., insulin)
      (c) _____ (Nitrobid paste)
      (d) Drops (liquid medication administered by dropper)
      (e) Percentages are used to measure mixes for _____ _____ or _____
   iv. Adult and pediatric dosages are based on various factors:
      (a) _____ in pounds or kilograms
      (b) _____
      (c) Diseased state of patient
      (d) Concentration of drug
F. Dosage Calculations
    i. Formulas are used to calculate adult and pediatric drug dosages.
   ii. One formula used is:

$$\frac{\text{Available strength}}{\text{Amount to give}} = \underline{\hspace{2cm}}$$

_____

_____

_____

_____

_____

_____

iii. Another formula is D/H × Q:

_____

_____

_____

_____

_____

_____

G. Calculating Dosages
  i. _____ or _____ _____ can be used to con-
      vert dosages.
  ii. Metric system is most commonly used.

_____

_____

  iii. MAs need to be familiar with both systems of measurement.
III. Administration Safety, Drug Classifications, Controlled Substance Act

  A. Safety Rules in Medication Administration

_____

_____

  B. Six Rights
    i. Right _____

_____

_____

    ii. Right _____

_____

_____

    iii. Right _____

_____

_____

    iv. Right _____

_____

_____

_____

    v. Right _____

_____

_____

_____

    vi. Right _____

_____

_____

_____

IV. The Prescriptions and Routes of Administration
   A. The Prescription
      i. _____ document to be written in _____.
      ii. Some states allow other professionals to fill in a blank form under doctor's order
      _____
      _____
      iii. Only a physician can sign Schedule II, III, and IV drugs.
   B. Common Parts of the Prescription
      i. Patient's name and address, and the prescription date
      ii. _____: the symbol Rx, which means "take"
      iii. _____ drug name, form, and strength
      iv. _____: directions to pharmacist for amount of drug to be dispensed
      v. Placed on label
      vi. _____ information ("REPETATUR 0 1 2 3 PRN"): refill instructions for
      the physician to circle
      vii. Physician's signature and "Dispense as written" or "Substitute Generic Medication"
   C. Safeguarding the Prescription
   _____
   _____
   _____
   _____
   _____
   _____
   _____
   _____
   _____
   _____

   D. Forms of Drug Administration
      i. Solid forms include tablets
      _____
      _____
      ii. _____ (sustained release and caplet form)
      iii. Lozenges, suppositories (vaginal, _____ or _____)
      iv. Dermatological forms (creams and ointments, transdermal patches)
      v. Liquid forms include
      _____
      _____
      vi. Injectables in powder form (mixed prior to administration) or in ready-to-use liquid form
   E. Routes of Drug Administration
      i. Oral (swallowing)
      ii. _____ (under the tongue)
      iii. Transdermal
      iv. _____ (intradermal, subcutaneous, intramuscular, and intravenous,
      _____, inhalation, irrigation, instillation, rectal, topical)
   F. Parenteral Medications
      i. Transdermal
      _____
      _____

ii. Injectable

_____

_____

iii. Amount of medication and location site will determine the size of the needle and syringe.

G. Types of Syringes

    i. _____: very small calibration marking, allows minute 0.1cc injections

      (a) Mantoux and allergy tests

    ii. Insulin syringes are calibrated in Units.

_____

_____

    iii. The 3 cc/ml syringes are used for intramuscular injections.

_____

_____

KEY TERMINOLOGY REVIEW

Complete the following sentences using the key terms found at the beginning of the chapter.

1. Lucia decided to study _____ because she is fascinated with the effects of drugs on the human body.

2. The DEA monitors the management and administration of _____ _____.

3. This is also known as the nonproprietary name, _____ _____.

4. Some analgesics are available _____ _____ _____ because a prescription is not required for purchasing them.

5. The antihistamine medication has a/an _____ _____ of drowsiness even though it isn't the purpose of the medication.

6. This name of a drug is based on its chemical composition, _____ _____.

7. Pregnancy is often a reason that a drug should not be administered; this is known as a/an_____.

8. The _____ _____ of a drug always has the first letter capitalized, as well as a registered trademark symbol.

9. A/an _____ _____ may have a potentially life-threatening effect.

10. This is synonymous with the term medication, _____.

APPLIED PRACTICE

Complete the following exercises.

Basic Math Review

Do not use a calculator.

Note: Though basic math is not covered in the textbook, it is a helpful review to prepare you for dosage calculations.

A. Addition

1. 18 + 49 = _____   2. 142 + 730 = _____   3. 1799 + 283 = _____
4. 7839 + 943 + 41 = _____   5. 28845 + 83 =____

B. Subtraction

1. 75 − 52 = _____   2. 429 − 81 = _____   3. 1648 − 379 = _____
4. 612 − 419 = _____   5. 3527 − 274 =____

C. Multiplication

1. 9 × 3 = _____   2. 32 × 5 = _____   3. 815 × 4 = _____
4. 711 × 30_____   5. 3780 × 210 = _____

D. Division

1. 150/15 = _____   2. 1152/12 = _____   3. 450/60 =_____
4. 327/6 = _____   5. 825/50 =_____

Dosage Calculations

1. The physician orders digoxin 0.125 mg to be given to a patient. On hand is a vial of digoxin marked 250 mcg/ mL. How much should the medical assistant administer?

_____
_____
_____
_____
_____

2. The physician orders 500 mg of metformin to be given to a patient. On hand is a bottle of metformin that reads 1000 mg/tablet. How much should the medical assistant administer?

_____
_____
_____
_____
_____

3. The physician orders 125 mg of a medication. On hand is a bottle of the same medication that reads 500 mg/5 mL. How much should the medical assistant administer?

_____
_____
_____
_____
_____

4. The medication that the physician ordered reads 20 mg/kg/day. Your patient weighs 220 lbs. The physician wants the patient to take the medication b.i.d. in equal doses. How much will the patient be given at each dose?

_____
_____

_____

_____

_____

_____

5. The physician orders 40 mg of furosemide to be given to a patient. On hand is a bottle of furosemide that reads 20 mg/tablet. How much should the medical assistant administer?

_____

_____

_____

_____

_____

_____

LEARNING ACTIVITY: MULTIPLE CHOICE

Circle the correct answer to each of the questions below.

1. Which of the following is not included in Schedule II drugs?
   a. marijuana
   b. morphine
   c. cocaine
   d. Dilaudid

2. An injection into the fatty tissue under the skin is a/an _____ injection.
   a. intramuscular
   b. Z-track
   c. subcutaneous
   d. intradermal

3. The medication abbreviation for twice a day is
   a. b.i.d.
   b. t.i.d.
   c. prn
   d. q2h

4. The oral route of taking/giving medication is the safest route because
   a. it can be absorbed at a slow rate so that the patient can be prepared for any ill effects
   b. most patients aren't afraid to swallow pills or liquids
   c. it can be retrieved through emesis immediately if for some reason it is determined the patient shouldn't have taken it
   d. it will dissolve or coat the stomach quickly and avoids nausea

5. If bubbles are present in the syringe when you are drawing up,
   a. it is all right and you can proceed if they are very small
   b. tap the ampule neck
   c. tap the syringe with your finger or a pen to dislodge them and push only that air back into the vial
   d. push all the med back into the vial and start again as many times as necessary until you can draw with no bubbles

6. When an injectable medication is in powder form,

   a. mix it with enough tap water to make it thin enough to be injectable

   b. mix it with sterile water to make it thin enough to be injectable

   c. mix it with the correct amount of sterile diluent as stated on the label

   d. mix it with the amount and type of diluent that the doctor specifies

7. If the doctor orders 4 mg of a certain medication, and the vial states that there are 2 mg in 1 cc, how many cc would you give to deliver 4 mg?

   a. 2 cc

   b. 4 cc

   c. 6 cc

   d. 1/2 cc

8. If the doctor orders 1 dram of medication to be given and the vial states there is 1 mg in each cc, you must

   a. give 1 cc

   b. ask the doctor how to determine the number of cc

   c. call the pharmacy first and ask

   d. convert from apothecary to metric and then calculate the dosage

9. If a medication has been given in the office but it may have possible side effects a short time following administration, you should

   a. warn the patient to watch for those effects

   b. ask the patient to wait in the waiting room for a certain period of time

   c. make sure the patient has a driver to get him or her home

   d. tell the patient what those effects could be and to call in immediately if the effects appear

10. Documenting the administration of medication must include all of the following except:

    a. the name of the medication

    b. the strength of the medication

    c. the side effects that could occur

    d. the route the medication was given

CRITICAL THINKING

Answer the following questions to the best of your ability. Use the textbook as a reference.

1. You have received a physician's order to administer 1 mg of a medication to a patient. It is a medication that is injected into the muscle. As soon as you have given the medication, you realize you measured 1 ml instead of calculating 1 mg. What would you do?

   _____

   _____

   _____

   _____

   _____

2. A patient has finished seeing the doctor and on her way out, she asks the MA for a sample of Motrin, which is an OTC medication. The MA gives her two packages but does not document this and does not ask the doctor, because the MA felt that since Motrin is an OTC medication, getting it without an order would be appropriate. Is this appropriate and if not, why?

_____

_____

_____

_____

3. A regular patient has come in wanting a new prescription for a medication she has taken for many years, because she is out of refills. The physician is not in the office today, but after checking the medical record and noting that it is the patient's usual medication, the MA calls in a new prescription to the pharmacy and makes a note to have the doctor write the order in the chart when she returns. Is this an appropriate action for the MA, since she used critical thinking to check the chart and felt sure the physician would approve it? Explain your answer.

_____

_____

_____

_____

4. Explain why IV infusion of medication is the most dangerous method to administer medication and *must* be the right med, strength, and amount. Errors with this route can cause serious problems. All routes of medication administration *must* be done accurately, but there are specific reasons why this route is more risky than the others.

_____

_____

_____

_____

5. Although a very small amount of bubbles or air injected into the muscle or the subcutaneous tissue would not be harmful, *the MA must never do it*. Explain why it is not acceptable to have even tiny bubbles within the medication inside the syringe.

_____

_____

_____

_____

_____

RESEARCH ACTIVITY

Use Internet search engines to research the following topics and write a brief description of what is found. It is important to visit reputable Web sites.

1. Visit www.rxlist.com. Navigate through the site and determine how the information on this site could best be used by patients. How could a patient benefit from this Web site?

CHAPTER 28
Vital Signs

CHAPTER OUTLINE

General review of the chapter:

   A. Introduction
   B. The Medical Assistant's Role in the Initial Clinical Visit
   C. Vital Signs
      i. Temperature
     ii. Pulse and respiration
    iii. Blood pressure
    iv. Weight and height
   D. Preparing the Patient for Physical Examination
      i. Gowning
     ii. Draping
    iii. Positioning the patient

STUDENT STUDY GUIDE

Use the following guide to assist in your learning of the concepts from the chapter.

  I. The MA's Role in the Initial Clinical Visit

    A. The MA will gather vital signs and the patient's history.
      i. The MA will observe the patient's:
        (a) Cooperation
        (b) _____ condition
        (c) Alertness
        (d) Level of _____
        (e) Presence of _____
     ii. The MA will then prepare the patient for examination by:

       _____

       _____

       _____

 II. Vital Signs

    A. Vital Signs and Overall Health
      i. Vital signs give insight to a patient's _____.
     ii. Vital signs include:

       _____

       _____

       _____

     iii. Vital signs are compared to normal ranges for diagnosis, prognosis, and course of treatment.
    B. Body Temperature
      i. Changes in _____ temperature can indicate illness.

ii. The _____ regulates heat production and loss.

iii. Glucose produces heat during the _____ process.

iv. Heat is lost through the skin by:

(a) _____

(b) _____

(c) _____

(d) _____

(e) Heat is lost through _____ and elimination of _____ and _____.

v. Methods of Obtaining Body Temperature

_____

_____

_____

_____

vi. Types of fevers

(a) _____: body temperature fairly constant and above the patient's normal baseline

(b) _____: Fluctuating body temperature remains above normal.

(c) _____: Fluctuating body temperature returns to normal, then rises again.

(d) _____: Fever returns after an interval of several days of normal temperature.

vii. Causes for lowered body temperature:

_____

_____

_____

_____

_____

_____

C. Pulse

i. As a health indicator:

(a) The pulse is a/an _____ beat of an artery caused by heart _____.

(b) It provides a picture of heart's pumping action, rate, rhythm, and volume.

(c) Normal BPM is _____ times per minute.

(d) Deviations are called _____.

(e) Refer to Table 28-3 in your textbook for average pulse rates by age.

ii. Pulse sites include:

_____

_____

_____

_____

iii. Factors affecting heart rate and rhythm:

(a) _____: Infants and children have more rapid heartbeat, elderly have slower rate.

(b) _____: Females often have a faster heartbeat than men.

(c) Exercise and physical activity increase heartbeat.

(d) _____: Larger people have faster heartbeats.

(e) _____ conditions: People who exercise vigorously have slower rate.

(f) Medications can _____ or _____ heart rate.

(g) Presence of disease or illness

(h) _____

(i) Depression

(j) _____ disease

(k) Hypothyroidism slows heart and hyperthyroidism causes rapid heartbeat.

D. Respiration
   i. As a health indicator:
     (a) Process of breathing that consists of _____ (inhaling oxygen)
     (b) _____ (exhaling carbon dioxide)
     (c) Rate, depth and rhythm are assessed for _____, further testing, or treatment.
     (d) Respiration rate is taken by _____ the number of breaths taken in one minute.
   ii. Factors that affect respiratory rate:
     (a) _____ reactions
     (b) Exercise, obstructed airway
     (c) _____, anger, pain, shock
     (d) Fever
     (e) Hemorrhage, _____, drugs
     (f) High _____, decrease or increase of _____ _____ in blood.

E. Blood Pressure
   i. As a health indicator:
     (a) Measurement of circulated _____ and _____ exerted on vessel walls by the pumping action of the heart
     (b) Pressure varies with the _____ and _____ phases of the heart.
     (c) _____ blood pressure lead to complications.
     (d) Deviations in pressure help determine a/an _____ and _____.
   ii. Measuring blood pressure
     (a) Sphygmomanometer and _____ to hear systolic and diastolic pressure
     (b) _____ _____ is the period of _____ pressure (when the heart contracts it forces blood against arterial walls).
     (c) _____ _____ is the period of lowest pressure, when the ventricles relax.
   iii. Blood pressure values:
     (a) See Tables 28-5 and 28-6
     (b) Hypertension:

_____

_____

     (c) Hypotension:

_____

_____

   iv. Korotkoff sounds
     (a) Sound of _____ walls _____ as air is removed from a BP cuff:
       (i) Phase 1:

_____

                    (ii) Phase 2: _____

_____

_____

                    (iii) Phase 3: _____

_____

_____

                    (iv) Phase 4: _____

_____

_____

                    (v) Phase 5: _____

_____

_____

_____

          v. Mensuration
               (a) The measurement of _____ and _____ is termed
                    mensuration.
               (b) Weight changes can indicate nutritional or _____ problems.
               (c) Decrease in_____ could be spinal compression.
               (d) Infants and children who fail to grow could be considered problematic.
III. Patient Preparation and Examination Techniques

     A. Patient Preparation: Gowning

_____

_____

_____

_____

     B. Patient Preparation: Draping

_____

_____

_____

_____

     C. Patient Preparation: Positioning
          i. Fowler's:

_____

_____

          ii. Supine:

_____

_____

          iii. Prone:

_____

_____

iv. Lithotomy:

_____

_____

v. Right/left lateral recumbent:

_____

_____

vi. Sims':

_____

_____

D. Examination Assessment Methods
   i. _____: visual exam of internal and external organs
   ii. _____: examination with touch of hands for size, tenderness
   iii. _____: listening to body parts for abnormalities (heart, lungs, GI tract)
   iv. _____: percussion reflex hammer, tapping fingertips on body for sound
   v. _____: measuring patient weight and height
E. Assisting with the Physical Exam
   i. MAs will help, depending on physician preference and office policy.
   ii. Assist with patient _____ and give instructions for _____ and _____
   iii. Watch for_____ pain or _____ during exam
   iv. Assist physician with equipment or specimens if collected
F. MA Duties in Recurrent Office Visits
   i. Rooming the patient in the proper exam room
   ii. Taking a brief history to include:

_____

_____

   iii. Measure

_____

_____

   iv. Update _____ _____ with _____ and findings
   v. Prepare patient for physical exam

KEY TERMINOLOGY REVIEW

Write a sentence using the selected key terms in the correct context.

1. Aural:

_____

_____

2. Auscultation:

_____

_____

3. Conduction:

_____

_____

4. Convection:

_____

_____

5. Inspection:

_____

_____

6. Mensuration:

_____

_____

7. Percussion:

_____

_____

8. Radial:

_____

_____

9. Systolic:

_____

_____

10. Turgor:

_____

_____

APPLIED PRACTICE

Follow the directions as instructed with each question below.

1. A patient who has a normal baseline temperature of 98.6 has had the following average body temperatures over the past 5 days: **Day 1: 101.2°F, Day 2: 100.1°F, Day 3: 98.6°F, Day 4: 99.0°F, Day 5: 101.3°F.** How would you describe this fever? Explain your answer.

_____

_____

2. Your patient is a 43-year-old female. Her blood pressure is 157/92. What is the patient's pulse pressure? Is the pulse pressure normal? Explain your answer.

_____

_____

_____

3. You are preparing a new patient for a physical examination. Because the patient has recently moved from a European country, he would like the medical assistant to tell him his body temperature in Celsius rather than Fahrenheit. When obtaining his temperature, the thermometer reads 99.0°F. How does this convert to Celsius? What is the conversion formula?

_____

_____

_____

_____

LEARNING ACTIVITY: FILL IN THE BLANK

Using words from the list below, fill in the blanks to complete the following statements. **Note:** *Some terms are used in more than one statement.*

assess	medical condition	respirations
auscultates	nares	rhythm
bladder	otoscope	sitting erect
bowel sounds	pelvic exams	speculum
depth	percussion	tuning fork
Fowler's	physical examination	underlying organs
hearing	pulse	volume
lightly but sharply	rate	vision
lithotomy	rectal	visual acuity

1. A/an _____ temperature is taken only when the patient's _____ dictates it.

2. The three aspects to note when taking _____ are _____, _____, and _____.

3. The three aspects to note when taking a/an _____ are _____, _____, and _____.

4. _____ refers to the physician's tapping the fingertips _____ against various areas of the body to _____ the size and location of _____.

5. The _____ position is used for _____ and pap smears.

6. Emptying the _____ makes the patient feel more comfortable during the _____.

7. The ears are examined with a/an _____, usually with a disposable _____; a larger _____ can be attached to the otoscope to examine the _____.

8. When the physician _____ the abdomen, he or she is listening to _____.

9. The _____ position is when the patient is _____ on the table.

10. The _____ is used to assess _____, and _____ is the assessment of the clarity of a patient's _____.

CRITICAL THINKING

Answer the following questions to the best of your ability. Use the textbook as a reference.

1. During a patient clinical visit, whether for a physical or other reason, the MA visually inspects the patient. Think of what may be visible about the patient that the MA may note.

_____
_____
_____
_____

2. If a patient walks in without an appointment and presents as extremely short of breath (SOB) and appears weak, do you think that you should spend the time doing weight, height, and all the vitals before alerting the doctor of the patient's immediate condition? Explain your answer.

_____
_____
_____

3. If a patient is not able to be in the knee-chest position due to a physical limitation, such as a back problem, what alternative position would work for a rectal examination?

_____
_____
_____

4. A 9-year-old child comes into the office with a temperature of 99.0° F orally, a pulse of 116, respiration of 24, and blood pressure of 112/58. Circle the vitals that are out of normal range. In those that do not have a range stated in the textbook, look on the Internet or in another textbook and list all vital normal ranges on an index card. State briefly in your own words why two people can have different vital sign measurements and still both will be considered normal.

_____
_____
_____
_____

5. You are assisting a physician with a physical exam. You have prepared all the supplies and have any equipment ready. The patient is a female and will be having a pelvic exam with the physical exam. Although the physician does not need you to assist him, you are expected to be present with the doctor anyway. State why the MA would be present in this situation. Would the same be true if the patient were a male? Would the same be true if the doctor were a female and the patient were a male?

_____
_____
_____
_____

RESEARCH ACTIVITY

Use Internet search engines to research the following topics and write a brief description of what is found. It is important to visit reputable Web sites.

1. Choose a health condition related to a vital sign (hypertension, obesity, etc.). Research informational Web sites related to your chosen condition. What type of information is included in the informational Web sites? How can this information be useful for patients?

CHAPTER 29
Minor Surgery

CHAPTER OUTLINE

General review of the chapter:

A. Introduction
B. The MA's Role in Office Surgery
C. Surgeries Performed in the Medical Office
D. Implied and Informed Consent
E. Preoperative Care and Patient Preparation
F. Assisting During Minor Surgery
G. Recovery/Postoperative Care

STUDENT STUDY GUIDE

Use the following guide to assist in your learning of the concepts from the chapter.

I. The Medical Assistant and Minor Surgery

A. The Medical Assistant's Role in Minor Surgery
    i. MAs assist physicians in various ways with minor surgery:
       (a) Obtaining _____ approval
       (b) _____ forms
       (c) Ordering supplies
       (d) Cleaning or _____ instruments
    ii. Preoperative, intraoperative, and postoperative duties

_____

_____

_____

_____

_____

_____

_____

_____

_____

_____

_____

B. The Medical "Scrub" Assistant
    i. Set up _____ field
    ii. _____ surgical scrub
    iii. Sterile gowning
    iv. Gloving or _____ the _____ with gloving
    v. Handing the instruments to the physician, draping, and cutting

C. The "Circulating" Medical Assistant
   i. Considered _____ not sterile
  ii. Obtains supplies, equipment, and sterile packs
 iii. Completes necessary _____
 iv. Identifies _____, sends to laboratory
  v. Positions patients, adjusts lights

II. Minor Surgery and Consent Forms
  A. Minor Surgery in the Medical Office
    i. Surgical procedures in the medical office often take _____ to complete.
   ii. These include:

_____

_____

_____

_____

_____

_____

_____

_____

_____

_____

  B. Informed Consent
    i. Unlike "implied consent" a patient must give "informed consent" for minor surgery.
   ii. Physician explains _____, _____, _____, and possible negative outcomes
  iii. When patient fully understands, they sign informed consent form
  C. Consent Forms
    i. Consent forms generally include:
     (a) Consent for a specific or _____ _____ during the surgery
     (b) Disclosure of potential risks
     (c) Consent to _____
     (d) Consent to dispose of tissue removed
     (e) Consent for _____ or recording of procedure
     (f) Consent for student or qualified medical professional to observe
     (g) Patient's _____, if known
     (h) Nature and purpose of the proposed treatment or procedure
     (i) _____ and _____ of the proposed treatment or procedure
     (j) Alternative treatments
     (k) Risk and benefits of the alternative treatment or procedure
     (l) Risks and benefits of _____ _____ or undergoing a treatment or procedure

III. Preparing for Minor Surgery
  A. The MA's Duties during Preoperative Care

_____

_____

_____

_____

_____

_____

B. Preparing the Room for Minor Surgery
    i. Confirm room is clean and surfaces disinfected
    ii. Wash hands before handling _____ _____
    iii. Check _____ dates on sterile packets
    iv. Sterile packets should be opened, instruments dropped on stand and covered
    v. Exam and surgical tables should have clean paper.
C. Surgical Instruments
    i. Surgical instruments are generally classified by function:
    ii. _____
    iii. _____
    iv. _____
    v. Typically made of steel, rustproof, stain-proof, heat-resistant and durable
D. The Surgical Tray

_____
_____
_____
_____

E. Clamping and Grasping Instruments
    i. Used for clamping blood vessels
    ii. Include two-pronged forceps, ring or sponge forceps, and hemostats
F. Cutting Instruments
    i. Used to _____ _____
    ii. _____ or _____ may be used.
    iii. Both may vary based on size and shape of blade.
G. Scopes, Speculums, Probes, and Trocars
    i. _____ or _____ explore the inside of the body cavity.
    ii. Probes are used to explore wounds and cavities; blunt point
    iii. Trocar: hollow _____ used to withdraw fluids
    iv. Punches are used to remove small samples of tissue.

IV. During and Post Surgery

A. Positioning and Draping
    i. Sterile drapes of _____ or paper are used to provide a sterile environment.
    ii. Fenestrated drapes:

_____
_____

    iii. MA positions patient on table and drapes the patient appropriately
    iv. Check for comfort, warmth, and dignity
B. Anesthesia
    i. Can cause a partial or complete loss of sensation
    ii. If used to alter _____, the patient is carefully monitored
    iii. A/an _____ _____ cart must be stocked and close to the surgical area.
C. Local Anesthesia
    i. Local anesthesia causes loss of sensation in a specific area.

_____
_____
_____
_____
_____

D. Assisting During Minor Surgery
    i. Provide _____ support for patients and answer questions.
    ii. Ask about _____ to _____, especially anesthesia.
    iii. Record vital signs.
    iv. Passing instruments to the physician
    v. Open _____ instrument packages.
E. Suture Materials
    i. Absorbable suture material dissolves in the body in _____ days
       (a) _____ _____ (catgut), synthetic materials like polyglycolic acid, polyglactin 910
    ii. Nonabsorbable sutures are used permanently in deep tissue and need to be removed.

    _____

    _____

F. Postoperative Care Duties
    i. Support the patient after a surgical procedure.
    ii. Clean skin, _____ _____, and dress site.
    iii. Help patient sit up or get dressed if needed.
    iv. Vital signs taken and recorded
    v. Review _____ surgical instructions with patient and _____
G. Postoperative Patient Teaching
    i. Instructions should be given orally and in written form.
    ii. Make sure patients can _____ instructions with accuracy.
    iii. Postoperative instructions include:

    _____

    _____

    iv. Chart vital signs, patient condition, understanding of instruction, method of discharge, and person accompanying patient.
H. Wounds
    i. Internal or external damage to skin
    ii. An open wound exposes the underlying tissue.

    _____

    _____

    iii. When the skin is not broken it's considered a closed wound.
       (a) Contusions or bruises
I. Stages of Wound Healing
    i. Inflammatory phase

    _____

    _____

    ii. Granulation phase

    _____

    _____

    iii. Contraction phase

    _____

    _____

J. Dressings and Bandages
    i. Provide a/an _____ _____ _____ against infection
    ii. Keep area clean and absorb drainage
    iii. Reduce discomfort by keeping area secure and prevent friction
    iv. Observations of _____, _____, _____, drainage, and healing should be charted.

KEY TERMINOLOGY REVIEW

Match the selected key terms with the definitions below.

a. abrasion	**k.** elective surgery
b. anesthesia	**l.** electrocautery
c. approximation	**m.** emergency surgery
d. avulsion	**n.** granulation
e. biopsy	**o.** hemostat
f. closed wound	**p.** incision
g. contraction	**q.** laceration
h. cutting	**r.** open wound
i. dissection	**s.** optional surgery
j. distal	**t.** punctures

_____ 1. Obtaining a representative tissue sample for microscopic examination.

_____ 2. Away from center.

_____ 3. A hole or wound made by a sharp, pointed instrument.

_____ 4. Scraping away of the surface by friction.

_____ 5. Requiring immediate medical or surgical evaluation or treatment.

_____ 6. Trauma to the underlying tissue without a break in the skin or mucous membrane or exposure of the underlying tissue.

_____ 7. Cauterization using a variety of electrical modalities to create thermal energy.

_____ 8. Break in the skin or mucous membrane that exposes underlying tissues.

_____ 9. Joining together of surgical wound edges.

_____ 10. Cutting into smaller parts for study and analysis of each part.

_____ 11. A wound or irregular tear of the flesh.

_____ 12. Using a knife or surgical scissors to separate or divide tissues.

_____ 13. Process of forcibly tearing off a part or structure of the body.

_____ 14. A treatment or surgical procedure not requiring immediate attention and therefore planned at the patient's or provider's convenience.

_____ 15. Surgery is not medically relevant; denial for surgery will have no adverse effects on the patient's health.

_____ 16. A cut made with a knife, electrosurgical unit, or laser especially for surgical purposes.

_____ 17. Process of drawing up or thickening of a muscle fiber.

_____ 18. Instrument used to stop blood flow.

_____ 19. Fleshy projections formed on the surface of gaping wound that is not healing by first intention or indirect union.

_____ 20. Partial or complete loss of sensation.

APPLIED PRACTICE

Follow the directions as instructed with each question below.

1. Label the surgical instruments on page 282 with their correct names.

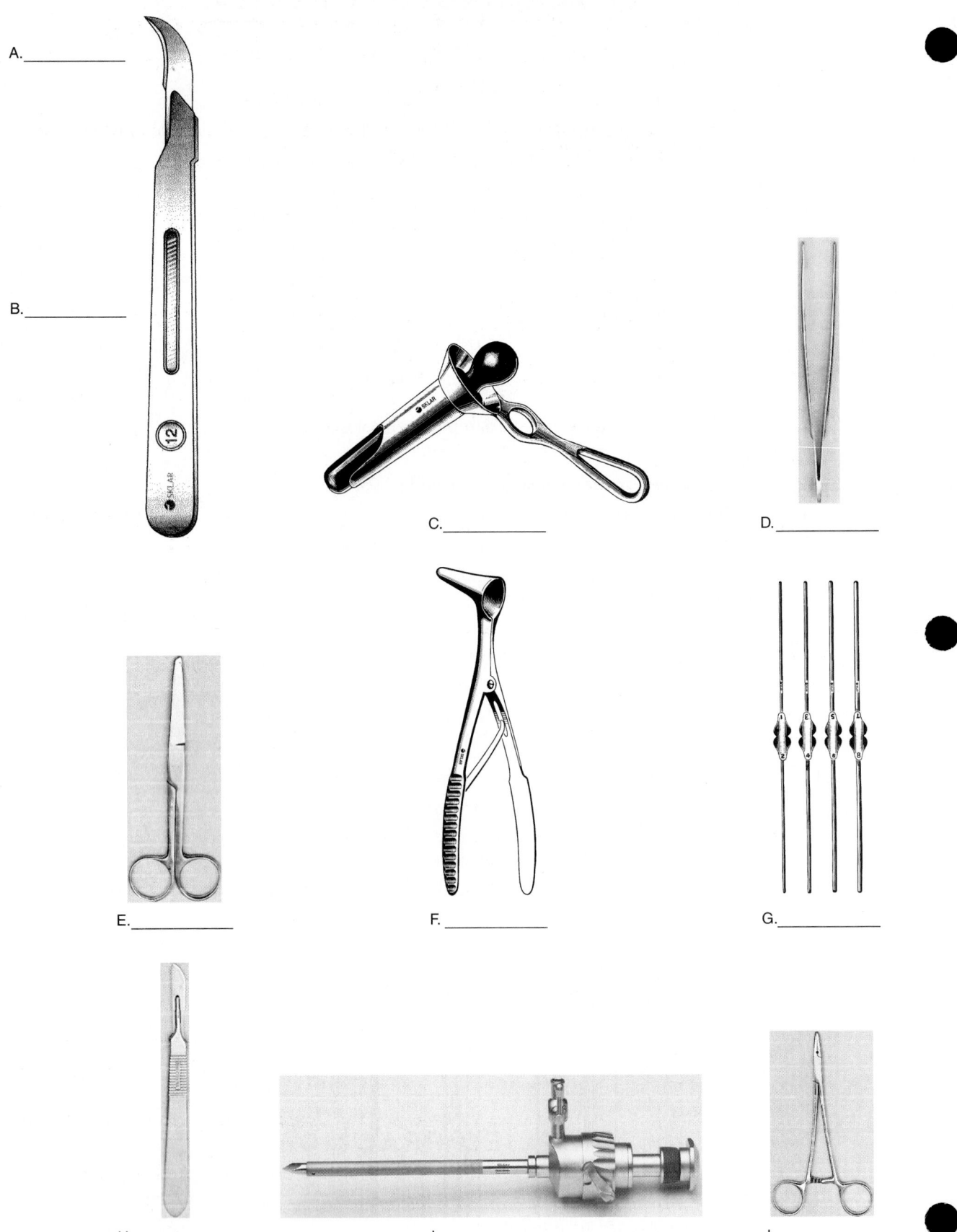

A. _____

B. _____

C. _____

D. _____

E. _____

F. _____

G. _____

H. _____

I. _____

J. _____

LEARNING ACTIVITY: MULTIPLE CHOICE

Circle the correct answer to each of the questions below.

1. Wound healing occurs in three major phases. Which of the following is the phase in which a scar begins to lighten and small blood vessels are absorbed?

   a. inflammatory
   b. granulation
   c. contraction
   d. fibroblastic

2. Which two of the following are alternatives to suture wound closures?

   a. wire staples
   b. dressing and bandage
   c. cartridge
   d. adhesive skin closure strips

3. When removing a dressing, the chapter states five main signs to assess the wound. Which one of the following is not one of those signs?

   a. color
   b. edema
   c. pain
   d. approximation

4. A fenestrated drape is one that

   a. can be connected to other drapes to cover a large area
   b. always has a plastic backing
   c. is always made of muslin
   d. none of the above

5. The textbook discusses surgical instruments in three major categories by their function. Which of the following is not one of those three categories?

   a. clamping and grasping
   b. repair and restructure
   c. dilating, probing, and visualizing
   d. cutting

6. The three basic steps of skin preparation include all of the following except:

   a. Apply antiseptic solution to the surgical area.
   b. Scrub with an antiseptic soap and rinse.
   c. Air dry the skin prior to cleansing.
   d. Shave as necessary.

7. Which of the following is not one of the indications of infection as discussed in your text?

   a. warmth
   b. odor of drainage
   c. hardness at surgical site
   d. decreased drainage

8. Sutures on the face are usually removed in

   a. 3–5 days.
   b. 1–3 days.
   c. 5–10 days.
   d. 0 days; absorbable suture is used on the face to minimize scarring.

9. The medical assistant working in the room with the physician for a minor surgical procedure could be (circle all that apply):

   a. circulating and sterile
   b. circulating and nonsterile
   c. preparatory and semisterile
   d. assisting and sterile

10. It is typically considered to be the job of the MA during a minor surgery to maintain and keep close by the (circle all that apply):

    a. drug tray

    b. emergency cart

    c. emergency lighting

    d. fire extinguisher

CRITICAL THINKING

Answer the following questions to the best of your ability. Use the textbook as a reference.

1. After rubbing the top of an anesthetic vial with alcohol, you invert the vial so that the physician may withdraw the appropriate amount of medication into the syringe. The physician accidentally touches the needle to the metal rim rather than the rubber stopper. Would the needle then be contaminated? Explain your answer.

   _____

   _____

   _____

   _____

   _____

2. In the same scenario as in question 1, you are holding the vial, and the physician accidentally sticks your finger instead of the rubber section. Are you at risk of being infected with a disease? Why or why not?

   _____

   _____

   _____

   _____

   _____

3. Patient instructions should be given both orally and in writing. Many errors can be made by the patient if instructions are not clear. Come up with a scenario of something harmful that could result if a patient did not have any written instructions and did not remember the oral instructions provided by the physician or medical assistant.

   _____

   _____

   _____

   _____

4. During a sterile cyst removal procedure, the physician reaches up to scratch her head briefly. She is wearing a surgical cap and no visible body fluids are on her gloves. Take some time and think through this scenario. Has the sterile procedure been compromised? If so, indicate your thoughts in paragraph form.

   _____

   _____

   _____

   _____

5. **Scenario:**

A patient has had general anesthesia during a minor surgical procedure today. He has been monitored appropriately during the recovery period without any indications of a problem. The patient seems to be fully awake and vitals are all normal. With some assistance, the patient does well sitting up and getting off the table. The patient seems to understand and is able to repeat post-op instructions back to you correctly. According to office policy, the patient may be discharged. However, the patient does not have a driver to take him home. You ask him if there is someone who can pick him up, and if not you would be happy to call a taxi. The patient states he is fine and can drive and insists he must get home to feed his pets. You ask him to wait a while longer but he refuses and leaves the office, insisting he is fine.

Part 1: On a separate page, chart this incident as you would in a medical record.

Note to Student: The chart note should have the date and time on the left side, followed by your note in narrative format. At the end, sign your first initial, your last name, and your title, "MA."

Part 2: Three hours later the office receives a phone call from a local hospital. The patient was just killed in a motor vehicle accident on his way home from your office. The hospital wants to know his condition when he left your office. Does your chart note cover all details that would likely relieve your office of legal liability for his death? Underline things in your chart note that would be supportive of your, the doctor's and the practice's defense.

_____

_____

_____

_____

RESEARCH ACTIVITY

Use Internet search engines to research the following topics and write a brief description of what is found. It is important to visit reputable Web sites.

1. Research one surgical procedure listed in Table 29-1 of your textbook. Why is the procedure performed? How is the procedure performed? What instruments would be required to perform this procedure?

_____

_____

_____

_____

_____

_____

_____

_____

_____

_____

_____

_____

CHAPTER 30
Diagnostic Procedures

CHAPTER OUTLINE

General review of the chapter:

    A. The Medical Assistant's Role in Diagnostic Testing
    B. Clinical Laboratory Improvement Amendments (CLIA)
    C. Regulations and Laboratory Safety
       i. Joint Commission on the Accreditation of Healthcare Organizations
      ii. Safe Medical Devices Act
    D. Hospital Laboratory Setting
    E. The Physician Office Laboratory
    F. Ordering Diagnostic Tests

STUDENT STUDY GUIDE

Use the following guide to assist in your learning of the concepts from the chapter.

  I. The MA's Role in Diagnostic Procedures

    A. Schedule tests
    B. Maintain _____ or _____ of results
    C. Record or log calibrations
    D. Assist with _____ records
    E. Obtain _____
    F. Following state regulations and under supervision MAs can:

    _____

    _____

    _____

    _____

    _____

    _____

    G. When using diagnostic equipment:

    _____

    _____

    _____

    _____

    _____

    _____

  II. Clinical Laboratory Improvement Amendments (CLIA)

    A. Passed by U.S. Congress in _____ to establish _____ standards for all _____ testing
    B. Ensures accuracy, reliability, and timeliness of patient test results

C. Health and Human Services requires any lab that examines "…materials derived from the human body fluids for diagnosis, prevention, or treatment…" to be certified.

D. CLIA Requirements
   i. _____
   ii. _____
   iii. _____
   iv. _____

E. Types of CLIA Tests
   i. _____
   ii. _____
   iii. _____

F. Waived Tests
_____
_____
_____
_____
_____
_____
_____
_____

G. PPMP Tests
_____
_____
_____
_____
_____
_____
_____
_____

H. Moderate Complexity Tests
_____
_____
_____
_____
_____
_____
_____
_____

I. High-Complexity Tests
_____
_____
_____

_____
_____
_____
_____
_____

J. Quality Control and Quality Assurance

_____
_____
_____
_____
_____
_____
_____
_____

K. Quality Control for Testing:
  i. Checking _____ on supplies and _____ reagents
  ii. _____ and performing _____ checks on equipment
  iii. Maintaining and documenting maintenance on equipment
  iv. Running and documenting _____ of each test for consistency

III. Regulations and Laboratory Safety

  A. _____: monitors the safety, medical relevance and clinical performance of equipment

  B. _____: enforces legal and proper disposal of hazardous chemical and biological materials

  C. _____: monitors health care workers and patients with use of personal protective equipment, training, and maintenance of chemicals used in medical setting

  D. General Safety Guidelines

_____
_____
_____
_____
_____
_____
_____
_____
_____
_____

  E. JCAHO

_____
_____
_____
_____
_____

F. Safe Medical Devices Act

_____

_____

_____

_____

_____

_____

_____

_____

_____

_____

IV. The Hospital Laboratory Setting
  A. A hospital laboratory is divided into areas based on the type of work they perform:

  _____

  _____

  _____

  B. Clinical tests require automated procedures that provide improved quality assurance.
  C. Diagnostic Laboratory Testing
    i. Blood tests check:

    _____

    _____

    _____

    ii. Hematology studies include:

    _____

    _____

    _____

    iii. Microbiology identifies microorganisms in blood, urine, stool, throat, or other body fluids.
    iv. Sensitivity to antibiotics is determined by a culture and sensitivity (C&S).

    _____

    _____

    _____

    v. Blood serum studies determine antigen-antibody reaction.
    vi. Serology tests check for disease associated with immune disorders.

    _____

    _____

    _____

    vii. Cytology testing analyzes cells from the body to determine abnormalities.
V. The POL and Ordering of Diagnostic Tests
  A. The Physician's Office Laboratory:
    i. MAs are trained _____, on the job, and by _____ to use equipment.
    ii. Safety and CLIA guidelines must be followed.
    iii. Equipment includes centrifuges, microscopes, autoclaves, and electronic equipment:

    _____

    _____

_____

_____

_____

_____

B. The Physician's Order for Tests
    i. Verbal or written request given to MA for _____ and _____
   ii. Preprinted forms or requisitions used with:

_____

_____

_____

_____

_____

_____

_____

_____

C. Precertification

_____

_____

_____

_____

_____

_____

_____

_____

_____

_____

D. MAs coordinate and schedule outside testing.

_____

_____

_____

_____

_____

_____

_____

_____

_____

_____

E. Screening and Test Followup
     i. Reference labs return results to medical offices.
    ii. Medical assistants _____ with normative values.
   iii. _____ are flagged for physician review.
   iv. All action, intervention, or _____ is charted.
    v. Verify with physician before _ever_ giving test results to patients

KEY TERMINOLOGY REVIEW

Write a sentence using the vocabulary terms in the correct context.

1. Centrifuge:

   _____

   _____

2. Glucometer:

   _____

   _____

3. Hematocrit:

   _____

   _____

4. Hemoglobin:

   _____

   _____

5. Photometer:

   _____

   _____

APPLIED PRACTICE

Follow the directions as instructed with each question below.

1. Using the information in the following scenario, correctly fill out the laboratory requisition on the following page.

Scenario

Dr. Mark Jefferson has ordered routine blood work that includes an FBS (fasting blood sugar) and a Hemoglobin, A1C. The patient chart reads:

Walters, Aiden S.
08-12-1956
03/15/20xx 10:30 am Ht: 72" Wt: 192 lbs. T: 98.4° F P: 76 bpm BP: 132/88
cc: Pt. presents to office for his 3 mo diabetic check-up. He states he has been feeling fine, and is continuing to take Glucophage 500 mg bid. Pt. states he hasn't had any food or drink since 9:00 P.M. last evening. --------------------- *Karla Mailor, RMA (AMT)*

Mr. Walters resides at 8399 West Main Street, Springfield, Pennsylvania 11110. His telephone number is 814-555-9877. His Social Security number is 123-45-6798. Dr. Jefferson would like the results faxed to 814-555-3678.

Lab Services

Patient instructions
and map on back

PHYSICIAN ORDERS

Patient _____ _____ ____ D.O.B. _____
Last Name   First   M.I.

M ☐ Patient
F ☐ SS# _____ — _____ — _____

Address _____ City _____ Zip _____ Phone # _____

Physician _____
ATTACH COPY OF INSURANCE CARD

Diagnosis/ICD-9 Code _____
(Additional codes on reverse)

Date & Time of Collection:
_____
Drawing
Facility _____

☐ 789.00 Abdominal Pain   ☐ 414.9 Coronary Artery Disease (CAD)   ☐ 244.9 Hypothyroidism
☐ 285.9 Anemia (NOS)   ☐ 250.0 DM (diabetes mellitus)   ☐ 272.4 Hyperlipidemia
                             ☐ 780.7 Fatigue/Malaise   ☐ 401.9 Hypertension
                             ☐ 272.0 Hypercholesterolemia   ☐ 483.9 URI (upper respiratory infection)

☐ ROUTINE   ☐ PHONE RESULTS TO: # _____
☐ ASAP   ☐ FAX RESULTS TO: # _____
☐ STAT   ☐ COPY TO: _____

HEMATOLOGY	CHEMISTRY	CHEMISTRY	MICROBIOLOGY

HEMATOLOGY
☐ 1021 CBC, Automated Diff (incl, Platelet Ct.)
☐ 1023 Hemoglobin/Hematocrit
☐ 1020 Hemogram
☐ 1025 Platelet Count
☐ 1150 Pro Time Diagnostic
☐ 1151 Pro Time, Therapeutic
☐ 1155 PTT
☐ 1315 Reticulocyte Count
☐ 1310 Sed Rate/ Westergren

URINE
☐ 1059 Urinalysis
☐ 1082 Urinalysis w/Culture if indicated
   Urine-24 Hr _____ Spot _____
   Ht. _____ Wt. _____
☐ 3033 Creatinine
☐ 3036 Creatinine Clearance (also requires blood)
☐ 3095 Protein
☐ 3096 Sodium/Potassium
☐ Microalbumin 24 Hr_____ Spot_____

SEROLOGY
☐ 8020 ANA (Antinuclear Antibody)
☐ 8040 Mono Spot
☐ 3494 Rheumatoid Factor
☐ 8010 RPR
☐ 5365 Rubella

CHEMISTRY
☐ 5550 Alpha Fetoprotein, Prenatal
☐ 3000 Amylase
☐ 3153 B12/Folate
☐ 3156 Beta HCG, Quantitative
☐ 3321 Bilirubin, Total
☐ 3324 Bilirubin, Total/Direct
☐ 3009 BUN
☐ 3159 CEA
☐ 3348 Cholesterol
☐ 3030 Creatinine, Serum
☐ 3509 Digoxin (recommend 12 hrs, after dose)
☐ 3515 Dilantin
☐ 3168 Ferritin
☐ 3193 FSH
☐ 3066 ▼ Glucose, Fasting
☐ 3061 Glucose, 1st Post 50 g Glucola
☐ 3075 ▼ Glucose, 2nd Post Glucola
☐ 3060 Glucose, 2nd Post Prandial (meal)
☐ 3049 ▼ Glucose Tolerance Oral GTT
☐ 3047 ▼ Glucose Tolerance Gestational GTT
☐ 3650 Hemoglobin, A1C

Additional Tests _____

CHEMISTRY
☐ 5232 HBsAg
☐ 3175 HIV (Consent required)
☐ 3581 Iron & Iron Binding Capacity
☐ 3195 LH
☐ 3590 Magnesium
☐ 3527 Phenobarbital
☐ 3095 Potassium
☐ 3689 Pregnancy Test Serum (HCG, qual)
☐ 3653 Pregnancy Test, Urine
☐ 3197 Prolactin
☐ 3199 PSA
☐ 3339 SGOT/AST
☐ 3342 SGPT/ALT
☐ 3093 Sodium/Potassium, Serum
☐ 3510 Tegretol
☐ 3551 Theophylline
☐ 3333 Uric Acid

MICROBIOLOGY
Source _____
☐ 7240 Culture, AFB
☐ 7200 Culture, Blood x _____
☐ Draw interval _____
☐ 7280 Culture, Fungus
☐ Culture, Routine
☐ 7005 Culture, Stool
☐ 7010 Culture, Throat
☐ 7000 Culture, Urine
☐ 7300 Gram Stain
☐ 7353 Occult Blood x _____
☐ 7365 Ova & Parasites x _____
☐ 7400 Smear & Suspension (includes Gram Stain/Wet Mount)
☐ 7060 Rapid Strep A Screen (____)
☐ 7065 Rapid Strep A Screen only
☐ 7030 Beta Strep Culture
☐ 5207 GC by DNA Probe
☐ 5130 Chlamydia by DNA Probe
☐ 5555 Chlamydia/GC by DNA Probe
☐ 7375 Wright Stain, Stool

PANELS & PROFILES

☐ ✗ **3309 CHEM 12**
Albumin, Alkaline Phosphatase, BUN, Calcium, Cholesterol, Glucose, LDH, Phosphorus, AST, Total Bilirubin, Total Protein, Uric Acid

☐ ▼ **3315 CHEM 20**
Chem 12, Electrolyte Panel, Creatinine, Iron, Gamma GT, ALT, Triglycerides

☐ ▼ **3357 CARDIAC RISK PANEL**
Cholesterol, HDL, LDL, Risk Factors, VLDL Triglycerides

☐ ✗ **3042 CRITICAL CARE PANEL**
BUN, Chloride, CO2, Glucose, Potassium, Sodium

☐ **3046 ELECTROLYTE PANEL**
Chloride, CO2, Potassium, Sodium

☐ ▼ **3399 EXECUTIVE PANEL**
Chem 20, Iron, Cardiac Risk Panel CBC, RPR, Thyroid Cascade

☐ **5242 HEPATITIS PANEL, ACUTE**
HAVIgMAb, HBsAg, HBsAb, HBcAb, HCVAb

☐ ▼ **3355 LIPID MONITORING PANEL**
Cholesterol, Triglycerides, HDL, LDL, VLDL, ALT, AST

☐ **3312 LIVER PANEL**
Alkaline,Phosphatase, AST, Total Bilirubin, Gamma GT, Total Protein, Albumin ALT

☐ ✗ **3083 METABOLIC STATUS PANEL**
BUN, Osmolality (calculated), Chloride, CO2 Creatinine, Glucose, Potassium, Sodium, BUN/Creatinine, Ratio, Anion Gap

☐ ✗ **3376 PANEL B**
Chem 12, CBC, Electrolyte Panel

☐ ▼ **3382 PANEL D**
Chem 20, CBC, Thyroid Cascade

☐ ✗ **3385 PANEL F**
Chem 12, CBC, Electrolyte Panel, Thyroid Cascade

☐ ▼ **3391 PANEL G**
Chem 20, Cardiac Risk Panel, CBC, Thyroid Cascade

☐ ▼ **3393 PANEL H**
Chem 20, CBC, Cardiac Risk Panel, Rheumatoid Factor, Thyroid Cascade

☐ ▼ **3397 PANEL J**
Chem 20, Cardiac Risk Panel

☐ **5351 PRENATAL PANEL**
Antibody Screen, ABO/Rh, CBC Rubella, HBsAg, RPR
☐ 1059 with Urinalysis Routine
☐ 1062 with Urinalysis w/Culture if indicated

☐ ✗ **3102 RENAL PANEL**
Matabolic Status Panel, Calcium, Phosphorus

☐ **3188 THYROID CASCADE**
TSH, Reflex Testing

▼ – patient **required** to fast for 12-14 hours
✗ – patient **recommended** to fast 12-14 hours

LAB USE ONLY
☐ SST   ☐ PLASMA
☐ PURPLE   ☐ SERUM
☐ YELLOW   ☐ SWAB
☐ BLUE   ☐ SLIDES
☐ GREEN   ☐ DNA PROBE
☐ GREY   ☐ B. CULT BTLS
☐ URINE
☐ BLACK
☐ OTHER: _____
RECV. SPECIMEN: ☐ FROZEN
☐ AMBIENT   ☐ ON ICE

Special Instructions/Pertinent Clinical Information _____

Physician's Signature _____   Date _____
These orders may be FAXed to: 449-5288   LAB   7060-500 (7/96)

Requisition form for outside laboratory

© 2010 Pearson Education, Inc.

Diagnostic Procedures **293**

2. Answer the following questions based on information found on the laboratory requisition on page 293:

a. What is the test number for each of the lab tests ordered?

_____

b. What diagnosis and ICD-9 code should be used?

_____

c. Assume the patient also complained of a sore throat, and Dr. Jefferson decided to perform and send a throat swab for a strep screening. *What test would be ordered? What is the number of the test that would be ordered? What would be an appropriate diagnosis to support the recommendation of this test?*

_____

_____

_____

LEARNING ACTIVITY: MULTIPLE CHOICE

Circle the correct answer to each of the questions below.

1. There are five types of CLIA certificate. Which of the following is not one of those types?

a. Certificate of Registration
b. Certificate of Waiver
c. Certificate of Comparison
d. Certificate for PPMP

2. Which of the following fall under the Hematology Department of a lab? (Circle all that apply.)

a. white blood cell count
b. glucose level
c. hemoglobin and hematocrit
d. a BUN level

3. A glucometer uses a/an _____ to reflect the light through the patient sample to determine the test result.

a. urinometer
b. photometer
c. lightometer
d. focusometer

4. Lab test results may be sent to the physician by (circle all that apply):

a. phone
b. fax
c. regular mail
d. e-mail

5. What laboratory area would a throat specimen go to based on the information in this chapter of your textbook?

a. chemistry
b. microbiology
c. hematology
d. immunology

6. When calling a patient about lab results or a request to return to the clinic to discuss them, you may get an answering machine. Which of the following are appropriate to leave on that machine?

a. your name
b. your phone number
c. your office or doctor's name
d. what tests the results are for (not the results themselves)

7. Which of the following choices are true about a reference laboratory? (Circle all that apply.)

   a. It is under the same regulations and guidelines as a POL.
   b. It can perform high-level testing.
   c. It is independently owned.
   d. It cannot have contracts with insurance providers and managed care providers.

8. Laboratories performing waived tests only apply for a

   a. Certificate of Accreditation
   b. Certificate of Compliance
   c. Certificate for PMPP
   d. Certificate of Waiver

9. Those who do the fewest amount of waived tests are (circle all that apply):

   a. medical assistants
   b. physicians
   c. medical lab technologists
   d. medical lab technicians

10. An example of quality control would be (circle all that apply):

   a. drawing blood from the patient
   b. confirming that the patient has followed the required preparation
   c. checking the accuracy of a glucometer
   d. selecting the appropriate container or system to collect the sample in

CRITICAL THINKING

Answer the following questions to the best of your ability. Use the textbook as a reference.

1. As you are ordering supplies for the office, you see a flyer in the mail for a sale on syringes and needles that are not safety devices. Would you try to save money on supplies or order the more expensive safety syringes and needles? Explain the reasons for your decision.

   _____
   _____
   _____
   _____

2. Your physician verbally (for now) gave you an order for a lab test that required a 7 ml purple top tube of blood, which you have already drawn. Now you cannot recall which test the physician wanted, and she has already left the office for the day. What are two ways you could find out? How can you prevent this from happening in the future?

   _____
   _____
   _____
   _____

3. You have scheduled a test at an outside agency for a patient who is not in the office at this time. You call the patient to tell her that you were able to get it booked for tomorrow at noon and that she should fast after midnight tonight. The patient becomes upset, stating that she is elderly and cannot fast until noon and that she would not have a ride to the test tomorrow as her son is working then. What could you have done differently to avoid this problem?

_____

_____

_____

_____

_____

4. You are working in an office and precepting a medical assisting student extern. A patient who is in her seventh month of pregnancy comes in, and you want the student to room the patient and perform the prenatal duties, but she doesn't do a urine glucose and protein dipstick. When asked, she tells you it is because there was no written order from the doctor. Explain in your own words and as if you were talking to the student what a standing order is.

_____

_____

_____

_____

_____

5. Your physician ordered a bone marrow biopsy to be done on a patient, which you scheduled and assisted with about three months ago. It is brought up today when the patient called the billing department. Someone came to you saying the patient was very angry because he has been billed for the procedure. He states his insurance company told him there was no precertification obtained prior to the procedure so it will not pay. You check the chart and realize you did not call to obtain the precertification before scheduling the biopsy. Consider some things you could do at this point (not what you would say to the patient) that are not specifically listed in the textbook but that seem to be logical steps to resolve this problem.

_____

_____

_____

_____

_____

RESEARCH ACTIVITY

Use Internet search engines to research the following topics and write a brief description of what is found. It is important to visit reputable Web sites.

1. Provide Internet research time for students to visit the JCAHO Web site and find the answer to the following questions:
   a. Name three types of programs or facilities they accredit.
   b. Review information about the Patient Safety Practices.
   c. Review information about Universal Precautions.
   d. What types of certification programs does JCAHO offer?

CHAPTER 31
Microscopes and Microbiology

CHAPTER OUTLINE

General review of the chapter:

    A. Medical Terminology
    B. The MA's Role in Specimen Collection
    C. Microscopes
        i. Types, structures, and use
    D. Microbiology
    E. Preparing Specimens
    F. Specimen Collection, Storage, and Transport

STUDENT STUDY GUIDE

Use the following guide to assist in your learning of the concepts from the chapter.

I. The MA's Role in Medical Specimen Collection

    A. Medical assistants participate in _____testing.
    B. Duties include:

        _____

        _____

        _____

        _____

    C. Accurate specimen collection ensures accurate results.

II. Microscopes

    A. Types of Microscopes
        i. _____: most common, with dark specimen against light background
        ii. _____: thickness provides contrast to see specimen
        iii. _____: light deflected from specimen to see image on dark background
        iv. _____: light rays illuminated on specimen with dark background
        v. _____: views ultramicroscopic organisms on a screen
    B. Structures of the Microscope
        i. Oculars:

        _____

        ii. Objectives:

        _____

        iii. Oil immersion object:

        _____

iv. Arm and focus control:

_____

v. Light source:

_____

vi. Stage:

_____

vii. Substage:

_____

C. Using the Microscope

_____

_____

_____

_____

_____

_____

_____

_____

_____

_____

_____

_____

_____

III. Microorganisms
  A. Microorganism Nomenclature
    i. Prokaryotes:

_____

    ii. Eukaryotes:

_____

    iii. Viruses:

_____

_____

  B. The Binomial System
    i. Binomial system used for _____ and _____ microorganisms
    ii. First name represents _____ and is always _____
    iii. Second name represents _____ name and is in _____
    iv. Both names are _____.
  C. Normal Flora

_____

_____

_____

_____

_____

  D. Pathology of Disease
    i. _____ is the ability of an organism to cause _____.
    ii. Pathogens cause damage to _____ directly or indirectly from
       _____.

iii. _____ pathogens cause disease when introduced into a/an _____ _____.

iv. _____ pathogens cause disease when immunity is _____.

E. Bacteria

i. Bacteria are classified by _____ or _____ and by _____ _____.

ii. Gram reaction is identification as positive or negative based on whether the organism stains.

iii. Bacteria varieties usually do not stain and gram-positive organisms retain the color.

F. Common Bacteria

i. *Staphylococcus aureus* found in foodborne illnesses, conjunctivitis, toxic shock syndrome, and urinary tract infections.

ii. *Streptococcus agalactiae* is associated with neonatal infections, vaginal infections, and UTIs.

iii. *Escherichia coli (E. coli)* is the most common cause of UTIs but can also be in foodborne illnesses.

G. Parasites

i. Parasites live off hosts' vital nutrients but do not contribute to its survival.

ii. Host cell is either _____ or totally _____ from _____

iii. Transmission of parasites requires:

_____

_____

_____

_____

iv. Common parasites: _____, _____, and _____

v. Most common symptoms of parasite infection:

_____

_____

H. Viruses

_____

_____

_____

_____

_____

_____

_____

_____

_____

IV. Specimens

A. Specimen Smear Sources

_____

_____

_____

_____

_____

_____

B. Steps for a Specimen Smear

_____

_____

_____
_____
_____
_____
_____
_____
_____
_____
_____
_____
_____
_____

C. Swab Specimen Smear
   i. _____ and turn the _____ across the slide.
D. Loop and Petri Dish Specimen Smear
   i. Gather _____ water with a sterile inoculating loop.
   ii. _____ specimen with _____ on the slide.
   iii. _____ loop over a/an _____.
E. Loop and Liquid Specimen Smear
   i. Dip _____ inoculating loop in the _____ until covered with a film.
   ii. Touch film to center of _____ and allow slide to _____.
   iii. Hold and _____ the slide through _____ several times.
F. Gram Staining
   i. Gram staining identifies small and almost colorless bacteria.
   ii. This procedure identifies if the bacteria are _____ or _____.

   _____
   _____

   iii. A physician will make an initial diagnosis and then, using the information from the gram stain, determine an appropriate medication.
   iv. Gram staining has four basic steps:

   _____
   _____
   _____
   _____
   _____
   _____
   _____
   _____

G. Wet Mount Slides
   i. There are three wet mount slide preparation methods:

   _____
   _____
   _____
   _____
   _____
   _____

_____

_____

   ii. Stool specimens are tested for:
      (a) Enteric pathogens
      (b) Parasitic pathogens
      (c) Occult blood

_____

_____

_____

_____

_____

   iii. Parasite stool testing

_____

_____

_____

_____

_____

_____

_____

_____

  H. Fecal Occult Blood Testing

_____

_____

_____

_____

_____

_____

_____

  I. Culture and Sensitivity Testing
    i. Refers to process of _____ a specimen of _____ or
    _____
    ii. After cultivation it's examined for pathogenic bacteria.
  J. Specimen cultures are processed in four steps:
    i. **Inoculation:**

_____

    ii. **Incubation:**

_____

    iii. **Inspection:**

_____

    iv. **Identification:**

_____

K. Sensitivity refers to how sensitive the organism is to selected drugs
   i. Two types of sensitivity testing:
    (a) _____

_____

L. Urinalysis
   i. Three methods to collect urine for urinalysis
    (a) _____

_____

_____

M. Clean-Catch Urine Collection

_____

_____

_____

_____

_____

_____

_____

_____

_____

_____

_____

_____

_____

N. Specimen Collection Time
   i. _____ urine must be tested within _____ hour of collection.
   ii. The specimen may be _____ for up to _____ hours.
   iii. Urine culture specimen may be refrigerated up to _____ without compromising results.

KEY TERMINOLOGY REVIEW

Use terminology words throughout the chapter to correctly complete the sentences below.

1. The _____ is the eyepiece of the microscope.

2. Because the microorganism was _____, it required the use of an electron microscope in order to be viewed.

3. _____ tests blood serum for the presence of antibodies.

4. The study of fungi, yeast, and molds is called _____.

5. _____ inhabits nonsterile major body systems.

6. A/an _____ microscope has two eyepieces.

7. Bacteria that lack an organized nucleus and cytoplasm are classified within this group of microorganisms: _____.

8. This is a method of classifying bacteria according to shape _____.

9. _____ have organized nuclear materials and organelles.

10. A specialized branch of microbiology that studies viruses is called _____.

APPLIED PRACTICE

Follow the directions as instructed with each question below.

1. Label the parts of the microscope pictured below:

1. _____
2. _____
3. _____
4. _____
5. _____
6. _____
7. _____
8. _____
9. _____
10. _____
11. _____
12. _____
13. _____
14. _____
15. _____
16. _____

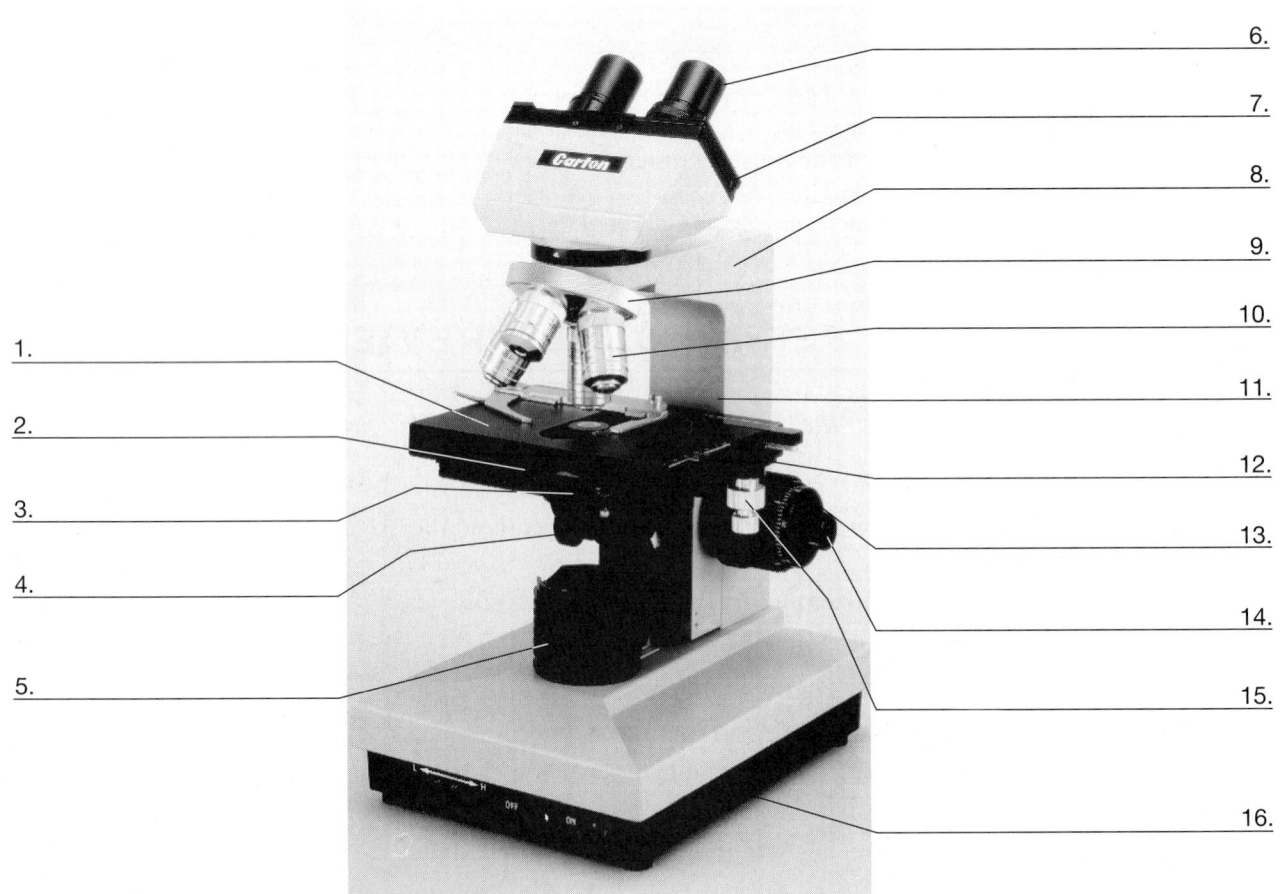

FIGURE 31-1   Binocular microscope

LEARNING ACTIVITY: TRUE/FALSE

Indicate whether the statement is true (T) or false (F).

_____ 1. A binocular microscope has one ocular lens.

_____ 2. The condenser is located on the substage of a microscope.

_____ 3. Oil immersion is used with the 10× lens to increase the power to 100×.

_____ 4. *E. coli* can cause a bladder infection (or other UTI).

_____ 5. There are three types of microscopes in addition to the five listed in your textbook.

_____ 6. Viruses are ultramicroscopic.

_____ 7. There are two focus knobs—for low power and high power.

_____ 8. The bacteria *Staphylococcus aureus* is always on our skin as normal flora.

_____ 9. When you are finished working with a microscope, you must clean the lenses with any soft cloth or paper.

_____ 10. Viruses carry DNA or RNA.

CRITICAL THINKING

Answer the following questions to the best of your ability. Use the textbook as a reference.

1. In the clinic, you are collecting urine from a patient using a catheter. As you are inserting the catheter, it slips from your hands and touches the patient's leg. What would you do and why?

_____

_____

_____

_____

2. A patient has been instructed to collect three stool specimens for occult blood. The patient brings the specimens into the office but tells you he was not able to do them on different days, and they were all collected on the same day. Is this acceptable? Why or why not?

_____

_____

_____

_____

3. You need to prepare a wet mount and set it up on the microscope for the doctor. As you look through the high power lens, it appears to be cloudy and has a lot of artifacts. When you move the slide slightly, you notice that the artifacts do not move with the slide. What do you think the problem could be? What would you do to correct this?

_____

_____

_____

4. If a patient had been treated with antibiotics for 10 days for a bladder infection and yet the infection was still present after the course of medication, what test do you think the physician might order at this point? Why?

_____

_____

_____

_____

5. You are preparing a specimen smear for a microbiological examination by the doctor. You heat-fix the slide but you realize you have heated it too much as it becomes hard to hold. What does this do to the specimen if this happens and what would you do?

_____

_____

_____

_____

_____

RESEARCH ACTIVITY

Use Internet search engines to research the following topics and write a brief description of what is found. It is important to visit reputable Web sites.

1. MRSA (Methicillin resistant *Staphylococcus aureus*) has become a very real threat not only to health care workers, but the general population. Visit www.cdc.gov and research the following topics:
   a. Provide a brief description of MRSA.
   b. What are some other multi–drug resistant organisms (MDROs)?
   c. In your opinion, what can be done to prevent the transmission of these organisms?

_____

_____

_____

_____

_____

_____

_____

_____

_____

_____

_____

_____

CHAPTER 32
Hematology and Chemistry

CHAPTER OUTLINE

General review of the chapter:

A. The MA's Role in Hematology and Chemistry
B. The Anatomy and Physiology of Blood
C. Blood Collection Equipment and Procedures
   i. Blood collection tubes
   ii. Order of draw
   iii. Venipuncture
   iv. Capillary puncture
   v. Transporting specimens
D. Performing Basic Laboratory Testing
E. Blood Chemistry Testing

STUDENT STUDY GUIDE

Use the following guide to assist in your learning of the concepts from the chapter.

I. The MA's Role and Responsibilities in Blood Collection
   A. The MA's Role in Hematology and Chemistry
      i. The MA must understand basic anatomy and physiology of _____.
      ii. Perform phlebotomy
      iii. Must know methods of _____ and _____ blood collection
      iv. Follow proper procedures of blood draws
   B. Blood Collection Responsibilities
      i. Properly _____ the patient
      ii. Review his/her order
      iii. Complete lab _____
      iv. Know which tube to use and proper amount of blood needed to test
      v. Use proper _____ during blood collection
II. The Anatomy and Physiology of Blood
   A. Components of Blood
      i. Plasma: _____ of blood content
      ii. Cellular components:
        (a) Erythrocytes: _____ of blood volume
        (b) Leukocytes and _____ (buffy coat) less than 1%
   B. Plasma

_____

_____

_____

_____

_____

C. White Blood Cells

    i. _____: most common and defend body against infection, especially bacterial

    ii. _____: second most common in adults and first in children; aid immune defense against viruses

    iii. _____: largest cells and play role in cell-mediated immunity

    iv. _____: function in allergic or inflammatory responses

    v. _____: least number of cells and react in allergic states

D. Platelets

    i. _____: cells found in blood

    ii. Critical for _____ and forming blood _____ to stop bleeding

    iii. Low platelet count means blood will not _____

    iv. Functions in _____: when the body spontaneously stops bleeding

    v. Agglutination is when the platelets _____ or aggregate to form a _____ or clot.

E. Blood Cell Formation

    i. Starts in _____ _____ marrow with _____ cells

    ii. Stem cells grow into blast cells that become erythrocytes, platelets, or leukocytes.

    iii. White blood cells function as part of the body's _____ defense

    iv. Hematopoietic system is responsible for _____ of all blood cells

    v. Blood disorders (_____) are failure of cell differentiation or development.

F. Immunohematology

    i. Study of antigens, antibodies, and their interaction

    ii. This is necessary knowledge for: _____.

    iii. Antigens recognize foreign substances or organisms to stimulate antibody reaction.

    iv. Antigen-antibody reactions can be _____.

III. Blood Collection

A. Equipment Used in Blood Drawing

_____

_____

_____

_____

_____

B. Color Coded Blood Draw Tubes

    i. Colors indicate type of additive in the tube

    ii. Additives include:

      (a) **Anticoagulants:**

_____

_____

      (b) **Clot activators:**

_____

_____

      (c) **Preservatives:**

_____

_____

C. Order of Draw
    i. The type of _____ ordered determines the tube that will be used.
    ii. Culture blood draws are done first to prevent _____.
    iii. Tubes containing anticoagulants or clot activators are second due to _____ sensitivity.
    iv. Order of draw will prevent thromboplastin release from cells during venipuncture.
    v. The Clinical and Laboratory Standards Institute (CLSI) has a recommended order of draw.
    vi. Color-top tubes should be drawn in the following order:

_____

_____

_____

_____

_____

_____

_____

_____

_____

_____

_____

D. Venipuncture
    i. Different methods of draws allow for the choice of _____ _____ and length.
    ii. Needle gauge: indicates the needle's _____
    iii. The larger the gauge number, the smaller the needle is in diameter.
    iv. The most common gauge sizes are _____.
E. Methods of Collecting Venous Blood Samples
    i. Evacuated tube system:

_____

_____

    ii. Syringe and needle:

_____

_____

    iii. Winged infusion set (butterfly) method:

_____

_____

F. Common Venipuncture Sites
    i. "_____ _____" triangular area below the elbow
    ii. Median cubital vein is preferred due to _____ size and well anchored
    iii. _____ vein harder to find and moves easily
    iv. Basilic vein close to _____ artery
    v. Dorsal wrist and hands veins acceptable sites
G. Capillary or Dermal Collection
    i. When small amount of blood is needed, dermal capillary collection is performed
    ii. Small children, infants, or adults whose veins are hard to find require capillary or dermal puncture.
    iii. Recommended for:

_____

_____

H. Capillary Puncture Equipment
    i. Trigger releasing, disposable, self-contained _____
    ii. Other equipment:

    _____

    _____

    iii. Document method being used
    iv. Elements of blood differ significantly if venipuncture or capillary draw is used.
I. Transporting Blood Specimens
    i. Sedimentation rates should be performed within _____ of collection.
    ii. Specimen should be in a/an _____ container.
    iii. Containers should be carried in a/an _____ bag for transport to lab.
    iv. Specimens should be placed in designated location for lab pickup

IV. Blood Testing, Chemistry, and Blood Typing
    A. Hematology Tests

    _____

    _____

    _____

    _____

    B. Diagnostic Information
        i. Hemoglobin and hematocrit indicative:

        _____

        _____

        ii. Hematocrit:

        _____

        _____

        _____

        _____

    C. The Physician's Office Laboratory

    _____

    _____

    _____

    _____

    _____

    D. Manual Blood Testing
        i. Manual blood cell tests may include:

        _____

        _____

        _____

        _____

    E. Blood Chemistry Tests
        i. Contribute to clinical diagnoses
        ii. Common tests:

        _____

        _____

        iii. Some chemistry tests are _____ diagnostic tools and others measure serious disease.

    iv. A/an _____ panel is when a lab combines commonly ordered groups of tests.

    v. Sometimes the test panels are organized based on organ function.

F. Automated Chemistry Analyzers

    i. Maintained and operated by _____ _____

    ii. Sophisticated calibration and quality control protocols

    iii. Designed for use in _____ or _____ laboratory settings

    iv. Programmed for specific organ panels, chemistry profiles, or individual chemistry tests

G. Blood Typing

    i. Specially trained technologist performs immunohematology testing in a lab

    ii. Some POLs offer blood typing tests.

    iii. Basis for blood typing is _____

      (a) This is when the blood type group antigen and its corresponding antibody come together.

    iv. When they unite, _____ results.

H. Blood Types

    i. _____ blood has A antigens and anti-B antibodies.

    ii. _____ blood has B antigens and anti-A antibodies.

    iii. _____ blood has both A and B antigens but lacks antibodies, so is a "universal recipient." These people can receive type A or B blood.

    iv. _____ blood has neither A nor B antigen, but it does have anti-A and anti-B antibodies.

    v. _____ blood is also known as a "universal donor" because it can be transfused to any patient regardless of blood type.

      (a) This is possible because it lacks antigens to interact with antibodies in type **A**, **B**, or **AB** blood.

KEY TERMINOLOGY REVIEW

Use a dictionary and the textbook to define the following key terms.

1. Agglutination:

    _____

    _____

2. Anticoagulant:

    _____

    _____

3. Coagulation:

    _____

    _____

4. Diluent:

    _____

    _____

5. Dyscrasia:

    _____

    _____

6. Erythrocytes:

_____

_____

7. Hematology:

_____

_____

8. Hemostasis:

_____

_____

9. Immunohematology:

_____

_____

10. Leukocytes:

_____

_____

11. Phagocytic:

_____

_____

12. Phlebotomist:

_____

_____

13. Phlebotomy:

_____

_____

14. Plasma:

_____

_____

15. Serum:

_____

_____

16. Spectrophotometric:

_____

_____

17. Thrombocytes:

_____

_____

18. Venipuncture:

_____

_____

APPLIED PRACTICE

Using the information found in the chapter, answer the questions following the scenario below.

Scenario

Julie Turner is working as a clinical medical assistant. A patient, Hector Olanski, comes in for a blood draw. The physician's order reads as follows:

COOK FAMILY MEDICINE
(188) 555-1111

Patient: Hector Olanski   DOB: 7-3-1938
                                 Date: 3-22-20xx

 PT\INR and CBC

Dx: (1) Heparin monitoring (E934.2)
    (2) Phlebitis of lower extremities (451.2)

Dr. Liam Cook

While gathering supplies, Julie grabs a lavender top tube, a red top tube, and a light-blue top tube.

1. a. Did Julie collect the right tubes for Mr. Olanski's blood draw? Why or why not? Explain your answer based on each color-top tube of blood Julie collected.

    b. What would be the correct order of draw?

    c. Are there any additives in the tubes that Julie is using for the blood draw? If so, explain which additives are used (based on color-top tube) and the action of the additive.

2. Fill in the label below according to how Julie should label each of Mr. Olanski's tubes of blood.

LEARNING ACTIVITY: MULTIPLE CHOICE

Circle the correct answer to each of the questions below.

1. Which two of the following terms mean the same thing? (Circle both terms.)

    a. venipuncture
    b. phlebotomy
    c. capillary puncture
    d. antecubital

2. The tourniquet in a hand draw should be about _____ above the wrist.

    a. 2 inches
    b. 3 inches
    c. 4 inches
    d. 5 inches

3. Quality control assessment in basic laboratory testing includes all of the following except:

    a. check of supplies
    b. check of reagents
    c. reporting needlesticks
    d. test performance

4. A blood hematocrit is defined as the volume of _____ in a given volume of blood and is usually measured as a percentage of the total blood volume.

    a. WBCs
    b. RBCs
    c. platelets
    d. serum

5. The most common site for a blood draw is _____.

    a. wrist
    b. hand
    c. foot
    d. antecubital fossa

6. A blood draw should be done with the needle bevel up and at a _____ degree angle.

    a. 10
    b. 20
    c. 30
    d. 40

7. Which of the following blood types is known as the universal recipient?

    a. A
    b. B
    c. AB
    d. O

8. Which of the following is not a reason to use a capillary puncture?

    a. The patient is too young for a draw in the antecubital area.
    b. Adults have difficult veins to find.
    c. The patient is too nervous about the pain of an antecubital draw.
    d. A small amount of blood is required.

9. Which three of the following are methods of measuring an ESR?

    a. Zeta
    b. Peta
    c. Westergren
    d. Wintrobe

10. When performing a WBC and platelet count, you will use two of the items listed below (circle both terms):

    a. Unopette
    b. Accu-Check
    c. glucometer
    d. hemacytometer

LEARNING ACTIVITY: TRUE/FALSE

Indicate whether the statement is true (T) or false (F).

_____ 1. A large red-top glass tube has no additive but only a clot activator in it.

_____ 2. In relation to blood, agglutination means clumping.

_____ 3. Capillary puncture is also called dermal puncture.

_____ 4. Sometimes charting may not be required for phlebotomy because laboratory processing documentation is sufficient.

_____ 5. Wait until all blood tubes have been collected before asking the patient to release his or her fist.

_____ 6. The National Committee for Clinical Laboratory Standards (NCCLS) has instituted a recommended order of draw to minimize the effects of additive carryover.

_____ 7. MCV, MVHV, and MCV are used to differentiate specific types of anemia.

_____ 8. When drawing blood, you should not promise the patient that the procedure will not hurt.

_____ 9. Always ask the patient if he or she has an allergy to latex when preparing to put on a tourniquet, as many are made of latex.

_____ 10. Type O blood is known as the universal donor.

CRITICAL THINKING

Answer the following questions to the best of your ability. Use the textbook as a reference.

1. A patient needs to have blood drawn for an ESR and a glucose level. The patient is extremely nervous and worried about the pain she will experience with a blood draw and asks if you can "stick her finger" instead. Will that work in this scenario? Tell why or why not.

_____

_____

_____

_____

2. You have drawn three tubes of blood in a gray top, a lavender top, and a green top. You filled the lavender top first, then the gray top, then the green top. Is this the correct order of draw? If not, what could possibly happen because of this?

_____

_____

_____

_____

3. A patient has come in today for a blood draw to check her cholesterol level. She is 78 years old, has fragile skin, and her veins are impossible to see. Which method of phlebotomy would you use on this patient and why?

_____

_____

_____
_____
_____

4. A patient needs a blood draw today but presents with a rash on both antecubital fossas, and you do not want to draw in this compromised area of skin. What would be your next choice of site and why?

_____
_____
_____
_____
_____

5. Your next patient for phlebotomy today is a 6-year-old child. What special considerations are appropriate for this patient?

_____
_____
_____
_____
_____

RESEARCH ACTIVITY

Use Internet search engines to research the following topics and write a brief description of what is found. It is important to visit reputable Web sites.

1. Visit The Clinical and Laboratory Standards Institute at www.clsi.org. Navigate through the Web site and identify reasons why the site would be beneficial for medical assistants working in the clinical or physician's office laboratory.

_____
_____
_____
_____
_____
_____
_____
_____
_____
_____
_____
_____
_____

CHAPTER 33
Urology and Nephrology

CHAPTER OUTLINE

General review of the chapter:

    A. Introduction
    B. The MA's Role in Urology and Nephrology
    C. Anatomy and Physiology of the Urinary System
    D. Renal Diseases
    E. Diagnostic Procedures
    F. Urinalysis
    G. The Male Reproductive System

STUDENT STUDY GUIDE

Use the following guide to assist in your learning of the concepts from the chapter.

    I. The Medical Assistant's Role in Urology and Nephrology

    A. Patient's medical history
    B. Obtain _____ _____
    C. Collect urine specimens
    D. _____ _____ testing
    E. Some _____ examination of urine specimens
    F. Catheterization requires _____ _____.

    II. Anatomy and Physiology of the Urinary System

    A. Structures of the Urinary System
        i. Kidney, ureter, _____ _____, and _____
        ii. Renal arteries supply the kidney with blood.
        iii. The blood circulates through to filter out toxins such as _____, _____, _____, and _____.
        iv. The two portions of the kidney are:

            _____

            _____

            _____

            _____

        v. 1 million microscopic tubules in each kidney called _____
        vi. Nephrons collect the urine, which is sent to the _____.
        vii. Ureter delivers urine to the _____
        viii. The _____ is where the both the ureter and urethra exist within the bladder.
        ix. Bladder:

            _____

            _____

x. Muscle contraction of the bladder expels urine through _____
_____

B. Urine Formation: The Nephron
   i. The nephron consists of five parts which function in urine formation:

_____
_____
_____
_____
_____

C. Urine Formation: Contributing Functions
   i. There are five contributing functions to the production of urine:

_____
_____
_____
_____
_____

III. Renal Diseases and Urinary Tract Infections
   A. **Acute Glomerulonephritis**

_____
_____
_____
_____

   B. _____ (_____ _____) **Glomerulonephritis**
      i. Also called Goodpasture's syndrome
      ii. Acute onset progresses to _____ and renal failure, which has poor progno-
          sis unless diagnosed early.
   C. **Chronic Glomerulonephritis**
      i. Membranous glomerulonephritis:

_____
_____
_____

      ii. Membrano-proliferative glomerulonephritis:

_____
_____
_____
_____

   D. **Acute Renal Failure**

_____
_____
_____

E. **Chronic Renal Failure**

_____

_____

_____

_____

F. **Nephrotic Syndrome**
   i. Generally develops when worsening _____ is accompanied by circulatory problems, such as_____
   ii. Often progresses to chronic renal failure

G. **Polycystic Kidney Disease**
   i. Slowly progressive disease that affects both kidneys
   ii. Multiple cysts form on dilated _____ and collecting ducts, resulting in

   _____ _____.

   iii. Most cases are inherited, or following long-term chronic kidney disease and/or

   _____.

   iv. No cure

   v. _____ _____
      (a) Often a sequela to diabetes mellitus
      (b) Cellular membranes of glomeruli harden or sclerose
      (c) Infectious process often involved

H. **Urinary Tract Infections**
   i. **Urethritis**

_____

_____

_____

_____

_____

   ii. **Cystitis**

_____

_____

_____

_____

   iii. **Acute pyelonephritis/nephritis**

_____

_____

_____

_____

   iv. **Chronic pyelonephritis**

_____

_____

_____

_____

v. Uremia

_____

_____

_____

_____

IV. Renal Dialysis and Renal Disorders
 A. Renal Dialysis
  i. Temporary treatment when a person has _____ _____
   _____ _____ (ESRD)
  ii. There are two different methods of dialysis:
   (a) Hemodialysis
   (b) Peritoneal dialysis
 B. Hemodialysis

_____

_____

_____

_____

_____

_____

_____

_____

_____

_____

_____

 C. Peritoneal Dialysis
  i. Dialyzing fluid is infused into peritoneum through a catheter
  ii. Three methods:
   (a) Continuous ambulatory peritoneal dialysis:

_____

_____

   (b) Continuous cycling peritoneal dialysis (CCPD):

_____

_____

   (c) Intermittent peritoneal dialysis:

_____

_____

 D. Neurogenic Bladder and Urinary Incontinence
  i. Lack of control over _____ of urine or _____ to start
   urinating
  ii. _____: insult or injury to nerve supply controlling bladder
  iii. _____: inability to control release of urine
 E. Obstructive Urinary Disorders
  i. Prevent the flow of urine from the urinary tract
  ii. The kidney becomes _____ and _____ with urine.
   (a) This is called _____.
  iii. The kidney will return to normal state once obstruction is removed

iv. Renal calculi obstruction:

_____
_____
_____
_____
_____

v. Bladder calculi:

_____
_____
_____
_____
_____

vi. Cysts:

_____
_____
_____
_____

F. Kidney or Ureter Cancer

_____
_____
_____
_____
_____

G. Bladder Cancer

_____
_____
_____
_____
_____

V. Urinalysis, Specimen Collection, and Diagnostic Assessment
   A. Urinalysis
      i. A/an _____ test commonly used to diagnose urinary tract infections
      ii. A/an _____ _____ _____ urine test must be collected.
      iii. If invasive tests are required for diagnosis they are performed using radiography.
      iv. Further specialized testing for _____ function may be necessary.
   B. Urine Specimen Collection
      i. There are various forms of urine collection:

_____
_____
_____
_____

_____

_____

C. Factors in Specimen Collection
   i. Correct and complete labeling is required.
   ii. Label must have _____ _____, _____, and
          _____ _____ of collection.
   iii. Best sample is fresh urine; otherwise it should be _____ or
          _____.
          (a) Must be tested within 1–2 hours
   iv. Preservation kits are available for transportation to other facilities.

D. Contamination

_____

_____

_____

_____

_____

_____

E. The 24-Hour Specimen

_____

_____

_____

_____

_____

F. Catheterization

_____

_____

G. Characteristics of Urine
   i. Determined by the _____, _____, _____,
          pH, and specific gravity
   ii. Normal urine will be yellow and clear.
   iii. The more hydrated a person is the _____ the urine will be.
   iv. Cloudy urine does not always signify _____.
   v. Fresh, normal urine will have a faint characteristic odor and a 5.0-8.0 pH balance.
   vi. Specific gravity is the measure of specific volume of urine to volume of water.

H. Chemical Test Strips
   i. Checks liver and kidney function

_____

_____

   ii. Test strips have chemicals that react with urine to produce predictable color change.
   iii. Colors are compared to a manufacturer's chart and reported.
          (a) Reflectance spectrophotometry is when a machine performs this task.
   iv. Strip reactions happen quickly and should be read within _____ to
          _____.
   v. Quality control tests should be performed every 24-hour testing period, or when a new
          dipstick container is opened.
   vi. Strips should be kept in _____ _____.

vii. Tests on chemical strips include:

_____

_____

_____

_____

_____

_____

viii. Disease indications by tests:
   (a) _____ _____ urine disorder or fluid status change
   (b) _____: acid-base disorders or urinary tract infections
   (c) Protein:

   _____

   _____

   (d) Microalbumin:

   _____

   _____

   (e) Glucose:

   _____

   _____

   (f) _____: diabetic ketoacidosis, starvation, disorders with severe vomiting and diarrhea
   (g) Blood:

   _____

   _____

   (h) Ascorbic acid: treatment with vitamin C
   (i) Bilirubin: _____ and _____ disease
   (j) Urobilinogen: hemolysis, _____
   (k) Nitrite: infection with gram-negative organisms
   (l) _____: infection of genitourinary system
ix. Microscopic Urinalysis
   (a) A centrifuge is used to separate the soluble from the insoluble material found in urine.
   (b) _____ settles at the bottom and is examined with a low or high power microscope.
   (c) Elements seen microscopically may indicate urinary or systemic disease.

   _____

   _____

   _____

   _____

   (d) Microscopic findings may include:

   _____

   _____

   _____

   _____

   _____

   _____

VI. The Male Reproductive System
   A. Structures of the Male Reproductive System
      i. Penis:

      _____

      _____

      _____

      _____

      ii. Scrotum:

      _____

      _____

      _____

      _____

      iii. _____: _____: carries sperm
      iv. _____: _____: produces alkaline fluid that becomes semen
         to transport sperm
      v. Prostate gland
      vi. Prostatic urethra: descends from urinary bladder
      vii. _____ or bulbourethral gland: produces mucous for semen
      viii. Urinary meatus: opening for semen to be expelled

   B. Disorders of the Male Reproductive System
      i. Diseases or disorders of the prostate gland

      _____

      _____

      _____

      _____

      _____

      _____

      ii. Causes of male infertility

      _____

      _____

      _____

      _____

      _____

      _____

      iii. Testicular disorders

      _____

      _____

      _____

      _____

      _____

      _____

KEY TERMINOLOGY REVIEW

Match the key terms to their definitions below.

a.	aliquot	**k.**	prodromal
b.	billirubin	**l.**	proteinuria
c.	cystitis	**m.**	pyuria
d.	electrolytes	**n.**	renal
e.	hematuria	**o.**	sequela
f.	incontinence	**p.**	turbidity
g.	jaundice	**q.**	ureter
h.	nocturia	**r.**	urethra
i.	oliguria	**s.**	urinary bladder
j.	polyuria	**t.**	urinary meatus

_____ 1. Inflammation of the urinary bladder.

_____ 2. Tube leading from urinary bladder to outside the body.

_____ 3. Pertaining to the initial stage of a disease.

_____ 4. Yellow color in the skin and mucous membranes.

_____ 5. Pertaining to the kidney.

_____ 6. Cloudiness, lack of clarity.

_____ 7. Presence of abnormally large amounts of protein in the urine.

_____ 8. External sphincter of the urethra.

_____ 9. Increased urine output at night.

_____ 10. Substance formed by the breakdown of hemoglobin.

_____ 11. Receptacle for urine that has been manufactured by the kidneys.

_____ 12. Involuntary leakage of urine or feces.

_____ 13. Ionized substances in blood, cells, and tissues.

_____ 14. Excessive urine production and frequent, urgent, and excessive urinary output.

_____ 15. Pus in the urine.

_____ 16. Outcome.

_____ 17. Tube leading from the kidney to the urinary bladder.

_____ 18. Blood in the urine.

_____ 19. Diminished urine output.

_____ 20. Representative sample of a well-mixed specimen.

APPLIED PRACTICE

Using the information found in the chapter, answer the questions following the scenario below.

Scenario

Mr. Bai Feng, born 8-13-66, presents to the office today with a fever of 99.7° F, noticeable beads of sweat on his brow, and complaints of right-sided pain in his lower back. He states "I am in so much pain I can't stand up straight and I feel like I always have to urinate." A urine specimen is obtained for urinalysis and shows ++ for blood in the urine as well as other abnormalities. His urine specimen is sent to the laboratory for further testing.

1. Based on his urinalysis and symptoms, what would a likely diagnosis be? (Keep in mind a Medical Assistant never diagnoses a patient; this is your opinion based on information found in the textbook.)

     _____

     _____

2. Below is the label that was affixed to Mr. Feng's urine specimen:

FENG, BAI
DOB: 8-13-1966   DATE: 7/18/20xx

     What piece of important information is missing? Why is it important for this to be on the label?

     _____

     _____

     _____

3. Draw a picture of the urinary system (kidneys, ureters, urinary bladder, urethra). Circle the area of the urinary system that is likely to be the causative factor for Mr. Feng's pain.

LEARNING ACTIVITY: FILL IN THE BLANK

Using words from the list below, fill in the blanks to complete the following statements.

15 and 40	bladder and urethra	catheterization
20 and 35	cancer	cleaned
abnormal	catheter	color

color change
discomfort or pain
genitals
life-threatening
pathogens
physical

physiological
reagent pad
red or red-brown
specific gravity
STDs
sterility

testicular self-exam
urethra and meatus
urinalysis
urine components
water
water balance

1. Although the _____ are normally sterile, a urine specimen can be contaminated with microorganisms from the lower portion of the _____.

2. The patient should feel no _____ after the _____ is removed.

3. Each _____ on a chemical test strip is saturated with chemicals that react with _____ to produce a predictable _____.

4. _____ is the measurement of a specific volume of urine to an equal volume of _____.

5. As with a female patient, it is imperative that the male patient's _____ be appropriately and thoroughly _____ before _____ to prevent the introduction of _____.

6. A refractometer is used to determine the _____ of urine in the _____ portion of a/an _____.

7. The most common set of _____ shades of color of urine is _____.

8. One of the _____ functions of the kidneys is maintaining the body's _____ by adjusting the amount or water in the urine.

9. Untreated _____ are spread unknowingly, can cause _____, and may even become _____.

10. Testicular _____ is relatively common between the ages of _____, although males between the ages of _____ should perform a monthly _____.

CRITICAL THINKING

Answer the following questions to the best of your ability. Use the textbook as a reference.

1. You drew blood for a PSA after the patient has been examined by the physician. What is wrong with this?

   _____

   _____

   _____

   _____

2. If you were working in a fertility clinic within a urology practice, you would undoubtedly have preprinted history forms specifically designed to elicit reproductive and fertility-related information. When the patient has the initial evaluation, the MA would go over the form with the patient after he or she has completed it, or would ask the questions and complete the form with the patient. Although this is not discussed in your textbook specifically, think of five questions that might be on that form.

   _____

   _____

_____

_____

_____

3. Imagine this scenario: You are a female. You have completed your externship and have been hired by a urology clinic in your first full-time medical assistant position. You are directed by the physician to instruct a patient in performing a testicular self-exam. You are suddenly nervous about doing this to a real patient even though you have practiced this in your medical assisting program with other students. Describe in one or two paragraphs how you would feel and what you would do or tell yourself to bolster your own comfort and confidence.

_____

_____

_____

_____

4. You are to instruct a 68-year-old female patient in the collection of a 24-hour urine specimen. Explain this, in your own words, as if you were speaking to the patient. Avoid medical terms that the patient may not understand very well but avoid treating the patient as if she were a child.

_____

_____

_____

_____

5. You have collected a clean-catch urine specimen from Mrs. Gonzalez, a long-time patient, and you have already performed the physical assessment of the color, odor, and clarity. Following are the results of your chemical testing. Fill in the normal value for each, circle those that are abnormal as if flagging them for the physician, and then state the possible reasons for the abnormal results.

	Your Results on Mrs. Gonzalez	Normal Value	Possible Causes
Color	orange-red		
Clarity	cloudy		
pH	7.8		
Specific gravity	1.026		
Protein	++ or positive		
Glucose	0		
Ketones	0		
Bilirubin	0		
Urobilinogen	4		
Blood	+		
Leukocytes	++++		
Nitrite	0		

RESEARCH ACTIVITY

Use Internet search engines to research the following topics and write a brief description of what is found. It is important to visit reputable Web sites.

1. Visit www.kidney.org. As you navigate through the site, what information would be helpful to provide a patient who is in need of a kidney transplant? What information is available for health care technicians? How could this Web site be beneficial for a urology/nephrology office?

   _____

   _____

   _____

   _____

   _____

   _____

   _____

   _____

   _____

   _____

   _____

   _____

   _____

   _____

   _____

   _____

   _____

   _____

   _____

   _____

   _____

   _____

   _____

   _____

   _____

   _____

   _____

CHAPTER 34
Medical Imaging

CHAPTER OUTLINE

General review of the chapter:

A. Medical Terminology
B. The MA's Role in Medical Imaging
C. Radiology
D. Equipment
E. Safety Precautions and Patient Protection
F. Limited-Scope Radiography
G. Scheduling Radiographs
H. Assisting with an X-Ray
    i. Patient preparation and instructions
I. Preparation of the X-Ray Room
J. Filing and Loaning Radiographic Records

STUDENT STUDY GUIDE

Use the following guide to assist in your learning of the concepts from the chapter.

I. Medical Imaging and the MA's Role

  A. Medical Imaging
    i. Includes radiology, sonography, _____, computed tomography (CT), _____ _____ _____ (MRI), and nuclear medicine
    ii. _____ are used in MRI instead of radiation to obtain a three-dimensional view of body parts.
    iii. Tomography scans body parts in _____ or _____ for three-dimensional image
    iv. Radiology uses radiographs or developed X-ray film to take pictures of the body.

  B. The MA's Role in Medical Imaging
    _____
    _____
    _____
    _____
    _____
    _____

II. Radiology

  A. Radiography
    i. Study of viewing the human body through various methods
    ii. X-rays utilize _____.
    iii. Small _____ of _____ travel in waves at the speed of light.

iv. _____

v. _____

B. Diagnostic Radiography

_____

_____

_____

_____

_____

_____

_____

C. Radiography and Contrast Medium

_____

_____

_____

_____

_____

_____

D. Fluroscopy
   i. _____
      (a) Organs examined include: heart, stomach, intestines, and fallopian tubes
   ii. Projects visual images on a/an _____ vs. _____
   iii. Myelography uses _____ and _____ methods to examine the spinal _____ space.

E. Computed Tomography

_____

_____

_____

_____

_____

F. Magnetic Resonance Imaging

_____

_____

_____

_____

_____

_____

_____

_____

_____

G. Sonography

_____

_____

_____

_____

_____

_____

H. Nuclear Medicine

_____

_____

_____

_____

_____

_____

III. Radiology Equipment and Radiation Protection
   A. Equipment
     i. Expensive

     _____

     ii. Four major components to the X-ray machine:
       (a) Tube: _____
       (b) Table: _____
       (c) Control panel: _____
       (d) Generator: _____

   B. Portable or Fluoroscopic Equipment

   _____

   _____

   _____

   _____

   C. Radiation Protection
     i. Prolonged exposure can cause biological changes:

     _____

     ii. Safety guidelines:
       (a) _____ : radiation exposure "as low as reasonably achievable"
       (b) Physician must _____ _____ against benefit derived from procedure
       (c) Patient must always be protected with _____ _____ barriers
     iii. _____ for women of childbearing age:

     _____

   D. Radiation Protection
     i. _____: length of exposure should be as short as possible
     ii. _____ : maximum distance between the tech and radiation source at all times
     iii. _____: lead aprons, lead gloves, thyroid shielding
     iv. Employees must wear radiation badge: _____

IV. Limited-Scope Radiography, Scheduling, Room Preparation, Radiographic Terms
    A. Limited-Scope Radiography
        i. Limited _____ and _____ of X-ray procedures
        ii. Usually upper and lower extremities, chest and some skull procedures
        iii. Only allowable under _____ and _____ of a/an
        _____

    B. Radiographic Scheduling

        _____

        _____

        _____

        _____

        _____

        _____

        _____

        _____

    C. Room Preparation

        _____

        _____

        _____

        _____

        _____

        _____

        _____

    D. Body Positions
        i. _____ = placement of the body or body part
        ii. _____ = sitting or standing
        iii. _____ = in a reclining position or lying down
        iv. _____ = lying down position
        v. _____ = lying on the left side, recumbent
        vi. _____ = lying on the right side, recumbent
    E. Body Movements
        i. _____ = lying face up
        ii. _____ = lying face down
        iii. _____ = lying on the left side
        iv. _____ = lying on the right side
        v. _____ = body or body part placed at a 90-degree angle
        vi. _____ = body or body part placed at less than a 90-degree angle
        vii. _____ = decreasing the angle between two bones; bending at the joint
        viii. _____ = increasing the angle between two bones; straightening at the joint
        ix. _____ = moving a body part away from the midline of the body
        x. _____ = moving a body part toward the midline of the body
        xi. _____ = turning a body part toward the outside
        xii. _____ = turning a body part toward the inside
        xiii. _____ = turning the palm of the hand upward
        xiv. _____ = turning the palm of the hand downward
V. Patient Education and Patient Preparation
    A. Mammography
        i. Appointment one week after menses, when the breasts are less tender.

ii. The patient should not wear:

_____

_____

B. Upper GI/Barium Swallow
    i. Light evening meal
    ii. _____ hours prior to X-rays
    iii. Procedural steps:

_____

_____

_____

_____

C. Lower GI
    i. Examine the _____ for disease or disorders.
    ii. Preparation (day prior):

_____

_____

_____

_____

_____

    iii. Day of procedure:

_____

_____

_____

_____

    iv. Procedure:

_____

_____

_____

_____

D. IVP
    i. Patient gowns and empties bladder prior to exam
    ii. An initial X-ray may be taken with the patient in a/an _____.
    iii. An IV is started and contrast medium injected.
    iv. _____
    v. The patient is asked to urinate again, and a final X-ray is taken.
    vi. _____

E. Cholecystogram
    i. Radiographic examination of the _____ to diagnose disease or disorders
    ii. Preparation (day prior):

_____

_____

_____

_____

_____

_____

iii. Preparation (day of):

_____

_____

iv. Procedure:

_____

_____

KEY TERMINOLOGY REVIEW

Match the correct medical term with the definition listed below.

a.	angiography	**h.**	radiation
b.	arthrography	**i.**	radiography
c.	cholecystography	**j.**	radiolucent
d.	echocardiogram	**k.**	radiopaque
e.	fluoroscopy	**l.**	sonography
f.	mammogram	**m.**	ultrasound
g.	myelography	**n.**	X-rays

_____ 1. Radiographic study in which structures are visualized in motion.

_____ 2. Radiant energy.

_____ 3. Radiograph of the vessels usually with contrast medium.

_____ 4. Radiograph of the gallbladder.

_____ 5. Use of high-frequency sound waves to project an image.

_____ 6. Capable of obstructing the passage of X-rays.

_____ 7. This type of sonogram allows for viewing of the internal structures of the heart.

_____ 8. Study or practice of radiology using X-rays.

_____ 9. Use of ultrasound waves to view internal body structures.

_____ 10. Radiograph of breast tissue.

_____ 11. Radiograph of the spinal cord using contrast medium.

_____ 12. Form of electromagnetic radiation that travels in waves at the speed of light.

_____ 13. Easily penetrated by X-rays.

_____ 14. Radiographic examination of a joint.

APPLIED PRACTICE

Follow the directions as instructed with each question below.

1. Use information from the patient's chart listed below to answer the following questions:

Epley, Marguerite V.

11-24-1941

3/18/XX 2:15 pm   Ht: 5'5"   Wt: 115 lbs   T: 98.6°F   P: 90 bpm   BP: 136/88

cc: Pt. presents to office with rt. lower leg pain, after falling while getting out of her bathtub. Pt. rates

the pain a 6 on a scale of 1-10. Rt. lower leg appears to be swollen and without bruising at this time.

--- *Jerry Li, CMA (AAMA)*

Scenario

Dr. Jefferson wants Jerry, the CMA (AAMA), to perform an X-ray of Ms. Epley's lower right leg. The order reads:

> PT: Marguerite Epley   DOB: 11/24/1941
>
> Rt. lower leg X-ray. AP and lateral views.
>
> Dx: R/O Fx (*Diagnosis: Rule Out Fracture*)

a. According to Mrs. Epley's height and weight, which appears to be average, how would you describe her body shape (habitus)?

_____

b. Dr. Jefferson ordered an AP view. What does this mean?

_____

c. How do you think Jerry should position the patient for the lateral view?

_____

d. If Jerry were to position Mrs. Epley lying face up on the table and flat on her back, what body position would this be?

_____

e. List some of the protective barriers Jerry would implement during the X-ray.

_____

_____

LEARNING ACTIVITY: FILL IN THE BLANK

Using words from the list below, fill in the blanks to complete the following statements.

allergic
allowed in your state
childbearing age
computed tomography (CT)
dissecting planes
education
equal or unequal
expose and develop film

front and back
front to back
iodine or shellfish
nuclear medicine
positioning
pregnant
radioactive
safety precautions

sonography
swallows or is injected
target tissue or organ
three-dimensional
training
vertically

1. In nuclear medicine, the patient either _____ with a/an _____ material called a tracer that is absorbed by the _____.

2. Related to limited-scope radiology: After the appropriate _____ and if it is _____, you may be asked to _____ in addition to preparing the patient.

3. The coronal plane divides the body into _____ portions.

4. The sagittal plane divides the body _____ into _____ right and left sections.

5. In the anteroposterior view (AP), the central ray is directed from _____.

6. Any female of _____ must be asked if she could be _____.

7. Regarding patient preparation and instructions for an IVP: This procedure should not be performed on a patient who is _____ to _____.

8. Medical imaging is a specialty that encompasses radiology, _____, fluoroscopy, _____, magnetic resonance imaging (MRI), and _____.

9. Computed tomography can scan a body part in _____ or "slices," then assemble them to produce a/an _____, 360-degree image.

10. The medical assistant's role in medical imaging may involve patient _____, preparation, and _____, scheduling, and following _____.

CRITICAL THINKING

Answer the following questions to the best of your ability. Use the textbook as a reference.

1. You have placed a patient on the table for an X-ray and notice that the lead strip around the table has a few very small cracks in it. What should you do?

   _____

   _____

   _____

   _____

   _____

2. A 22-year-old female patient needs to have an X-ray of her shoulders. What must you remember to ask this particular patient that you may not ask all patients?

_____

_____

_____

_____

3. Mr. Abdul has come in for a cholecystogram. As you put the patient into the room, you verify that he has followed the preparation instructions of taking iodine the day before and then NPO this morning. He looks surprised and then admits he forgot to take the iodine. What would you do?

_____

_____

_____

_____

4. A patient comes to the front desk and does not have an appointment. She wants to get a copy of a mammogram she had at the clinic about 12 years ago. What can you tell this patient?

_____

_____

_____

_____

5. Your next patient has come in for an MRI and answers no to your question of whether he has any metal or a pacemaker implanted in his body. As the patient removes his shirt to put on a gown, you notice he has a bright-colored tattoo on his posterior right flank. What should you say?

_____

_____

_____

_____

RESEARCH ACTIVITY

Use Internet search engines to research the following topics and write a brief description of what is found. It is important to visit reputable Web sites.

1. Research your state's laws regarding limited-scope radiography. Would you be allowed to practice limited-scope radiography as an MA with proper training and supervision?

_____

_____

_____

CHAPTER 35
Cardiology and Cardiac Testing

CHAPTER OUTLINE

General review of the chapter:

A. Introduction
B. The Medical Assistant's Role in Cardiology
C. The Anatomy and Physiology of the Heart
D. Diseases and Disorders of the Heart
    i. Diagnostic tests
    ii. Electrocardiogram
    iii. Holter monitor
    iv. Stress testing
    v. Echocardiogram
    vi. Thallium scan
    vii. MUGA scan
E. Identifying Arrhythmias/Dysrhythmias

STUDENT STUDY GUIDE

Use the following guide to assist in your learning of the concepts from the chapter.

I. The MA's Role in a Cardiology Office

  A. Routinely perform _____ in physician's office
  B. Knowledge of anatomy and physiology of heart required
  C. Knowledge of _____ _____ system of heart important
  D. Understand interpretation of rhythm strip
  E. Prepare Patients for Cardiac Testing

_____

_____

_____

_____

_____

_____

II. Anatomy and Physiology of the Heart

  A. Circulation of Blood
    i. The heart is a muscle that pumps blood throughout the body.
    ii. The _____ atrium receives _____ blood via the inferior and superior vena cava.
    iii. The blood passes through the _____ valve into the right ventricle, through the _____ valve and into the pulmonary arteries.

iv. The oxygen-_____ blood is transported through the pulmonary arteries, where a gas exchange takes place via the pulmonary alveolar-capillary network.

v. Oxygen is transferred to the blood and carbon dioxide is removed in the _____.

vi. This is removed in the _____ process via the _____.

vii. Oxygen-rich blood returns through the pulmonary _____ to the left _____.

viii. Upper left chamber of the heart pumps blood through _____ valve into the _____ ventricle.

ix. Aortic valve blood passes through the _____ coronary arteries of the heart, carotid arteries of the _____, and other circulatory arteries.

x. Blood goes through the _____ and _____ vena cava and returns to the right _____.

B. Layers of the Heart

_____

_____

_____

_____

C. The Myocardium

i. Myocardium is cardiac muscle cell containing _____ filaments.

ii. The actual _____ of myocardial tissue is what causes blood to flow.

D. Electrical Conduction of the Heart

_____

_____

_____

_____

_____

_____

_____

_____

_____

_____

_____

_____

_____

_____

E. The SA Node

i. The SA node is also called the _____ of the heart.

(a) This is where the _____ system begins.

ii. The SA node initiates electrical impulses that begin the process of _____ and _____ of cardiac cells.

iii. Depolarization is the _____ (or systole) of the heart.

iv. Repolarization is the _____ (or diastole) of the heart.

III. Coronary Artery Disease

A. Plaque buildup in the arteries is called _____.

B. Over time plaque increases and hardens the artery.

C. Blood flow is severely restricted when arteries become _____ or
   _____.

D. Ischemia =

   _____

   _____

E. Infarction occurs when there is complete _____.

F. Symptoms of CAD

   _____

   _____

   _____

   _____

IV. "Heart Attacks"

   A. There are two types of heart attacks:

   _____

   _____

   _____

   _____

   B. Myocardial ischemia
      i.   Reduced blood flow to the myocardium
      ii. Causes _____-type pain
      iii. If circulation is restored within _____ it may be reversed.

   C. Sudden cardiac death occurs when the conduction system suffers an insult, causing a/an
      _____ arrhythmia.

   _____

   _____

   _____

   _____

   _____

   _____

   D. Risk Factors
      i. Nonmodifiable risk factors:

   _____

      ii. Modifiable risk factors:

   _____

   E. Angina
      i.   _____-type pain felt when experiencing a cardiac problem
      ii. Usually down the _____ arm, to the left _____ and the
           right chest and arm
      iii. Immediate medical attention required to rule out _____
      iv. Intervention treatment includes:

   _____

   _____

   F. Myocardial Infarction
      i. Obstruction of myocardial tissue results in a myocardial infarction.
      ii. Ischemia occurs if blood is not restored within 6 hours.

iii. Ischemia caused by:

_____

_____

_____

_____

iv. Intervention:

_____

_____

_____

_____

G. Follow-Up Care/Tests
   i. Visit with a cardiovascular surgeon
  ii. Office visits including:

_____

_____

_____

_____

iii. Other conditions are assessed:

_____

_____

iv. If all assessments check out as normal, rehabilitation is discussed and scheduled.

H. Sudden Cardiac Arrest
   i. Ischemia in the _____ path
  ii. Lethal arrhythmia that causes the heart to stop
 iii. Causes:

_____

_____

_____

_____

iv. If _____ and _____ efforts are immediately applied, the victim may be resuscitated.

V. Hypertension

A. Known as the _____
B. Symptoms include:

_____

_____

C. Treatment

_____

_____

_____

_____

_____

_____

_____

_____

_____

_____

VI. Congestive Heart Failure
   A. Symptoms

_____

_____

_____

_____

_____

_____

   B. Treatment

_____

_____

_____

_____

_____

_____

   C. Pulmonary Edema

_____

_____

_____

_____

_____

_____

VII. Cardiomyopathy
   A. A noninflammatory disease of the _____
   B. Rarely is there an identifiable cause of the disease.
   C. Myocardial muscle thickens and the ability to pump blood is affected.
   D. Two types:
      i. _____
      ii. _____
   E. Walls of the heart become _____.
   F. Caused by increased workload of the myocardium
   G. Muscle fibers are stretched and chambers are dilated.
   H. Heart compensates and chambers enlarge to stretch even more: _____.
   I. Symptoms of _____ _____

_____

_____

_____

_____

   J. Treatment includes:

_____

_____

_____

_____

K. Hypertrophic Cardiomyopathy
  i. Wall of the heart _____ due to abnormal growth, usually in left
     _____
  ii. Causes difficulty in contraction and relaxation, thus blood flow diminishes
  iii. Symptoms include:

  _____

  _____

  iv. _____ _____ can result from occasional chaotic
      heartbeats
  v. Common in asymptomatic young males
  vi. Symptoms will appear after _____ _____.
  vii. Diagnosis includes echocardiograms and auscultation of heart sounds
  viii. Treatment is designed to inhibit lethal arrhythmias.

VIII. Cardiac Arrhythmias
  A. Heart automatically initiates an impulse that originates in the SA node.
  B. Numerous conditions cause interruptions of the impulse; _____
     _____.
  C. Classifications of Arrhythmia

  _____

  _____

  _____

  _____

  _____

  _____

  D. Arrhythmia Resulting from Point of Origin

  _____

  _____

  _____

  _____

  E. Arrhythmia Resulting from Conduction Disturbance
    i. Conduction of the impulse is _____ or has abnormal delays.
    ii. Blockage is categorized.

  _____

  _____

  _____

  _____

  F. Arrhythmia Resulting from Consistency of Impulse
    i. Impulses that have the same point of origin are called _____.
    ii. Various origination points are called multifocal.
    iii. ECG identifies _____ arrhythmias which are lethal.
    iv. Atrial rhythms originate in atria, ventricular rhythms in the ventricles.
    v. Sinus rhythms originate in the _____ node, nodal rhythms in the
       _____ node.

G. Arrhythmia According to Prognosis
   i. Seriousness or prognosis is another method of arrhythmia classification.

   _____

   _____

   _____

   _____

   ii. Death-producing arrhythmias require immediate and aggressive intervention.
H. Arrhythmia Treatment
   i. Antiarrhythmic drugs
      (a) Medication controls the _____ and does not address the
          _____ cause.
      (b) Frequent assessment until condition clears or symptoms disappear
   ii. Pacemakers or internal defibrillators

   _____

   _____

IX. Infective Heart Diseases and Disorders

   A. Caused by Bacteria, Viruses, Fungi or Parasites
   B. Endocarditis
      i. _____ infections that cause heart chamber lining and valve surfaces to
         _____

      ii. Usually occurs on the _____ side of the heart
      iii. _____

      iv. Heart murmurs are heard if the left side cannot completely close.
      v. Symptoms

      _____

      _____

      _____

      _____

   C. Myocarditis
      i. Cardiac muscle inflamed due to a/an _____ _____ or
         _____.

      ii. Symptoms

      _____

      _____

      iii. Treatment includes _____ for infection and _____ to con-
           trol the arrhythmias.
   D. Pericarditis
      i. Sac of the pericardium becomes inflamed
      ii. Results from infection, inflammation, or other conditions
      iii. Symptoms

      _____

      _____

      iv. _____ is the most common treatment.
   E. Rheumatic Fever or Disease
      i. Usually follows a sore throat caused by:

      _____

      ii. Valves/endocardium become inflamed and bacteria grow and form endocardial scar tissue.

    iii. Leads to valvular _____ and/or _____

    iv. Symptoms

               _____

               _____

    v. Prevention is the best _____.

X. Valvular Disorders

  A. Any of the heart valves can be affected by disease or disorder

  B. There are four different valves of the heart:

        _____

        _____

        _____

        _____

  C. When a valve fails to close completely it's called _____.

  D. When a constriction causes the valve to fail it's called _____.

  E. Mitral Valve Disorder

        _____

        _____

        _____

        _____

        _____

        _____

        _____

XI. Vascular Disorders

  A. Phlebitis

        _____

        _____

        _____

        _____

  B. Thrombophelbitis

        _____

        _____

        _____

        _____

        _____

  C. Embolisms

        _____

        _____

        _____

        _____

        _____

D. Deep Vein Thrombosis

_____

_____

_____

_____

_____

_____

E. Arteriosclerosis and Atherosclerosis

_____

_____

_____

_____

_____

_____

F. Aneurysm

_____

_____

_____

_____

_____

_____

G. Raynaud's Disease

_____

_____

_____

_____

_____

_____

H. Berger's Disease

_____

_____

_____

_____

_____

_____

XII. Cardiac Testing
    A. The Electrocardiogram
        i. Equipment that measures the _____ activity of the heart
        ii. Recording called electrocardiogram (ECK or EKG)
        iii. Indicates _____ areas of the myocardium that helps diagnose cardiac
           _____
        iv. Electrocardiograph prints a record of the heart's electrical activity.

v. _____ = cardiac monitor displaying heart's electrical responses on screen
vi. _____ are placed on patient, who is connected to the electrocardiograph.
B. 12-Lead EKG
   i. Measures different planes of the _____
   ii. _____ is the most important.
   iii. Shows the P waves of the heart and is recorded on the rhythm strip
   iv. Limb leads: _____
   v. Augmented leads are: _____
   vi. Precordial leads: _____
C. The Holter Monitor
   i. _____ heart monitor patients can use at home
   ii. Noninvasive way to measure _____ in day-to-day activities
   iii. Patients must avoid _____ and record all major events in a diary.
   iv. Patients return after _____ for equipment to be removed.
   v. Results are interpreted by a/an _____.
D. Stress Testing
   i. For patients with cardiac history or cardiovascular surgery
   ii. Test measures the patient's heart while on a controlled _____
      _____
   iii. A/an _____ is performed _____ to stress test and respiration
      is monitored
E. The MA's Role in Stress Testing
   i. Medical assistants _____ stress testing equipment and patients.
   ii. MAs must make sure the patient understands:
      _____
      _____
      _____
      _____
F. Echocardiogram
   i. Ultrasound of arteries, _____, _____, pulmonary
      veins/arteries, and superior vena cava
   ii. Visualizes _____ thickness, position, and movements of cardiac structures
   iii. _____ test that uses a transducer and gel to help the sound waves enter body
   iv. Tests:
      _____
      _____
      _____
      _____
      _____
   v. MAs do not perform this test, but assist the patient and/or technician.
G. Thallium Scan
   i. A/an _____ infusion of the radioisotope _____ is used to
      assess myocardial perfusion.
   ii. At the _____ of the stress test, thallium is infused.
   iii. A/an _____ camera is used to take pictures of the _____.
   iv. Ischemic or diseased portions of heart do not absorb the thallium.
   v. Helps determine possible prognosis of myocardial condition
H. MUGA Scan
   _____
   _____

XIII. Cardiac Rhythms

    A. Normal Sinus Rhythm (NSR)

    B. Sinus Bradycardia

    C. Sinus Tachycardia

    D. Atrial Fibrillation (A-fib)

    E. Atrial Flutter

    F. Supraventricular Tachycardia (SVT)

    G. Paroxysmal Atrial Tachycardia (PAT)

    H. Premature Atrial Contractions (PACs)

    I. Premature Junctional Rhythms (PJC)

    J. Bundle Branch Block (BBB)

    K. First-Degree AV Block

L. Second-Degree Heart Block I, Mobitz Type I

_____

_____

M. Premature Ventricular Contractions (PVCs)

_____

_____

N. Unifocal PVCs

_____

_____

O. Multifocal PVCs

_____

_____

P. Ventricular Tachycardia (V-tach)

_____

_____

Q. Ventricular Fibrillation (V-fib)

_____

_____

R. Asystole

_____

_____

KEY TERMINOLOGY REVIEW

Write a sentence using the selected vocabulary terms in the correct context.

1. Angina:

_____

_____

2. Artifact:

_____

_____

3. Dysphasia:

_____

_____

4. Depolarization:

_____

_____

5. Embolism or emboli:

_____

_____

6. Focus or foci:

_____

_____

7. Palpitations:

_____

_____

8. Precordial lead:

_____

_____

9. Sinoatrial node:

_____

_____

10. Stenosis:

_____

_____

11. Stent:

_____

_____

12. Systole:

_____

_____

13. Tachycardia:

_____

_____

14. Thrombosis:

_____

_____

15. Unifocal:

_____

_____

APPLIED PRACTICE

Follow the directions as instructed with each question below.

1. Read the following scenario and answer the corresponding questions.

Scenario

Carmen DiStefano, CMA (AAMA) is working with Dr. Juarez. Dr. Juarez has instructed Carmen to perform an EKG on Mr. Capstone in exam room #3. When Carmen reviews the chart she reads the following information.

| | | | Capstone, Kevin. |
| | | | 06-14-1942 |

04/14/20XX 1:15 pm   Wt: 234 lbs   T: 99.0°F   P: 118 bpm   R: 22, labored   BP: 140/92

cc: Pt. has gained 20 lbs since 3/01/xx. Pt states that he has been SOB with pain near the center of his chest and says "I can't seem to get enough sleep." Pt had difficulty walking to the examination room from waiting room. -- *Carmen DiStefano, CMA (AAMA)*

a. Based on his signs and symptoms, what cardiovascular disease does this resemble?

_____

_____

b. Label on the figure below where Carmen should place the precordial leads:

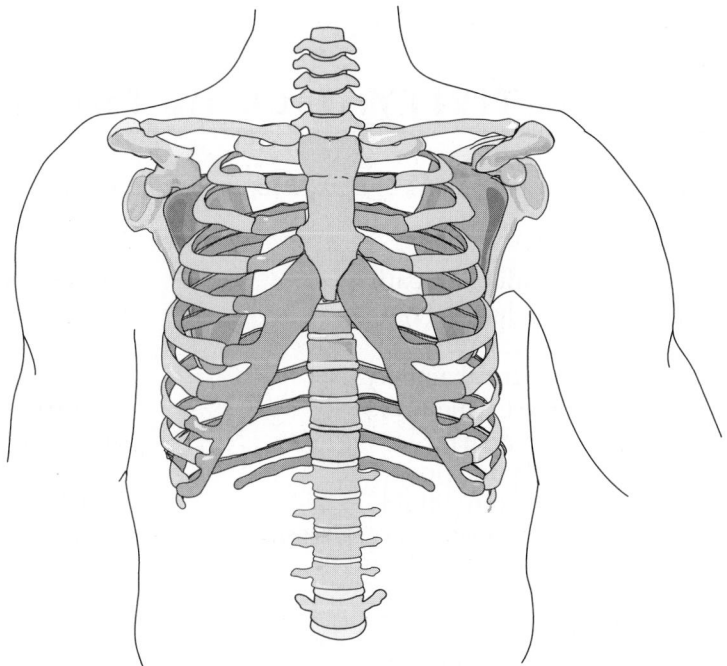

FIGURE 35-1 The precordial leads

c. Create a normal EKG waveform and label isoelectric lines and the P, Q, R, S, T waves.

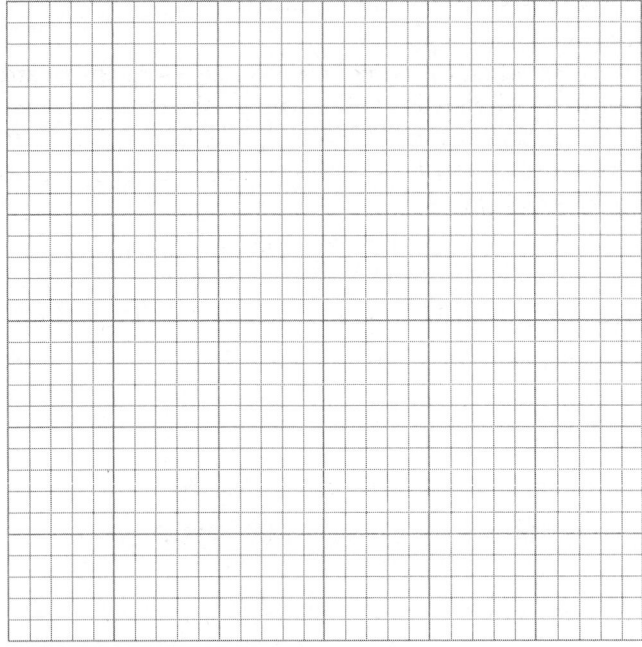

FIGURE 35-2   ECG waveforms

LEARNING ACTIVITY: FILL IN THE BLANK

Using words from the list below, fill in the blanks to complete the following statements.

24-hour period
abnormal EKG
angina-type pain
aorta and the coronary vessels
arm or groin
arrest
arrhythmia
bacterial infection
cardiac condition
catheter
chambers

CHF
conduction path
conduction system
contractility
electrical activity
heart structures
hemorrhage
inflammation
interstitial fluid
life-threatening situation
massive insult

noninvasive
pacemaker
portable
reduced blood flow
sinoatrial (SA) node
standstill
surfaces
trauma
visual
workload

1. An echocardiogram provides a/an _____ concept of the _____ coordinated with the _____ and the _____ of the myocardium.

2. Myocardial ischemia is the result of _____ to the myocardium, which causes _____.

3. Pulmonary edema follows _____ as the lungs fill with _____ and pressure builds in the lung tissue, increasing the _____ of the heart.

4. An electrocardiogram is a recording of the _____ of the heart.

5. The medical assistant performing EKGs must know when to alert the physician to an _____ or a/an _____.

6. The conduction system originates in the _____, also known as the _____.

7. Sudden cardiac arrest occurs when the conduction system of the myocardium sustains a/an _____, such as ischemia in the area of the essential cardiac _____, a lethal _____ that causes cardiac _____, electrocution, major _____ to the chest and heart, massive _____, drug overdose, respiratory _____, and drowning.

8. Endocarditis, a/an _____ of the lining of the heart _____ and valve _____, is usually the result of a/an _____.

9. During a cardiac catheterization, a/an _____ is threaded through an artery in the _____ to the _____ and dye is injected into the vessels.

10. A Holter monitor is a/an _____ form of monitoring that allows _____ recording of the patient's _____ over a/an _____.

CRITICAL THINKING

Answer the following questions to the best of your ability. Use the textbook as a reference.

1. You are working at the front desk and looking out at the patients who have been waiting for their appointments. One man appears to be holding his left hand in front of his chest, he seems to be SOB, and his face looks sweaty or clammy. What is your first thought about this patient? Describe what the danger signs are to you even though the patient has not come up to the desk to voice a complaint about how he is feeling. What might you ask the patient and how would you handle that?

_____
_____
_____
_____

2. You are performing an EKG. As it is printing, you notice that there is a normal waveform and complex but the beats per minute are over 100. What do you think the problem could be? Use the information from Table 35-10, Cardiac Rhythms, to speculate on what the doctor might diagnose.

_____
_____
_____
_____

3. You are doing a history on a new patient and the patient states that she often feels that her heart has "skipped a beat." Review the information on identifying arrhythmias and dysrhythmias, then state what this may be. Then define what this condition is.

_____
_____
_____

4. What would you do if a patient fell in the waiting room and had no pulse? Explain in detail.

5. You need to perform an EKG on an elderly female patient, but she seems to be nervous or fearful. What are some of the signs the patient might exhibit that lead you to the conclusion she is fearful of the EKG? How would that fear affect the EKG?

RESEARCH ACTIVITY

Use Internet search engines to research the following topics and write a brief description of what is found. It is important to visit reputable Web sites.

1. Visit www.americanheart.org and navigate through the Web site. Pay particular attention to the link entitled For Healthcare Professionals. Explain what information you think is most useful in this section and why.

CHAPTER 36
Pulmonology and Pulmonary Testing

CHAPTER OUTLINE

General review of the chapter:

   A. Introduction
   B. The Medical Assistant's Role in Pulmonology
   C. Anatomy and Physiology of the Pulmonary System
      i. The upper airway
      ii. The lower airways
      iii. Pulmonary physiology
   D. Diseases and Disorders of the Pulmonary System
   E. Pulmonary Assessment and Diagnosis
   F. Inhalers and Nebulizers
   G. Oxygen Therapy

STUDENT STUDY GUIDE

Use the following guide to assist in your learning of the concepts from the chapter.

  I. The MA's Role in Pulmonology
    A. _____
    B. _____
    C. _____
    D. _____

  II. Anatomy and Physiology of the Pulmonary System
    A. Anatomy of the Upper Airway
      _____
      _____
      _____
      _____

    B. Anatomy of the Lower Airway
      i. _____ cavity:
        _____
        _____
      ii. Pleural cavity: formed by the _____
        _____
        _____

    iii. _____: membrane covering lungs

_____

_____

    iv. Trachea divides into right and left _____.

    v. The bronchi divide into bronchioles.

    vi. Bronchioles have clusters of air sacs called _____.

C. Pulmonary Physiology

    i. Main components include:

_____

_____

_____

_____

    ii. Physical mechanics include _____ and _____.

D. Mechanics of Gas Exchange

    i. Law of _____ is the basis of gas mechanics.

    ii. Diffusion is when molecules move across a membrane from an area of
_____ concentration to an area of _____ concentrations.

    iii. Lungs exchange _____ and _____ through diffusion.

    iv. _____-rich blood circulates from the right side of the heart to the lungs.

    v. During inhalation blood enters the lungs and the oxygen diffuses into the carbon-dioxide-rich blood to raise the oxygen level.

    vi. Excess carbon dioxide is _____.

    vii. The oxygen-rich blood returns to the left side of the heart for various organs and tissues in the body.

III. Diseases and Disorders of the Pulmonary System

A. Upper Respiratory Diseases and Disorders

_____

_____

_____

_____

_____

_____

B. Classification of Lower Respiratory Diseases and Disorders

_____

_____

_____

_____

C. Chronic Obstructive Lung Disease

    i. Collective name for long-term lung diseases that block the airway

    ii. Caused by:

_____

_____

    iii. Secondary conditions include chronic _____ and _____.

    iv. Treatment:

_____

_____

    v. Asthma, acute bronchitis, and pneumonoconiosis are also included.

D. Infectious and Inflammatory Disorders
  i. Pathogenic microorganisms such as bacteria and viruses cause inflammation.
  ii. Disorders include:

  _____

  _____

  _____

  _____

E. Malignancies
  i. Cancer of the lung(s) and larynx
  ii. Symptoms are similar to a/an _____ _____.
  iii. _____ growth blocks the respiratory airway, decreasing oxygen flow.
  iv. Smokers and/or people with family history require support and education for a healthy lifestyle.
F. Mechanical Insults
  i. _____

  ii. _____

  iii. Pneumothorax: lungs partially or completely collapse
  iv. _____: blood accumulation in pleural cavity which restricts lung expansion
  v. Hemopneumothorax: _____ and _____ accumulate, causing collapse of the lung(s)
IV. Pulmonary Assessment and Diagnosis
  A. Symptoms of Pulmonary Disorders or Disease
    i. Sounds:

    _____

    _____

    _____

    _____

    ii. Cyanosis
    iii. Cough:

    _____

    _____

    iv. Sputum: may be blood-tinged (hemoptysis) or yellow/green (indicates infection)
    v. Chronic respiratory conditions:

    _____

    _____

    _____

    _____

  B. Respiratory Breathing Patterns

  _____

  _____

  _____

  _____

  C. Pulmonary Function Tests
    i. Assess the performance of the _____ system
    ii. Confirm, evaluate and/or manage diagnosed pulmonary disorders

iii. Several types of PFTs exist, which include:

_____

_____

D. Spirometry

_____

_____

_____

_____

_____

E. Chest X-Rays
   i. Noninvasive
   ii. Help diagnose or screen for:

_____

_____

F. Arterial Blood Gases (ABGs)
   i. Used to analyze the acid/base balance of blood in acute and chronic respiratory conditions
       including:

_____

_____

G. Pulse Oximetry
   i.   Noninvasive screening of _____ _____ of tissues
   ii. Analyzes symptoms of cardiac, circulatory, or respiratory distress
   iii. Such conditions include:

_____

_____

_____

_____

H. Methacholine Challenge Test
   i.   Used in the diagnosis and treatment of _____
   ii. Patient inhales _____ and increasing amounts of methacholine and
        undergoes _____
   iii. PFTs assess the reaction of the _____ airways and the effect on the
        _____ _____.

I. Additional Diagnostic Tests
   i.   _____ _____ used to diagnose respiratory infections, such
        as pneumonia
   ii. _____ sputum samples diagnose lung carcinoma (malignant tumor).
   iii. Acid-fast bacilli (AFB) sputum samples are used in culture testing for pulmonary
        tuberculosis.
   iv. Blood tests for _____ level reveals inadequate, excessive, or toxic medication
        levels
   v.   Sweat test is performed to confirm diagnosis of _____
        _____
   vi. _____ is an invasive procedure for visualizing the bronchial tree, clearing
        mucous obstructions, and obtaining a biopsy.
   vii. Other diagnostic tests include the peak flow test and Mantoux test.

V. Treatment for Pulmonary Disorders
    A. Inhalers and Nebulizers
        i. Treat obstructive airway disorders
        ii. _____
        iii. Inhalers are small and portable.
        iv. Allow patient to _____-_____ medication
        v. _____ deliver fine particles of medication via compressed air through a
        mask and tubing.
        vi. Nebulizers are usually used in a hospital but also in _____
        _____ settings.
    B. Oxygen Therapy
        i. Administered for three reasons

        _____
        _____
        _____
        _____

        ii. Administered through nasal cannula (nasal prongs) and a portable oxygen tank
        iii. Safety considerations:

        _____
        _____
        _____
        _____

KEY TERMINOLOGY REVIEW

Match the correct medical term with the definition listed below.

a.	alveolus	**m.**	hemothorax
b.	asthma	**n.**	hepatotoxicity
c.	bronchiole	**o.**	immunocompetence
d.	bronchitis	**p.**	intradermal
e.	bronchodilator	**q.**	noninvasive
f.	bronchus	**r.**	orthopnea
g.	diaphragm	**s.**	ototoxicity
h.	dyspnea	**t.**	pneumothorax
i.	emphysema	**u.**	pulmonary function testing
j.	eupnea	**v.**	septum
k.	hemopneumothorax	**w.**	tachypnea
l.	hemoptysis		

_____ 1. Airway less than 1 mm in diameter.

_____ 2. Primary muscle of breathing; separates chest and abdominal cavities.

_____ 3. Normal breathing.

_____ 4. Body's ability to fight infection.

_____ 5. Harmful effects of drugs on nerves or organs in the ear.

_____ 6. Lung disease characterized by wheezing and shortness of breath; often caused by an allergic response.

_____ 7. Disease of chronic airway obstruction (COLD) in which air is trapped; usually caused by either smoking or heredity.

_____ 8. Coughing up sputum containing blood.

_____ 9. Pertaining to a procedure or technique that does not require entry into the body through incision or inserting an instrument.

_____ 10. The collection of air or gas in the pleural cavity that causes the lung to partially or completely collapse.

_____ 11. Testing performed to evaluate air flow and lung volume.

_____ 12. Microscopic air sacs that are the primary unit of gas exchange in the lungs.

_____ 13. Between the layers of the skin.

_____ 14. One of two primary airways that branch into the lungs.

_____ 15. Accumulation of blood and air in the pleural cavity; resulting in the partial or complete collapse of the lung.

_____ 16. Lung disease characterized by large volumes of pulmonary secretions and air trapping; can be chronic or acute in nature.

_____ 17. Harmful effect of drugs on the liver.

_____ 18. A thin wall dividing the two sides of the interior nose.

_____ 19. The ability to breathe only in a standing or upright sitting position.

_____ 20. Accumulation of blood and fluids in the pleural cavity that limit the expansion of the lung.

_____ 21. Difficulty breathing.

_____ 22. Rapid breathing.

_____ 23. Medication that dilates the walls of the bronchi.

APPLIED PRACTICE

Follow the directions as instructed with each question below.

1. Read the scenario and answer the questions that follow.

Scenario

It is a slow day at Fairview Family Practice where you are working as a clinical medical assistant. As you return files to the front office for filing, you see a woman rushing through the front door of the reception area. She states that her teenage son is in the car and suddenly began to have an asthma attack as they were driving. Two of your colleagues rush outside with the mother to assist in transporting the boy to an exam room. At the same time you inform the physician of the situation. He asks that you gather "necessary" supplies to assist him in assessing and treating the boy.

   a. What signs and symptoms would the boy exhibit during a severe asthma attack?

   _____

   _____

   _____

b. What "necessary" supplies would you gather?

_____

_____

c. What steps might the physician take to assess and treat the boy?

_____

_____

_____

2. Label the structures of the respiratory system on the figure below.

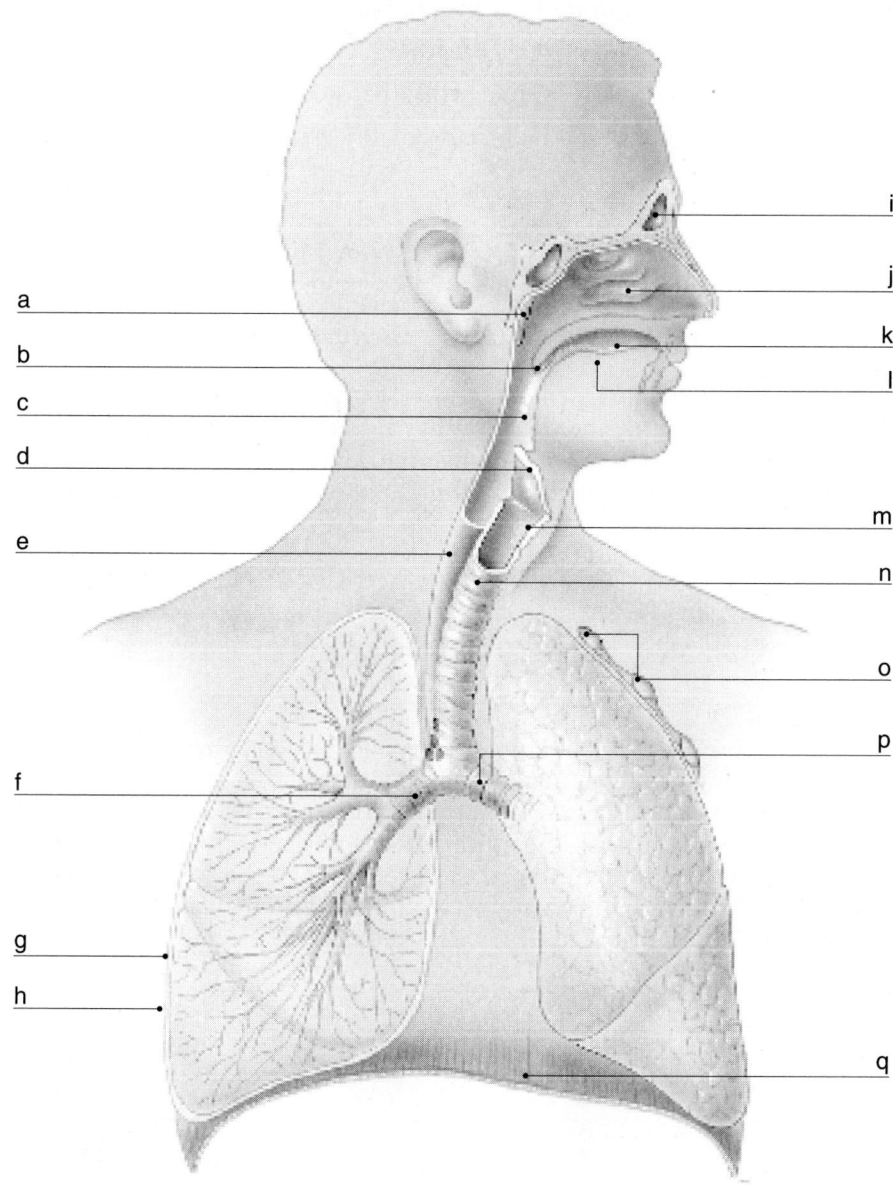

The respiratory system

LEARNING ACTIVITY: TRUE/FALSE

Indicate whether the statement is true (T) or false (F).

_____ 1. Oxygen is a prescription drug that is administered only with a physician's order.

_____ 2. The upper airway consists of the nose and the adjacent zone of the pharynx.

_____ 3. Mucous is a thick fluid secreted by membranes.

_____ 4. Saliva begins digestion in the mouth.

_____ 5. The Mantoux test is used to screen patients for contact with or presence of the active disease state of TB.

_____ 6. Acute rhinitis is the most common URI.

_____ 7. The pulse oximeter uses an infrared light to measure oxygen in the tissues.

_____ 8. The acronym ABCD stands for airway, breathing, cardiovascular, defibrillation.

_____ 9. A peak flow meter can detect an asthma attack before symptoms occur.

_____ 10. The Mantoux test is administered by intradermal injection of petrified protein derivative (PPD).

CRITICAL THINKING

Answer the following questions to the best of your ability. Use the textbook as a reference.

1. You have prepared an intradermal Mantoux test for a patient who is elderly. You check both anterior forearms to select a site for the injection but find that both of her arms are covered in a heat rash. Where else could this test be administered? The Internet, medical dictionaries and encyclopedias, and various patient care and/or clinical books are good sources to research this if you need help.

_____

_____

_____

_____

_____

2. You have been asked to help a young patient and her mother with a nebulizer treatment for the child. The child is in such respiratory distress that you work quickly to get it prepared and started. About five minutes into the treatment, you realize you did not perform a PFT on the patient for a baseline prior to starting the nebulizer and medication. Although this is not covered in the textbook, use critical thinking skills to determine what you would do. You may even offer more than one possible course of action.

_____

_____

_____

_____

_____

3. A patient has been put on home oxygen therapy, and you have set up the delivery of the equipment. You have instructed the patient on the use and maintenance of the equipment. Instruct the patient about safety around oxygen; write your answer as if speaking to the patient.

_____

_____

_____

_____

_____

4. A patient needs to start using an inhaler at home on a daily basis. The patient has rheumatoid arthritis and cannot hold the inhaler the usual way. What would you do or how would you teach this patient to use the inhaler?

_____

_____

_____

_____

_____

5. You have a patient with obstructive lung disease who wants to know why he has a hard time breathing. This person has a form of COLD that doesn't allow him to exhale very much. Explain briefly here, as if explaining to the patient, why he feels so short of breath.

_____

_____

_____

_____

_____

RESEARCH ACTIVITY

Use Internet search engines to research the following topics and write a brief description of what is found. It is important to visit reputable Web sites.

1. Visit www.lungusa.org. What information do you think will be most useful in regard to patient education? What is "hidden" asthma, and what age group does it commonly affect? How can this information be useful to patients?

_____

_____

_____

_____

_____

_____

_____

_____

_____

CHAPTER 37
EENT

CHAPTER OUTLINE

General review of the chapter:

A. Introduction
B. The Medical Assistant's Role in the EENT Practice
C. The Anatomy and Physiology of the Eye
   i. Disorders and diseases of the eye
   ii. Diagnostic procedures
D. The Anatomy and Physiology of the Ear
   i. Disorders and diseases of the ear
   ii. Diagnostic procedures
   iii. Ear treatments
E. The Anatomy and Physiology of the Nose
   i. Disorders and diseases of the nose and nasal passages
   ii. Diagnosis and treatment
F. The Anatomy and Physiology of the Throat
   i. Diseases of the mouth and throat
   ii. Diagnosis and treatment

STUDENT STUDY GUIDE

Use the following guide to assist in your learning of the concepts from the chapter.

I. The MA's Role in EENT and Other EENT Health Care Practitioners

A. The MA's Role in the EENT Practice
   i. Obtaining and recording vital signs and patient history
   ii. Testing _____ acuity
   iii. Performing _____
   iv. Performing eye and ear _____ and _____
B. EENT Physicians
   i. _____ : eye diseases and conditions
   ii. _____ : ear, nose, and throat diseases and conditions
   iii. _____ : ear and throat diseases and disorders
   iv. _____ : throat diseases and disorders
   v. _____ : nose diseases and disorders
   vi. _____ : ear diseases and disorders
C. Other EENT Health Care Providers
   i. Optometrists and _____ are not _____.
   ii. Patients are referred to an ophthalmologist if _____ is suspected.
   iii. _____ are trained to examine eyes, test visual acuity, and prescribe contact lenses.
   iv. _____ are trained to grind lenses, insert lenses into frames, and fit eyeglasses.

II. The Eye
   A. Anatomical Structures of the Eye
      i. Eyebrows, _____, _____, frontal orbital sockets, conjunctiva, and the mucous membrane covering the eyeball
      ii. Three layers of tissue in the eyeball:

      _____

      _____

      _____

   B. Eye Tissues
      i.   _____: the fibrous white tissue on the outside of the eyeball
      ii. Vascular tunic or choroids: thin layer of tissue that contains blood vessels, lymphatics, and intrinsic eye muscles
      iii. Iris and ciliary body are in the _____ layer.
      iv. _____ transmits images to the brain via the optic nerve.
      v.   Humors help maintain the eye's internal _____ and fill the globe of the eye.
      vi. The _____ regulates the light that enters the eye and displays the eye _____.
      vii. The _____ nerve sends the image to the thalamus.
      viii. Intrinsic muscles are the colored portion of the eye membrane.
   C. Eye Muscles
      i.   Superior rectus muscle: moves the eye to look _____
      ii. Inferior rectus muscle: moves the eye to look _____
      iii. Lateral rectus muscle: moves the eye _____ (corner to corner)
      iv. Medial rectus muscle: moves the eye _____ (to the middle)
      v.   Superior oblique muscle: rolls the eye as it looks _____ and to the _____
      vi. Inferior oblique muscle: rolls the eye as it looks _____ and to the _____
   D. Eye Disorders and Diseases
      i.   Refractive disorders include any type of disruption to the light path in the eye.
           (a) Variations of refractive errors include:

           _____

           _____

           _____

           _____

      ii. Infectious disorders include:

           _____

           _____

           _____

           _____

      iii. Degenerative disorders include:

           _____

           _____

           _____

           _____

      iv. Disorders are also caused by insult or injuries from foreign bodies.

E. Diagnostic Eye Equipment
    i. Ophthalmoscope: used to examine the _____ and other internal structures of the eye
    ii. _____ _____: used to examine and perform specialized procedures within the front of the eye
    iii. Eye spud: used to remove a/an _____ _____ or rust ring from the cornea
    iv. _____: used to measure intraocular pressure
    v. Snellen chart: measures _____ visual acuity
    vi. Jaeger chart: measures _____-_____ acuity

III. The Ear
    A. Anatomical Structures of the External Ear
    _____
    _____
    _____
    _____
    _____
    _____

    B. Anatomical Structures of the Middle Ear
    _____
    _____
    _____
    _____
    _____
    _____

    C. Anatomical Structures of the Inner Ear
    _____
    _____
    _____
    _____
    _____
    _____

    D. Diseases and Disorders of the Outer Ear
        i. Impacted _____
            (a) Earwax hardens and compacts, causing hearing loss.
        ii. _____ _____
            (a) Inflammation of outer ear (swimmer's ear) causes impaired hearing
        iii. Foreign bodies
            (a) Injury from _____ or _____ going into ear canal; causes impaired hearing
    E. Diseases and Disorders of the Middle Ear
        i. Otosclerosis
    _____
    _____
    _____

ii. Ruptured tympanic membrane

_____

_____

_____

iii. Otitis media

_____

_____

_____

F. Diseases and Disorders of the Inner Ear
i. Labyrinthitis

_____

_____

_____

_____

ii. Menière's disease

_____

_____

_____

_____

iii. Nerve trauma

_____

_____

_____

_____

G. Diagnostic Hearing Procedures
i. Audiologists perform audiometry to measure patient's hearing:

_____

_____

_____

_____

_____

_____

H. Instruments to Assess the Ear
i. _____: handheld device to visualize inside of ear
ii. _____ _____: used to examine the external auditory canal and eardrum
iii. _____ _____: magnifies the tympanic membrane
iv. Tuning fork

IV. The Nose

A. Anatomical Structures of the Nose
i. Nasal septum separates the interior nose, which has three zones:
(a) **Vestibular zone:**

_____

_____

_____

(b) **Olfactory zone:**

_____

_____

_____

(c) **Respiratory zone:**

_____

_____

_____

    ii. Sinuses: surround nose inside of skull

B. Diseases and Disorders of the Nose

    i. Upper respiratory tract infections:

_____

_____

_____

    ii. Epistaxis:

_____

_____

_____

    iii. Foreign bodies:

_____

_____

_____

    iv. Nasal polyps:

_____

_____

_____

    v. Rhinitis:

_____

_____

_____

    vi. Septal defects:

_____

_____

_____

    vii. Sinusitis:

_____

_____

_____

V. The Throat

A. Anatomy of the Throat

    i. _____: located above soft palate; includes tonsils (adenoids) and Eustachian tube

    ii. _____: portion visible when mouth is open; palatine tonsils, oral cavity, teeth, tongue and taste buds, cheeks, and salivary glands

iii. _____: above vocal cords, lingual tonsils, epiglottis, which is the cartilage that prevents liquids from entering the airway

iv. Vocal cords:

_____

_____

_____

B. Diseases of the Mouth and Throat

_____

_____

_____

_____

_____

_____

KEY TERMINOLOGY REVIEW

Match the selected key terms to their definitions below.

a.	acuity	**i.**	optician
b.	audiologist	**j.**	optometrist
c.	audiometry	**k.**	otic
d.	cerumen	**l.**	otologist
e.	decibel	**m.**	purulent
f.	intraocular	**n.**	tinnitus
g.	laryngologist	**o.**	vertigo
h.	ophthalmologist		

_____ 1. Unit for measuring the intensity of sound.

_____ 2. Physician who specializes in the treatment of eye diseases and disorders.

_____ 3. Physician who specializes in the treatment of ear diseases.

_____ 4. Containing pus.

_____ 5. Professional trained to assess hearing levels.

_____ 6. Ringing in the ears.

_____ 7. Within the eye.

_____ 8. Pertaining to the ear.

_____ 9. Earwax.

_____ 10. Measuring and testing hearing acuity.

_____ 11. Keenness or sharpness.

_____ 12. Physician specializing in disorders and diseases of the throat.

_____ 13. Trained professional who grinds lens, inserts the lens into frames, and fits the patient's glasses.

_____ 14. Licensed professional who examines eyes, tests for visual acuity, prescribes and adapts lens for patients.

_____ 15. Dizziness.

APPLIED PRACTICE

Read the scenario below and answer the questions that follow.

Activity 1

Scenario

Shawn is working as a medical assistant at a local family practice. Rajan Avuri is a 17-year-old patient being seen for a driver's license physical exam. As part of the exam, Shawn tests Rajan's vision with a Snellen Eye chart similar to the Snellen eye chart below. Shawn asks Rajan to cover his right eye and read line 8. Rajan reads the following letters from left to right "D, E, F, P, O, T, E, C." Shawn asks Rajan to continue and read line 9. Rajan reads the following letters from left to right "L, E, P, O, D, R, O, T."

Shawn then asks Rajan to uncover his right eye and cover his left eye for assessment. Beginning with line 8, Rajan reads the following letters from left to right "D, E, F, R, O, T, E, C." Rajan is not able to distinguish any letters on the lines below number 8.

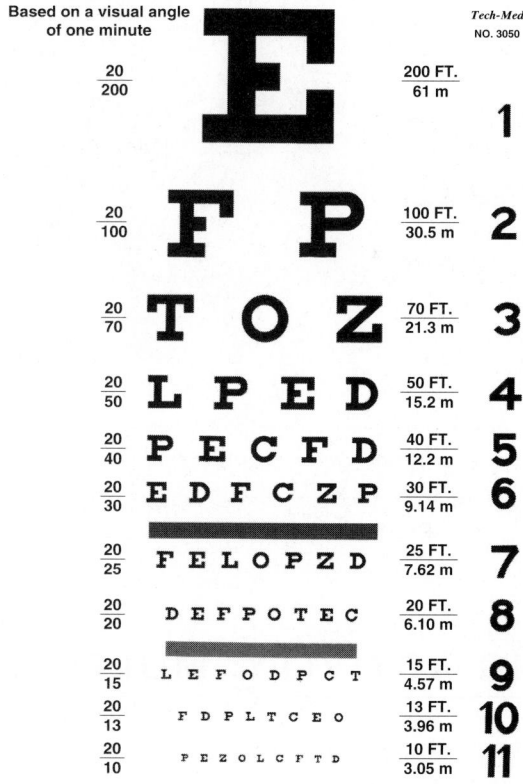

Snellen chart

1. How should Shawn record Rajan's vision in his left eye? Explain your answer.

_____

_____

_____

_____

2. How should Shawn record Rajan's vision in his right eye? Explain your answer.

_____

_____

_____

_____

Activity 2

Label the structures of the ear.

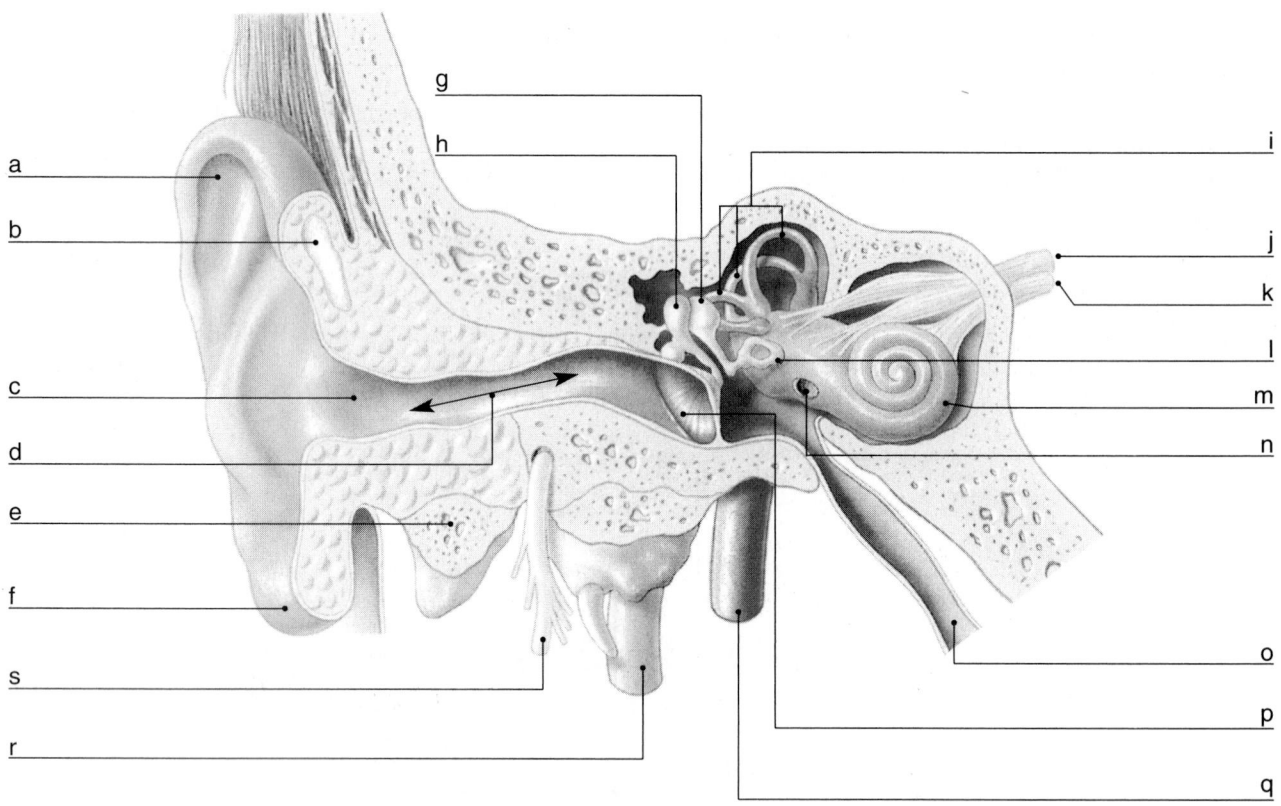

LEARNING ACTIVITY: MULTIPLE CHOICE

Circle the correct answer to each of the questions below.

1. Which physician would prescribe adaptive lenses?
   a. ophthalmologist
   b. otologist
   c. optometrist
   d. rhinologists

2. Which instrument measures intraocular pressure?
   a. ophthalmoscope
   b. tonometer
   c. slit lamp
   d. otoscope

3. Bright light reduces pupil size as the circular muscle of the _____ contracts.

   a. choroid
   b. cornea

   c. retina
   d. iris

4. Items used to cover one eye while testing the other eye during a Snellen visual acuity test include (circle all that apply):

   a. card
   b. occluder

   c. spud
   d. spatula

5. The outer or external ear is comprised of the (circle all that apply):

   a. auricle
   b. pinna

   c. external auditory canal
   d. cerumen

6. Which tasks does the medical assistant perform in an EENT practice? (Circle all that apply.)

   a. performing audiometry
   b. performing tonometry

   c. performing eye and ear irrigations
   d. testing visual acuity

7. The chonchae are the nasal bones located in the most interior portion of the nose; their purpose is to (circle all that apply):

   a. warm the air
   b. soften the palate

   c. filter air inhaled by trapping particles
   d. humidify air before it reaches the respiratory zone

8. One of the three types of color *deficiency* is

   a. protanopia
   b. myopia

   c. Daltonism
   d. Ishihara

9. Which of the following are functions of the sinuses? (Circle all that apply.)

   a. to reduce the weight of the eyeballs
   b. to reduce the weight of the skull

   c. to enhance phonation
   d. to produce vocal sounds

10. The three tiny bones or ossicles in the middle ear are:

   a. otosclerosis
   b. malleus

   c. stapes
   d. incus

LEARNING ACTIVITY: TRUE/FALSE

Indicate whether the statement is true (T) or false (F).

_____ 1. Humors of the eye are watery fluids that help maintain the eye's internal pressure.

_____ 2. The laryngopharanyx is just above the soft palate.

_____ 3. The two types of color blindness are achromatic vision and Daltonism.

_____ 4. Drops used to stain the eyes for an ophthalmological exam are called fluorescein.

_____ 5. Cerumen can block the passage of sound waves to the external ear.

_____ 6. An eye patch may be ordered to keep the eyelid from passing back and forth over the cornea.

_____ 7. Hearing tests include tuning fork testing.

_____ 8. The holes in the nose are known as nares.

_____ 9. Labyrinthitis is also known as otitis media.

_____ 10. An eye spud is used to remove a foreign particle or rust ring from the retina.

CRITICAL THINKING

Answer the following questions to the best of your ability. Use the textbook as a reference.

1. You need to perform a Snellen visual acuity test and an Ishihara color vision test per the physician's orders. You do not have an occluder or the Ishihara plates. Which of the tests, if any, could you still perform using a different item and what replacement item(s) can you use?

   _____

   _____

   _____

   _____

   _____

2. If a patient called in for an appointment for possible hearing loss, which specialist would the physician likely suggest for the patient be referred to?

   _____

   _____

   _____

   _____

   _____

3. In the case study for this chapter, answer the following questions:

   a. What is the likely treatment the physician will order for the 4-year-old girl with sand in her eye?

      _____

      _____

   b. Who would likely perform the Snellen visual acuity test on the college student?

      _____

      _____

   c. What specialist would be most appropriate to see the 3-year-old boy with a toy stuck in his nose?

      _____

      _____

4. You work for an optometrist in the optical department of a large medical center. The provider sees a patient and performs tonometry only to find the intraocular pressure reading is very high. What specialist would the optometrist refer this patient to for the IOP?

_____

_____

_____

_____

5. You are asked by the physician to perform an ear irrigation on a 12-year-old patient because the tympanic membrane cannot be seen due to a large amount of cerumen. How will you know when the irrigation is completed?

_____

_____

_____

_____

RESEARCH ACTIVITY

Use Internet search engines to research the following topics and write a brief description of what is found. It is important to visit reputable Web sites.

1. Visit different Web sites that deal with speech and hearing loss. What information could be found to help families with speech and hearing deficiencies? What Web sites did you find most useful? Could these sites be beneficial to staff members of an EENT practice, and, if so, why?

_____

_____

_____

_____

_____

_____

_____

_____

_____

_____

_____

CHAPTER 38

Immunology and Allergies

CHAPTER OUTLINE

General review of the chapter:

    A. Introduction
    B. The Medical Assistant's Role in Immunology and Allergy
    C. The Anatomy and Physiology of the Immune System
    D. Diseases and Disorders of the Immune System
        i. Immunodeficiency diseases
        ii. Autoimmune diseases
        iii. Hypersensitivity and allergic reactions

STUDENT STUDY GUIDE

Use the following guide to assist in your learning of the concepts from the chapter.

  I. The MA's Role in an Immunology Office

    A. Obtain the patient's _____.
    B. Take _____.
    C. Instruct the patient about removing clothing, provide a gown and drape, and help the patient with gowning if necessary.
    D. Assist the immunologist or allergist with the examination and procedures.
    E. Watch for signs of _____ when allergy _____ injections are given.
    F. Instruct patient about _____.
    G. Stress the importance of keeping followup appointments.

  II. The Immune and Lymphatic Systems

    A. Anatomy and Physiology of the Immune System
        i. Immune system protects against bacterial and viral infections
        ii. Several barrier mechanisms exist:

        _____

        _____

        _____

        _____

        _____

        iii. _____ are substances that produce _____ allergic reactions.
        iv. Antigens are _____ _____ (proteins) that evoke allergic responses.
        v. When antigens enter the body, the immune system _____, _____, or _____ them.

380

B. The Immune Response
    i. _____ produces T-cell lymphocytes

    _____

    _____

    _____

    ii. _____ produces B-cell lymphocytes
    iii. _____ utilizes chemical, vascular, and leukocyte activities.

    _____

    iv. _____ begins when inflammation does not adequately handle infection.

    _____

C. The Lymphatic System
    i. _____ are filtered here.
    ii. Substances in the _____ portion of _____ activate the
        _____ response.
    iii. Transfusion reaction or tissue rejection may result after a transplant.
    iv. With a transplant, long-term use of medication suppresses the inflammatory response and
        prevents tissue rejection.
D. Anatomy of the Immune System
    i. Primary organs:

    _____

    ii. Secondary organs:

    _____

    _____

E. Leukocytes
    i. _____ leukocytes react to infection and protect cells from damage.
    ii. _____ are the first line of defense in _____.
    iii. _____ are attracted to cells and parasites then erode walls of the invading
        organism.
    iv. _____ are important in _____ reactions in the allergic
        response.
    v. _____ are responsible for the antigen-antibody response and sensitization,
        or memory, of cells to previous antigen exposure.
F. Types of Immunity
    i. Natural immunity is _____.

    _____

    ii. Acquired immunity is _____.

    _____

    iii. _____ _____: long-term or lifelong immunity
    iv. _____ _____: short-term

    _____

    _____

III. Immune System Diseases and Disorders
   A. Immunodeficiency Disease

      _____

      _____

      _____

      _____

      _____

      _____

      _____

   B. _____ _____: The body fails to recognize its own cells and develops self-antigens to destroy foreign cells.
   C. _____ and _____ reactions are caused by foreign substances.
   D. All areas of the body can be affected by autoimmune diseases.
   E. Other body systems and disorders related to autoimmunity:

      _____

      _____

      _____

      _____

      _____

      _____

      _____

IV. Allergies
   A. An allergy is the body's response to a/an _____ _____:
      i. This results in _____ or _____.
   B. Allergies result from the repeated _____.
   C. Examples include:

      _____

      _____

      _____

      _____

   D. Anaphylaxis
      i. _____ reaction to repeated allergen exposure
      ii. Can occur due to:

      _____

      _____

      _____

      _____

      _____

E. Diagnostic Allergy Tests
    i. _____ : injecting a small amount of potential antigen under the skin
    ii. _____ : putting a patch soaked with potential antigen on the skin
    iii. _____ : putting the potential antigen into a scratch made on the skin
    iv. _____ : to check for RBCs, platelets, and WBCs, including B and
        T lymphocytes

KEY TERMINOLOGY REVIEW

Write a sentence using selected vocabulary terms in the correct context.

1. Allergen:

    _____

    _____

2. Dysphagia:

    _____

    _____

3. Dysphasia:

    _____

    _____

4. Eechymosis:

    _____

    _____

5. Hemolytic:

    _____

    _____

6. Immunodeficiency:

    _____

    _____

7. Intrinsic factor:

    _____

    _____

8. Petechiae:

    _____

    _____

9. Reactive:

    _____

    _____

10. Subcutaneous:

    _____

    _____

APPLIED PRACTICE

Follow the directions as instructed with each question below.

1. Identify the structures of the lymphatic system on the picture below.

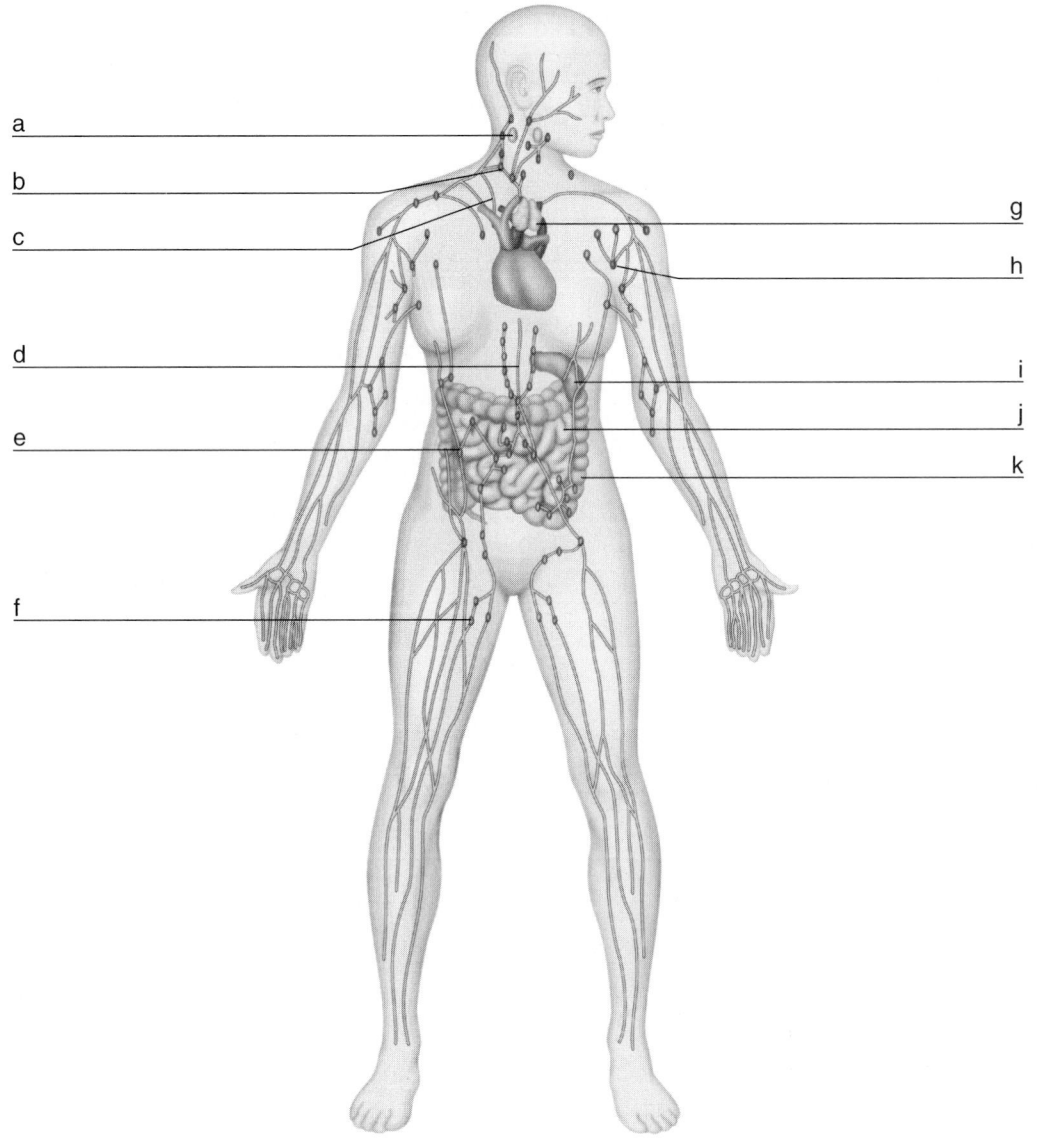

The lymphatic system

a. _____

b. _____

c. _____

d. _____

e. _____

f. _____

g. _____

h. _____

i. _____

j. _____

k. _____

LEARNING ACTIVITY: MULTIPLE CHOICE

Circle the correct answer to each of the questions below.

1. Which of the following are part of the four components of the body's immune system? (Circle all that apply.)

   a. humoral
   b. cell-mediated
   c. specific
   d. nonspecific

2. Aspirin has three actions, while acetaminophen has only two of those same actions. Which of the following choices is the action that aspirin has but acetaminophen does not?

   a. antipyretic
   b. analgesic
   c. hemopoietic
   d. anti-inflammatory

3. Which of the following are methods of diagnostic allergy testing? (Circle all that apply.)

   a. skin patch
   b. scratch testing
   c. ESR
   d. intradermal

4. A severe and prolonged form of asthma that can be life threatening is called

   a. asthma anaphylaxis
   b. anaphylaxis asthmaticus
   c. status asthmaticus
   d. status anaphylaxis

5. Which of the following are common food allergies as listed in your textbook? (Circle all that apply.)

   a. fish
   b. peanut butter
   c. lobster
   d. walnuts

6. Which statement is false in relation to HIV/AIDS transmission prevention strategies?

   a. Maintain a monogamous relationship.
   b. Avoid food that has been touched or prepared by someone with AIDS.
   c. If you get a tattoo, be sure a new needle is used.
   d. Use condoms.

7. Which of the following is not one of the five types of leukocytes discussed in this chapter of your textbook?

   a. monocytes
   b. eosinophils
   c. macrophages
   d. polymorphonuclear

8. Which of the following is not one of the three general categories of immune system diseases and disorders?

    a. hypersentivity and allergy reactions   c. autoimmune disorders

    b. genetic disorders   d. immunodeficiency diseases

9. The thymus gland decreases in size and function from _____ and on.

    a. birth   c. mid-adulthood

    b. early childhood   d. puberty

10. The primary set of organs in the immune system are: (circle all that apply)

    a. bone marrow   c. thymus gland

    b. liver   d. tonsils

CRITICAL THINKING

Answer the following questions to the best of your ability. Use the textbook as a reference.

1. Review and recall Standard Precautions (discussed in another chapter—look this up if necessary). Would you do any additional preparation when drawing blood from an AIDS patient than you would from another patient? Explain your answer.

    _____

    _____

    _____

    _____

2. You are in the clinic and two patients come to the front desk without appointments. Both are having breathing difficulties. One patient has just mowed his lawn and is extremely congested in both nose and airways. The other patient has just come from lunch at a Thai restaurant next door. She had taken about three bites of her food and then her tongue and throat became itchy. It progressed quickly and now her tongue is starting to swell. Which patient must be seen first and why?

    _____

    _____

    _____

    _____

3. Make a list with a column for your children, yourself, your parents, and each of their parents. If this is not possible in your family, try to use at least three people you know who are related to each other. Fill in the any allergies that each person has. Observe similarities among family members as it is common for allergies to run in families.

    _____

    _____

    _____

    _____

4. A patient has been coming in weekly for allergy injections. You have just administered her dose as prescribed by the physician, and you have asked her to wait in the office for about 20 minutes for observation before she leaves. Answer the following questions:

a. Why would you want the patient to wait for a while before leaving?

_____

_____

b. What symptoms might the patient exhibit within the 20 minutes?

_____

_____

5. A patient has just been diagnosed with several allergies. It is her first visit and you are providing patient education and various instructions. How would you explain (in layman's terms) what antigens and allergens are to the patient?

_____

_____

_____

_____

_____

RESEARCH ACTIVITY

Use Internet search engines to research the following topics and write a brief description of what is found. It is important to visit reputable Web sites.

1. Choose an autoimmune disease to research that is of most interest to you. Identify signs and symptoms of the disease, how diagnosis is made, and treatment options. Also research support groups, societies, or foundations that relate to the autoimmune disease you have chosen to research. *It is important to cite the Web sites where information is found.*

_____

_____

_____

_____

_____

_____

_____

_____

_____

_____

_____

_____

_____

_____

CHAPTER 39
Dermatology

CHAPTER OUTLINE

General review of the chapter:

    A. Introduction
    B. The Medical Assistant's Role in Dermatology
    C. The Anatomy and Physiology of the Skin
    D. Diseases and Disorders of the Skin
    E. Cancerous Skin Conditions
    F. Miscellaneous Skin Conditions

STUDENT STUDY GUIDE

Use the following guide to assist in your learning of the concepts from the chapter.

  I. The MA's Role in Dermatology

    A. _____
    B. Vital signs
    C. Instructions and help with gowning
    D. _____
    E. Medication instructions
    F. _____

  II. Anatomy and Physiology of the Integumentary System

    A. The integumentary system includes:

_____

_____

_____

_____

_____

_____

_____

_____

    B. Functions of the integumentary system:
       i. Acts as a/an _____ for _____
      ii. Regulates _____
     iii. Protects against _____
      iv. Senses _____, _____, and _____
       v. Synthesizes vitamin D from sunlight
      vi. Excretes _____ in _____

C. Layers of the Skin
    i. Epidermis, dermis, and subcutaneous tissue
       (a) Epidermis:

_____

_____

_____

_____

_____

       (b) Dermis:

_____

_____

_____

_____

       (c) Subcutaneous tissue:

_____

_____

_____

    ii. Skin appendages:

_____

_____

_____

_____

_____

_____

III. Diseases and Disorders of the Skin

   A. Dermatitis
     i. An inflammation on or in the layers of skin
     ii. Dermatitis can be _____ or _____.
     iii. Types of dermatitis

_____

_____

_____

_____

_____

   B. Psoriasis: chronic, noninfectious, and inflammatory
     i. Congenital
     ii. Unknown _____ or _____

iii. Symptoms of psoriasis:

_____
_____
_____
_____

iv. _____: exposure to UV light, steroid cream, antihistamines, and
chemotherapy

C. Infectious Skin Disorders

_____
_____
_____
_____
_____
_____

D. Fungal Skin Conditions
    i. _____:

_____
_____
_____
_____
_____
_____

    ii. _____:
        (a) Affects scalp
        (b) Lesions: round, scaly, itchy
        (c) Antifungal cream to reduce fungus and help healing
        (d) Oral antifungal drugs when antifungal creams are not recommended
    iii. _____:
        (a) Affects hairless body skin
        (b) Transmitted by infected animals, including cats
        (c) Symptoms:

_____
_____
_____
_____

    iv. _____:
        (a) Affects groin area and inner part of upper thigh
        (b) Symptoms:

_____
_____
_____

        (c) Antifungal cream reduces fungus and promotes healing.
        (d) Oral antifungal drugs given when antifungal creams are not recommended.

v. _____:
    (a) Affects the feet and is common in athletes
    (b) Cracks and blisters between the _____ and on _____
         of the feet
    (c) Symptoms:

_____

_____

_____

_____

E. Parasitic Skin Diseases
    i. Parasite itch mite causes _____ and _____.
    ii. Location of the infestation determines the name.
    iii. _____ (*Pediculus humanus capitis*) are common in children and easily
         spread via hats, combs, brushes, and coatrooms.
    iv. *Pediculus humanus pubis* or _____ are spread through sexual contact.
F. Pigmentation Disorders
    i. Disease involving pigmentation of skin:

_____

_____

_____

G. Benign Neoplasms
    i. Do not _____ surrounding tissues, metastasize, spread or cause symptoms.
    ii. May affect _____ _____
    iii. Includes:

_____

_____

_____

IV. Cancerous Skin Conditions

A. _____(BCC)
B. _____(SCC)
C. _____
D. Most common and most curable when _____ _____
E. Most common risk factor is unprotected sun exposure
F. Diagnosis: ABCD Rule
    i. A = _____

    ii. B = _____

    iii. C = _____

    iv. D = _____

G. Prevention

_____

_____

_____

_____

_____

_____

_____

V. Miscellaneous Skin Conditions

   A. Cellulitis

   _____

   _____

   _____

   B. Folliculitis

   _____

   _____

   _____

   C. Alopecia

   _____

   _____

   _____

   D. Hirsutism

   _____

   _____

   _____

   E. Lyme disease

   _____

   _____

   _____

KEY TERMINOLOGY REVIEW

Match the correct medical term with the definition listed below.

a.	appendage	**h.**	integumentary system
b.	cauterization	**i.**	keratin
c.	collagen	**j.**	lesion
d.	cryosurgery	**k.**	melanin
e.	dermatitis	**l.**	melanocytes
f.	dermatologist	**m.**	neuralgia
g.	dermatophytoses	**n.**	sebaceous glands

_____ 1. Skin inflammation.

_____ 2. Anything attached to a larger or major body part.

_____ 3. Pigment (color) in the skin and hair.

_____ 4. A physician that specializes in the treatment of skin disorders and conditions.

_____ 5. Small glands in the dermis that secrete sebum.

_____ 6. Tough protein substance found in hair, nails, and horny tissue.

_____ 7. Destruction of tissue with a caustic, electric current, hot iron, or by freezing.

_____ 8. Freezing lesions with nitrous oxide.

_____ 9. Tissue abnormality that when associated with skin, is on or within the skin tissue.

_____ 10. Superficial fungal infections of the skin and its appendages.

_____ 11. Cells that produce melanin.

_____ 12. Fibrous connective tissue.

_____ 13. The skin and its supporting structures.

_____ 14. Sharp, stabbing, or burning pain that occurs along the course of a nerve.

APPLIED PRACTICE

Follow the directions as instructed with each question below.

1. Using information found in the textbook, fill out the table below regarding infectious skin disorders.

Disorder	Symptoms	Diagnosis	Treatment
Furuncles/carbuncles			
Herpes zoster			

Impetigo			
Herpes simplex			

2. Label the figure of the nail bed below.

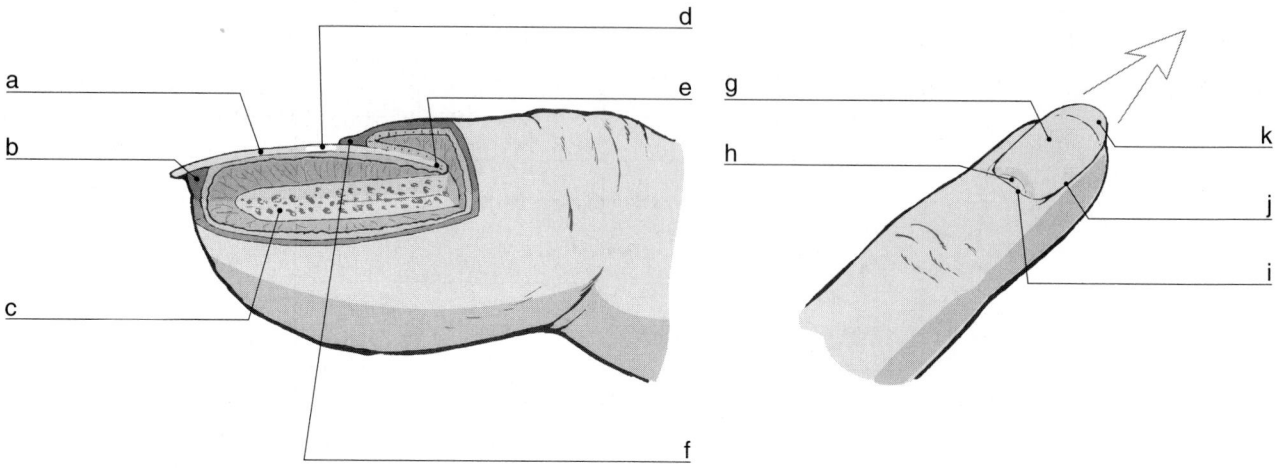

Nail bed and structure

LEARNING ACTIVITY: FILL IN THE BLANK

Using words from the list below, fill in the blanks to complete the following statements

ABCD
appearance
blood and lymph
common
connective tissue
curable
cushions
dehydration
dermis
diagnosed early

rule fat
generalized illness
hair growth
heat and cold
inflammation and infection
insulation
irritations or lesions
microorganisms
nails
nerve

cells polycystic
Staphylococcus
subcutaneous
subcutaneous tissue
support
sweat and sebaceous
toxins
temperature
tumors
vitamin D

1. Skin cancers are initially diagnosed according to their _____. Malignant melanoma is identified by the _____.

2. The integumentary system includes the _____, hair, and _____ glands.

3. Skin cancers are the most _____ type of cancer as well as the most _____ when _____.

4. The skin serves as a barrier to prevent _____ and other foreign bodies from entering; regulate _____; protect against _____; be an environmental sensor, including pain, temperature, and touch; synthesize _____ from sunlight; and excrete _____ in perspiration.

5. The dermis contains _____ vessels, _____ cell endings, and skin _____ organs.

6. Hirsutism is a condition of excessive _____, which may be caused by _____ ovaries or _____ of the adrenal glands and ovaries.

7. A break in the defense system of the skin may result in _____ as well as localized _____.

8. Cellulitis is a condition of _____ of the skin and subcutaneous tissue commonly caused by _____.

9. Sweat glands are located in the _____ and the _____.

10. The innermost layer of skin, the _____ tissue, is made up of _____ and _____ and acts as _____ for the body; provides protection against extreme _____ and against heat loss; and _____ and protects underlying structures.

CRITICAL THINKING

Answer the following questions to the best of your ability. Use the textbook as a reference.

1. As you are assisting an elderly patient get into a gown for an examination, you notice she has a dime-sized mole with an irregular border on her back. You realize the patient likely cannot see it and may be unaware of it. Would you mention it to the patient or only to the physician? State the reason for your answer.

   _____
   _____
   _____
   _____
   _____

2. Go to the Internet and locate a reputable site that provides pictures of various skin conditions, including lice. Draw a picture of head lice and state how this condition is treated.

3. What possible advice could you give to a patient who has had a skin cancer removed today and works daily as a lifeguard in the sun?

   _____
   _____
   _____
   _____
   _____

4. A female patient comes in for an examination for excessive dark hair she has developed in the last six months or so. She asks you what it is and what can be done for it, but she has not seen the physician yet. What would you say to this patient at this time?

   Hint: The answer is not specifically in the book and will require your current knowledge and critical thinking skills regarding the medical assistant's scope of practice.

   _____
   _____
   _____
   _____
   _____

5. Although not specifically stated in the text, what precautions would you recommend to a patient who has an infectious skin disorder to prevent it from spreading?

_____

_____

_____

_____

_____

RESEARCH ACTIVITY

Use Internet search engines to research the following topics and write a brief description of what is found. It is important to visit reputable Web sites.

1. Visit the Skin Cancer Foundation at www.skincancer.org. After reviewing the Web site, answer the following questions:
   a. What "Prevention" information do you find most interesting, and why?
   b. After reading "Skin Cancer Facts," which facts do you find most surprising?
   c. What can you do to further reduce your risk of developing skin cancer?

_____

_____

_____

_____

_____

_____

_____

_____

_____

_____

_____

_____

CHAPTER 40
Endocrinology

CHAPTER OUTLINE

General review of the chapter:

    A. Introduction
    B. The Medical Assistant's Role in Endocrinology
    C. Anatomy and Physiology of the Endocrine System
    D. Endocrine Glands
        i. Pituitary gland disorders
       ii. Thyroid gland disorders
      iii. Parathyroid disorders
      iv. Disorders of the pancreas
       v. Adrenal gland disorders

STUDENT STUDY GUIDE

Use the following guide to assist in your learning of the concepts from the chapter.

   I. The MA's Role in an Endocrinology Office

    A. Obtain and record vital signs.
    B. Patient history and reason for visit
    C. Obtain _____ and _____ specimens.
    D. Perform blood _____ tests.
    E. Instructions for _____, _____, and _____
    F. _____ regarding preparation for _____ testing

  II. The Endocrine System

    A. The Endocrine and Nervous Systems
        i. Autonomic system is part of the _____ _____ and controls

           _____ _____

           _____

           _____

       ii. Endocrine system tells the body how to _____ with _____

           _____

           _____

    B. Endocrine Glands

      _____

      _____

      _____

      _____

      _____

      _____

      _____

      _____

C. Endocrine Gland Dysfunction

    i. _____: too much of hormone is being excreted

    ii. _____: too little of hormone is being excreted

    iii. Hormones control body functions:

    _____

    _____

III. Anatomy and Physiology of the Endocrine System

  A. Anatomy

    i. **Pituitary gland**

      (a) Located in _____ of _____ in the _____

      (b) Anterior lobe and posterior lobe

      (c) Controlled by _____

      (d) Releases _____ hormones

    ii. **Thyroid gland**

      (a) Contains _____ lobes in the _____ on both sides of

      _____

      (b) Secretes thyroxine (**T3**), triiodothyronine (**T4**), and calcitonin

      (c) T3 and T4 are under the control of _____; stimulate cell
      _____ and are essential for energy and cell building and repair.

    iii. **Parathyroid gland**

      (a) _____ glands attached to surface of thyroid gland

      (b) Parathyroid hormone (**PTH**) affects _____ levels in the blood.

      (c) In conjunction with _____, maintains appropriate calcium levels in
      the body

    iv. **Pancreas gland**

      (a) _____ and _____ gland

      (b) Endocrine produces _____ and glucagons in islets of

      _____.

      _____

      _____

    v. **Adrenal glands**

      (a) _____ glands on upper surface of each _____

      (b) Adrenal medulla (inner portion) works with _____ nervous system to
      produce _____ and norepinephrine

      (c) Adrenal cortex (outer portion) produces corticosteroids, mineral corticoids, gluco-
      corticoids, _____, _____, and progestins

    vi. **Thymus gland**

    _____

    _____

    _____

    _____

    vii. **Pineal gland**

    _____

    _____

    _____

    _____

    _____

B. Physiology
  i. **Pituitary (anterior lobe)**
     (a) Growth hormone:

     _____

     _____

     (b) _____ _____ _____: stimulates secretion
         of thyroid hormones
     (c) Adrenocorticotropic hormone: glucocorticocoid secretion
     (d) _____ _____ stimulates estrogen secretion and follicle
         development and sperm maturation
     (e) LH: stimulates _____, corpus luteum development, secretion of
         _____

  ii. **Pituitary (posterior lobe)**
     (a) antidiuretic hormone: absorbs _____, elevates _____
         _____ and volume
     (b) _____: stimulates uterine contractions, milk ejection and contractions
         of the prostate

  iii. **Thyroid**
     (a) thyroxiine (T3):

     _____

     (b) triiodothyronine (T4):

     _____

     (c) calcitonin:

     _____

  iv. **Parathyroid**
     (a) parathormone (PTH): increases _____ removal from the bones
     (b) mineralocorticoids (aldosterone): stimulates reabsorption of _____ in
         kidney tubules, accelerates loss of potassium ions from _____
     (c) _____ (cortisol, corticosterone, cortisone): influences metabolism of
         food, exhibits anti-inflammatory effect
     (d) gonadocorticoids (androgens, estrogens, progestins): possible support of
         _____ _____

  v. **Adrenal medulla**

     _____

     _____

     _____

     _____

  vi. **Pancreas islets**

     _____

     _____

     _____

     _____

  vii. **Thymus**

     _____

     _____

  viii. **Pineal gland**

     _____

     _____

ix. Ovaries

_____

_____

_____

_____

x. Testes

_____

_____

_____

IV. Endocrine Gland Disorders

  A. Pituitary Gland Disorders
- i. Pituitary considered _____
- ii. Controlled by the _____ via the anterior _____ gland
- iii. Releases tropic hormones to control or stimulate other gland activity
- iv. _____: overstimulation of growth hormone after growth period
- v. _____: underproduction of growth hormone
- vi. _____: diminished release of vasopressin or antidiuretic hormone

  B. Thyroid Gland Disorders
- i. _____ is an enlargement of the thyroid gland.
  - (a) Also known as a/an _____
  - (b) Caused from inadequate amounts of _____ in diet
  - (c) _____ cannot secrete hormones if body lacks _____
  - (d) If enlargement isn't stopped it will compromise the airway.
  - (e) Treatment includes iodine supplements and/or surgical removal of overgrowth of tissue
- ii. _____ is an underproduction and undersecretion of thyroid hormones.
  - (a) Causes slow metabolic rates, low T3, T4, pale, cool skin, slow heart rate, lethargy, decreased appetite, weight gain, intolerance to cold, and possible goiter
  - (b) Treatment is life-long hormone replacement therapy
    - (1) Hashimoto's disease:

      _____

      _____

      _____

    - (2) Myxedema:

      _____

      _____

      _____

    - (3) Cretinism:

      _____

      _____

      _____

- iii. _____ caused from oversecretion of thyroid hormones
  - (a) Also known as _____ _____
  - (b) Symptoms may include:

    _____

    _____

    _____

(c) Treatment:

_____

_____

_____

C. Parathyroid Gland Disorders
    i. _____ causes low serum calcium levels: called _____
        (a) Symptoms:

_____

_____

_____

        (b) Treatment:

_____

_____

_____

    ii. _____ caused from excessive production and secretion of parathyroid
       hormone: called _____
        (a) Symptoms:

_____

_____

_____

        (b) Treatment:

_____

_____

_____

D. Glucose Metabolism Disorders
    i. The pancreas is a/an _____ and _____ gland.
    ii. Digestive process requires _____

_____

_____

_____

_____

_____

_____

_____

_____

_____

E. Types of Diabetes
    i. _____: insulin-dependent diabetes mellitus
    ii. _____: non-insulin dependent diabetes mellitus
F. Insulin-dependent diabetes mellitus
    i. Usually occurs before age _____ with _____onset
    ii. Referred to as _____-_____ diabetes
    iii. _____ does not secrete insulin

iv. Insulin _____ or _____ pump is required

v. Complication of diabetes is _____ and _____

G. Hypoglycemia

   i. Symptoms:

_____

_____

_____

   ii. Causes:

_____

_____

_____

   iii. Sudden decrease in insulin levels causes insulin shock

   iv. Life threatening and requires immediate intervention

H. Hyperglycemia

   i. Symptoms:

_____

_____

_____

   ii. Causes:

_____

_____

_____

   iii. Diabetic coma occurs when blood sugar levels rise well above the normal range of
_____.

   iv. Treatment includes _____ and _____.

I. Gestational Diabetes Mellitus

_____

_____

_____

_____

_____

_____

J. The MA's Role with Diabetic Patients

   i. Instructions on _____ _____ (if within state scope of practice)

   ii. Use of _____

   iii. Record keeping of daily blood _____ _____

   iv. _____ _____

   v. Dietary plans, glucose monitoring, medication instructions, followup appointments

   vi. Signs and side effects of hyper/hypoglycemia

K. Adrenal Gland Disorders

   i. Cushing's Syndrome

_____

_____

_____

_____

_____

_____

_____

_____

ii. Addison's Disease

_____

_____

_____

_____

_____

_____

KEY TERMINOLOGY REVIEW

Write a sentence using the vocabulary terms in the correct context.

1. Endocrine glands:

_____

_____

2. Exocrine glands:

_____

_____

3. Gluconeogenesis:

_____

_____

4. Hormones:

_____

_____

5. Hypothalamus:

_____

_____

APPLIED PRACTICE

Follow the directions as instructed with each question below.

1. Using the information from the following patient charts, correctly identify the possible endocrine gland disorder based on the patient's signs and symptoms.

					Mikovich, Anya
					10-26-1982

04/02/20xx   3:45 pm   Wt: 134 lbs   T: 98.6°F   P: 104 bpm, bounding   BP: 118/78

cc: Pt. presents to office complaining of insomnia, she states "I can't sleep, and have been sweating a lot recently. I always feel hot." She is displaying exophthalmos, and has lost 6 lbs since her last visit 3 months ago, though she claims she hasn't been trying to lose weight.------------ *Adam Bello, RMA*

a. Anya's possible endocrine disorder:

_____

					Booker, Melvin
					07-01-1968

04/03/20xx   11:30 am   Wt: 250 lbs   T: 99.0°F   P: 84 bpm, bounding   BP: 130/88

cc: Pt. presents to office due to abdominal pain × 3 weeks, he states "I am always thirsty, and my mouth is always dry." + for increased urination, and skin appears dry and warm to the touch. --------------------

-- *Josie Schmitt, MA*

b. Melvin's possible endocrine disorder:

_____

2. Label the endocrine glands on the picture shown below.

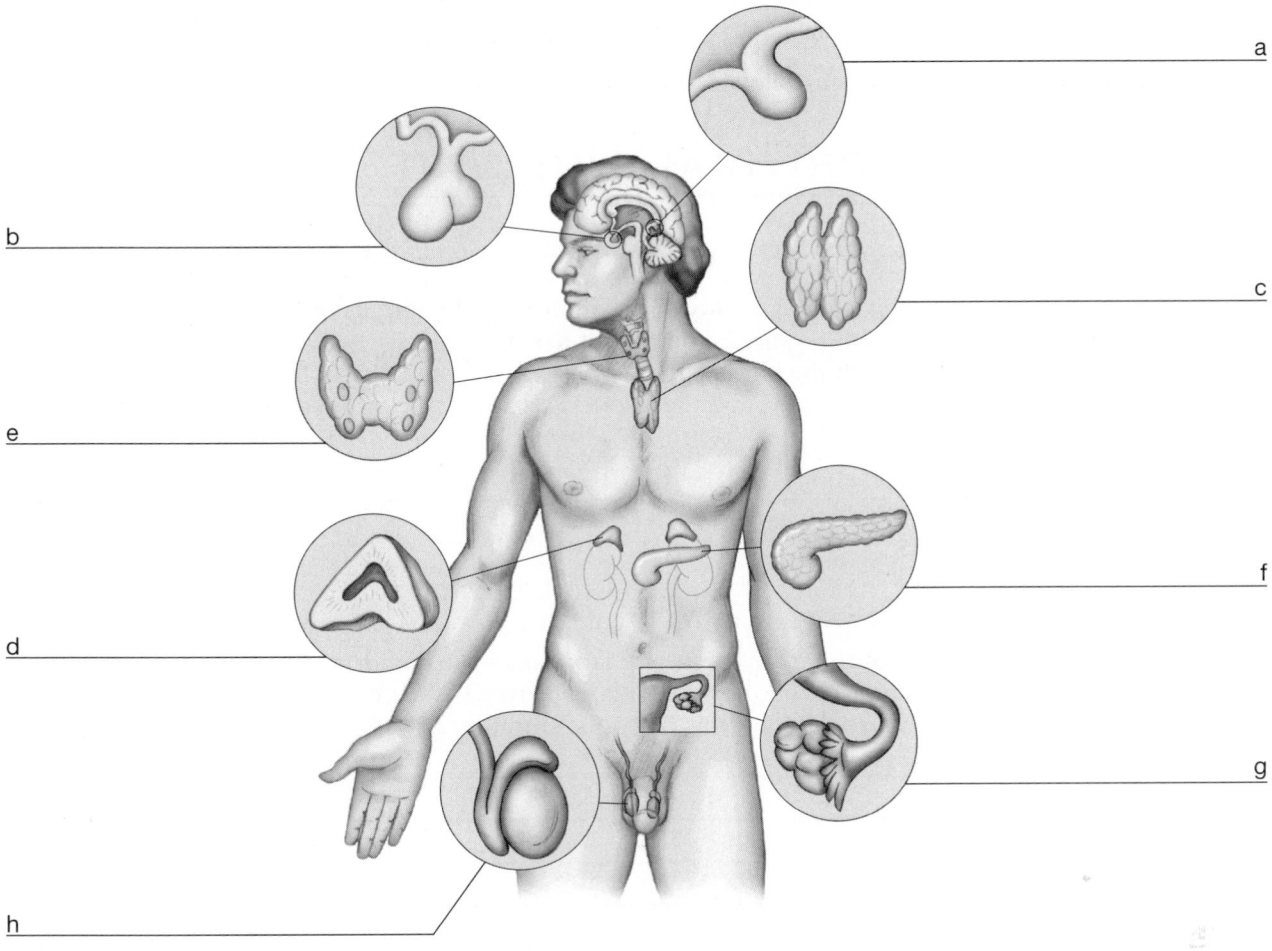

b _____

e _____

d _____

h _____

a _____

c _____

f _____

g _____

Endocrine glands scattered throughout the body

LEARNING ACTIVITY: TRUE/FALSE

Indicate whether the statement is true (T) or false (F).

_____ 1. The hypothalamus controls the activity of the gland by releasing factors to the anterior pituitary gland.

_____ 2. Endocrine disorders are the result of too much or too little of a particular hormone being stimulated or released.

_____ 3. Gestational diabetes is a form of diabetes that has its onset during adult age instead of childhood.

_____ 4. Myxedema is a severe or acute hypothyroid state in adults that may lead to hypoglycemia, among other things.

_____ 5. The pancreas is both an endocrine and an exocrine gland.

_____ 6. Cushing's syndrome is caused by the hyposecretion of adrenocortical secretions.

_____ 7. The opposite of hypoglycemia is insulin shock.

_____ 8. The two control systems of the body are the gastrointestinal and endocrine systems.

_____ 9. The thyroid gland requires iron in the diet in order to function properly.

_____ 10. Hypoparathyroidism causes low serum sodium levels.

CRITICAL THINKING

Answer the following questions to the best of your ability. Use the textbook as a reference.

1. You have a 28-year-old female patient who is four months pregnant. She has come in stating she has symptoms of diabetes—her OB physician found that her urine glucose was high and sent her to your endocrinology office. Although the physician always diagnoses and orders tests, what do you think the first step will be for this patient? State the two tests that may be ordered by the provider.

   _____

   _____

   _____

   _____

2. A pregnant patient who is overdue for going into labor may need a hormone to help stimulate the process of uterine contractions. What hormone may be given? What endocrine gland would produce this hormone naturally? What else does this hormone stimulate?

   _____

   _____

   _____

   _____

3. In the case study in your textbook, what are the three things that this patient could control that may help his physical condition?

   _____

   _____

   _____

   _____

4. In the case study in the textbook, the patient seems to be in denial or at least resistant to lifestyle changes. Once you have given the patient all the education possible in your office, what are the three resources listed at the end of the chapter that would be most appropriate for him to contact?

   _____

   _____

   _____

   _____

5. Consider the same case study and answer this question with your opinion. There are no specific right answers for this, but please give your opinion using your critical thinking skills. If the patient tells you during the patient education that he refuses to change lifestyle, what would you do or say?

_____

_____

_____

_____

_____

RESEARCH ACTIVITY

Use Internet search engines to research the following topics and write a brief description of what is found. It is important to visit reputable Web sites.

1. Visit www.diabetes.org. Research information as to how diabetes plays an ethnic and cross-cultural role. What facts do you find most surprising regarding this topic? How prevalent is diabetes within your ethnic race or culture?

_____

_____

_____

_____

_____

_____

_____

_____

_____

_____

_____

_____

_____

CHAPTER 41
Emergency Care

CHAPTER OUTLINE

General review of the chapter:

- A. Introduction
- B. The Medical Assistant's Role in Emergency Care
- C. Emergency Resources
  - i. EMS
- D. Medical Office Preparedness
  - i. Emergency equipment and supplies
- E. Emergency Intervention

STUDENT STUDY GUIDE

Use the following guide to assist in your learning of the concepts from the chapter.

I. Emergency Care: Roles Played and Supplies Needed

  A. The MA's Role in Emergency Care
- i. MAs must be familiar with _____ and _____ emergency plans.
- ii. Regular reviews for plans are necessary to stay up to date.
- iii. Standard policy is to treat the "_____ _____."
- iv. Performing the Heimlich Maneuver, _____, and _____
- v. Bandaging and manipulating _____ _____
- vi. Immobilizing _____, _____, and _____

  B. The Role of EMS in Emergency Care
- i. Provide on-the-scene _____ and treatment.
- ii. Prepare a victim with injuries, trauma, or illness for _____.
- iii. Transport the victim to the emergency facility.
  - (a) Transportation can be done via _____, _____, or a/an _____

  C. The Emergency Crash Cart
- i. MAs often responsible for _____ the crash cart
- ii. Crash cart is easily accessible for immediate use
- iii. Usually rolled to wherever patient is located

  D. Standard Crash Cart Supplies

_____

_____

_____

_____

_____

_____

_____

_____

_____

_____

   E. Medical Drug Box Contents
      i. Activated _____, _____ and epinephrine
     ii. Instant _____, _____, and _____
    iii. Normal saline, sodium bicarbonate, spirits of ammonia, and local anesthetics

II. Cardiac Arrest
   A. Causes of cardiac arrest

_____

_____

_____

_____

_____

_____

   B. CPR Protocol
      i. _____ vary by age group.
     ii. Always call EMS immediately if person _____
    iii. General rules:
       (a) "_____ first" for unresponsive adults
       (b) "_____ first" for unresponsive children and infants
          (1) 9-1-1 is called after _____ minutes.
   C. CPR in Children and Infants
      i. Do not perform _____ _____.
     ii. Do not _____ babies:

_____

_____

    iii. Infants should be _____ or _____ on the feet.
    iv. If no response, the airway should be opened by tilting the head backward.
     v. If they do not start breathing, _____ should be performed.
    vi. Age varies for _____ _____ location, compression techniques, and rescue breathing rate.
   D. American Heart Association Guidelines
      i. Check for a pulse.
     ii. _____ and _____ of skin
    iii. Victim movement
    iv. If a pulse is not present CPR should be performed.
     v. If a second person is available they should monitor compression quality.
   E. Automated External Defibrillator
      i. _____ _____ if performed within minutes of cardiac arrest.
     ii. Defibrillator corrects electrical_____, which is common cause of arrest
    iii. AED gives _____ _____ to rescuer for easy use
    iv. Not applied to infants
     v. Can be used with children 1-8 years after one minute of CPR
   F. Chest Pain Emergencies
      i. Patients with chest pain should sit and _____ _____.
     ii. Notify _____ and the physician.
    iii. Administer _____ per office protocols.

     iv. If patient has nitroglycerin it should be taken (administered with _____).

     v. Tablets can be given every _____ _____ until the pain subsides.

  G. Symptoms of Cardiac Arrest

_____

_____

_____

_____

_____

_____

_____

_____

  H. Patients Calling into the Medical Office with Chest Pain

     i. Keep the patient on the _____ while help is sought.

     ii. Get the caller's name and location, and inform him or her that you are calling _____.

     iii. Stay on the line with them while _____ _____ calls EMS.

     iv. Let the person know when services will arrive.

     v. Do not _____ _____ until EMS has arrived.

III. Respiratory Distress

  A. Causes of Respiratory Distress

_____

_____

_____

_____

_____

_____

  B. Signs and Symptoms of Respiratory Distress

_____

_____

_____

_____

_____

_____

_____

_____

  C. Shortness of Breath (SOB)

     i. Immediate care required

     ii. Make sure the person can _____,

_____

     iii. Question patient about cause and onset of symptoms

  D. Hyperventilation

     i. _____, _____ breathing or rapid, shallow breathing

     ii. Carbon dioxide in blood _____.

      iii. Blood vessels dilate and blood pressure is lowered.

      iv. Treat using oxygen mask, blocking one nostril, or breathing in a paper bag.

  E. Chronic Obstructive Pulmonary Disease

      i. Diseases include:

_____

_____

_____

_____

      ii. Unable to expel carbon dioxide because air is trapped in lungs

  F. Pulmonary Edema

      i. Fluid accumulates in the lungs and alveoli, causing swelling.

      ii. Symptoms include:

_____

_____

_____

_____

_____

_____

      iii. Make sure the patient is _____ _____ and call the physician.

      iv. If ordered give the patient _____ and then call EMS.

IV. Shock

  A. The Body's Response to Shock

      i. Something causes insufficient _____ _____.

      ii. Cardiovascular system _____ and shock results

      iii. Necessary nourishment and blood do not get supplied to tissues and organs.

      iv. Leads to _____ if not treated immediately

  B. Common Causes of Shock

_____

_____

_____

_____

_____

_____

_____

_____

_____

_____

  C. Symptoms of Shock

_____

_____

_____

_____

_____

_____

D. Handling Shock Patients
  i. Get _____ and _____ treatment to prevent death.
  ii. Lie the patient down.
  iii. Keep patient _____
  iv. Verify there is a/an _____ _____ for breathing.
  v. Monitor vital signs and control any bleeding.
  vi. Emotionally support the patient.
E. Anaphylactic Shock
  i. Certain substances cause _____ _____ in the body.
  ii. Physiological reactions lead to allergic anaphylactic shock.
  iii. Causes include medications, _____ _____, or allergy to latex gloves.
  iv. Symptoms include:

  _____

  _____

  _____

  _____

  _____

  _____

  v. Treating anaphylactic shock:

  _____

  _____

  _____

  _____

V. Bleeding and Wounds
  A. Arterial Bleeding
    i. Copious _____ red blood that bleeds rapidly and spurts similar to a heartbeat
    ii. Must be controlled immediately by applying direct pressure to the _____ _____ or _____ _____
    iii. Elevate injured part higher than _____ to slow bleeding
    iv. Bandage wound and call EMS
  B. Venous Bleeding
    i. Blood is _____ in color and flows at a/an _____ rate.
    ii. Direct pressure to wound usually stops the blood flow.
    iii. Use _____ bandage and add new bandages if bleeding through occurs.
    iv. _____ _____ remove the original bandage
    v. Pressure bandage will help control bleeding
  C. Internal Bleeding
    i. May be _____ or _____
    ii. Bruising or discoloration of the skin is common indication
    iii. Symptoms include:

    _____

    _____

    iv. If not treated, shock may occur.
  D. Precursors of Shock Due to Internal Bleeding

    _____

    _____

    _____

_____

_____

_____

_____

_____

E. Types of Open Wounds
    i. Abrasions
    ii. Avulsion
    iii. Amputation
    iv. Lacerations
    v. Incisions
    vi. Punctures

F. Open Wounds
    i. Integrity of skin is _____
    ii. Wound must be cleaned to prevent infection
    iii. The bacillus *Clostridium tetany* can enter the body through open wounds.
    iv. Patients may need a/an _____ _____ if immunization is not up to date
    v. Tetanus (_____) affects the central nervous system and causes muscle spasms.
    vi. Tetanus can cause _____ but tetanus immunization can prevent this.

G. Abrasions
    i. Include:

_____

_____

_____

    ii. Underlying tissue is exposed and outer layer of skin is _____ away.
    iii. Nerve endings are exposed, causing pain.

H. Avulsions
    i. Skin or tissue is torn away.
    ii. Common with _____ or motor vehicle accidents
    iii. Cleanse gently with soap and water.
    iv. Put skin back in place.
    v. Apply _____ and _____.

I. Amputation
    i. Immediately gather body part, clean with sterile saline, and wrap with moist gauzes
    ii. Store in a/an _____ _____ and keep on ice.
    iii. Cover the person's injured body part and seek immediate treatment for best recovery.

J. Lacerations
    i. Typically have _____ edges
    ii. Skin and underlying tissue are torn.
    iii. Bleeding will occur if blood vessels are torn.
    iv. Clean with soap and water.
    v. Treat with:

_____

_____

_____

K. Incisions
    i. Treated the same way as lacerations.
    ii. Incisions are cut with a smooth edge from a/an _____ or _____ object.

iii. Doctor may provide surgical treatment such as:

_____

_____

_____

L. Puncture Wounds

_____

_____

_____

_____

_____

M. Impaled Objects

_____

_____

_____

_____

_____

N. Contusions

_____

_____

_____

_____

_____

_____

VI. Thermal Insults
   A. Burns
      i. _____ = flames, fire, radiation, steam, hot liquids, or objects
      ii. _____ = acids, bases, or caustics
      iii. _____ = electrocution, lightning
      iv. _____ or _____ = sunburn, chemotherapy
   B. Classification of Burns
      i. First-degree burns affect the _____.
      ii. Second-degree or _____ _____ burns affect the
      _____ and _____.
      iii. Third-degree or full-thickness burns involve all the layers of skin including:

_____

_____

_____

      iv. Infants, children under 5, and adults over 55 are at greater risks for complications.

    v. The _____ of _____ is used to determine percentage of body burned

       (a) Face, hands, feet, or genitals require special care.

    vi. Singeing of eyebrows, nasal or facial hair, along with charring or soot may indicate _____ _____.

C. Treatment of Burns

    i. Stop active burning with _____.

       (a) Except electrical burns: Do not touch patient until the electricity is turned off

    ii. Immerse injured body part in cool water or cover with gauze soaked in saline.

    iii. When cooled, cover with dry bandages.

    iv. Flush _____ _____ with water until burning subsides and care is available.

    v. Electrical or lightning burn victims may go into _____ _____ and require CPR.

    vi. Monitor cardiac and respiratory functions for shock and blood pressure fluctuations.

D. Frostbite

    i. Caused by:

_____

_____

    ii. Soft tissue is frozen.

    iii. Skin becomes numb, loses all sensation, and eventually turns white.

    iv. Results in tissue death

E. Treatment of Frostbite

_____

_____

_____

_____

_____

F. Heat Exhaustion

    i. Body is depleted of _____ and _____ due to strenuous activity.

    ii. Symptoms:

_____

_____

_____

    iii. Remove from heat source and _____ the patient down; water should be sipped and cool compresses used.

    iv. Prevent with salt tablets and drinking plenty of water before, during, and after activities.

G. Hyperthermia

    i. Overexposure to hot temperatures for extended time

    ii. Mild shock occurs from the loss of _____ and _____ in perspiration.

    iii. Symptoms:

_____

_____

_____

_____

iv. Remove from heat immediately.
v. Remove clothing to cool down as soon as possible
vi. Use a/an _____ _____ or _____
_____ to cool patient
vii. Call EMS if heat stroke is suspected.
viii. Monitor vital signs and cardiac status.
H. Hypothermia
i. Overexposure to _____ or _____ _____
ii. Causes the core body temperature to drop below _____
iii. Symptoms:

_____

_____

_____

iv. Warm patient by removing cold clothes and applying warm blankets, heat packs, and warm liquids

VII. Other Emergency Situations
A. Musculoskeletal Injuries
i. Fractures
(a) Simple fractures:

_____

_____

(b) Open or compound fractures pierce the skin or tear it open by external force.
(c) Bone can break in three ways:

_____

_____

ii. Strains and Dislocations
(a) Pulled muscles results in strains
(b) A/an _____ pulled away from a/an _____ is considered to be dislocated.
(c) Dislocations must be reduced and the bone reinserted into the joint.
(d) _____ needed to diagnose sprain, strain, or dislocation and rule out a/an _____
B. Allergic Reactions
i. Range from itching, to hives, to anaphylaxis
ii. Symptoms:

_____

_____

_____

iii. Treat by removing the allergen or victim from the environment
iv. If ordered, administer a prescribed steroid or histamine-induced reaction.
C. Neurological Emergencies
i. Examples:

_____

_____

_____

_____

_____

ii. Treating Neurological Emergencies
    (a) Require special care not typically available in doctors' offices
    (b) Place patient in a/an _____ or _____-
        _____ position
    (c) Perform _____ _____ and call EMS.
    (d) Watch for signs of shock and record vital signs along with level of consciousness.
iii. Basic Neurological Exam

_____

_____

_____

_____

_____

D. Acute Abdominal Pain
    i. Location of pain can be indicative of underlying problem
    ii. Upper right quadrant:

_____

    iii. Lower right quadrant:

_____

    iv. Back or flank region (retroperitoneal):

_____

    v. Pelvis:

_____

_____

_____

E. Hyper- and Hypoglycemia
    i. Can result in diabetic coma or insulin shock
    ii. Hypoglycemia has great risks:
        (a) Patients act _____, have cold clammy skin, and are anxious or combative.
        (b) Blood sugar drops so low brain cells begin dying.
        (c) Starts when blood sugar levels are below _____
        (d) A drop below _____ places patient in grave danger
F. Treatment of Hypoglycemia

_____

_____

_____

_____

G. Hyperglycemia

_____

_____

_____

_____

_____

_____

H. Poisoning
  i. Overdoses may be accidental or intentional.
  ii. Four ways poison is introduced into the body:

  _____

  _____

  _____

  _____

  _____

  iii. Poison Control
    (a) Available all over the United States 24 hours a day, seven days a week
    (b) Registered nurses, _____, and _____ available
    (c) Followup contact is made within _____ of the first call.
    (d) Be prepared to provide:

  _____

  _____

  _____

  _____

I. Foreign Bodies in the Eye

  _____

  _____

  _____

  _____

  _____

  _____

VIII. Emergency Psychosocial Situations and Emergency Preparedness
  A. Psychosocial Situations

  _____

  _____

  _____

  _____

  _____

  _____

  B. Handling Psychosituations
    i. _____ or _____ abuse are reportable by law.
    ii. Reporting domestic violence varies by _____ _____.
      (a) Patients requesting no legal involvement must have wishes honored
    iii. Specific_____ are designed for rape and sexual abuse.
    iv. Be sensitive to victims' needs and support them emotionally.
    v. Deal with intoxicated individuals or persons with rage sensitively and diffuse the situation.
  C. Emergency Preparedness
    i. A medical assistant should be well versed in emergency preparedness.
    ii. Emergencies may be either man-made or natural disasters.
      (a) Natural disasters may include:

  _____

  _____

iii. Planning ahead
   (a) The Federal Emergency Management Association suggests the following:
       (1) _____
       (2) _____
       (3) _____
       (4) _____
       (5) _____
       (6) _____

iv. Man-made Disasters
   (a) May include:

   _____

   _____

   _____

   _____

v. Bomb threats
   (a) If there is a call made regarding a bomb threat, try to ask the caller:
       (1) _____
       (2) _____
       (3) _____
       (4) _____
       (5) _____

vi. Biological agents and nuclear blasts
   (a) Biological agents can be delivered via:

   _____

   _____

   (b) A medical office may choose to have a high efficiency particulate air filter installed.
   (c) In the event of a nuclear blast take immediate cover _____
       _____ and lie flat on the ground with your head covered

KEY TERMINOLOGY REVIEW

Match the selected key terms to their definitions below.

a. abrasion	g. hyperglycemia	m. laceration
b. Ambu bag	h. hypertension	n. patent
c. anaphylaxis	i. hyperthermia	o. sepsis
d. avulsion	j. hypoglycemia	p. status epilepticus
e. cyanosis	k. hypothermia	q. venous
f. epistaxis	l. incision	

_____ 1. Condition in which blood glucose is below normal.

_____ 2. Severe allergic reaction.

_____ 3. Open wound with smooth edges made with a knife or other sharp object.

_____ 4. Bluish tint in skin or mucous membrane.

_____ 5. Open wound in which skin and underlying tissue are torn and skin integrity is broken.

_____ 6. Open wound in which the outer layer of skin is scraped away.

_____ 7. Febrile state characterized by pathogens in the bloodstream.

_____ 8. Condition in which body temperature is below normal.

_____ 9. Continued elevation of blood pressure above normal.

_____ 10. Open.

_____ 11. Bag-valve-mask unit used to provide ventilation to a nonbreathing patient.

_____ 12. Condition in which body temperature is much higher than normal for a prolonged period of time.

_____ 13. Pertaining to blood vessels that carry blood toward the heart.

_____ 14. Condition in which blood glucose is elevated above normal.

_____ 15. Continuous seizure activity.

_____ 16. Nosebleed.

_____ 17. Severe allergic reaction.

APPLIED PRACTICE

Using your textbook, answer the questions that follow each scenario below.

Scenario A

Tasha has recently been hired as a clinical medical assistant for a brand new family practice. She has been asked to stock the emergency crash cart and make sure it is ready in the case of an emergency. This is what she found:

CRASH CART INVENTORY LIST

- Alcohol pads
- Blood pressure cuffs and a sphygmomanometer
- Stethoscope, scissors, gauze, and pressure bandages
- Sterile gloves, needles, syringes
- Pen and paper
- Oxygen tank: flow meter and wrench
- Airways, tubing
- Oxygen masks: adult and pediatric
- Ambu bags
- Variety of resucitation masks
- IV fluids in 500 mL bags
- Hemostats
- Tourniquets
- Alcohol preps
- IV tubing (collapsible)

---

1. Based on the inventory list, what are some items that Tasha should add to the crash cart?

_____
_____
_____
_____

Scenario B

Sascha is employed at Community Urgent Care. A 47-year-old male patient has been brought to the facility. His right index finger was torn off of his hand while he was working on a piece of farming machinery. His coworker has driven him to the medical facility and has the dismembered finger in an empty coffee container.

2. What type of injury has this man sustained?

_____

3. How should Sascha handle the dismembered finger?

_____
_____
_____
_____
_____

Scenario C

Later in the day at Community Urgent Care, Sascha encounters a 36-year-old female patient who is presenting with a liquid chemical burn entirely covering the front and back of her right arm. Residue from the liquid chemical remains on the patient's arm.

4. What will the first step likely be for treating this patient? Explain your answer.

_____
_____
_____
_____

5. Because the patient's skin was extremely sensitive to the chemical agent, the physician has diagnosed a second-degree burn on the front and back of the patient's arm. According to the rule of nines, what percentage of her body has been affected?

_____

LEARNING ACTIVITY: TRUE/FALSE

Indicate whether the statement is true (T) or false (F).

_____ 1. An AED is not used on an infant.

_____ 2. Having a crash cart in the facility has legal liability issues for the practice.

_____ 3. Lock jaw is also known as an avulsion.

_____ 4. Establishing a baseline assessment of a head injury patient is often done using the Glasgow Coma Scale.

_____ 5. The pulse of an infant is taken on the carotid artery.

_____ 6. To prevent accidental or careless exposure, do not eat, drink, or touch your face during emergencies without first washing your hands.

_____ 7. A bolus of food is the most common object that adults choke on.

_____ 8. If direct pressure for bleeding does not stop the flow, a tourniquet must then be applied by a physician.

_____ 9. Usually an animal bite must be reported to the local animal control department.

_____ 10. In an emergency, if a person can wheeze, make a high-pitched sound, cough, or speak, do not take any action.

LEARNING ACTIVITY: FILL IN THE BLANK

Using words from the list below, fill in the blanks to complete the following statements.

105° F	dressings	ligaments
advice	EMS	massage
bright red	exposure	overdose
bruising	flushing	perspire
chemical	gentle stream	poisoning
cleansed	hard	pressure
contamination	healing	rub
copious	heart	strains
darker in color	immobilize	tendons
direct pressure	infection	underlying tissues
dislocations	insidious	water
distally to proximally		

1. Arterial bleeding is usually _____, rapid, _____, and often spurts. Venous bleeding is slower, _____, and can usually be controlled by _____.

2. An individual experiencing heat stroke usually fails to _____ and has a body temperature of _____ or higher.

3. Internal bleeding may be obvious or _____. _____ or discoloration of the skin may be an indication of bleeding in the _____.

4. Open wounds must be _____, and most wounds require some type of dressing to promote _____ and prevent _____.

5. Bandages are used to anchor _____ in place, prevent _____ of a recent wound or surgical site, support and _____ injured extremities, and may be used to apply _____ to slow and/or stop bleeding.

6. If tissue has been frozen and is _____ to the touch, call _____ or the physician. Never _____, squeeze, or _____ frozen tissue.

7. Musculoskeletal injuries involve bones, muscles, _____ and _____ and include fractures, _____, sprains, and _____.

8. Poison Control Centers offer emergency _____ concerning accidental _____ and _____; this service is usually provided at no charge.

9. To help venous blood flow return to the _____, always apply bandages _____, or far to near.

10. If a liquid chemical is the cause of a burn, remove it from the skin by _____ with copious amounts of _____. If it is a dry or powdery _____, it should be carefully wiped from the victim while avoiding _____ to yourself or bystanders, then flush the area with a copious but _____ of water.

CRITICAL THINKING

Answer the following questions to the best of your ability. Use the textbook as a reference.

1. A patient has presented to the front desk without an appointment and is obviously SOB. Her lips and fingertips appear a bit cyanotic. She seems weak and needs to be seated somewhere quickly. What would you do?

   _____
   _____
   _____
   _____
   _____

2. A patient who is sitting in the waiting room comes to the front desk with epistaxis, and the blood flow is very heavy. What would you do?

   _____
   _____
   _____
   _____
   _____

3. A patient's wife comes up to the front desk with some questions for the MA before her husband is seen. She asks how she could tell if her husband has or is having a stroke. How would you explain a CVA's signs and symptoms? (You are not diagnosing but simply giving the signs and symptoms in general.)

   _____
   _____
   _____
   _____
   _____

4. Why must you wash your hands after taking off gloves? Won't the gloves keep your skin clean so that you do not have to wash every time? Explain this in your own words.

   _____
   _____
   _____
   _____

5. If you come upon an unconscious person who you did not witness collapse, what should you do first? Would your answer be the same or different if the person was a 6-month-old infant?

   _____
   _____
   _____

RESEARCH ACTIVITY

Use Internet search engines to research the following topics and write a brief description of what is found. It is important to visit reputable Web sites.

1. Use the Internet to reference specific Web sites that can be useful when planning for emergency situations. What Web sites did you find most useful and how would a MA be able to use these sites to plan for emergency preparedness?

   _____

   _____

   _____

   _____

   _____

   _____

   _____

   _____

   _____

   _____

   _____

   _____

   _____

CHAPTER 42
Gastroenterology and Nutrition

CHAPTER OUTLINE

General review of the chapter:

    A. Introduction
    B. The MA's Role in the Gastroenterology Office
    C. The Anatomy and Physiology of the Gastrointestinal System
        i. Functions of the gastrointestinal system
    D. Diseases and Disorders of the GI Tract
    E. Nutrition
    F. Diagnosis and Treatments of GI Disorders

STUDENT STUDY GUIDE

Use the following guide to assist in your learning of the concepts from the chapter.

  I. The MA's Role in a Gastroenterology Office

    A. Obtaining and recording the patient's medical _____ and _____

        _____

    B. Assisting the physician as needed

    C. Gowning and specimen collection _____

    D. Arranging appointments for _____ tests and _____

    E. Providing _____ information and instructions _____ diet.

    F. Providing information for community _____ _____ and

        _____ support

  II. Anatomy and Physiology of the Gastrointestinal Tract

    A. The GI System

        i. Contains the _____ canal and _____ organs

        ii. Alimentary structures:

            (a) Upper gastrointestinal tract (UGI)

            (b) Lower gastrointestinal tract (LGI)

    B. Structures of the Upper GI

_____

_____

_____

_____

_____

_____

C. Structures of the Lower GI

_____

_____

_____

_____

_____

_____

D. The Small Intestine

_____

_____

_____

E. The Large Intestine

_____

_____

_____

_____

_____

_____

F. Accessory Organs

_____

_____

_____

_____

_____

G. Functions of the GI System

_____

_____

_____

_____

H. Alimentation
    i. Provides _____ to the body
    ii. Elimination rids the body of _____ _____.
    iii. Steps involved in alimentation:

_____

_____

_____

_____

_____

III. Diseases, Disorders, and Conditions of the GI Tract
  A. Conditions:
     i. Inflammatory conditions
     ii. _____ conditions
     iii. Infectious disorders
     iv. Disorders due to increased or decreased peristalsis
     v. Circulatory and _____ disorders
     vi. Congenital disorders
     vii. _____ disorders
     viii. Neoplasms
     ix. _____ invasion
     x. Food poisoning
     xi. Constipation
     xii. Diarrhea
     xiii. Paralytic obstruction
     xiv. _____
  B. Anatomical and Congenital Anomalies
     i. Diverticulosis
     ii. _____ reflux disease
     iii. _____ hernia
     iv. Organic obstructions
     v. _____ hernia
  C. Infectious Conditions
     _____
     _____
     _____
     _____
     _____
     _____

  D. Inflammatory Disorders
     _____
     _____
     _____
     _____
     _____
     _____
     _____
     _____
     _____
     _____
     _____

  E. Malignancies
     _____
     _____
     _____
     _____
     _____
     _____

F. Vascular Related Conditions
    i. _____ varices
    ii. Hemorrhoids

IV. Nutrition
    A. Basic components of food:
        i. _____
        ii. _____
        iii. _____
        iv. _____
        v. _____
        vi. _____

    B. Carbohydrates:
    _____
    _____
    _____
    _____

    C. Proteins
        i. Amino acids are the _____ _____ of protein.
        ii. They assist in building and renewing body tissues.
        iii. There are _____ amino acids.
    _____
    _____
    _____
    _____

    D. Fats
        i. Triglyceride fats include saturated, unsaturated and polyunsaturated fats.
          (a) Saturated fats are usually derived from _____ sources.
          (b) Unsaturated fats generally come from _____ sources.
          (c) _____ fats come from fish and corn, soybean and safflower oils.
          (d) Monosaturated fats are found in _____, _____, and
              _____.

    E. Lipoproteins
        i. Simple proteins that combine with lipid components, including _____,
          _____, and _____
        ii. High-density lipoprotein (HDL) and low-density lipoprotein (LDL) are a transport
          medium that carries fats in the bloodstream.
          (a) HDL:
    _____
    _____
          (b) LDL:
    _____
    _____

    F. Water
        i. The human body is _____ water.
        ii. The human body can live longer without _____ than it can
          _____.

iii. Many body processes require water:

_____

_____

_____

_____

G. Vitamins
    i. Required for _____, _____, and _____
    ii. Classified as fat soluble and water soluble
    iii. _____ vitamins include A, D, E, and K.
    iv. _____ are B complex and C.
    v. Vitamins A, C, and E are considered _____.

H. Minerals
    i. Contribute to _____ development and repair
    ii. Occur naturally in nature
    iii. Essential to every cell for regulatory processes:

_____

_____

_____

_____

I. Dietary Fiber
    i. Found in food:
      (a) Plants, fruits, vegetables, grains, and legumes
    ii. Fiber is a form of _____ the body does not digest.
    iii. Adequate amount in daily diet maintains proper intestinal health and prevents disease

V. The Importance of Nutrition and Food Allergies

A. Food Guide Pyramid
    i. Developed to help Americans maintain healthy eating habits
    ii. Guide shows the number of servings for different types of food groups necessary to meet daily nutritional needs
    iii. Food pyramids are different depending on _____ groups, _____ groups, and persons with medical needs.

B. Effects of Nutritional Deficiencies
    i. Single effect:

_____

_____

_____

_____

    ii. Seesaw effect:

_____

_____

_____

_____

    iii. Cascading effect:

_____

_____

_____

_____

C. Nutritional Deficiencies
   i. Seen in:

_____

_____

   ii. People with dental problems:

_____

_____

_____

_____

D. Caloric Intake
   i. Harmful cultural, economic, and lifestyle factors affect caloric intake:
     (a) _____ celebrate with food.
     (b) Low-income groups buy larger amounts of _____.
     (c) Busier lifestyles _____ _____ and eat more fast food.

E. Alcohol and Nutrition
   i. Small amounts may have therapeutic benefits.
   ii. In general, alcohol interferes with _____.
   iii. Contributes to _____ and other medical problems
   iv. Too much alcohol accumulates as fat and may eventually cause _____.
   v. Prevents enzyme use for other necessary nutritional reactions
   vi. Long-term use can cause malnutrition, _____, _____, cancer, _____, and _____.

F. Altered Nutritional Status
   i. As people age, nutritional status diminishes:

_____

_____

_____

_____

_____

_____

_____

   ii. Diseases due to an altered nutritional status include:

_____

_____

_____

_____

_____

_____

_____

_____

G. Food Allergies
   i. Symptoms can range from _____ to _____ (itching to anaphylaxis).

ii. Common food allergies in adults include:

_____

_____

_____

_____

iii. Common food allergies in children include:

_____

_____

_____

_____

H. Food Allergy Determination
   i. A physician will perform a detailed _____ _____.
   ii. The patient is asked to keep a detailed _____ _____.
   iii. _____ diets are based on the absence of food, and thus, the absence of symptoms.
   iv. _____ _____ testing may be performed.
   v. Blood tests may also be performed to measure the presence of IgE.

VI. Divisions of the Abdomen and Diagnostic Procedures

A. Clinical Divisions of the Abdomen
   i. The Right Upper Quadrant (RUQ)

_____

_____

_____

_____

_____

_____

   ii. The Right Lower Quadrant (RLQ)

_____

_____

_____

_____

_____

   iii. The Left Upper Quadrant (LUQ)

_____

_____

_____

_____

_____

   iv. The Left Lower Quadrant (LLQ)

_____

_____

_____

_____

_____

_____

B. Anatomical Divisions of the Abdomen
   i. Right and left _____ regions
  ii. _____ region
 iii. Right and left lumbar regions
  iv. _____ region
   v. Right and left _____ regions
  vi. _____ region

C. Diagnostic Procedures

_____

_____

_____

_____

_____

_____

_____

_____

_____

_____

_____

_____

D. The Colonoscopy
   i. Determines the _____ and _____ of the colon
  ii. American Cancer Society recommends everyone over the age of _____ be screened.
 iii. Checks for _____, _____, _____, and abscesses within the colon.

E. The Sigmoidoscopy
   i. Evaluates lower gastrointestinal disorders; tumors, positive fecal occult blood tests, bleeding, polyps, or suspected cancer
  ii. Exam provides a visual of the _____, _____, _____ intestine, and appendix.

F. Special Diets
   i. Examples of special diets include:

_____

_____

_____

_____

_____

_____

KEY TERMINOLOGY REVIEW

Match the selected key terms to their definitions below.

a. absorption
b. alimentation
c. bolus
d. chyme
e. complete protein
f. dyspepsia
g. dysphagia

h. elimination
i. emesis
j. emulsification
k. hematemesis
l. incomplete protein
m. intrinsic factor
n. jaundice

o. melena
p. metabolism
q. obesity
r. peristalsis
s. saturated fats
t. triglycerides

_____ 1. Protein containing all the essential amino acids.

_____ 2. Passage of digested food products through the wall of the intestine into the bloodstream.

_____ 3. Yellowing of skin and mucous membranes resulting from deposit of bile.

_____ 4. Rhythmic, involuntary, wave-like motion in the hollow tubes of the body that assists the passage of contents.

_____ 5. Vomiting of blood, an indication of bleeding in upper GI tract.

_____ 6. Fats derived from animal sources that are solid at room temperature.

_____ 7. Regurgitation of partially digested food from the stomach; vomit.

_____ 8. Black, tarry stools.

_____ 9. Mass of masticated food that is swallowed.

_____ 10. Difficulty swallowing.

_____ 11. Protein lacking one or more of the essential amino acids.

_____ 12. Expulsion of waste products from the body.

_____ 13. Process of changing nutrients from food into substances for anabolic or catabolic activity.

_____ 14. Mixture of partially digested food and enzymes that enters the small intestine.

_____ 15. A glycoprotein secreted by the parietal cells of the gastric mucosa.

_____ 16. Chief form of fat found in foods.

_____ 17. Excess body weight 20 to 30 percent above average for gender, age, and height, with abnormal amounts of body fat.

_____ 18. Painful digestion.

_____ 19. Transformation of ingested particles of fat into small globules with bile.

_____ 20. Entire process of providing nourishment to the body that includes mastication, swallowing, digestion, and absorption.

APPLIED PRACTICE

Read the scenario below and then, using your textbook, answer the questions that follow.

Scenario

Emily is a medical assistant working for Dr. Wyn, a gastroenterologist. Melody Hoffstettler is the first patient of the day. Melody has been experiencing left upper quadrant pain. She has recently started vomiting small amounts of blood. The physician makes a note in Melody's chart that states "there seems to be a slight distension in the patient's abdomen."

1. Melody is exhibiting signs/symptoms of what inflammatory disease of the gastrointestinal tract?

   _____

2. Melody's pain has been in the upper right quadrant of the abdomen. What main and accessory organs are found here?

   _____

   _____

   _____

   _____

3. Assume, rather, that Melody presents to the office with severe onset of pain in her right lower quadrant. What is this a classic symptom of?

   _____

4. Based on your above answer, which of the nine clinical divisions of the abdomen would be affected?

   _____

5. Label the anatomical structures of the figure on page 437. Try to recall the structures from memory without the help of your textbook.

   a. _____

   b. _____

   c. _____

   d. _____

   e. _____

   f. _____

   g. _____

   h. _____

   i. _____

   j. _____

   k. _____

   l. _____

   m. _____

   n. _____

   o. _____

   p. _____

   q. _____

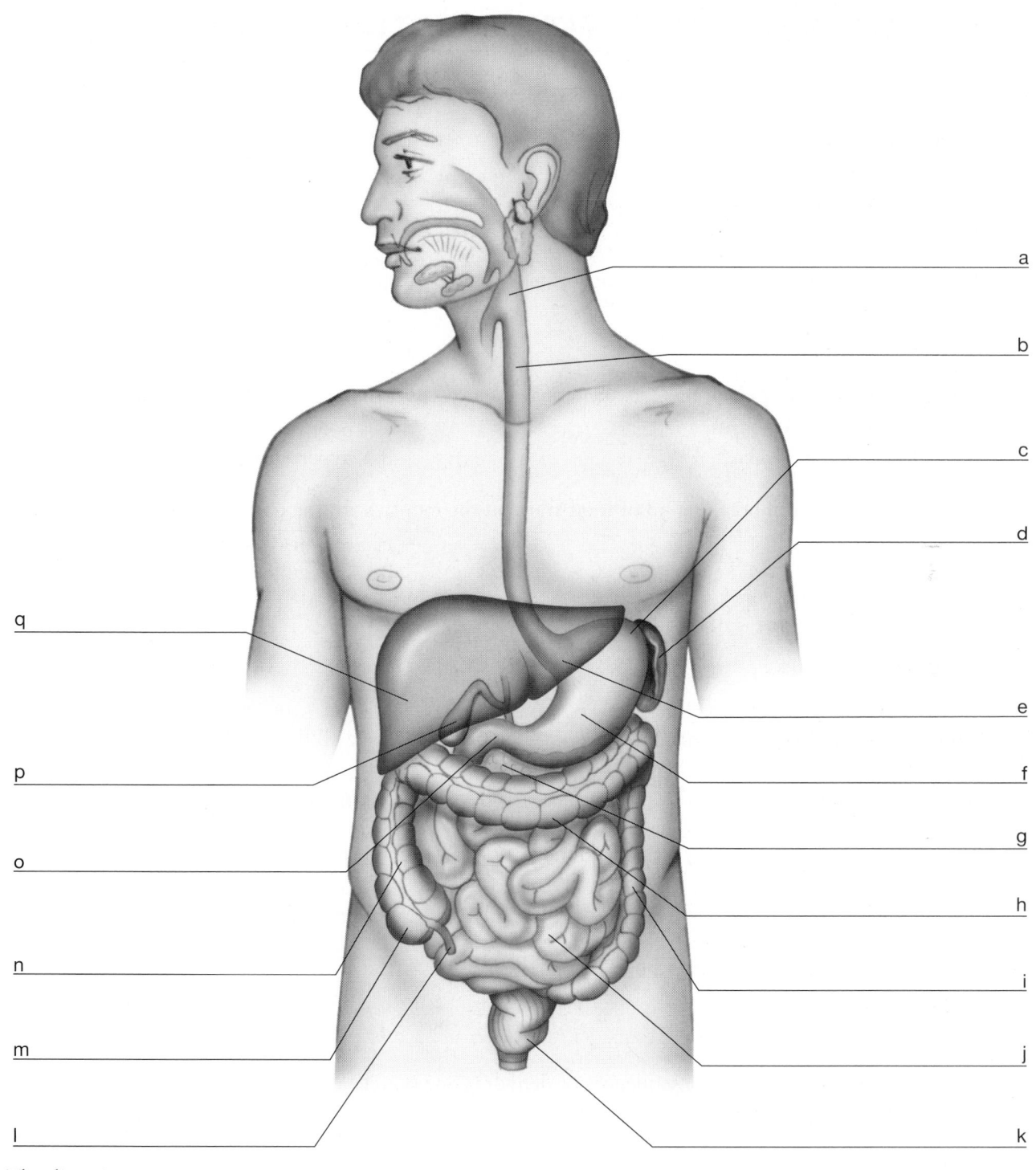

a

b

c

d

q

e

p

f

o

g

h

n

i

m

j

l

k

The digestive system

LEARNING ACTIVITY: MULTIPLE CHOICE

Circle the correct answer to each of the questions below.

1. Which of the following are not common-sense treatments of nausea as discussed in your text? (Circle all that apply.)
   - a. Keep eyes open.
   - b. Drink flat carbonated soft drinks.
   - c. Drink clear liquids.
   - d. Increase fiber in the diet.

2. Which of the following food choices are complex carbohydrates? (Circle all that apply.)
   - a. fruit
   - b. whole grains
   - c. honey
   - d. potatoes

3. Which of the following disorders may benefit from a therapeutic diet? (Circle all that apply.)
   - a. diabetes mellitus
   - b. hypercholesterolemia
   - c. polyps
   - d. hypertension

4. The initial mechanical breaking up of food starts in the mouth with the (circle all that apply):
   - a. tongue
   - b. pharynx
   - c. salivary glands
   - d. mandible

5. Which of the following is not a complete protein?
   - a. eggs
   - b. whole grains
   - c. meat
   - d. fish

6. Which of the following are warning signs of GI problems? (Circle all that apply.)
   - a. melenoma
   - b. hematemesis
   - c. coffee-ground emesis
   - d. flatulence

7. Which of the following is a layer of the alimentary canal? (Circle all that apply.)
   - a. serosa
   - b. submuscular
   - c. mucosa
   - d. muscularis

8. Which of the following activities burns the most calories?
   - a. swimming
   - b. tennis
   - c. aerobics
   - d. running

9. Which of the following are consequences of dehydration? (Circle all that apply.)
   - a. increased blood volume
   - b. hypotension
   - c. increased urine production
   - d. possible hypovolemic shock

10. Which of the following is not located in the lower right quadrant of the abdomen?
   - a. cecum
   - b. appendix
   - c. spleen
   - d. right ureter

LEARNING ACTIVITY: TRUE/FALSE

Indicate whether the statement is true (T) or false (F).

_____ 1. Energy released from the metabolism of proteins, fats, and carbohydrates is measured in units of kilograms.

_____ 2. LDLs transport fats from body cells to the liver for disposal.

_____ 3. Bright red blood in the stools is an indicator of gastric cancer.

_____ 4. A good post-op diet is the clear liquid diet.

_____ 5. Water, fluids, and electrolytes are absorbed mainly in the large intestine.

_____ 6. A person's religion can play a role in his or her nutrition.

_____ 7. In a heart-healthy diet, avoid tuna packed in oil.

_____ 8. Carbohydrates are the body's primary source of energy and are found primarily in breads, cereals, pasta products, rice, fruit, and potatoes.

_____ 9. Lipids (fats) are a primary source of energy.

_____ 10. For rapid absorption of a medication without the risk of GI upset, you must inject medication.

CRITICAL THINKING

Answer the following questions to the best of your ability. Use the textbook as a reference.

1. A patient has just been given some medication rectally and has been kept in the office for about 30 minutes. She is experiencing some sleepiness and dizziness, and her sister will be driving her home. Educate the patient about any side effects she may experience.

_____

_____

_____

_____

2. Mr. McNeill is experiencing constipation and has called in for advice on how to deal with this. Try to recall what you have read in this chapter of your textbook and use your common sense to list a few things that may help. After you have done that, check the book and review items you may have not learned yet.

_____

_____

_____

_____

3. You take a call from a patient who had a sigmoidoscopy earlier today. She is complaining of excess gas. What suggestions can you give her to give her some relief at home until she can pass the gas?

_____

_____

_____

4. From your own understanding, without reviewing the textbook first, explain why HDL lipoproteins are considered the good cholesterol and LDL lipoproteins are considered the bad cholesterol.

_____

_____

_____

_____

_____

5. The patient, Millie Stewart, is chatting while you are getting her ready for an exam. She tells you she has tried every kind of diet and many have worked well and rapidly, but the weight always comes back. Ms. Stewart explains that she has decided that she is just supposed to be 20 pounds overweight and she isn't going to diet any more; she is going to enjoy her food and her life. How would you respond to this? Consider that the information on Fad Diets under Tips for Success in your textbook is a resource for you to follow while working in a GI office. Plan your answer and write it out based on the information you know or deduce. You can check the book later, but respond to this using your common sense and critical thinking.

_____

_____

_____

_____

_____

RESEARCH ACTIVITY

Use Internet search engines to research the following topics and write a brief description of what is found. It is important to visit reputable Web sites.

1. Visit www.mypyramid.gov. As you navigate through the site, take note of specific items that can be useful as patient education. Make your own MyPyramid Plan and explain what is recommended for your specific body type. What information do you find particularly useful within this Web site?

_____

_____

_____

_____

_____

_____

_____

_____

_____

_____

_____

_____

CHAPTER 43
Orthopedics and Physical Therapy

CHAPTER OUTLINE

General review of the chapter:

    A. Introduction
    B. The Medical Assistant's Role in Orthopedics and Physical Therapy
    C. Anatomy and Physiology of the Musculoskeletal System
        i. Bones
       ii. Muscles
    D. Common Musculoskeletal Diseases and Disorders
    E. Diagnostic Procedures
    F. Treatment of Musculoskeletal Conditions in the Orthopedic Office

STUDENT STUDY GUIDE

Use the following guide to assist in your learning of the concepts from the chapter.

  I. The MA's Role in an Orthopedic Office

    A. Obtaining and recording medical history
    B. _____ and _____ symptoms
    C. Assisting the physician throughout the exam
    D. Placing _____ films on radiograph
    E. Gowning instructions and assistance
    F. Arranging _____ for other tests and procedures
    G. Providing _____ devices
    H. Instructing patients and family members on proper _____ _____
        and thermodynamic treatments
    I. Providing community resources information

 II. Anatomy and Physiology of the Musculoskeletal System

    A. Divisions of the Skeletal System
        i. _____ section contains:

            _____

            _____

       ii. _____ section contains:

            _____

            _____

    B. Bones of the Body
        i. _____
       ii. _____

iii. _____

iv. _____

C. Bone Tissue
   i. Periosteum cartilage covers bone.

   _____

   _____

   ii. Osteoblasts are within cartilage and assist with bone tissue formation.

   _____

   _____

D. Joints
   i. A joint is the point where two bones meet
      (a) _____ = cartilaginous joints that are slightly movable
      (b) _____ = fibrous joints with no movement
      (c) _____ = synovial joints that are freely movable

E. Synovial Joints
   i. _____ (shoulders and hips)
   ii. _____ (junction of metacarpal joint and first phalanx of each finger)
   iii. _____ (wrist and ankle)
   iv. _____ (knee, elbow)
   v. _____ (radius and ulna in arm)
   vi. _____ (metacarpal bone of thumb and wrist)

F. Range of Motion
   i. Range of motion is abbreviated _____.
   ii. Refers to the full degree of movement that a joint is capable of
   iii. Exercises or treatments are given to increase the ROM in cases of injury or atrophy.

G. Anatomy and Physiology of Muscles
   i. Muscles facilitate movement by contracting and relaxing.
   ii. Three kinds of muscle tissue in the body:

   _____

   _____

H. Functions of Muscles

   _____

   _____

   _____

   _____

   _____

   _____

   _____

   _____

I. Muscle Movement
   i. _____ muscles cause voluntary movement.
      (a) Throwing a ball
   ii. _____ muscles cause involuntary movement.
      (a) Cardiac muscle pumping

J. Neuromuscular Function
   i. Synaptic gap lies between the _____ cell and the _____ cell
   ii. A stimulus causes the release of _____.
   iii. Neurotransmitters excite and prompt a response from the muscle fiber or cell.

      iv. This causes _____ impulses across the entire muscle cell.

      v. Which results in _____ of the muscle

III. Diseases and Disorders of the Musculoskeletal System

    A. Classification of Orthopedic Diseases and Disorders

        i. Anatomical structures

_____

_____

        ii. Type of conditions

_____

_____

    B. Congenital Disorders

_____

_____

_____

_____

    C. Myasthenia Gravis: loss of muscle strength

    D. Degenerative disorders or diseases occur at various stages of life.

_____

_____

    E. _____: softening of bone with deformities

    F. Infectious Musculoskeletal Conditions

_____

_____

_____

_____

    G. Neoplasia

_____

_____

_____

_____

    H. Fractures

        i. Fractures compromise the integrity of bone structure.

        ii. Types vary based on:

_____

_____

    I. Types of Fractures

_____

_____

_____

_____

_____

_____

_____

J. Soft-Tissue Injuries
   i. _____: caused by insult to muscles, tendons, or ligaments around a joint
   ii. _____: overstretched muscles, tendons, or ligaments
   iii. _____: bones displaced or separated from a joint
   iv. _____ is an incomplete or partial dislocation.
   v. Severed tendons are lacerated or an acute tear to surrounding tissue.
   vi. _____ is total or partial removal of a limb or digit.

K. Diagnostic Procedures for Musculoskeletal Injuries

_____

_____

_____

_____

_____

L. Splints, Braces, and Casts
   i. _____ is the correction of a fracture and realigning the bone fragments.
   ii. External manipulation or open _____ manipulation is used.
   iii. Splints, braces or casts are usually used with fractures.
   iv. Ambulatory devices, _____ or _____, may be required.
   v. Splints prevent the movement of body parts.
   vi. Braces are more _____ and support weak muscles or joints.
   vii. Casts are solid, rigid, cylindrical casings that immobilize joints or body parts.
   viii. Plaster used in past, today casts are made of synthetic fiberglass, polyester, or cotton

M. Cast Application

_____

_____

_____

_____

_____

_____

_____

_____

_____

IV. Physical Therapy Modalities

A. _____
   i. Cold therapy _____ blood vessels.
   ii. Slows circulation
   iii. Reduces swelling, inflammation, and pain
   iv. Common forms include cold compresses, ice-filled _____, or ice _____.

B. Thermotherapy
   i. _____ therapy increases blood flow to an area.
   ii. Provides comfort and healing
   iii. Common sources include hot soaks, compresses, lights or heating pads.

C. _____ therapy improves joint flexibility, muscle tone, strength, and mobility.

D. Hydrotherapy utilizes _____ exercises.
E. Massage stimulates circulation and promotes healing.
F. Range of motion exercises improve flexibility and mobility.
G. Ultrasound vibrates tissues, generates _____, and promotes _____.

H. Ambulatory Aids

_____

_____

_____

_____

_____

I. Prostheses in Orthopedics

_____

_____

_____

_____

_____

_____

_____

_____

KEY TERMINOLOGY REVIEW

Use a dictionary and highlighted terms in the textbook to define the following terms.

1. Amphiarthrosis:

_____

_____

2. Arthritis:

_____

_____

3. Articular:

_____

_____

4. Atony:

_____

_____

5. Atrophy:

_____

_____

6. Axillary:

_____

_____

7. Body mechanics:

_____

_____

8. Bursa (plural: bursae):

_____

_____

9. Bursitis:

_____

_____

10. Cartilage:

_____

_____

11. Cast:

_____

_____

12. Compress:

_____

_____

13. Cryotherapy:

_____

_____

14. Diarthrosis:

_____

_____

15. Endosteum:

_____

_____

16. Hematopoiesis:

_____

_____

17. Ligament:

_____

_____

18. Neoplasia:

_____

_____

19. Orthopedics:

_____

_____

20. Osteoblast:

_____

_____

21. Periosteum:

_____

_____

22. Prosthesis (plural: prostheses):

_____

_____

23. Range of motion:

_____

_____

24. Reduction:

_____

_____

25. Soak:

_____

_____

26. Splint:

_____

_____

27. Synarthrosis:

_____

_____

28. Tendon:

_____

_____

29. Tetany:

_____

_____

30. Thermodynamics:

_____

_____

31. Thermotherapy:

_____

_____

APPLIED PRACTICE

Follow the directions as instructed with each question below.

1. Read the following scenario and answer the corresponding questions.

Scenario

It is a busy Monday morning and you are working as a clinical MA at an orthopedic office. Rachel, an administrative MA, has just informed you that an emergency appointment was just scheduled for Miles Sampson, a teenager who injured his lower leg while participating in a soccer game during gym class. He is currently en route to the office.

The following information is charted:

Sampson, Miles

12-05-1994

04/08/20xx   10:30 am   Ht: ----   Wt: ----   P: 90 bpm   BP: 130/88

cc: Pt. states that he was playing soccer when a classmate tripped him and fell on his lower Rt. leg. Pain is rated as an 8, he describes the pain as "extreme." Rt. lower leg appears bruised and swollen, an ice pack has been applied --- *Your name, MA*

Dr. Stephanie Walters has ordered AP and lateral views of the lower right leg. There appears to be a transverse fracture of the Rt. tibia.

a. Draw a picture of how this transverse fracture may appear on an X-ray.

b. Would this be a simple or compound fracture? Explain why.

_____

_____

c. Assume that your clinic applies fiberglass casts. List the supplies that are needed to prepare for a fiberglass cast application.

_____

_____

_____

_____

_____

d. What would the patient do immediately after the cast has been applied?

_____

_____

LEARNING ACTIVITY: MULTIPLE CHOICE

Circle the correct answer to each of the questions below.

1. Bones are classified according to structure, and four are listed in your textbook. Which of the following is not one of the four structure classifications?
   a. flat
   b. round
   c. short
   d. long

2. Your text includes five classifications of common musculoskeletal diseases and disorders. Which of the following are included in these classifications as stated in the book? (Circle all that apply.)
   a. congenital
   b. malignant
   c. infectious
   d. degenerative
   e. traumatic

3. Arthritis is the inflammation and degeneration of joint structures. Which of the following is not a form of arthritis?
   a. osteoarthritis
   b. rheumatoid arthritis
   c. bursitis
   d. gouty arthritis

4. Which of the following is a diagnostic procedure that could diagnose/confirm intervertebral disc disorders?
   a. electromyogram
   b. arthrogram
   c. bone scan
   d. myelogram

5. Involuntary muscles are controlled by the
   a. autonomic nervous system
   b. peripheral nervous system
   c. sympathetic nervous system
   d. parasympathetic nervous system

6. Which of the following types of fracture usually does not require surgical intervention at an emergency or urgent care center?
   a. displaced
   b. greenstick
   c. avulsed
   d. compound

7. There are three types of muscle tissue in the body. Which of the following are not one of those three types? (Circle all that apply.)

   a. tendon

   b. cartilage

   c. cardiac

   d. smooth

8. Trauma to the musculoskeletal system does *not* include insults in the form of:

   a. fractured bones

   b. insults to muscles

   c. soft-tissue insults to ligaments and tendons

   d. arthritis

9. A complete or partial dislocation is called a

   a. manipulation

   b. laceration

   c. subluxation

   d. displacement

10. Degeneration of the neuromuscular system is discussed briefly in your textbook under The Contraction of Muscle Cells, and three examples of diseases in this category are given. Which of the following is not one of the three?

    a. Parkinson's disease

    b. muscular dystrophy

    c. atrophy

    d. multiple sclerosis

CRITICAL THINKING

Answer the following questions to the best of your ability. Use the textbook as a reference.

1. Consider that you have a 7-year-old male patient with a fractured ankle. He is full of energy and seems to be the type who will be running around in his cast and be pretty hard on it. Which casting material would you choose for this child and why? (The answer is not in the book; use your reasoning or critical thinking and decide on your answer.)

   _____

   _____

   _____

   _____

2. Review the case study at the beginning of this chapter in the textbook. Explain why the X-ray may not show a fracture of a bone.

   _____

   _____

   _____

   _____

3. You were at the scene of an injury to a 14-year-old female who had fallen off of her bike. You can see that a portion of her flesh and a piece of bone has been torn away and is lying in the dirt at the edge of the sidewalk. Should you save that piece of tissue and if so, how would you prepare/store it until it can be given to a doctor?

   _____

   _____

_____

_____

_____

4. Without looking back at the material right now, picture that you are working in an orthopedic office and a 19-year-old college football player has been brought into the clinic by his coach. He has been seen by the doctor, and X-rays have been taken and looked at by the doctor. He was diagnosed with a strain, and you are preparing him for application of a cast by the technician. The patient insists he has a sprain, not a strain, and asks that you explain to him the difference between the two. From your memory of the material, write your answer. Then go back and check the book and write a correct answer if yours differs.

_____

_____

_____

_____

_____

5. A patient calls in and has questions after reading her cast care written instructions. She asks how she is supposed to apply ice to the injury when she has a cast on over the injury. What patient education/instruction would you give her?

_____

_____

_____

_____

_____

RESEARCH ACTIVITY

Use Internet search engines to research the following topics and write a brief description of what is found. It is important to visit reputable Web sites.

1. Research new materials and advances being made in prosthetics. What information do you find most interesting and why?

_____

_____

_____

_____

_____

_____

_____

_____

_____

_____

CHAPTER 44
Obstetrics and Gynecology

CHAPTER OUTLINE

General review of the chapter:

A. The Medical Assistant's Role in the OB/GYN Office
B. The Anatomy and Physiology of the Female Reproductive System
C. The Menstrual Cycle
D. Contraception
E. Pregnancy and the Birth Process
F. Gynecological Diseases and Disorders
G. Routine Assessment
H. Diagnostic Procedures
I. Treatment Modalities

STUDENT STUDY GUIDE

Use the following guide to assist in your learning of the concepts from the chapter.

I. Introduction and the MA Role in the OB/GYN Office

  A. Introduction
    i. Specialization of women's issues

    _____

    _____

    ii. Gynecology focuses on the _____ _____ system.
    iii. Obstetrics focuses on _____ and _____.
    iv. Obstetrician is the physician that works with women during childbirth

  B. The MA Role in an OB/GYN Office
    i. Obtain patient history and vital signs
    ii. Assist physicians with pelvic exams, pap smears, and specimen collection.
    iii. Prenatal visits require:

    _____

    _____

    iv. The presence of the MA is often required during physician examinations.

II. Anatomy and Physiology of the Female Reproductive System

  A. _____: two small almond-shaped glands produce ova (eggs)
  B. Fallopian tubes: structure ova take to _____.
  C. Uterus: hollow _____-shaped organ in the pelvis where fertilized _____ are implanted
    i. Three layers:

    _____

    _____

D. Vagina: extends from vaginal opening to the cervix
E. Cul-de-sac: highly sensitive area behind the _____
F. Vulva: name of the female external genitalia
    i. Labia majora: _____
    ii. Labia minora: _____
    iii. _____ gland: lubrication gland
    iv. _____: erectile tissue
    v. Perineum: area between the vaginal orifice and _____
G. The Female Breasts
    i. _____ glands that develop during puberty
    ii. Nonfunctional until the end of _____
    iii. Used to breast-feed infants
    iv. _____ is produced until the mother's milk comes in.
    v. Contain:

_____

_____

III. The Menstrual Cycle
A. _____ changes stimulate the onset of menses and the menstrual cycle.
B. Hormones control the development, _____, and release of ova.
C. When fertilization does not occur, the _____ lining is shed.
D. Normal menstrual cycle is one lunar month, or _____.
E. Menses is the _____ day of the cycle and lasts for about _____ days.
    i. Endometrial lining is shed in a bloody fluid
F. Once complete, the hormonal cycle begins the repair of this lining for _____ days.
G. On the 14th day, _____ hormone causes ovulation to occur.
H. Ova move through fallopian tube for a duration of five days.
I. Endometrium _____ in preparation for a fertilized egg
J. If fertilization does not occur, menses begins.
K. Menopause

_____

_____

_____

_____

_____

L. Menstrual Disorders
    i. Dysmenorrhea: _____
    ii. Amenorrhea: _____
    iii. Menorrhagia: _____
    iv. Metrorrhagia: _____
    v. Mittelschmertz: _____
    vi. Premenstrual syndrome: _____
M. Treatment of Menstrual Disorders

_____

_____

_____

_____

IV. Contraception
  A. Types of Birth Control
      i. Barrier method
     ii. Chemical contact
    iii. Hormonal control
     iv. Intrauterine devices
      v. Periodic sexual abstinence
     vi. Surgical sterilization
  B. Barrier Methods of Birth Control

  _____
  _____
  _____
  _____
  _____
  _____

  C. Spermacides

  _____
  _____
  _____
  _____
  _____

  D. Hormonal Contraceptives

  _____
  _____
  _____
  _____
  _____

  E. Intrauterine Device

  _____
  _____
  _____

  F. Sexual Abstinence
      i. Avoiding sexual intercourse during the fertile period of the menstrual cycle
     ii. Signs of fertility include:

  _____
  _____
  _____
  _____

  iii. Very _____ method of birth control

  iv. Only acceptable method in some _____

 G. Sterilization and Tubal Ligation

  i. Surgical procedures

  ii. Tubal ligation done with _____

_____

_____

_____

_____

  iii. In males the vas deferens is cauterized in the vasectomy procedure.

 H. Infertility

  i. Health status of the mother is tested comprehensively

_____

_____

_____

_____

  ii. When pregnancy does not occur, in-vitro fertilization may be attempted.

V. Pregnancy and Childbirth

 A. Pregnancy

  i. Stages of pregnancy start with _____.

  ii. Ovum is released from ovary and fertilized by male sperm in fallopian tube

  iii. A/an _____ is formed.

  iv. As it divides and grows, it becomes an embryo.

  v. Embryo implants itself in the endometrium

  vi. With perfect conditions it will grow to a fetus.

  vii. Normal gestational period is _____, or _____ the date of conception

  viii. EDD = _____ _____ _____

  ix. EDC = _____ _____ _____

 B. Childbirth

_____

_____

_____

_____

 C. Obstetrical History

_____

_____

_____

_____

 D. Routine Obstetrical Procedures and Tests

_____

_____

_____

_____

_____

_____

E. Patient History for Prenatal Visits
  i. Date of _____ _____ _____ (LMP)
  ii. Age of onset of menses
  iii. _____ and duration of periods
  iv. Pain during menstruation
  v. Total number of _____
  vi. Number of live births
  vii. Number of stillbirths
  viii. Number of _____ or abortions
  ix. Age of cessation of menses
  x. Surgical procedures if any
  xi. History of any sexually transmitted diseases
  xii. Dates of last _____ and pap smear
  xiii. Medications, including birth control
  xiv. Method of _____
  xv. Breastfeeding if there is a history of pregnancy
  xvi. _____ _____

F. Pregnancy Complications
  i. _____ _____: nausea and vomiting
  ii. Spontaneous abortion or miscarriage: unknown _____ resulting in bleeding and termination of pregnancy
  iii. _____ or _____ pregnancy: embryo implants somewhere other than uterus; causes severe pain
  iv. Premature labor and delivery
  v. _____ mole: conception error causing abdomen to grow without fetal heart tones
  vi. Toxemia: _____ during the pregnancy resulting in _____
  vii. Pre-eclampsia or eclampsia: milder versions of toxemia without symptoms of convulsions
  viii. _____ _____: placenta implanted across the cervical os or low in the uterus
  ix. Abruptio placenta: placenta prematurely _____

G. Monitored Conditions during Pregnancy
  _____
  _____
  _____
  _____

H. Breast Feeding
  i. Very personal choice to each mother
  ii. Advantages to both breast feeding and formula feeding
  iii. Mother's milk provides _____ to diseases.
  iv. Assures proper _____ and _____
  v. Essentially free and readily available
  vi. Requires mother to have a/an _____ _____
  vii. Mother must be readily available to feed.

I. Formula Feeding
  _____
  _____
  _____
  _____

VI. Diseases and Disorders of the Female Reproductive System
   A. _____ _____: no known etiology and can cause abdominal pain
   B. Pelvic inflammatory disease: caused by _____ with symptoms of pelvic pain
   C. _____: endometrial tissue displaced into the pelvis
   D. _____ _____: benign fibrous growths that cause heavy periods and pelvic pain
   E. Vaginitis: caused by _____ *Trichomonas*; _____, foul-smelling discharge
   F. _____ _____: uterus drops into the vaginal orifice
   G. _____: downward displacement of the urinary bladder into the vagina
   H. _____: downward displacement of the rectum into the vagina
   I. Ovarian cancer has an unknown _____.
   J. Uterine or endometrial cancer: unknown etiology linked to overexposure to estrogen
   K. Cervical cancer: linked to overexposure to _____ _____ virus
   L. Labial cancer: occurs in females over the age of _____ with an unknown etiology.
   M. Vaginal Bleeding
      i. Main symptom in any female reproductive-related disorder or disease
      ii. _____
      iii. If present in young girls it can be a symptom of _____ _____.
      iv. In postmenopausal women it may indicate a/an _____ _____ or pathology.
      v. During pregnancy prompt medical attention should be sought.
      vi. Assessment of Vaginal Bleeding

      _____
      _____
      _____
      _____
      _____
      _____

   N. Sexually Transmitted Diseases
      i. Contracted by sexual contact, via _____, _____, or _____ _____.
      ii. Referred to as STDs
      iii. Occur in both males and females
      iv. Commonly seen in the OB/GYN office
      v. Bacterial STDs

      _____
      _____
      _____
      _____
      _____
      _____

      vi. Viral STDs

      _____
      _____

_____

_____

O. Breast Disorders and Diseases
    i. Prone to various conditions:

    _____

    _____

    ii. Diminutive size
    iii. Massive size
P. Fibrocystic Changes

    _____

    _____

    _____

    _____

Q. Breast Cancer
    i. A/an _____ is the most common sign of cancer.
    ii. Can be found early with monthly self-breast exams
    iii. Mammograms are recommended after the age of _____.
    iv. _____ are performed to determine if lump is benign or malignant
    v. Treatment includes chemotherapy or _____.
R. Breast Surgeries
    i. Breast reduction is performed on women with large breasts.

    _____

    _____

    ii. Breast augmentation not covered by insurance
         (a) Considered cosmetic
VII. Diagnostic Assessment

    A. Pap tests
        i. Routine pelvic and Pap tests are recommended:

        _____

        _____

        _____

        _____

    B. Obtaining a complete history
    C. Measuring weight, height, blood pressure, and temperature
    D. Collecting a/an _____ sample
    E. Assessing vaginal bleeding
VIII. Diagnostic Tests

    A. _____
    B. _____
    C. _____
    D. _____
    E. _____
    F. _____

IX. Treatment Modalities

    A. _____ and _____: cervix is dilated and the lining of the uterus is
        scraped with a curette after a miscarriage
    B. Laparoscopy views _____ structures, _____ or removes organs

C. Tubal ligation is the cauterization of fallopian tubes to prevent pregnancy.
D. Abdominal or _____ hysterectomies remove the female uterus.
E. A/an _____: the removal of one ovary
F. _____: the removal of one fallopian tube
G. Surgery is used for a prolapsed uterus, and to repair a/an _____ or
_____.
H. Episiotomies are incisions in the perineum to facilitate the delivery of an infant.
I. Psychological Issues
    i. Patients should be listened to compassionately.
    ii. Many issues are faced by patients and families.

_____

_____

_____

_____

_____

_____

_____

KEY TERMINOLOGY REVIEW

Write a sentence using the selected vocabulary terms in the correct context.

1. Amniocentesis:

_____

_____

2. Colostrum:

_____

_____

3. Effacement:

_____

_____

4. Fundal Height:

_____

_____

5. -gravida:

_____

_____

6. Menarche:

_____

_____

7. Ovum:

_____

_____

8. -para:

_____

_____

9. Postpartum:

_____

_____

10. Zygote:

_____

_____

APPLIED PRACTICE

Follow the directions as instructed with each question below.

1. Read the following scenario and answer the corresponding questions.

   Scenario

   Today, Patty, an RMA (AMT), is working with Dr. Susan Antolik. Dr. Antolik specializes in obstetrics and gynecology. Dr. Antolik's next patient is Sally McNally, age 32 y. The following dialogue is exchanged between Patty and Sally.

   Patty, RMA (AMT): "What brings you to the office today Ms. McNally?"

   Sally McNally: "My period is late and I just don't feel right. I am also due for my annual exam."

   a. What should Patty ask Sally next?

   _____

   b. What type of specimen should Patty collect?

   _____

   c. What would Patty likely do with the specimen?

   _____

   d. If Dr. Antolik chooses to perform a pelvic exam and Pap test, what supplies would Patty need to assemble before the examination?

   _____

   _____

   _____

LEARNING ACTIVITY: FILL IN THE BLANK

Using words from the list below, fill in the blanks to complete the following statements.

38	cervix	counselors or other professionals
266	color	date of confinement
after	compassion	effacement
age and sex	conception	estrogen-progestin
amount lost	congenital	examinations
blood	contact numbers	fertilization
blood tests	contraception	gynecological
breast cancer	contractions	menstrual flow

needs
not successful
permanent
physician
positive

semen
sensitive
sexually transmitted diseases
subsequent routine

their families
ultrasound examination
vagina
vaginal secretions

1. In a normal delivery, the _____, or mouth of the uterus, dilates and begins _____, and uterine _____ propel the fetus through the _____ and into the external environment.

2. When a patient reports abnormal vaginal bleeding, even an unusually heavy _____, the actual _____, as well as its _____, must be determined.

3. Both OB and GYN offices care for patients with contagious diseases that are transmitted through sexual contact, commonly referred to as _____ or venereal diseases. STDs may be experienced by either males or females and are transmitted during sex by _____, _____, and _____.

4. Many psychologically _____ issues are addressed in the OB/GYN office. It is important to listen with _____ to patients and _____ as they present with various problems.

5. The normal gestational period is _____ days, or _____ weeks, from the date of _____. The expected date of delivery is also called the estimated _____.

6. Recent studies on hormone replacement therapy (HRT) suggest that this therapy, especially the _____ combination, increases a woman's risk for _____.

7. The use of ultrasound during a pregnancy, as well as to assess _____ conditions, is becoming more common. The _____ of the fetus and possible _____ conditions are often determined during a/an _____.

8. Keep in mind that not every pregnancy is a planned or _____ event. Be sympathetic to the patient's _____ and have appropriate _____ available for reference to _____.

9. The first prenatal appointment takes more time than _____ visits and includes several _____, manual _____, and consultation with the _____.

10. A tubal ligation is a/an _____ form of _____, as it prevents the sperm from meeting the egg for _____. Reversal is generally _____, and there are recorded instances of females conceiving _____ a tubal ligation.

CRITICAL THINKING

Answer the following questions to the best of your ability. Use the textbook as a reference.

1. A patient, 18-year-old Maria Riojas, has come in with a chief complaint of bleeding between periods. This will be her third GYN visit since menarche, and she is still quite apprehensive about the exams and getting undressed. She says she hopes the doctor won't have to do a pelvic exam today; she just wants a stronger or different birth control pill. Her friend told her she has breakthrough bleeding because she is on the wrong pill. What would you say to the patient?

_____

_____

_____

2. Considering the case study in your textbook for this chapter, if the patient is encouraged by the physician to take the hormone replacement anyway but the patient refuses, does it mean she will develop a disease or problem from not taking it? What is the worst thing for the patient if she does not take treatment of any kind?

_____

_____

_____

_____

3. A patient has come in and from her patient health history, you find she has had three abortions in the past and is now pregnant for the fourth time. She is scheduled for a prenatal workup today. Your personal morals are against abortion, but you know that abortions can be therapeutic (by choice or for medical reasons) or spontaneous (miscarriage), and you don't know which type her abortions were. What, if any, of your personal beliefs can be conveyed to the patient? Would you say anything about her OB history?

_____

_____

_____

_____

4. A patient comes in with her husband, and she asks that he be allowed to come into the exam room with her. When you ask her to disrobe, she looks hesitant then looks at her husband and doesn't move to take the gown and drape. What do you anticipate is happening? What should you do?

_____

_____

_____

_____

5. A patient who is 6 months pregnant calls in saying that she has been bleeding a little (just spotting) all morning and wanted to let the doctor know. She wants an appointment for Thursday and today is Monday. What would you say?

_____

_____

_____

_____

RESEARCH ACTIVITY

Use Internet search engines to research the following topics and write a brief description of what is found. It is important to visit reputable Web sites.

1. Research information about the HPV vaccine. Imagine the physician you work for has asked you to create a brochure on information related to the vaccine. List items that you believe are important to outline in the brochure.

_____

_____

_____

_____

_____

_____

_____

_____

_____

_____

_____

_____

_____

_____

_____

CHAPTER 45

Pediatrics

CHAPTER OUTLINE

General review of the chapter:

    A. Introduction
    B. The MA's Role in Pediatrics
    C. Physical, Developmental, and Emotional Growth of a Child
    D. Routine Visits (Well-Baby Checks)
    E. Common Pediatric Diseases and Disorders
        i. Common contagious diseases of childhood
        ii. Congenital neurological disorders/neural tube defects
        iii. Congenital heart conditions
        iv. Blood disorders
        v. Other conditions
    F. Diagnostic Procedures

STUDENT STUDY GUIDE

Use the following guide to assist in your learning of the concepts from the chapter.

  I. Introduction and the MA's Role in a Pediatric Office
    A. Introduction
        i. Pediatrician:

        _____

        _____

        ii. Pediatric evaluations assure proper growth and development.

        _____

        _____

        iii. Regular inoculations are done with _____-_____ visits.
    B. The MA's Role in a Pediatric Office
        i. Obtain the child's _____ and _____ history.
        ii. Take vital signs, measure, and _____ growth.
        iii. Assist the physician during the physical examination and treatment.
        iv. Help the parent restrain the child if necessary.
        v. Obtain a urine specimen, and administer _____ _____ and
        _____.

  II. Physical and Development Stages of Childhood
    A. Stages
        i. Fetus or embryo =

        _____

        _____

       ii. Neonates or newborns =

_____

_____

      iii. Infant =

_____

_____

      iv. Toddler =

_____

_____

      v. Preschool children =

_____

_____

      vi. School age =

_____

_____

      vii. Adolescence =

_____

_____

B. Factors Affecting Physical Growth

_____

_____

_____

_____

_____

_____

C. Prenatal Factors Influencing Growth
      i. A mother's _____ or _____ use
      ii. Smoking
      iii. _____ injury
      iv. Poor diet
      v. Infection with _____

D. Growth Charts
      i. Developed by the National Center for Health Statistics (NCHS)
      ii. Also by the CDC's National Center for Chronic Disease Prevention and Health Promotion Office

E. Standard Medical Growth Charts

_____

_____

_____

_____

_____

_____

III. Well-Child Visits

A. Procedures for Well-Child Visits
      i. Measuring _____ and _____
      ii. Measuring _____ and _____ _____

   iii. Taking temperature, pulse, respirations and, in older children, blood pressure

   iv. Testing range of motion (ROM) of limbs, head, and neck

   v. Testing _____ reaction

   vi. Checking _____, _____, and _____

   vii. Checking cardiac and respiratory status

   viii. _____ the abdomen

 B. Well-Child Visits for Older Children

_____

_____

_____

_____

_____

_____

 C. Importance of Growth Measurement

   i. Includes newborn length, weight, and _____ _____

   ii. Evaluates the child's _____ patterns

   iii. Abnormal patterns warrant further assessment and diagnosis.

 D. Child Immunizations

   i. Prevent epidemics of diseases

   ii. U.S. children are routinely inoculated.

   iii. Immunized against:

_____

_____

   iv. American Academy of Pediatrics (AAP) recommends booster injections among college students

 E. Side Effects of Immunizations

_____

_____

_____

_____

_____

_____

 F. The Immunization Record

   i. Documentation in the record includes:

    (a) _____, type, and site of each immunization

    (b) Manufacturer, _____ _____, and date of expiration of the immunization product

    (c) Parents' _____

    (d) _____ of the person administering the shot

IV. Childhood Diseases and Disorders

 A. Contagious Childhood Diseases

_____

_____

_____

_____

_____

_____

B. Neural Tube Defects
  i. Spinal fusion disorders

  _____

  _____

  _____

  _____

  ii. Cranial fusion disorders

  _____

  _____

  _____

  _____

C. Congenital Heart Defects
  i. Causes
    (a) Developmental _____
    (b) Failure of fetal _____ to convert to normal _____
        _____ after birth
    (c) Easily identified with ultrasound testing
    (d) Two types of heart conditions: acyanotic and cyanotic

  _____

  _____

  _____

  _____

  _____

  _____

  ii. Blood disorders

  _____

  _____

  _____

  _____

D. Common Childhood Conditions
  i. _____ _____ syndrome
  ii. "Crack babies": born to mothers who used crack cocaine during pregnancy
  iii. Helminthes or parasitic intestinal worms
  iv. _____ (roundworm) and _____ (pinworm) infestations

V. Pediatric Diagnostic Procedures
  A. Common Diagnostic Procedure
    i. _____
    ii. _____
    iii. _____
    iv. Culture and sensitivity (C&S)
    v. Additional diagnostic procedures:

  _____

  _____

  _____

  _____

B. Restraint Positions for Child Examinations
    i. Ear examination

    _____

    _____

    _____

    _____

    _____

    ii. Ears, eyes, nose, and throat exam

    _____

    _____

    _____

    _____

    _____

    iii. Mummy restraint

    _____

    _____

    iv. A papoose board

    _____

    _____

C. Pediatric Urine Collection
    i. For newborns, infants, or toddlers who need to provide a sample
    ii. Genitals are cleansed properly.
    iii. A/an _____ _____ is attached around the genitals.
    iv. A diaper is worn and the child is encouraged to _____
        _____.
    v. Diaper (collection bag) is _____ _____.
D. Tests Requiring Pediatric Urine Specimens

    _____

    _____

    _____

    _____

    _____

    _____

    _____

    _____

    _____

    _____

KEY TERMINOLOGY REVIEW

Write sentences using the key terms below within their correct context.

1. Acyanotic:

    _____

    _____

2. Cyanotic:

_____

_____

3. Fontanelle:

_____

_____

4. Lavage:

_____

_____

5. Pediatrician:

_____

_____

6. Pediatrics:

_____

_____

APPLIED PRACTICE

Read the scenario below and then, using your textbook, answer the questions that follow.

Scenario

Sandra Norwood has brought her son, Micah, into the office for his 6-month well-baby visit. Austin Shwartz is the medical assistant working with Sandra and Micah. From reading Micah's chart, Austin knows that Micah has had two doses of the following vaccines; HepB, Rota, DTaP, Hib, and PCV. *(Micah's chart entry for today's visit appears below)*

Norwood, Micah

04-23-20xx

10/30/20xx   9:30 am   Wt: 21 lbs   length: 27¼"   Head Circumference: 17½" Chest

Circumference: 18". cc: mother states "Micah is here for his 6-month check up and immunizations." ---

--- *A. Shwartz, RMA (AMT)*

---

1. Using the growth chart found in the textbook and the information noted above in the chart entry, determine the percentile for Micah's length-for-age and weight-for-age:
   a. Length-for-age percentile: _____
   b. Weight-for-age percentile: _____

2. Using the immunization schedule found in the textbook and the information stated in the scenario, what vaccines would Micah be eligible to receive?

   (**Note:** Immunizations are *only* given based upon a physician's order.)

   _____

   _____

   _____

   _____

3. Of the vaccines that you listed above, state which have the option to be given at a later month. Explain your answer.

   _____

   _____

   _____

   _____

LEARNING ACTIVITY: FILL IN THE BLANK

Using words from the list below, fill in the blanks to complete the following statements.

Note: *Some terms may be used in more than one statement.*

Allen	illnesses	reactions
allergies	importance	respiratory or cardiac
CDC	important	route
circumcision	medical history	rubeola
diagnose	not routinely	side effects
E	parent or guardian	Snellen
effects	parotitis	spoons or cups
fifty	patterns	storage
first three years	PDR	surgically removed
five	pertussis	transfer
frequency	pharmacist	truthful
German measles	physical development	vaccine package insert
growth records	potentially painful	varicella
hospital		

1. Part of your patient instruction in administering liquid medications will be to stress the _____ of measuring with the _____ supplied by the _____ or the manufacturer.

2. Never tell a child "This will not hurt" when a/an _____ procedure is about to be done. Always be _____. Reassure the _____ about the procedure.

3. For immunizations, review the information from the _____ or from other sources, such as a/an _____ or the _____. Know the purpose of the medication, precautions, potential side _____ or adverse _____, correct _____ for administration, and _____ requirements.

4. Thanks to routine preventive inoculations, the common contagious diseases of childhood are far less prevalent now than they were _____ years ago. These diseases include chicken pox (_____), measles (_____), rubella (_____), mumps (_____), whooping cough (_____), polio, and diphtheria.

5. Measuring growth and keeping _____ for the pediatric patient is _____. The physician uses growth _____ to observe normal _____ or _____ diseases.

6. A procedure usually performed in the _____ shortly after birth is _____, in which the foreskin on an infant boy is _____.

7. Head circumference is measured during the _____ of life. Infant chest circumference is _____ measured, except when _____ abnormalities are suspected.

8. Immunizations have dramatically reduced the _____ of many childhood illnesses and the _____ of disease to other children and adults. But it is important to alert the _____ to potential _____.

9. When children require a vision check, you will use a/an _____ chart (when the child can recognize shapes but not directions), a/an _____ chart (when the child knows directions but not the alphabet), or a/an _____ chart (when the child knows the alphabet, around _____ years old).

10. Before any immunization, it is important to obtain the _____ from the _____. Ask about any known _____ or recent _____.

CRITICAL THINKING

Answer the following questions to the best of your ability. Use the textbook as a reference.

1. If you needed to give an injection in the vastus lateralis muscle to a 9-month-old, and the child was crying and kicking, what could you do to ensure safety and proper administration? List a few ideas that would be appropriate.

   _____
   _____
   _____
   _____
   _____

2. You have an order to obtain blood for a test for a patient, who is a 4 1/2-year-old girl here with her father. She starts to get tears in her eyes when you approach, and the father tells her to quit that crying or he'll tell the MA to stick her a second time. What would you do?

   _____
   _____
   _____
   _____

3. You have a parent of a 3-month-old baby who calls in two to three times per day, extremely anxious and worried over every little thing and leaving messages with questions for the doctor. When you get the advice from the physician and return her calls, she keeps talking in detail for long periods of time. This is her first child, and she has no family in town to help her through this time of learning how to care for an infant. Everyone in the office is aware of her neediness and many feel some annoyance at the amount of time and attention this one patient requires. How would you handle the continuing phone calls? What would you do and/or say?

   _____
   _____

4. The MA should document immunizations on the patient's chart and on the parent's copy of the child's immunization record. Considering other types of documentation you have learned in your program so far, think of two examples of other places that immunization documentation may be needed (depending on the type of practice and the office policies). This is not stated in this chapter, so use prior knowledge, common sense, and critical thinking to find examples.

_____

_____

_____

_____

_____

5. A parent brings in a child and a jar with a urine specimen in it. The parent thought the urine might be needed, and explained that it is so difficult to keep her child on a urine pediatric collection bag, so she collected the specimen about three hours ago and has kept it refrigerated. Would this urine be useful? Provide your reason why or why not.

_____

_____

_____

_____

_____

RESEARCH ACTIVITY

Use Internet search engines to research the following topics and write a brief description of what is found. It is important to visit reputable Web sites.

1. Visit www.cdc.gov/vaccines. What information do find would be most helpful for health care professionals? How could a pediatric office benefit by using materials found on this Web site?

_____

_____

_____

_____

_____

_____

_____

_____

_____

_____

_____

CHAPTER 46
Neurology

CHAPTER OUTLINE

General review of the chapter:

    A. Introduction
    B. The Medical Assistant's Role in Neurology and Neurosurgery
    C. The Anatomy and Physiology of the Nervous System
    D. Assessing the Neurological System
    E. Disorders and Diseases of the Central Nervous System
    F. Diseases of the Peripheral Nervous System

STUDENT STUDY GUIDE

Use the following guide to assist in your learning of the concepts from the chapter.

  I. Introduction and the MA's Role in Neurology

    A. Neurology
       i. Study and treatment of diseases of the nervous system
      ii. Neurologist treats diseases and conditions of the nervous system
    B. Neurological Conditions
       i. Traumatic insult to the

        _____

        _____

      ii. Presence of a/an _____ body
     iii. Tumor or _____ in these structures
     iv. Pressure from _____ hemorrhage
      v. Provide pain relief from tremors of Parkinsonism
    C. The MA Role in Neurology
       i. Obtain a preliminary history and information pertaining to the current visit
      ii. Assess and record _____ _____
     iii. Assist with patient examination
     iv. Provide _____
      v. Confirm appointments, schedule, and obtain _____ for tests

 II. Anatomy and Physiology of the Nervous System

    A. The Nervous System
       i. _____ and _____ stimuli are coordinated in the body by the nervous system.
      ii. This system initiates a/an _____ response.
     iii. For example, the body automatically constricts blood vessels to reduce heat loss when it is in a cold environment.
     iv. _____ is the ability of the body to adjust to internal and external changes and function at an optimum level.

B. The CNS and PNS
    i. Central nervous system (CNS)

_____

_____

    ii. Peripheral nervous system (PNS)

_____

_____

C. The Central Nervous System
    i. Contains _____ and _____ cord
    ii. Controls the peripheral nervous system
    iii. Integrates _____ between the two divisions
    iv. Cranium and vertebral column protect brain and spinal cord
    v. _____ forms a watertight sheath around the spinal cord

D. Layers of the Meninges
    i. _____ _____ (tough outer membrane)
    ii. Arachnoid meninges (middle _____ web section)
    iii. _____ mater (thin innermost layer)
    iv. Cerebrospinal fluid cushions and protects brain/spinal cord

E. Major Areas of the Brain
    i. Cerebrum manages:

_____

_____

_____

_____

    ii. Interprets _____ muscle and _____ activities
    iii. Outer cerebrum contains gray matter and houses neuron cell bodies
    iv. Cerebellum coordinates motor activities:

_____

_____

_____

_____

    v. Brain stem regulates:

_____

_____

_____

F. The Peripheral Nervous System
G. The PNS consists of:
    i. Cranial nerves
    ii. _____ nerves
    iii. Autonomic system

_____

_____

H. Cranial Nerves
    i. Originate from the base of the brain
    ii. Named for the location of origin and what it controls
    iii. Distribute nervous system impulses to head and neck

iv. Controls

_____

_____

v. The 12 cranial nerves include:
   (a) _____: smell
   (b) _____: vision
   (c) _____: eye movement
   (d) _____: eye movement
   (e) _____: sensations of head and chewing
   (f) _____: abduction of eye
   (g) _____: facial expression, taste
   (h) _____: balance and equilibrium
   (i) _____: sensations and movement of the tongue
   (j) _____: sensations and movement of organs supplied
   (k) _____: shoulder movement
   (l) _____: tongue movements

I. Spinal Nerves
   i. _____ of spinal nerves
   ii. Originate from the spinal cord
   iii. Carry impulses to the brain

J. Neurons
   i. _____: functional unit of the nervous system.
   ii. Neurons are composed of _____.
   iii. _____ _____: houses the nucleus
   iv. _____
   v. Axon: sends impulses away from the cell body to other neurons
   vi. Dendrites: receive impulses from other neurons and are carried to the cell body

K. Structures of a Neuron
   i. _____ neurons: have a very thin, almost nonexistent sheath
   ii. _____ can cause inflammation and symptoms such as a slow or altered gait, altered speech or mental process, or inability to control movements.
   iii. Dendrites and axons have _____ fiber tissue called white matter.
   iv. Nerve cell body tissue is called gray matter.

L. Types of Neurons
   i. _____: carry impulses toward the brain and spinal cord
   ii. _____: carry impulses away from the CNS to the muscles
   iii. Interneurons: relay information within the _____
   iv. Neurotransmitters are chemical messengers of the electrical impulses across the synaptic gap.

M. Divisions of the Nervous System
   i. Voluntary, somatic system is consciously controlled
   ii. Involuntary, or autonomic system, controls things that do not require conscious effort

_____

_____

_____

N. The Autonomic System
   i. Contains the sympathetic and parasympathetic system
   ii. Regulates all homeostatic functions

_____

_____

_____

_____

O. Sympathetic and Parasympathetic
    i. Sympathetic ("fight-flight")

_____

_____

    ii. Parasympathetic ("brakes") homeostatic nerves

_____

_____

P. Reflexes
    i. Protect body with automatic, rapid neuromuscular reactions to stimulus
    ii. Spinal reflexes do not involve coordination with the brain.
    iii. Spinal reflexes include:

_____

_____

    iv. Catching your balance

III. Assessing the Neurological System

A. Neurological Exams
    i. Determine deficits in numerous areas:

_____

_____

_____

_____

B. Neurological Assessment Techniques
    i. Observation
    ii. _____ _____
    iii. Monitoring overall behavior
    iv. Grip responses
    v. _____
    vi. Closing eyes while trying to touch nose with one finger
    vii. Balancing on one foot
    viii. Touching various parts of the body to determine sensitivity
    ix. _____
    x. Reflex hammers

C. Cranial Nerve Testing

_____

_____

_____

_____

D. The Glasgow Coma Scale
    i. Rapid standardized assessment
    ii. Tests:

_____

_____

_____

   iii. Three basic responses are tested:

_____

_____

_____

_____

   iv. Each response is assigned a numerical value.
    v. Three values provide an estimate of injury.
  E. Lumbar Puncture
    i. Tests the pressure within the _____ canal
   ii. Pressure measured with a manometer
  iii. Cerebral spinal fluid removed
   iv. Tested for red blood cells, _____, _____,
         _____ or microorganisms
    v. Helpful in diagnosis of central nervous system disorders and diseases

IV. Diseases and Disorders of the Central Nervous System

  A. Cerebrovascular Accidents
    i. Also called strokes
   ii. Usually caused by:

_____

_____

_____

_____

  iii. CVA symptoms:

_____

_____

_____

_____

  B. Transient Ischemic Attacks
    i. Temporary reduction of blood flow to the _____
   ii. Symptoms are similar to _____, but not as severe
  iii. Typically resolve within 24 hours
   iv. Can be a warning sign of possible impending CVA
  C. Epilepsy
    i. Chronic _____ disorder
   ii. _____ muscular contractions
  iii. Caused by various conditions such as:

_____

_____

_____

_____

_____

_____

_____

D. Tonic-Clonic Seizures
    i. Can be very severe
    ii. Patients experience an aura.
    iii. An aura can include distinct

_____

_____

_____

_____

    iv. Involve the whole body and are bilaterally symmetrical
    v. Person doesn't _____ tonic-clonic seizures

E. Petit Mal Seizures
    i. Only a few seconds of _____ is experienced.
    ii. Usually occurs with children
    iii. May go unnoticed, as it can appear as if they are staring into space.

F. Status Epilepticus Seizures
    i. Repetitive seizures occur in series.
    ii. Patient does not regain consciousness
    iii. Requires prompt _____ and _____ medical intervention

G. Parkinson's Disease
    i. Causes muscular _____, _____, and _____
    ii. Degenerative condition that is slow progressing and occurs later in life
    iii. Signs/symptoms include:

_____

_____

_____

    iv. The cause is unknown.
    v. _____ and anticholinergic drugs help minimize the effects of the disease.

H. Multiple Sclerosis
    i. Progressive destruction of the _____ _____ of the nerve
    ii. Transient motor and sensory disturbances occur.
    iii. _____ becomes impaired and _____ may weaken.
    iv. Linked to immune, viral, and genetic causes: exact *etiology* is unknown
    v. Adrenocorticotropic hormones are used to relieve symptoms.

I. Headache/Cephalgia
    i. Diffuse acute or chronic pain occurring in any part of the head
    ii. Typically caused from irritation of sensory nerve ending in the head or neck
    iii. Symptoms include:

_____

_____

_____

_____

    iv. Migraine headaches are intense, throbbing, and incapacitating.
    v. Prodromal symptoms include:

_____

_____

_____

_____

J. CNS Infections
    i. Include _____, _____, and _____

ii. Symptoms include:

_____

_____

_____

_____

iii. Quick progression of the disease causes _____ _____ (stiff neck), seizures, and loss of consciousness.

iv. Diagnosis includes patient history, _____ _____, _____ _____ and CSF analysis

v. Treatment involves drug therapy with antiviral agents, steroids, antipyretics, and anticonvulsants.

K. Meningitis

i. Viruses or bacteria that invade the _____

ii. The symptoms are similar to other CNS conditions.

_____

_____

_____

_____

iii. Vigorous treatment is required for this medical emergency.

L. Brain Abscesses

i. Infectious microorganisms migrate to the brain from other infections within the body.

ii. Examples of migrating infections include:

_____

_____

iii. Symptoms:

_____

_____

_____

_____

M. Brain Tumors

i. Grow from _____ cell development

ii. Can be _____ or _____

iii. Pressure is exerted on surrounding tissue, causing symptoms:

_____

_____

_____

_____

iv. Diagnosed by:

_____

_____

_____

_____

v. Treated with chemotherapy, radiation, and surgical removal

N. Head Trauma
   i. Common symptoms include:

   _____

   _____

   _____

   _____

   _____

   _____

   ii. A/an _____ is a collection of blood that forms above or between the
       _____.
   iii. In some cases, the _____ will resolve spontaneously without surgical
        intervention.
O. Concussions
   i. _____: skull takes the brunt of the impact to prevent injury to the brain
   ii. Symptoms:

   _____

   _____

   _____

   _____

   iii. Most _____ heal without long-term effects.
P. Contusions
   i. _____: occurs when blood vessels are ruptured due to a bruise in the brain
   ii. More severe than a concussion
   iii. Individuals may lose _____ from the intracranial pressure and symptoms
        of head injuries are present.
Q. Spinal Cord Injuries
   i. Fractured vertebrae, _____ _____, or other traumas to the
      vertebral column
   ii. When injury is present it creates pressure, or _____, on the spinal cord or
       nerves.
   iii. Paraplegia: spinal cord injury in the _____ regions:

   _____

   _____

   _____

   _____

   _____

   iv. Quadriplegia: spinal cord injuries in the _____ area
   v. Cause paralysis of the entire _____ and _____
   vi. Respiration is often impaired and patients require breathing assistance.
   vii. Diagnosis involves history of _____, observation, physical exam, neurolog-
        ical assessment, and imaging studies
   viii. Treatment focuses on reducing pressure on spinal cord and spinal nerves.
R. Disk Injuries
   i. Affect _____ disks
   ii. Either from trauma or _____ diseases
   iii. Common cause of back pain

      iv. Caused by:

    _____

    _____

    _____

    _____

      v. Degenerative diseases cause the disks to _____
     vi. Diagnosis comes from _____ studies, patient _____, and neurological exam
    vii. Course of treatment is usually determined by the extent of pain
  viii. Some disorders resolve spontaneously and others require surgical intervention.
  S. Sciatica
      i. _____ of the vertebral canal
     ii. Spinal cord compresses the connecting nerves and causes _____ and _____ leg pain
    iii. Symptoms include:

    _____

    _____

    _____

    _____

    iv. _____ and _____ contribute to this condition.

V. Diseases of the Peripheral Nervous System
  A. Bell's Palsy
      i. Bell's palsy affects the _____ _____ nerve that controls facial muscles.
     ii. Onset is typically _____.
    iii. Symptoms include unilateral _____ paralysis, awakening with one side of the _____ drooping; particularly the mouth
    iv. This sometimes follows a/an _____ infection; however, etiology is unknown.
     v. History, _____, duration of the condition, physical exam, and _____ are all used to diagnose this disorder.
    vi. _____ therapy is used for treatment: Some cases resolve spontaneously, others have indefinite side effects.
  B. Trigeminal Neuralgia
      i. Trigeminal neuralgia affects the area stimulated by the _____ and _____ nerves.
     ii. Unilateral with a sudden onset of extremely _____, _____, and intermittent pain
    iii. Diagnosed based on observation and exam; etiology is unknown
    iv. Treatment includes drug therapy and in extreme cases, _____ _____ of the nerves to stop the sensory impulses is performed.
  C. Shingles
      i. Shingles: caused by the _____ _____ _____ virus
     ii. Symptoms of intense pain and small blisters appear _____ on the body
    iii. Other symptoms include:

    _____

    _____

    _____

    _____

iv. This condition is only contagious to people who have not had a case of
_____.

v. Most cases resolve in less than a month.

vi. Drug therapy consists of

_____

_____

_____

_____

KEY TERMINOLOGY REVIEW

Match the correct medical term with the definition listed below.

a. affect   m. neurology

b. aura   n. neuron

c. cephalgia   o. neurotransmitter

d. clonic   p. nuchal rigidity

e. countercoup   q. palsy

f. decerbrate posture   r. paraplegia

g. decorticate posture   s. postictal

h. dermatome   t. prodromal

i. exacerbation   u. projectile vomiting

j. hemiparesis   v. pyogenic

k. innervate   w. quadriplegia

l. neuralgia   x. tonic

_____ 1. Injury in which traumatic impact on the head is strong enough to make the brain strike the opposite of the cranium and bounce back to strike the impacted side.

_____ 2. Loss of nerve and muscle function on one side of the body.

_____ 3. Study of the nervous system.

_____ 4. Warning of impending seizure.

_____ 5. Temporary or permanent loss of ability to control or make muscle movement.

_____ 6. Posture characteristic of brain injury in which the patient is rigid, with clenched fists, flexed arms, and extended legs.

_____ 7. Emotional expression associated with facial and body behaviors.

_____ 8. Chemicals that aid in the transmission of electrical impulses from one neuron to the next.

_____ 9. Vomiting with uncontrollable force.

_____ 10. Rigidity in the neck in which the head is bent forward toward the chest.

_____ 11. Increasing severity and recurrence of symptoms.

_____ 12. Altering muscle contraction and relaxation.

_____ 13. Specific area of skin stimulated by a segment of the spinal cord.

_____ 14. Nerve cell; basic unit of the nervous system.

_____ 15. Sharp nerve pain.

_____ 16. Pus-forming.

_____ 17. Loss of sensation and motor activity of the lower trunk and lower extremities.

_____ 18. Paralysis of the entire trunk and all four extremities.

_____ 19. Stimulate.

_____ 20. Pertaining to muscular tension.

_____ 21. Pertaining to the period immediately following a seizure.

_____ 22. Diffuse acute or chronic pain in any part of the head, commonly known as the headache.

_____ 23. Pertaining to symptoms during the period immediately preceding onset of a disease condition.

_____ 24. Posture characteristic of brain injury in which the patient is rigid, with clenched fists, flexed arms, and extended legs.

APPLIED PRACTICE

Read the scenarios below and answer the questions that follow.

Scenario 1

A 20-year-old female patient presents to your office with the following symptoms: headache × 3 days, temperature of 103.2° F, dizziness, and blurred vision. She said that since she woke up this morning she has not been able to move her head. In her medical chart, you make a note that "the patient states 'My neck is so stiff, I can't bend it.' Her head appears bent forward toward her chest."

1. What would you suspect the diagnosis might be based on her symptoms? (Medical assistants never make a diagnosis; this is a question of your knowledge of the signs and symptoms of various conditions.)

_____

2. What is the medical term for a stiff neck that is bent forward toward the chest?

_____

Scenario 2

A 59-year-old male patient presents to your office with observable right-sided facial drooping, specifically near the mouth. The patient states that he "woke up this way" and he "can't feel anything on the entire right side of my face."

3. What would you suspect the diagnosis might be based on his symptoms? (Medical assistants never make a diagnosis; this is a question of your knowledge of the signs and symptoms of various conditions.)

_____

4. What does treatment consist of for this condition?

_____

Scenario 3

As an administrative medical assistant, one of your duties is transcribing for the neurologists in the office where you work. Dr. Preston dictated notes on a patient he saw in the emergency room last night. He dictates "17-year-old male patient presents to the ER with suspected countercoup injury of the head with a 4-inch laceration on the right temporal region of his skull. Due to the extent of the contusion, the patient will remain hospitalized for observation for 48 hours."

5. How would you explain a "countercoup injury" in layman's terms?

   _____

   _____

6. What is the difference between a concussion and a contusion?

   _____

   _____

LEARNING ACTIVITY: MULTIPLE CHOICE

Circle the correct answer to each of the questions below.

1. There are three vascular conditions in the brain that can cause a cerebrovascular accident. Which of the following is not a cause of CVA?

   a. thrombus
   b. vessel rupture

   c. seizure
   d. embolus

2. Which two of the following would complete this statement: The _____, height, _____, and rate of brain waves on an EEG are unique to each person, like a brain "fingerprint."

   a. length
   b. rhythm

   c. strength
   d. pattern

3. Sciatica is also called

   a. a spinal cord injury
   b. Bell's palsy

   c. spinal stenosis
   d. paraplegia

4. Which of the following are disease(s) whose cause is unknown? (Circle all that apply.)

   a. Parkinson's disease
   b. TIA

   c. trigeminal neuralgia
   d. multiple sclerosis

5. A patient must follow certain pretesting instructions prior to having an EEG. Which of the following is not part of the patient instructions?

   a. Eliminate caffeine.
   b. Avoid smoking.

   c. Discontinue certain medications.
   d. Have a well-balanced dinner the night before the test, then nothing by mouth.

6. Which of the following are the two anatomical divisions of the nervous system?

   a. central nervous system
   b. autonomic nervous system

   c. peripheral nervous system
   d. brain and spinal cord

7. An epidural hematoma is

   a. above the dura mater
                   c. under the arachnoid meninges

   b. below the dura mater
                    d. a concussion

8. Which two of the following are not used in diagnosing epilepsy?

   a. MRI
                   c. CSF studies

   b. biopsy
                  d. recurrent seizure activity

9. Which of the following is not one of the common bacterial agents listed in your textbook as being a cause of meningitis?

   a. *Hemophilus influenzae type B*
            c. *Neisseria meningitis*

   b. *Streptococcus pneumoniae*
            d. *Staphlyococcus aureus*

10. Which of the following shows the correct conduction path of a nervous system impulse?

   a. dendrite, through nerve cell body, along axon, crosses synaptic gap, next dendrite
            c. dendrite, through nerve cell body, along axon, through nerve cell body, crosses synaptic gap, next dendrite

   b. dendrite, through axon, through nerve cell body, crosses synaptic gap, next dendrite
            d. dendrite, through axon, through nerve cell body, crosses synaptic gap, through the axon, next dendrite

CRITICAL THINKING

Answer the following questions to the best of your ability. Use the textbook as a reference.

1. A patient, a 57-year-old female named Katie Gilpatrick, has come in following an ER visit where she was diagnosed with a cerebrovascular accident. What are the three things that could have caused this stroke in the patient? Explain why a stroke only affects one side of the body.

   _____

   _____

   _____

   _____

2. A fellow health care worker comes to work and states she cannot do very much because she has a "migraine." She was out late last night at a party and states that the headache is not because she had some drinks. She hopes you will help her through the day by rooming some of her patients. She is incorrect in diagnosing herself with a migraine because it is a specific type of headache, and she has not been diagnosed with migraines by a physician. Explain why it is unlikely someone with a true migraine would be able to come to work and function even at a slow pace.

   _____

   _____

   _____

   _____

3. In the case study in this chapter, imagine that Milo does not have any blisters or lesions. Knowing that Milo had recently had varicella, what infectious condition of the central nervous system could Milo have? The medical assistant does not diagnose, but you should have knowledge of the signs and symptoms of various nervous system problems; use this knowledge to answer the question.

_____

_____

_____

_____

_____

4. A patient, a 28-year-old male who has paraplegia, has come in to the office for an exam. The physician needs the patient on the table to do a thorough exam. How will you get the patient on to the exam table, since he cannot stand or use the bottom half of his body at all? Explain possible transfers from his wheelchair to the table.

_____

_____

_____

_____

_____

RESEARCH ACTIVITY

Use Internet search engines to research the following topics and write a brief description of what is found. It is important to visit reputable Web sites.

1. Visit the Parkinson's Disease Foundation at www.pdf.org. Click on the "News and Events" tab on the top of the page, then select "Science News." Choose an article of interest and provide a summary of the information discussed within the article. What interested you most about this article?

_____

_____

_____

_____

_____

_____

_____

_____

_____

_____

_____

_____

CHAPTER 47
Mental Health

CHAPTER OUTLINE

General review of the chapter:

A. Introduction
B. The Medical Assistant's Role in the Mental Health Field
C. Mental Wellness
D. General Mental Disorders
E. Assessment and Diagnosis
F. Standard Treatments for Mental Disorders

STUDENT STUDY GUIDE

Use the following guide to assist in your learning of the concepts from the chapter.

I. Introduction and the MA's Role in the Mental Health Field

  A. The Field of Psychology
    i. Studies the _____ and _____ of the mind
    ii. Looks at how the mind relates to behaviors and the _____
    iii. Deals with normal and abnormal mental processes and behaviors
    iv. Focuses on the diagnosis, treatment, and _____ of mental disorders

  B. Psychologist
    i. _____ in psychology
    ii. Specialize in:

    _____

    _____

    _____

    _____

  C. Psychiatrist
    i. Medical doctor specializing in treatment of mental disorders
    ii. Treats by using:

    _____

    _____

    _____

    _____

  D. Other Mental Health Professionals

  _____

  _____

  _____

  _____

  _____

  _____

E. The MA's Role in Mental Health
   i. Administrative opportunities are plentiful.
   ii. Clinical assistance includes:
      (a) Measuring weight, vital signs
   iii. Completing forms, precertification, scheduling appointments
   iv. _____ collection

II. Anatomy and Physiology of Cognitive Functioning
   A. The Human Brain
      i. Contains many types of _____ and _____
      ii. Commands of the brain, body, and behavior are communicated via neurons and synapses.
      iii. Neurotransmitters transmit _____ impulses from one neuron to the next.
      iv. _____ to this conduction system _____ brain functions and behaviors.
   B. Cerebral Hemispheres
      _____
      _____
      _____
      _____

   C. The Mid-Portion of the Brain
      i. Relay system important to perception and pleasure
      ii. Hypothalamus is the master control for the autonomic system, _____ secretion, _____ _____, and emotions
      iii. _____ is the gateway for the passage of new memories, _____ _____, _____ _____, and recalling spatial relationships
   D. The Cerebellum and Brainstem
      i. Responsible for _____ and voluntary and involuntary muscle control
      ii. The _____ controls wakefulness, mental alertness, and levels of tiredness.
      iii. The _____: lowest part of the brainstem regulating heart rate, respirations, blood pressure, and reflexes, including coughing, sneezing, swallowing, and vomiting.

III. Mental Wellness
   A. State of being or _____ to _____ in healthy ways
   B. Elements of healthy wellness include:
      _____
      _____
      _____
      _____
      _____
      _____

IV. General Mental Disorders
   A. Schizophrenia
      i. Symptoms of schizophrenia
      _____
      _____
      _____
      _____
      _____

      ii. Etiology is unknown
      iii. Attributed to _____, _____, and _____

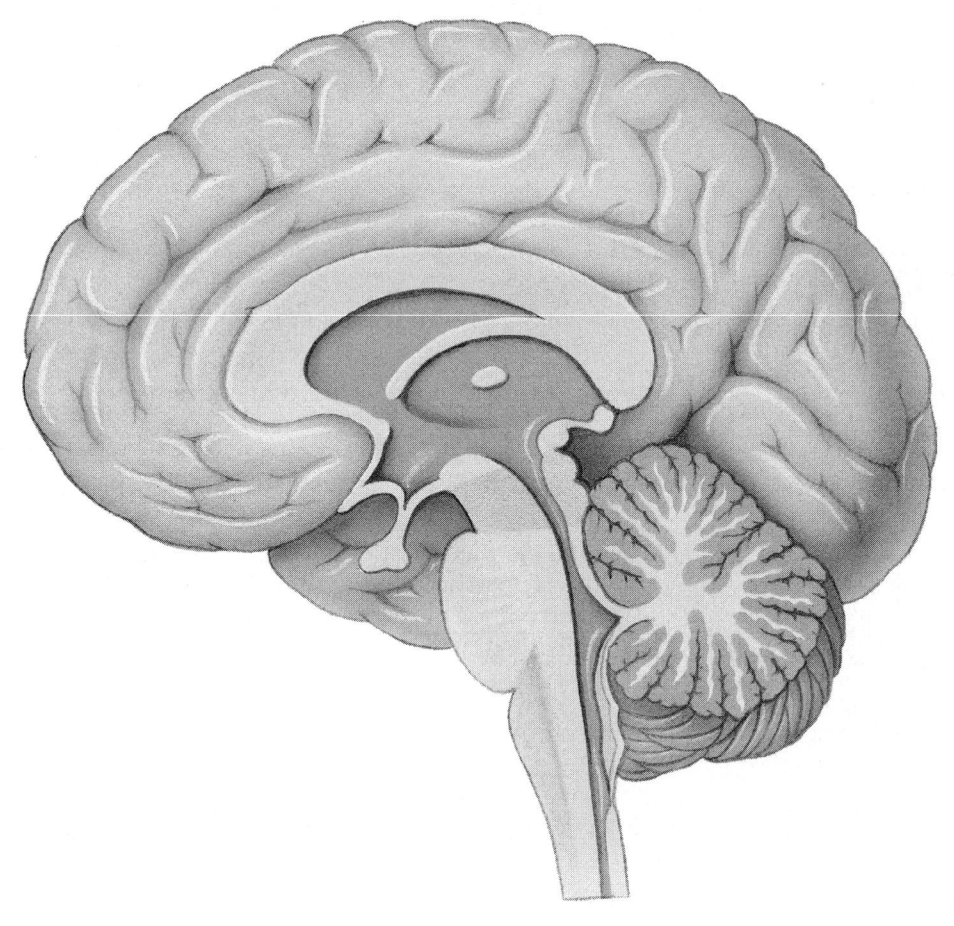

iv. Treated with antipsychotic medications to control symptoms:

_____

_____

B. Mood Disorders
   i. Depression
      (a) Symptoms:

_____

_____

_____

_____

      (b) Caused by imbalance of neurotransmitters (especially _____) or traumatic life experiences:

_____

_____

      (c) Treatment:
         (1) Antidepressants, monoamine oxidase inhibitors (_____), tricyclics, and selective serotonin reuptake inhibitors (_____).
   ii. Postpartum depression
      (a) Occurs after childbirth; may last for weeks or months
      (b) Symptoms:

_____

_____

_____

_____

_____

_____

      (c) Caused by sudden change in hormones and _____ _____

      (d) Symptoms must be monitored to prevent _____ or _____.

      (e) Commonly self-resolves or antidepressants can be prescribed
   iii. Seasonal affective disorder
      (a) _____ disorder occurs when sunlight is limited
      (b) Autumn and winter are common times of occurrence due to _____ _____.

      (c) Symptoms include:

_____

_____

_____

_____

      (d) Treatment:

_____

_____

_____

_____

   iv. Bi-polar/manic depressive disorder
      (a) Characterized by intense _____ _____

(b) "Manic phase":

_____

_____

(c) Depressive phase:

_____

_____

_____

_____

(d) Alterations in neurotransmitter levels are usually the cause of this disorder.
C. Personality Disorders
  i. Deviation from the standard patterns of appropriate behavior
  ii. Three categories of disorders:

_____

_____

_____

_____

  iii. Etiology is _____ but diagnosis should not be confirmed until adulthood
D. Odd Cluster
  i. Paranoid personality disorder: causes people to feel extremely distrustful and suspicious of others
  (a) Believe they are being exploited, deceived, or harmed by others
  ii. Schizoid personality disorder:

_____

_____

_____

_____

  iii. Schizotypical personality disorder is similar to schizoid personality disorder and the person is _____, _____, anxious, and depressed.
E. Dramatic Cluster
  i. Antisocial personality disorder

_____

_____

_____

_____

  ii. Borderline personality disorder

_____

_____

_____

_____

_____

_____

  iii. Histrionic personality disorder

_____

_____

_____

iv. Narcissistic personality disorder

_____

_____

_____

_____

_____

_____

F. Anxious Cluster
   i. Avoidant personality disorder

_____

_____

_____

_____

   ii. Dependent personality disorder

_____

_____

_____

_____

_____

_____

   iii. Obsessive-compulsive personality disorder

_____

_____

_____

_____

G. Anxiety Disorders
   i. Generalized anxiety disorder
     (a) Constant state of anxiety without _____
     (b) Constant worry and difficulty _____ _____
     (c) Symptoms include:
       (1) Difficulty sleeping, hypertension, diarrhea, and tense muscles
   ii. Panic disorder
     (a) Sudden onset of _____ and severe _____
     (b) Results in panic attacks, which are disabling at times
     (c) Feeling of impeding _____ or fear they are dying
     (d) Symptoms include:

_____

_____

   iii. Phobic disorder
     (a) Unusual fear or anxiety concerning a specific object, situation, or activity
     (b) In reality it does not present any _____.
     (c) The fear is so extreme, it controls the person's life.
     (d) Familiar phobias include:

_____

_____

_____

_____

    iv. Post-traumatic stress disorder
        (a) Characterized by _____ to a traumatic event
            (1) Such as a hurricane, war, fire, rape, or accident
        (b) Symptoms include:

_____

_____

_____

_____

_____

_____

        (c) Symptoms may be immediate or delayed.
H. Somatoform Disorders
    i. _____ _____
        (a) Traumatic situation usually precedes the conversion disorder
        (b) Physical symptoms:

_____

_____

_____

_____

    ii. Hypochondriasis
        (a) Causes people to report pain and have symptoms without a/an _____
            basis
        (b) People experience symptoms and pain even if the condition is _____
            _____.
        (c) Preoccupied with their health and move from _____ to
            _____ to find problem
        (d) Abnormal fixation on their health can affect their _____ or
            _____ lives
    iii. Factitious disorders
        (a) Purposefully or fraudulently claims to have a disorder for personal or
            _____ _____
        (b) _____ is the fake exaggeration of symptoms and complaints.

_____

        (c) _____ syndrome by proxy

_____

_____

_____

_____

I. _____ _____ Disorder
    i. Feeling of belonging to the opposite sex
    ii. Being uncomfortable and unhappy with their biological gender
    iii. Have low self-esteem, experience social isolation, and may take on the characteristics of
        the opposite sex
    iv. Often seek psychological counseling or sex-change therapy later in adulthood

J. Mental Retardation
   i. _____ growth of the child is stunted during _____ develop-
      ment, birth process, or _____ _____
      (a) Show lower than normal intellectual and interpersonal skills
      (b) Behavioral performance issues arise in the areas of self-care, hygiene, safety, self-
          direction, and communication difficulty
   ii. Caused by:

   _____

   _____

   _____

   _____

   _____

   iii. A cure is not possible because the compromised brain cells cannot be replaced or repaired.
K. Dementia
   i. Compromised _____ or _____ functioning that occurs
      after age 18
   ii. Caused by:

   _____

   _____

   _____

   _____

   iii. Interruption of blood flow contributes to dementia
   iv. Symptoms may be _____ or have a sudden onset.
L. Alzheimer's Disease
   i. Progressive degenerative disease of the brain
   ii. Reduces _____ and _____ functioning
   iii. Onset is usually after age _____ and is common in the aging
   iv. Diagnosis is difficult and currently there is not a cure.
   v. Current research is studying the _____ found on the _____
      of Alzheimer's patients
   vi. Signs of Alzheimer's disease

   _____

   _____

   _____

   _____

   _____

   _____

M. _____ Dementia
   i. Decreased blood flow to brain leads to decreased oxygenation and nutrition to brain
   ii. Caused by _____, narrow or stenosed arteries
   iii. These prevent normal oxygenation of cerebral tissue.
   iv. As the condition worsens, the patient loses interest in personal hygiene, appearance, and
       surrounding activities
   v. Symptoms of vascular dementia

   _____

   _____

   _____

_____

_____

_____

N. Head Trauma
    i. Causes _____ if it causes reduced blood flow to the brain
    ii. May be a closed or an open head injury
    iii. Can include

_____

_____

_____

_____

    iv. Symptoms similar to vascular dementia, only with an insidious onset of ischemia
O. Childhood Disorders

_____

_____

_____

_____

_____

_____

P. Substance Abuse
    i. Crosses all _____, _____, _____, and edu-
cational backgrounds
    ii. Involves alcohol of all types such as beer, wine, liquor, and spirits
    iii. Prescription drugs are commonly abused.

_____

_____

_____

_____

    iv. Illegally abused substances include:

_____

_____

    v. Abuse affects all social and family relationships.
    vi. Abusers have altered behaviors, _____ _____, and possible
medical problems
    vii. Greatest risk is the operation of _____ or motor vehicles while under the
influence
    viii. Treatment may include:

_____

_____

_____

_____

V. Assessment and Diagnosis

A. Initial _____ intake questionnaire
B. Mental status examination
C. A treatment plan

D. Treatment may include:

_____

_____

_____

_____

VI. Standard Treatment for Mental Disorders
    A. Chemical imbalances may be treated with drugs, psychotherapy, counseling, group therapy, stress reduction therapy, and _____ techniques.
    B. Inherited or genetic conditions do not have a course of treatment.
    C. Deprivation of oxygen and nutrition are treated with _____ care.

KEY TERMINOLOGY REVIEW

Match the correct medical term with the definition listed below.

a.	addiction	**j.**	psychiatry
b.	affect	**k.**	psychologist
c.	antidepressant	**l.**	psychology
d.	antipsychotic	**m.**	psychosis
e.	comorbid	**n.**	psychotherapeutic
f.	dementia	**o.**	psychotherapy
g.	dependence	**p.**	psychotropic
h.	phobia	**q.**	tolerance
i.	psychiatrist		

_____ 1. The diminished mental or cognitive function that has an onset after 18 years of age.

_____ 2. Alleviating symptoms of anxiety, depression, and psychosis.

_____ 3. The state of addiction to certain drugs.

_____ 4. Repetitive and dependent behavior usually involving legal or illegal substance abuse.

_____ 5. Medication used to treat depression.

_____ 6. Treatment of mental disorders with talk therapy or counseling.

_____ 7. Branch of medicine that deals with diagnosis, treatment, and prevention of mental disorders.

_____ 8. Requiring greater amounts of a substance to achieve the desired effect.

_____ 9. Science dealing with normal and abnormal mental processes and behavior.

_____ 10. Medication used to treat psychotic episodes.

_____ 11. Irrational, obsessive fear of an object, situation, or activity.

_____ 12. Affecting psychic function, behavior, experience, or emotions.

_____ 13. Abnormal mental coping of the individual who is out of touch with reality.

_____ 14. Medical doctor or physician specializing in the medical treatment of mental illness.

_____ 15. Denoting coexisting, unrelated medical diseases or conditions.

_____ 16. Specialist in the field of psychology, therapy, and research.

_____ 17. The observable emotional reaction associated with an experience.

APPLIED PRACTICE

Follow the directions as instructed with each question below.

1. Refer to the picture of the brain that was used in the study guide labeling activity. Now, using this same picture, color the parts of the brain as instructed below:

   a. This part of the brain is responsible for equilibrium. Effects of alcohol on this portion of the brain are seen in the staggering of an intoxicated person. Color or highlight this section *yellow*.

   b. This part of the brain controls wakefulness, mental alertness, and sleepiness states. Color or highlight this section *pink*.

   c. This part of the brain is a relay station and important to perception and pleasure. Color or highlight this section *green*.

   d. This part of the brain regulates the heart rate, respirations, blood pressure. Color or highlight this section *blue*.

LEARNING ACTIVITY: TRUE/FALSE

Indicate whether the statement is true (T) or false (F).

_____ 1. Some alcohol addicts have been known to go so far as to drink after-shave lotion.

_____ 2. Stuttering is a physical problem instead of a learning disorder.

_____ 3. A person with panic disorder often expresses the fear that he or she is dying.

_____ 4. Malingering is faking or exaggeration of symptoms and complaints.

_____ 5. Analgesics are over-the-counter drugs that are subject to abuse.

_____ 6. Psychology deals with diagnosis, treatment, and prevention of mental disorders.

_____ 7. Caffeine and nicotine are legal substances that can be abused.

_____ 8. Many mental disorders are caused by a chemical balance in the brain.

_____ 9. Mental retardation occurs as the result of an interruption in the intellectual growth of the child, either during prenatal development, the birth process, or after birth.

_____ 10. The patient should be included in or give input into the treatment plan.

LEARNING ACTIVITY: FILL IN THE BLANK

Using words from the list below, fill in the blanks to complete the following statements.
Note: Some terms may be used more than once.

absence	crying spells	impending
affect	daily living	implemented
anger	degenerative	insidious
behavior	deteriorate	judgment
brain	diagnose	medical
capacity to cope	educational	mental and physical
childbirth	emotions and thoughts	*Mental Disorders*
compromised brain cells	ethnic	psychological
concurrent	frequent phenomenon	psychosis
constructive	homeostasis	reference

relationships
repaired
safety
schizophrenia

social
society
state of being

Statistical
substance
visual or auditory

1. Patients going through _____ withdrawal and others with _____ problems may experience periods of _____ and angry behavior. Health care providers must be alert to _____ anger and use _____ approaches to help manage that anger and provide _____ for themselves, the patient, and others.

2. Substance abuse occurs among people from every _____, professional, _____, racial, and _____ background. The economic cost to _____ is immeasurable.

3. Disordered or disorganized thinking, inappropriate _____, unpredictable _____, and _____ hallucinations are all symptoms of _____.

4. Substances that have the capacity to alter _____, impair _____, and create _____ problems. Social and family _____ suffer and may _____.

5. The brain maintains the body's _____ by reacting to sensory inputs, including _____, with processing and interpretation.

6. The *Diagnostic and* _____ *Manual of* _____ *IV* (DSM-IV) is the _____ manual used by mental health providers to _____ a wide range of mental disorders.

7. Alzheimer's disease usually has a/an _____ onset, is a progressive _____ disease of the _____, and _____ functioning is reduced.

8. Mental wellness is a/an _____. It is not necessarily a/an _____ of mental problems but a/an _____ in healthy ways with the pressures of _____.

9. There is no cure or drug therapy for mental retardation, as the _____ cannot be replaced or _____. Any _____ mental disorders should be addressed and treatment options explored and _____.

10. Postpartum depression is a/an _____ in the first few days or weeks after _____. It ranges in severity from _____ or "new baby blues" through sadness and despair to _____, with potentially devastating outcomes.

CRITICAL THINKING

Answer the following questions to the best of your ability. Use the textbook as a reference.

1. Explain why the *Diagnostic and Statistical Manual of Mental Disorders IV* is used to diagnose patients with mental disorders. This is not stated in the book, but common sense and critical thinking skills should give you ideas.

_____

_____

_____

_____

_____

2. Referring to the case study in the textbook, what are some of the possible sources of assistance this family could benefit from if Yolanda were willing? The answer is not in the book. Read the case study carefully to determine their problems and needs. Then list what you feel would be potential resources and what they may offer. There is a wide range of appropriate things, so list as many as you can.

_____

_____

_____

_____

_____

3. Can you think of someone you know, have met, or that you know of whom you consider to be "mentally well"? Consider this carefully and decide on someone as your example. Don't state names or identifying personal information, but write a paragraph on why you feel this person is mentally well. (What are the traits or characteristics or actions, etc., that give you the impression of mental wellness?)

_____

_____

_____

_____

_____

4. If a patient mentions to you that she was thinking about suicide recently and asks you not to tell the doctor because she would "never really do it," what would you say or do? The answer is not in the book, but use knowledge from what you have learned in your program so far and your thoughts to formulate a few sentences for your answer.

_____

_____

_____

_____

_____

5. You have a patient who is a 4-month-old female infant, and the mother has come in today for test results on the child. The infant was diagnosed with mental retardation, and the mother was told by the physician that there is no treatment that will help the child. The mother is upset and wants to know why there is no treatment available when modern medicine can transplant hearts and do brain surgery. What will you tell her?

_____

_____

_____

_____

_____

RESEARCH ACTIVITY

Use Internet search engines to research the following topics and write a brief description of what is found. It is important to visit reputable Web sites.

1. Visit the National Mental Health America Web site at www.hmha.org.

   What information do you find most helpful on this site?
   How could patients with mental health issues benefit from this site?
   What ways could you become involved with National Mental Health America?

   _____

   _____

   _____

   _____

   _____

   _____

   _____

   _____

   _____

   _____

   _____

   _____

   _____

CHAPTER 48
Oncology

CHAPTER OUTLINE

General review of the chapter:

A. Introduction
B. The Medical Assistant's Role in the Oncology Practice
C. The Classification and Physiology of Cancers
D. Diagnostic Procedures
    i. Routine diagnostic screening
    ii. Tumor markers
    iii. Staging and grading malignant tumors
E. Cancer Treatment
F. Hospice and Emotional Support
G. The Cancer Prevention Lifestyle

STUDENT STUDY GUIDE

Use the following guide to assist in your learning of the concepts from the chapter.

I. Introduction to Oncology and the MA Role

  A. Oncology
    i. Studies _____ and _____
    ii. Characterized by _____ cellular growth
    iii. 500,000 deaths due to cancer each year in the United States
    iv. _____ cancer diagnoses a year
    v. There is extensive research into the origin and causes of this disease.

  B. The MA's Role in an Oncology Office
    i. Obtaining medical _____ and _____
    ii. Assisting oncologists with patient examination and procedures
    iii. _____ patient regarding clothing removal and gowning assistance
    iv. Providing patients with information on _____ _____
    v. Arranging appointments for other tests and procedures
    vi. _____

II. Classifications and Physiology of Cancers

  A. Malignant or Cancerous Growth
    i. In normal bodies cell _____ and _____ occurs at a controlled rate.
    ii. _____, uncontrollable reproduction of _____ cells exists in cancers and malignancies.
    iii. Abnormal cells advance quickly, _____ normal cells of _____.
    iv. Eventually healthy cells are forced out of their normal environment.
    v. Malignant tumors destroy local, adjacent, and distal sites of tissue and organs.
    vi. Total _____ is difficult in _____ and recurrence is a common.

B. Classifications of Malignance
   i. Primary site:

_____

_____

   ii. Metastasis:

_____

_____

   iii. Malignant neoplasms:

_____

_____

C. Neoplasms and Points of Origin
   i. Carcinoma:

_____

_____

   ii. Glioma:

_____

_____

   iii. Leukemia:

_____

_____

   iv. Lymphoma:

_____

_____

   v. Melanoma:

_____

_____

   vi. Sarcoma:

_____

_____

D. Benign Tumors
   i. _____ and resemble tissue of origin
   ii. Caused by a/an _____ growth
   iii. Cellular structure is close to adjacent cells.
   iv. Causes _____ of the surrounding tissues or no symptoms at all
   v. Can be removed surgically with little effect.
E. Possible Causes of Cancer

_____

_____

_____

_____

_____

_____

_____

_____

_____

_____

_____

III. Diagnostic Procedures
   A. Cancer Screening
      i. _____ detection, _____, and treatment are critical for
          _____ and cure.
      ii. Educate patients on signs and symptoms of cancer, as well as the benefits of early treatment.
   B. Routine Diagnostic Tests
      i. Cancer detection techniques:

      _____

      _____

      _____

      _____

      _____

      _____

      _____

      _____

   C. Cancer-Specific Routine Testing
      i. _____ screening: _____ screen of fecal matter for occult
          blood
      ii. Barium enemas or lower _____ X-ray
      iii. _____ screening (yearly after 40)
      iv. Pap smear and pelvic examinations: yearly in sexually active females
      v. PSA screenings and digital rectal examinations (yearly after _____)
   D. Tumor Markers
      i. _____ tools used to determine the progress of cancer treatment or
          _____ of a tumor
      ii. Markers are _____, _____ and other substances tumors
          released into _____.
      iii. Routine diagnostic examples include:

      _____

      _____

      _____

      _____

   E. Tumor Markings and Benign Conditions
      i. Certain conditions may elevate tumor markers:

      _____

      _____

      _____

      _____

   F. Malignancy Staging and Grading
      i. Used to determine the _____ and _____ course of treatment
      ii. Identifies the type of cancer and the degree to which it has metastasized
      iii. Numerous elements are evaluated:

      _____

      _____

G. TNM Staging:
   i. T:

_____

_____

_____

_____

_____

_____

_____

_____

_____

_____

   ii. N:

_____

_____

_____

_____

_____

_____

   iii. M:

_____

_____

_____

_____

_____

_____

H. Cancer Cell Differentiation
   i. Grading refers to the differentiation of the cancer cells.
   ii. Well differentiated cancer cells retain some of the _____ of the _____ cell.
   iii. Well differentiated signifies a better _____.
   iv. Cells that are _____ differentiated no longer _____ the cells of origin.
   v. When this occurs, cancer is usually in the more _____ stages.

IV. Cancer Treatment
 A. General
   i. Ideally, eradicates all abnormal cells from the body
   ii. Three main types of treatment:

_____

_____

   iii. Metastatic diseases cannot be cured but treatment extends quality of life.

B. Chemotherapy

_____

_____

_____

_____

_____

_____

C. Radioactive Treatment
    i. Radioactive materials injected or implanted into the body
    ii. Intended to _____ the tumor while _____ healthy tissue
    iii. Treatment is rarely localized to abnormal cells and some normal cells are affected.

_____

_____

    iv. Common side effects include:

_____

_____

_____

D. Surgical Treatment
    i. Goal is a/an _____ or _____ symptom control
    ii. Surgery only curative for _____ stage tumors
    iii. Helpful in the treatment of solid cancers and staging
    iv. Care must be taken to remove _____ amounts of _____ tissue when tumor is removed
    v. If appropriate margins are not achieved, a second surgery may be necessary.
    vi. _____ _____ are checked for invasion and removed if necessary.
    vii. Palliative surgery is achieved by:

_____

_____

_____

_____

E. Hormonal and Immunotherapy
    i. _____ and _____ cancer can be treated effectively with hormone therapy.
    ii. Advancements have been made and therapy may involve:

_____

_____

_____

    iii. Biotherapy: The body's immune system is built up with a combination of chemotherapy and radiation therapy

_____

_____

_____

_____

F. Cancer Vaccinations

_____

_____

_____

_____

_____

_____

G. Monoclonal Antibody
    i. Monoclonal antibody is an antibody clone _____ in a laboratory setting.
    ii. Developed to target certain _____ of cancer cells that are not found in _____ cells
    iii. Some antibodies are currently approved for use:
        (a) trastuzumab (breast cancer) and rituximab (lymphoma)

H. Immunotherapy
    i. _____ immunotherapy can be used as primary treatment
    ii. Often used as adjuvant, or assistive to other types of cancer treatment
    iii. _____: naturally occurring hormones
    iv. Regulate the growth and activity of blood and immune systems cells
    v. Used in nonspecific immunotherapy and to reduce the side effects of chemotherapy and radiation

I. Side Effects of Cancer Treatment
    i. Advances in cancer treatment have decreased the need for radical surgery.
    ii. Pain management exists with every stage and is handled with:

_____

_____

_____

    iii. Terminally ill patients are referred to hospice.
    iv. Treatment is just as toxic to the healthy cells as the toxic cells: Thus long-term treatment may be necessary.
    v. Some patients are predisposed to cancers:

_____

_____

    vi. Some side effects aren't seen for years.
    vii. Side effects can be more dramatic in _____.

_____

_____

J. Cancer Research Advances
    i. "Starving" a tumor:

_____

_____

_____

_____

_____

_____

    ii. Genetics also contribute to cancer:

_____

_____

_____

_____

iii. _____ _____ _____ : higher and more accurate
focused dose of neutron energy is also a recent advance.

K. The Impact of Cancer

_____

_____

_____

_____

_____

_____

L. Hospice Care
i. _____ ill patients can be cared for in the home or a home-like setting.
ii. Provides _____ and _____ care in the final stages of
illness.
iii. Hospice provides _____ care for terminally ill patients and family support.
iv. Pain management:

_____

_____

v. Disease is managed by:

_____

_____

vi. Hospice is provided by:

_____

_____

_____

_____

M. Cancer Prevention
i. _____ cause some types of cancer.
ii. Many predisposing factors to cancer are a result of lifestyle choices:

_____

_____

_____

_____

_____

iii. Steps to improve lifestyle:

_____

_____

_____

_____

_____

_____

KEY TERMINOLOGY REVIEW

Write a sentence using the selected vocabulary terms in the correct context.

1. Benign:

   _____

   _____

2. Cancer:

   _____

   _____

3. Chemotherapy:

   _____

   _____

4. Malignant:

   _____

   _____

5. Metastasis:

   _____

   _____

6. Neoplasm:

   _____

   _____

7. Oncology:

   _____

   _____

8. Remission:

   _____

   _____

9. Tumor:

   _____

   _____

10. Stenosis:

   _____

   _____

11. Tumor Marker:

   _____

   _____

APPLIED PRACTICE

Follow the directions as instructed with each question below.

1. Read the following scenario and answer the corresponding questions.

Scenario

Jane Wyngard presents to your office with complaints of a painful lump found under her left breast. This was discovered during her monthly self-breast exam. After an X-ray was performed, the physician ordered blood work including a CBC, liver function tests, and tumor markers. Soon after the lab results were received, Ms. Wyngard was scheduled for surgery to remove the tumor. The tumor was then sent for biopsy to a laboratory. The physician determined her breast cancer staging to be T2 N0 M0 Stage II.

a. What is the medical term for the X-ray Ms. Wyngard had performed?

_____

b. Would the physician have included tumor marker CD19-9 or CA125 as a part of Ms. Wyngard's blood work? Explain your answer.

_____

_____

c. What is the medical term for the surgical removal of a tumor from the breast?

_____

d. Explain what *T2 N0 M0 Stage II* means. Is this a good or poor prognosis? Explain your answer.

_____

_____

_____

LEARNING ACTIVITY: MULTIPLE CHOICE

Circle the correct answer to each of the questions below.

1. The term for cancer appearing in a secondary site elsewhere in the body is called:
   a. spreading
   b. metastasis
   c. malignant
   d. eradication

2. Carcinoma originates in _____ tissue.
   a. lymphoid
   b. stem cells
   c. basal
   d. epithelial

3. The "A" in the ABCDs of abnormalities in warts and moles stands for:
   a. asymmetry
   b. assimilation
   c. atrophy
   d. alimentary

4. There are three major methods of cancer treatment. Which of the following is *not* one of the three?
   a. chemotherapy
   b. staging and grading
   c. surgery
   d. radiation

5. The two goals of surgery for cancer as a treatment modality are (circle both):

   a. palliative

   b. to avoid radiation and chemotherapy

   c. cure

   d. avoid the negative margins

6. Two ways to screen for prostate cancer include (circle the two that are correct):

   a. barium enema

   b. PSA blood test

   c. digital rectal examination

   d. colonoscopy

7. Which of the following are a part of a healthy lifestyle to try to prevent cancer? (Circle all that apply.)

   a. Reduce intake of animal fat.

   b. Get an EKG.

   c. Apply sunscreen prior to sun exposure.

   d. Have your eyes checked.

8. Which of the following are early warning signs of breast cancer? (Circle all that apply.)

   a. positive occult blood test

   b. a depression or dimpling in the skin

   c. bloody or spontaneous discharge from the nipple

   d. swelling of the lymph nodes in the armpit

9. The "N" in malignancy staging by the TNM system stands for

   a. note size, depth, and location

   b. nodal involvement

   c. normal

   d. neurological involvement

10. Overexposure to the sun's UV rays raises the risk of three types of cancer. Which of the following is not one of the three types?

   a. squamous

   b. basal

   c. lymphoma

   d. melanoma

CRITICAL THINKING

Answer the following questions to the best of your ability. Use the textbook as a reference.

1. Sharyn Holliker (a 44-year-old female) was told today by the doctor the results of a biopsy performed three days ago. She has a benign tumor, and the doctor recommended removal to prevent it from pushing on surrounding tissues if/when it grows. The patient was fine when talking with the doctor, but a little later when you meet with her to arrange the surgery, she starts crying and states that she "doesn't think it is benign or else the doctor wouldn't want to remove it." She feels sure she really has cancer but that the doctor won't tell her the truth. What would you say or do? The answer is not specifically in your textbook; this will be your opinion and should be based on the knowledge you have gained in your studies so far.

_____

_____

_____

_____

_____

2. In the case study in this chapter of the textbook, what would you say to the patient, Ruth Dillan, if she asked you to explain how cancer runs in families? This answer is not specifically in the textbook, so use your critical thinking skills and current knowledge to determine the most appropriate answer.

_____

_____

_____

_____

_____

3. A patient named Claire has come in today for her annual checkup; she has been cancer free for six years now. A melanoma on her shoulder was removed with clear margins. She states she has no complaints, although you notice an open sore on her ankle. You casually ask her how long she has had it, as you put on the blood pressure cuff. She tells you she has had it for "weeks; I keep putting antibiotic ointment on it but it just doesn't go away." She confides she thinks it isn't healing because she keeps using some self-tanning cream even though it irritates the sore for a few minutes after she puts it on every day. What red flag would this raise to you? What would you say or do?

_____

_____

_____

_____

_____

4. Explain, as if giving patient education, what remission is in oncology. You may need to do research on the Internet or in other texts to complete your answer.

_____

_____

_____

_____

5. The following is a hypothetical situation involving a patient who is a smoker with lung cancer. There is not a particular right or wrong answer, but it is meant to help the student recognize his or her own feelings, which are usually not expressed in the office. You should picture yourself in this situation as realistically as you can, and then state what you would say or do using critical thinking and common sense.

Scenario

The patient is a 68-year-old male who was diagnosed 2 weeks ago with lung cancer caused by smoking. The patient is in the office today to discuss which treatment he has chosen from those offered last week by the physician. The patient, Mr. Holman, has been smoking since he was 14 years old and drinks about 6 beers per day. His wife passed away a few years ago, and he has no children. He tells you that he wants chemo but no radiation and that he won't quit smoking. He says that he has nothing left in life, and if drinking and smoking help him get through each day, he is too old to change it now. He thinks if he cuts down, at least the chemo will still be able to kill the cancer.

Write a paragraph on what you would likely say to this patient. Then, consider how you would feel personally about this particular scenario. Even though you cannot convey your personal morals and opinions to the patient, it is important that you acknowledge your true biases. Write a paragraph about how you feel about this situation (which you would hide from the patient for professionalism). What would you be thinking about this patient's choice? Would you feel differently if he had a different type of cancer? Would you feel differently if the patient had lung cancer, had never smoked, but was a heavy drinker and he refused to stop drinking?

_____

_____

_____

_____

_____

RESEARCH ACTIVITY

Use Internet search engines to research the following topics and write a brief description of what is found. It is important to visit reputable Web sites.

1. Visit www.cancer.gov. Research the clinical trials available for various forms of cancer. What are your thoughts regarding clinical trials? Also, research Complementary and Alternative Medicine (CAM) available for cancer patients. What forms of CAM would you find most beneficial and why?

_____

_____

_____

_____

_____

_____

_____

_____

_____

_____

_____

_____

CHAPTER 49

Geriatrics

CHAPTER OUTLINE

General review of the chapter:

    A. Introduction
    B. The Medical Assistant's Role in Orthopedics and Physical Therapy
    C. The Aging Process
        i. Physical aspects of aging
        ii. Social and psychological aspects of aging
        iii. Nutritional aspects of aging
        iv. Economic aspects of aging
    D. Cultural Views of the Aging
    E. Promoting Health Among the Elderly

STUDENT STUDY GUIDE

Use the following guide to assist in your learning of the concepts from the chapter.

  I. The MA's Role in the Geriatric Office

    A. _____

    B. _____

    C. _____

    D. _____

    E. _____

  II. Physical Changes of the Aging

    A. Dry, thin, and less _____ skin that tears easily
    B. _____ changes, aging spots appear
    C. Wrinkles begin to develop.
    D. Fat cells and collagen are lost, skin will _____.
    E. Men, generally, will lose their hair and women's breasts will sag.
    F. Effects on the cardiovascular system

_____

_____

_____

_____

_____

_____

_____

_____

_____

_____

G. _____ hypotension
H. Reduced motion and activity leading to aches and pains
I. _____ tone declines.
J. Joints become _____ and less _____.
K. Bones are at risk for _____ and breaking.
L. Natural deterioration causes people to be shorter and stoop.
M. _____, _____, _____ and feet are less limber.
   Fingers become stiff and joints are swollen.
N. Ability to taste _____ and _____ items declines.
O. _____ and _____ become impaired.
P. Sensations are diminished.
Q. _____ system declines
R. _____ system declines
S. _____ memory declines
T. GI tract has a tendency to _____.
U. Constipation
V. Bladder _____
W. _____ bladder, _____
X. Loss of _____ _____
Y. Enlarged prostate causing urinary retention, _____, or _____

III. Psychological, Social, Nutritional, and Economic Changes of the Aging

A. Psychological Changes

_____

_____

_____

_____

_____

_____

_____

_____

_____

_____

_____

_____

B. Social Changes
   i. Loss of _____ can affect social environment.
   ii. Common changes occur:

_____

_____

_____

_____

_____

_____

C. Social Organizations

_____

_____

_____

_____

_____

_____

D. Nutritional Changes

_____

_____

_____

_____

_____

_____

E. Economic Impact of Aging
   i. Retirement at age _____ is considered a rite of passage.
   ii. Retirement is often devastating because of the loss of:

   _____

   iii. Other major economic issues include health insurance, cost of medications, and Social Security.
IV. Medicare, Medigap, and Social Security
   A. Medicare
      i. Established in _____ for
         (a) People over 65
         (b) _____ _____
         (c) Individuals in the _____ _____ _____ disease (ESRD)
      ii. About a month before turning 65, people will start receiving information regarding benefits.
      iii. They become eligible the first day of the month they turn 65.
   B. Medicare Part D
      i. Started _____
      ii. Allows drug coverage to Medicare beneficiaries for a monthly premium
      iii. Anyone on Medicare is entitled to coverage: No one is denied.
      iv. _____.
      v. _____ and senior citizen organizations may offer assistance on choosing a plan.
   C. Medigap

   _____

   _____

   _____

   _____

   _____

   _____

   _____

   _____

   _____

   D. Social Security
      i. Implemented in _____ for supplemental retirement benefits at 65 years of age
      ii. Spouses of individuals eligible for Social Security benefits also qualify for benefits when they reach a qualifying age.

      iii. _____ and _____ are also eligible for some benefits.

      iv. A person must have contributed for at least _____ working quarters to be eligible.

      v. Medical assistants need to be aware of local financial services and listen to patients to ensure their needs are being met.

V. Cultural Views on the Aging

  A. Japanese Culture

_____

_____

_____

_____

  B. Latino Culture

_____

_____

_____

  C. Korean Culture

_____

_____

_____

_____

  D. American Indian Culture

_____

_____

_____

_____

  E. Dominant American Culture

_____

_____

_____

_____

VI. Health Promotion for the Aging

  A. Meals on Wheels programs

  B. _____

  C. Moderate exercise should be encouraged (approved by physician)

  D. Set up home for safety: rails in bathrooms, removal of rugs, lighting

  E. _____

  F. Handrails, shower benches, etc., elevated toilet seats

  G. _____

  H. _____

  I. Large print and audio books, helper dogs

KEY TERMINOLOGY REVIEW

Use terminology words throughout the chapter to correctly complete the sentences below.

1. After his stroke Mr. Liu experienced right-sided _____, losing the function of his right arm.

2. At the age of 90, Miriam DeJuan received a hearing aid. Her condition of hearing deficiency associated with age is known as _____.

3. Henry Atkinson decided to move into a/an _____ _____ _____ when he needed some medical attention but did not require 24-hour care.

4. Dr. Myer diagnosed Vivian with _____ _____ due to her decreased blood pressure when she changes positions from sitting to standing.

5. An automobile caused _____ in Anthony Michaleson, causing paralysis in his lower body.

6. Though MaryAnn has fond childhood memories, she often forgets what occurred the day before or even hours earlier. Thus, she is lacking _____ _____ _____.

7. _____ is visual deficiency associated with aging.

8. After completing his medical school training, Dr. Watson decided to concentrate in _____ because of his fascination with the aging process.

APPLIED PRACTICE

Follow the directions as instructed with each question below.

1. Read the following scenario and answer the questions that follow.

Scenario

Fredrick Alamar, age 73, presents to your office today for a physical and a flu vaccination. Upon obtaining his weight, it is apparent that Mr. Alamar has lost 18 pounds since his last visit two months ago, which was shortly after his wife died. You make a note of this in his chart. Prior visits to the office have shown Mr. Alamar to be in fairly good health for his age. He only takes metoprolol succinate for hypertension. As you obtain his blood pressure, Mr. Alamar removes his sweater. You notice scratches and bruising on his lower back. He states "I fell after stepping out of the bathtub. I have been falling down a lot more lately and I don't seem to have any strength." After noting this in his chart, you excuse yourself from the examination room, and inform the doctor of Mr. Alamar's changes since his last visit.

a. What are the likely causes for Mr. Alamar's significant weight loss?

_____

_____

b. What could be the cause of his recent lack of strength?

_____

_____

c. What things could be done to help Mr. Alamar at home?

_____

_____

d. The doctor may recommend a form of permanent care for Mr. Alamar. What options may be available for Mr. Alamar?

_____

_____

LEARNING ACTIVITY: MULTIPLE CHOICE

Circle the correct answer to each of the questions below.

1. The typical length of time between visits by a doctor to a patient at an extended care facility is:

   a. daily
   b. weekly
   c. monthly
   d. semi-monthly

2. Which of the following is not an assistive device to aid older individuals?

   a. handrails and grab bars
   b. throw rugs
   c. bathtub seat
   d. Velcro fasteners

3. In which of the following cultures is it considered shameful not to care for elderly parents?

   a. Chinese
   b. Indian
   c. Latino
   d. Korean

4. All older patients should be encouraged to document their wishes regarding:

   a. which community resources to refer them to
   b. the extent of medical intervention they want when they cannot speak for themselves
   c. arrangements for transportation to doctor appointments and shopping
   d. submitting their information to the Local Councils on Aging

5. Changes in metabolic rate are a condition of which system?

   a. endocrine
   b. cardiac
   c. integumentary
   d. gastrointestinal

6. Normal wear and tear and natural deterioration take their toll on spinal disks, and the individual may (circle all that apply):

   a. cause orthostatic hypotension
   b. stoop
   c. lose muscle tone
   d. become shorter

7. Which of the following are true statements? (Circle all that apply.)

   a. The process of aging has physiological aspects.
   b. The loss of hearing, taste, smell, and mobility can lead to depression.
   c. Changes in sensorimotor abilities improve how the elderly interact with their environment.
   d. The elderly undergo changes in their physical appearance.

8. Which of the following is not listed in your textbook as one of the three examples of factors that accelerate the aging process?

   a. disease
   b. stress

   c. depression
   d. lack of social interaction

9. Seborrheic keratosis is a condition of what system?

   a. endocrine
   b. cardiac

   c. integumentary
   d. gastrointestinal

10. Three changes to hearing (related to the nervous system) are listed in the textbook. Which of the following is not one of those three?

   a. delayed auditory response
   b. damage to ossicles

   c. sensoneural damage to auditory nerve
   d. decreased equilibrium

CRITICAL THINKING

Answer the following questions to the best of your ability. Use the textbook as a reference.

1. Your patient is an 82-year-old woman who is in fairly good health, but she is worried about money. She states that Medicare doesn't pay for enough things, and she wonders if you know of any other resources for her. What can you suggest to this patient regarding medical costs?

   _____

   _____

   _____

   _____

   _____

2. Because your patient, Mr. Bjorklund, has a diminished short-term memory, what can you do to ensure that any patient education you deliver will not be ignored because the patient forgot?

   _____

   _____

   _____

   _____

3. Mr. and Mrs. Holman, a married couple in their 70s, are both patients at your clinic and they are both in for their annual physicals today. The woman tells you in the hallway that her husband's driving is becoming a problem. She states he has bumped into a few planters and fences when parking and that he drifts out of his lane when driving. She asks that you not tell the doctor because it would be difficult if they did not have a car. What would you do?

   _____

   _____

   _____

   _____

4. A 68-year-old patient named Mrs. Royer has come in today because she is depressed. She says she used to have lots of friends and family but now she is alone. Make a list of possible reasons that this patient feels so isolated.

_____

_____

_____

_____

5. After you have practiced Procedure 31-1: Role-Play Sensorimotor Changes of the Elderly, write at least two paragraphs on how you felt, or what it was like, or even a list of the things you didn't realize before trying this. You can choose to write a paragraph each on two of the various aging conditions (loss of vision, paralysis, etc.), or you can write two paragraphs on the overall experience. There are no right or wrong answers in this critical thinking question. This is for you to explore and consider how your patients feel and what they have to deal with. This is a valuable experience.

_____

_____

_____

_____

_____

_____

_____

_____

_____

_____

RESEARCH ACTIVITY

Use Internet search engines to research the following topics and write a brief description of what is found. It is important to visit reputable Web sites.

1. Research additional "assistive aids" that can help elderly patients with their daily activities. What aids do you find most helpful? Which would you be most likely to recommend to future patients?

_____

_____

_____

_____

_____

_____

_____

_____

_____

_____

CHAPTER 50
Alternative Medicine

CHAPTER OUTLINE

General review of the chapter:

A. Introduction
B. Complementary and Alternative Medical Systems
   i. Alternative medicine
   ii. Ayurveda
   iii. Homeopathy
   iv. Naturopathy
   v. Acupuncture
C. Mind-Body Interventions
D. Biologically Based Therapies
E. Manipulative and Body-Based Methods
F. Energy Therapies

STUDENT STUDY GUIDE

Use the following guide to assist in your learning of the concepts from the chapter.

I. Introduction and the MA Role in Alternative Medicine

A. Complementary and Alternative Medicine (CAM)
   i. Not presently considered to be part of conventional medicine
   ii. Includes _____, _____, and _____ medicines
   iii. Alternative medicine is used in place of _____ medicine.
   iv. Complementary medicine works in _____ with conventional medicine.
   v. _____ medicine incorporates conventional, complementary, and alternative therapies to treat medical conditions.

B. Classifications of CAM
   i. Alternative medicine:

     _____

     _____

   ii. Mind-body intervention:

     _____

     _____

   iii. Biologically-based therapies:

     _____

     _____

   iv. Manipulative and body-based methods:

     _____

     _____

    v. Energy therapies:

_____

_____

  C. The MA's Role in Alternative Medicine
      i. Be knowledgeable about forms of CAM.
     ii. Include forms of CAM when taking a/an _____ _____.
    iii. Harmful interactions can occur between conventional and alternative medicine.
  D. Direct patient _____ regarding alternative therapy toward the physician.

II. Alternative Medicine

  A. Overview
      i. Origins in cultures around the world for centuries
     ii. Types of alternative medicine include:
        (a) _____
        (b) _____
        (c) _____
        (d) _____
  B. Ayurveda
      i. Sanskrit meaning *"knowledge of life"*
     ii. An ancient _____ healing practice
    iii. Focuses disease prevention by promoting _____ _____
        instead of _____ _____
     iv. Two basic operating principles
        (a) Principle 1:

_____

_____

        (b) Principle 2:

_____

_____

  C. Homeopathic Medicine
      i. Treatment stimulates the body's _____ system and _____ ability.
     ii. Natural remedies are made from plants, animals, or _____ substances.
    iii. Dosages are _____ in varying degrees and prescribed based on patient assessment.
  D. Naturopathic Medicine
      i. Treats psychological, physical, and genetic factors to assist the body in healing itself
     ii. Uses:

_____

_____

_____

_____

    iii. Practitioners are _____ primary care givers.
        (a) Complete _____ years of naturopathic medical school
        (b) Receive the Naturopathic Medicine (N.D.) degree
  E. Acupuncture
      i. Helps the body regulate _____ and _____ blood cell counts and raise _____ levels
     ii. Treatment:

_____

_____

_____

_____

   iii. Effective with conventional medicine against pain management, asthma, drug addiction (illegal, narcotic, alcohol, and nicotine), and strokes

   iv. Reimbursed by _____ _____ and _____

III. Mind-Body Intervention

  A. General

    i. Focuses on areas that directly affect physiological health

_____

_____

_____

_____

  B. Biofeedback

    i. Biofeedback teaches people how to relax, _____, and meditate.

    ii. A machine monitors

_____

_____

_____

_____

   iii. _____ signals help the patient learn to consciously control body responses.

   iv. Over time, a patient will learn biofeedback without the use of a machine.

    v. Useful with stress, migraines, depression, insomnia, and other conditions

  C. Aromatherapy

    i. Utilizes _____ _____ extracted from flowers and herbs

    ii. Practiced since ancient times

_____

_____

   iii. Affects the autonomic nervous system

    (a) Stimulates the release of chemicals that are responsible for relaxation and the reduction of pain.

  D. Essential Oils

    i. Can be prescribed for complaints such as:

_____

_____

_____

_____

    ii. _____ oil is used for muscle relaxation and pain relief.

   iii. _____ oil helps ease depression.

   iv. _____ oil and oil of _____ relieve congestion.

    v. Lavender oil relieves _____ and improves sleep.

   vi. _____ oil relieves nausea and aids in digestion.

   vii. Lemon, orange, and other citrus oils improve the _____ and _____ alertness.

  viii. Aromatherapy is a complementary therapy and should not be used as a substitute for conventional medical care.

   ix. Essential oils can be quite _____, and some carry _____ side effects.

IV. Manipulative and Body-Based Techniques
  A. General
     i. Utilize different modalities to treat patients
     ii. Bodywork: hands-on manipulation of the musculoskeletal system to promote

     _____

     _____

  B. Hydrotherapy
     i. Uses water to treat disease
     ii. Can be done using Jacuzzis, swimming pools, whirlpools, steam baths, etc.
     iii. Increases _____ and _____
     iv. Accelerates the _____ process
     v. Hydrotherapy is usually an addition to physical therapy.
  C. Chiropractic
     i. Uses _____ and _____ to promote health
     ii. Treatment corrects spinal misalignments causing pain, decreased agility, and illness.
     iii. In addition to vertebral manipulation, treatments include:

     _____

     _____

     iv. All states require chiropractors to be licensed:

     _____

     _____

  D. Reflexology
     i. Restores the body's natural _____ flow
     ii. Stimulates specific reflex points on the _____ or _____
     iii. Pressure is applied to these points to restore function.
     iv. No state licensing requirements currently needed for the practice of reflexology
     v. _____ program followed by a/an _____ and
        _____ exam are recommended.
  E. Massage
     i. Manipulation of muscle and soft tissue:

     _____

     _____

     ii. Can enhance the client's sense of well-being *if* done correctly
     iii. Types of massage include:

     _____

     _____

     iv. Not appropriate when patient:

     _____

     _____

     _____

     _____

V. Energy Therapies
  A. General
     i. Work with the electromagnetic fields that are believed to surround the human body
        (a) "Biofields"
     ii. Some energy therapies use hand manipulation:

     _____

     _____

     iii. It has not been scientifically proven that biofields exist.

B. Reiki
    i. A practitioner places his or her hands _____ or _____ a specific body area.
    ii. "_____" is transferred to the patient.
    iii. Believed to provide strength, harmony, and balance
    iv. Involves a total of _____ hand positions covering all body systems

C. Therapeutic Touch
    i. _____, holistic approach, to healing
    ii. Attempts to stimulate the receiver's own powers of recuperation
    iii. Based on the principle of a/an _____ exchange between people
    iv. Believed to

      _____

      _____

    v. Practitioners believe they have the ability to _____ health by sensing and _____ these energy fields.
    vi. Its positive effect may be a result of the positive energy generated by the practitioner.

KEY TERMINOLOGY REVIEW

Write a sentence using the selected vocabulary terms in the correct context.

1. Alternative Medicine:

    _____

    _____

2. Complementary Medicine:

    _____

    _____

3. Essential Oils:

    _____

    _____

4. Integrative Medicine:

    _____

    _____

LEARNING ACTIVITY: MULTIPLE CHOICE

Circle the correct answer to each of the questions below.

1. Which two of the following are the main reasons for homeopathic treatment as listed in your text?
    a. stimulate the immune system
    b. maintain a balance of three doshas
    c. treat psychological factors
    d. strengthen the body's healing processes

2. The three major areas of care under alternative medicine are (circle all three):
    a. integrative
    b. naturopathic
    c. alternative
    d. complementary

3. Mind-body interventions use techniques that enhance the mind's ability to influence body function and symptoms. For example, positive thinking, laughter, and personal contact help to release _____, which are natural anti-pain mediators.

   a. hormones
   b. endorphins

   c. potassium and sodium
   d. enzymes

4. Which of the following is *not* a form of hydrotherapy?

   a. hot tub
   b. moist heat pack

   c. sauna
   d. All of the above are forms of hydrotherapy.

5. Which of the following types of therapies does not use conventional medicine at all?

   a. integrative
   b. complementary

   c. alternative
   d. all of the above

6. Which herb has an anti-inflammatory property?

   a. ginseng
   b. ginkgo

   c. garlic
   d. goldenseal

7. Which of the following is not considered a natural substance that can be used as the basis for biologically based therapies?

   a. hormones
   b. essential oils

   c. vitamins
   d. herbs

8. Biofeedback includes three areas in which the patient is trained. Which of the following is not one of the three areas?

   a. relaxation
   b. meditation

   c. massage
   d. visualization

9. Homeopathic treatment involves the use of natural remedies made from:

   a. plant, animal, or mineral substances
   b. chemicals made from natural sources

   c. natural hormones
   d. regular household items such as vinegar and baking soda

10. Traditional Chinese medicine is listed under which of the categories of complementary and alternative methods?

   a. mind-body interventions
   b. energy therapies

   c. biologically based therapies
   d. alternative medicine

LEARNING ACTIVITY: FILL IN THE BLANK

Using words from the list below, fill in the blanks to complete the following statements.

acupuncture	disease process	healing process
blood chemistry	energy flow	health
blood pressure	flexibility and strength	herbs
concepts	hands-on manipulation	holistic
conventional medicine	heal itself	India

knowledge of life   practices   safety and effectiveness
mental   properties   spiritual
physiological health   psychological   traditional exercise
popular   relaxation   very thin needles

1. Ayurveda is an ancient healing practice that originated in _____. It means "_____."

2. Alternative medicine has become so _____, and in many instances so promising, that the government has created the National Center for Complementary and Alternative Medicine (NCCAM) to focus on the _____ of alternative therapies.

3. Bodywork is a broad term referring to the _____ of the musculoskeletal system to promote healing, _____, pain reduction, _____, and improved _____.

4. The focus of mind-body medicine is the ways in which a person's _____, emotional, social, and _____ health directly affect his or her _____.

5. Asian medical tradition has contributed several important _____ in alternative medicine, such as _____, acupressure, and the use of _____.

6. Herbs are chosen according to their _____ and are usually used in combination with other _____ treatments.

7. "Complementary and alternative medicine," as defined by NCCAM, "is a group of diverse medical and health care systems, _____, and products that are not presently considered to be a part of _____."

8. Naturopathy is an eclectic approach that helps the body _____ by treating _____, physical, and genetic factors in addition to the _____.

9. Acupuncture involves the insertion of _____ into predetermined sites to stimulate changes in heart rate, _____, brain activity, _____, and the immune and endocrine systems.

10. Hydrotherapy increases _____ and accelerates the _____. It can be used with individuals who cannot withstand the rigors of _____ programs.

CRITICAL THINKING

Answer the following questions to the best of your ability. Use the textbook as a reference.

1. As you take the patient history of a 22-year-old female patient, you ask her if she has been taking any herbal supplements or other natural remedies or receiving any alternative treatments. She looks very surprised and asks why you want to know that. She states that since her "herbal supplements are natural," they wouldn't interfere with any medications she is taking. You know this is a false statement, so explain to the patient why this information is important to the physician.

_____

_____

_____

_____

_____

2. A patient has come in today who would like to try Ayurvedic treatment, but she wants to know how to tell if it is worthwhile. She has researched on the Internet and cannot find the accrediting board(s) for the practice of Ayurveda medicine. What would you tell her?

_____

_____

_____

_____

_____

3. Today Mr. Arnold has an appointment. As you are noting his chief complaint, he mentions that he wants to know which herbs should be used to relieve anxiety. Which herbs would you recommend to him?

_____

_____

_____

_____

_____

4. Your patient, a widowed 59-year-old female named Marie DuLac, has been prescribed lymphatic massage. Although she said nothing to the physician, she now admits to you that she is very worried about having it. She is concerned that it will be painful or that it is dangerous compared to traditional massage. Write out the response/patient education you would give orally to her in the office during a visit.

_____

_____

_____

_____

_____

5. A father comes in with the patient, Paul, his 14-year-old son, who is joining a school sports team for the first time this year. Since Paul has weak knees and ankles, the provider has recommended sports massage, but the father is skeptical and feels this won't be beneficial to his son as much as aerobic or strength-building exercise. Educate the father on the benefits of sports massage.

_____

_____

_____

_____

RESEARCH ACTIVITY

Use Internet search engines to research the following topics and write a brief description of what is found. It is important to visit reputable Web sites.

1. Research more information about one of the following CAM therapies:
   - Ayurveda
   - Homeopathy
   - Reiki
   - Therapeutic Touch

Why did you decide to research your chosen topic?
What information do you find most interesting and useful?
Would you be or are you willing to try this form of CAM?

_____

_____

_____

_____

_____

_____

_____

_____

_____

_____

_____

CHAPTER 51
Competing in the Job Market

CHAPTER OUTLINE

General review of the chapter:

    A. Introduction
    B. The Externship Experience
    C. Writing an Effective Resume
    D. Preparing a Cover Letter
    E. Looking for Employment
    F. Completing Applications
    G. The Successful Interview

STUDENT STUDY GUIDE

Use the following guide to assist in your learning of the concepts from the chapter.

  I. The Externship Experience
    A. The Externship
        i. Every accredited MA program requires an externship experience lasting from
            _____ hours.
       ii. During an externship, medical assistant students are _____ in a medical
           office and should behave as _____:

          _____

          _____

          _____

          _____

      iii. The externship site is a forum for students to exercise their _____ and
           _____ skills.
      iv. Students benefit from this hands-on, real-world experience:

          _____

          _____

       v. If the externship is a/an _____ _____, the site may offer the
           student a position to work for the office.
    B. The MA Program Director
        i. The medical assistant program director is responsible for _____ students in
           appropriate _____ sites.
       ii. The program director will serve as a/an _____ for the student:

          _____

          _____

      iii. Most extern sites are well versed in the responsibilities of externships.

II. Seeking Employment
   A. A sub-par resume can sacrifice employment potential.
   B. Resumes should summarize:

   _____

   _____

   _____

   _____

   C. Items to include for a professional resume include:

   _____

   _____

   _____

   _____

   _____

   D. The Cover Letter
      i. Cover letters are often the link between _____ and _____

         _____.
      ii. They must be error free, accurate, and professionally presented.
      iii. Cover letters are critical job-searching tools:
         (a) They should accompany _____ _____, including those
             submitted via _____.
      iv. An effective cover letter includes a heading that contains:

      _____

      _____

      _____

      _____

      v. The cover letter should also include the reasons that the applicant is best suited for the
         position available.
   E. Seeking Employment
      i. Medical assistants may choose to look in the following places for employment:

      _____

      _____

      _____

      _____

      _____

      _____

III. The Interview
   A. Interview Dos
      i. Prepare prior to an interview which includes researching the medical office:
         (a) An applicant that is _____ about the interviewing office may stand out
             as a candidate for the position.
         (b) Arrive prepared with:

         _____

         _____

         _____

B. Interview Don'ts

_____

_____

_____

_____

_____

C. Dressing for the Interview
  i. Dressing for the interview is very important:

  _____

  _____

  _____

  _____

  _____

  ii. The applicant should have impeccable _____ _____.
D. Body Language
  i. Upon meeting the interviewer, the applicant should _____ and shake his or her hand.
  ii. Body language communicates a great deal to prospective employers:

  _____

  _____

  _____

  _____

IV. Interview Followup
  A. Interview followup increases the likelihood of hiring.
    i. This reminds employers of _____.
    ii. It allows the opportunity to ask _____, extend _____, and emphasize their interest in _____.
    iii. A handwritten or typed _____ note should be sent to the office _____ days after the interview.
  B. Changing Jobs
    i. When planning to change jobs, medical assistants should provide their current employer with at least _____ notice.
    ii. This should be in writing.
    iii. During the final two weeks, the MA should attend to his or her job duties as _____.
    iv. During the final days the MA must communicate the statuses of all his or her _____.
    v. The MA should also clean their workspace and return the office's items.
    vi. It is also suggested to request a/an _____ of _____ from the current employer.

KEY TERMINOLOGY REVIEW

Complete the sentences below with the correct key terms found at the beginning of the chapter.

1. Kevin prepared his _____ that would accompany his resume to the office manager of Elk Valley Medical Center.

2. Tamara, RMA (AMT), was a/an _____ for extern students at Elk Valley Medical Center. She was considered one of the best employees in the office for students to learn from.

3. The final phase of an accredited medical assisting program is the _____ that consists of hands-on training at a medical office.

4. Sally Henderson, CMA (AAMA) was Kevin's program director. She acted as his _____ when an issue arose with the office manager at Kevin's externship site.

5. Kevin carefully checked his _____ for grammatical and typographical errors prior to sending it out.

6. Wayne Anderson, the office manager at Elk Valley Medical Center, called Kevin to request a/an _____ after receiving his well written resume.

7. Shaundra, MA works as a/an _____ for externship students at her medical office. She answers any questions the student medical assistants may have.

APPLIED PRACTICE

Answer the following questions and complete the activities as instructed.

Assume that you are a recent medical assisting graduate preparing to enter the workforce.

1. You have recently received a phone call for an interview for Mountain View Health Care Center. How will you research the medical facility prior to your interview, and why is this important?

   _____

   _____

   _____

   _____

2. Considering your current wardrobe, which outfit would you choose to wear to your interview?

   _____

   _____

   _____

   _____

3. Practice filling out Mountain View Health Center's application for employment on pages 537 and 538.

   Note: For this activity, do not include your actual Social Security number, or the real address and telephone numbers of your references. This information should be made up.

APPLICATION FOR EMPLOYMENT

Mountain View Health Care Center is an equal opportunity employer and upholds the principles of equal opportunity employment. It is the policy of Mountain View Health Care Center to provide employment, compensation and other benefits related to employment based on qualifications and performance, without regard to race, color, religion, national origin, age, sex, veteran status or disability, or any other basis prohibited by federal or state law. As an equal opportunity employer, Mountain View Health Care Center intends to comply fully with all federal and state laws and the information requested on this application will not be used for any purpose prohibited by law. Disabled applicants may request any needed accommodation. This application is intended to allow you, the applicant, to provide Mountain View Health Care Center with the information and data so that your suitability and qualifications can be fairly determined for the position(s) for which you are applying. Please complete this application and answer all questions completely. Please print clearly in ink.

PLEASE PRINT CLEARLY—BE SURE TO SIGN THIS APPLICATION

Date

Name: Last   First   Middle

Social Security No.:   Home Phone:

Address:

No.   -   Street

City   State   Zip

Have you been previously employed by Mountain View Health Care Center?   ☐ Yes   ☐ No
If "Yes", when?   In what capacity?

How did you learn of the position for which you are applying:
☐ Newspaper/Print Advertisement   ☐ Friend/Relative   ☐ Employment Agency   ☐ Job Service   ☐ Radio/TV Advertisement

EMPLOYMENT DESIRED
Position(s) applied for
Shift Preferences: ☐ First Shift – Days   ☐ Second Shift – Evenings   ☐ Third Shift – Nights
☐ Full-time   ☐ Part-time If "Part time", number of shifts/hours desired:
Date available to start   Salary requested

PERSONAL HISTORY
Are you a United States citizen or do you have an entry permit which allows you to lawfully work in the U.S.?   ☐ Yes   ☐ No
    If applicable, Visa Type: Immigration No.:
Are you at least 18 years old?   ☐ Yes   ☐ No

Are you able to perform all of the duties required by the position for which you are applying, without endangering yourself or compromising the safety, health, or welfare of the Patients or other Staff Persons?   ☐ Yes   ☐ No
    If "No," please explain:

EDUCATION
Name and Location Of School   Graduation   Course of Study/
                                       Date   Degree Issued
High School

College

Other

LICENSURE/CERTIFICATION/REGISTRATION
    Type of License/Certification   Registration Number

List any special skills or qualifications which you posses and feel are relevant to health care and the position for which you are applying.

Sample employment application.

EMPLOYMENT HISTORY
Please give accurate and complete information. Start with present or most recent employer.

May we contact and communicate with your present employer?   ☐ Yes   ☐ No

Employer _____ Telephone No. _____

Address _____ Employed from   /   to   /

Name of Supervisor _____ Hourly Pay: Start _____ Last _____

Position and Responsibilities

Reason for Leaving

- -

Employer _____ Telephone No. _____

Address _____ Employed from   /   to   /

Name of Supervisor _____ Hourly Pay: Start _____ Last _____

Position and Responsibilities

Reason for Leaving

- -

Employer _____ Telephone No. _____

Address _____ Employed from   /   to   /

Name of Supervisor _____ Hourly Pay: Start _____ Last _____

Position and Responsibilities

Reason for Leaving

- -

MILITARY SERVICE

Branch _____ From _____ To _____

What were your duties?

Did you receive any specialized training?   ☐ Yes   ☐ No
If "Yes", describe:

REFERENCES
Names of friends or relatives, if any, currently employed by Mountain View Health Care Center.

Name _____ Address _____ Phone _____

Name _____ Address _____ Phone _____

Names of co-workers (no relatives) you have worked with and whom we may contact for a reference.

Name _____ Address _____ Phone _____

Name _____ Address _____ Phone _____

Please read the following statements completely and carefully before you initial and sign your name.

The Applicant HEREBY CERTIFIES that the answers given on this Application For Employment, including any statements or answers provided by the Applicant during interview, are true and correct. The Applicant fully authorizes Mountain View Health Care Center to contact any references, past and present employers, persons, schools, law enforcement agencies and any other sources of information which may be relevant to the Applicant and this Application For Employment. It is understood and agreed that any misrepresentation, false statement, or omission by the Applicant will be sufficient reason for rejection of the Application For Employment or for dismissal from employment at any time, without recourse or liability to Mountain View Health Care Center.

I have read, understand and agree to the above statement.   (Please initial here). _____

SIGN HERE _____   DATE _____

Sample employment application (*continued*)

LEARNING ACTIVITY: MULTIPLE CHOICE

Circle the correct answer to each of the questions below.

1. The _____ is a fellow medical assistant who will serve as a resource to the student medical assistant during the externship.

   a. office manager
   b. mentor
   c. physician
   d. none of the above

2. Which of the following is a responsibility of the student medical assistant during the externship?

   a. Be on time.
   b. Dress appropriately.
   c. Act in a professional manner.
   d. all of the above.

3. The medical assisting program director acts as a/an _____ for the student medical assistant while on externship.

   a. preceptor
   b. mentor
   c. advocate
   d. none of the above

4. When a student medical assistant has a concern about something at the extern site, to whom should the student bring the problem to attention?

   a. the medical assisting program director
   b. a coworker
   c. the student's spouse
   d. the dean of the college

5. Which of the following may be a reason why the medical assistant may not be called for an interview?

   a. The resume contains typographical errors.
   b. The resume contains grammatical errors.
   c. The resume contains crossed-out words and hand-written corrections.
   d. all of the above

6. Resumes should ideally be _____ pages in length.

   a. 2–3
   b. 1–2
   c. 3–4
   d. 4–5

7. A thank-you note should be sent to the potential employer after an interview within _____ days.

   a. 1–2
   b. 2–3
   c. 3–5
   d. 6–8

8. Which of the following are places a medical assistant might look for employment?

   a. the newspaper
   b. the local medical assisting program
   c. an employment agency
   d. all of the above

9. Which of the following is an interview "don't"?

   a. request parking validation
   b. arrive a bit early
   c. take notes
   d. all of the above

10. Which of the following is an appropriate dress code for an applicant going to a job interview?

    a. casual attire
    b. business suit
    c. scrubs
    d. any of the above

CRITICAL THINKING

Answer the following questions to the best of your ability. Use the textbook as a reference.

1. Willie Harrison is finishing his medical assisting training and is preparing for his externship experience. Willie's wife asks him what he will be doing during his externship. How might Willie answer her question?

_____

_____

_____

_____

_____

_____

2. Joann Felmer is a student in an administrative medical assisting course. She has been given an assignment to describe the benefits of the externship experience for the student medical assistant. How might Joann answer this question?

_____

_____

_____

_____

_____

_____

3. Corey Rubatino, CMA (AAMA), has recently been hired to work for Dr. Joe Cresanti. On Corey's first day, he has been asked by Dr. Cresanti to describe what is meant by practicing within his scope of practice. How might Corey answer this question?

_____

_____

_____

_____

_____

_____

4. Maggie Levinski, RMA (AMT), is the program director in an accredited medical assisting program. She is attempting to add additional extern sites to the program roster. When Maggie meets with a potential site, she is asked to explain the benefits of the externship to the extern site. How might Maggie answer this question?

_____

_____

_____

_____

_____

_____

5. Jason Ripper is a student medical assistant going out to his externship site for the first time. When he arrives at the site, the office manager asks Jason to sign a HIPAA agreement before Jason can begin work. Jason asks the office manager to explain why this form is needed. How might the office manager answer?

_____

_____

_____

_____

_____

RESEARCH ACTIVITY

Use Internet search engines to research the following topics and write a brief description of what is found. It is important to visit reputable Web sites.

1. Using the Internet and other sources, locate prospective job opportunities for medical assistants in your area. Which jobs appear most interesting to you? Explain why.

_____

_____

_____

_____

_____

_____

_____

_____

_____

_____

_____

_____

APPENDIX
Competency Check-Offs

Affective Behaviors

Affective behaviors are very important to the role of medical assisting. These behaviors display sensitivity to the patient, convey an understanding of laws and regulations, and also provide an overall professional component to the medical assisting profession.

The weighed competencies that are found in the student workbook vary slightly from the competencies found in the textbook. The competencies within the student workbook have placed an emphasis on these affective behaviors by showing them in a ***bold and italicized*** font. Not all procedures will have affective behaviors; affective behaviors will primarily be addressed during a procedure that involves direct patient contact.

Your instructors will be expecting to see these behaviors demonstrated during the performance of a procedure, as necessary. Failure to exhibit these affective behaviors will result in a loss of points associated with the point value of the given step. It is essential to review the weighted competencies found in the workbook prior to being tested and graded.

Procedure 2-1:

Adapting to Change

Objective: To adapt to change when given a new task within the time limit set by the instructor

Supplies: Notepad and pen

Affective Behaviors: Affective behaviors provide a professional approach to a skill that enhances the patient encounter. These behaviors may also display sensitivity to a patient's rights and enhance communication. Pay close attention to these skills, which will be in ***bold, italicized*** font.

Notes to the Student

_____

_____

_____

_____

_____

_____

Skills Assessment Requirements

Read and familiarize yourself with the procedure; complete the minimum practice requirements. Document each MPR using proper charting technique. Complete each procedure within a reasonable amount of time, with a minimum of 85 percent accuracy.

Name: _____

Date: _____

POINT VALUE ✦ = 3–6 points ⋆ = 7–9 points		**PRACTICE TRIAL**	**GRADED TRIAL # 1**	**GRADED TRIAL # 2**	**NOTES**
1. ✦	**Listen closely** as a new task is requested.				
2. ✦	Ask questions to clarify the request, if needed.				
3. ✦	Take notes about the task, if needed.				
4. ⋆	Begin working on the new task while **maintaining a positive and professional attitude.**				

Name: _____

Date: _____

Document: Enter the appropriate information in the chart below.

Grading

Points Earned	_____		
Points Possible	_____	27	27
Percent Grade (Points Earned/Points Possible)	_____		
PASS:	_____	❏ YES ❏ NO ❏ N/A	❏ YES ❏ NO ❏ N/A

Instructor Sign-Off

Instructor: _____ Date: _____

Procedure 4-1:

Prepare an Informed Consent for Treatment Form

Objective: Prepare an informed consent for treatment form correctly within the time limit set by the instructor.

Supplies: Informed consent for treatment form, blue or black ink pen, copy machine

Affective Behaviors: Affective behaviors provide a professional approach to a skill that enhances the patient encounter. These behaviors may also display sensitivity to a patient's rights and enhance communication. Pay close attention to these skills, which will be in **_bold, italicized_** font.

Notes to the Student

_____

_____

_____

_____

_____

_____

Skills Assessment Requirements

Read and familiarize yourself with the procedure; complete the minimum practice requirements. Document each MPR using proper charting technique. Complete each procedure within a reasonable amount of time, with a minimum of 85 percent accuracy.

Name: _____

Date: _____

POINT VALUE ✦ = 3–6 points ★ = 7–9 points		PRACTICE TRIAL	GRADED TRIAL #1	GRADED TRIAL #2	NOTES
1. ★	As the physician goes over the details of the upcoming procedure with the patient, fill in the informed consent form. The form must include: • The name of the procedure or treatment to be performed • The expected benefits of the procedure • Any possible risks of the procedure • Any accepted alternatives to the procedure and the risks or benefits associated with each • The fact that the patient may choose to forego the procedure and the possible risks or benefits associated with that choice **Doublecheck this information for accuracy.**				
2. ✦	Be certain the form lists the patient's name, birth date, and the place the procedure is to be performed (in office, hospital, etc.). **Doublecheck this information for accuracy.**				
3. ✦	Show the consent form to the physician for him/her to verify all information is correct.				
4. ★	After the physician has left the room, go over the form with the patient. If the patient has further questions about the procedure, have the patient wait in the treatment room while you ask the physician to return to answer the questions. If the patient has no further questions about the procedure, have the patient sign the consent form.				
5. ✦	Sign the consent form as a witness to the patient's signature.				
6. ✦	Go over any specifics with the patient about the procedure day, such as any restrictions to eating or drinking on the day of the surgery, or where the patient should park their car.				

Document: Enter the appropriate information in the chart below.

Grading

Points Earned	_____		
Points Possible	_____	42	42
Percent Grade (Points Earned/Points Possible)	_____		
PASS:	_____	❑ YES ❑ NO ❑ N/A	❑ YES ❑ NO ❑ N/A

Instructor Sign-Off

Instructor: _____ Date: _____

Procedure 4-2:

Obtaining Authorization for the Release of Patient Medical Records

Objective: Obtain an authorization to release information from a patient correctly within the time limit set by the instructor.

Supplies: Release-of-records authorization form, blue or black ink pen, copy machine

Affective Behaviors: Affective behaviors provide a professional approach to a skill that enhances the patient encounter. These behaviors may also display sensitivity to a patient's rights and enhance communication. Pay close attention to these skills, which will be in **_bold, italicized_** font.

Notes to the Student

_____

_____

_____

_____

_____

_____

Skills Assessment Requirements

Read and familiarize yourself with the procedure; complete the minimum practice requirements. Document each MPR using proper charting technique. Complete each procedure within a reasonable amount of time, with a minimum of 85 percent accuracy.

Name: _____

Date: _____

POINT VALUE ✦ = 3–6 points ★ = 7–9 points	PRACTICE TRIAL	GRADED TRIAL # 1	GRADED TRIAL # 2	NOTES
1. ★ When the patient states all or a portion of the patient's records is to be released to a third party, ask the patient to sign and date a release-of-records form.				
2. ✦ Verify the address where the patient would like the copies of the record sent.				
3. ✦ Verify the records the patient would like released. If the patient requests specific release dates, ask the patient to write those dates on the release-of-records form.				
4. ✦ Verify if the patient would like super-protected information (HIV/AIDS, mental health, drug or alcohol rehabilitation information, sexually transmitted disease information, or information about family planning), and ask the patient to check the appropriate box on the authorization form to allow the release of that information.				
5. ★ Identify which information in the medical record must be copied.				
6. ✦ Copy the appropriate documents from the medical record. **To protect patient privacy, verify all of the patient's medical record has been removed from the copy machine.**				
7. ✦ Send the copies to the requested location.				

Name: _____

Date: _____

Document: Enter the appropriate information in the chart below.

Grading

Points Earned	_____		
Points Possible	_____	48	48
Percent Grade (Points Earned/Points Possible)	_____		
PASS:	_____	❏ YES ❏ NO ❏ N/A	❏ YES ❏ NO ❏ N/A

Instructor Sign-Off

Instructor: _____   **Date:** _____

Procedure 4-3:

Respond to a Request for Copies of a Patient's Medical Record

Objective: Respond to a request for copies of a patient's medical record correctly within the time limit set by the instructor.

Supplies: Release-of-records authorization form, blue or black ink pen, copy machine

Affective Behaviors: Affective behaviors provide a professional approach to a skill that enhances the patient encounter. These behaviors may also display sensitivity to a patient's rights and enhance communication. Pay close attention to these skills, which will be in **_bold, italicized_** font.

Notes to the Student

_____

_____

_____

_____

_____

_____

Skills Assessment Requirements

Read and familiarize yourself with the procedure; complete the minimum practice requirements. Document each MPR using proper charting technique. Complete each procedure within a reasonable amount of time, with a minimum of 85 percent accuracy.

Name: _____

Date: _____

POINT VALUE ◆ = 3–6 points ★ = 7–9 points		PRACTICE TRIAL	GRADED TRIAL #1	GRADED TRIAL #2	NOTES
1. ★	Verify that the release-of-records form has been signed and dated by the patient or the patient's legal representative.				
2. ◆	***Carefully review the release form for any specific date or information requests.***				
3. ◆	Check if the patient has authorized release of super-protected information (HIV/AIDS, mental health, drug or alcohol rehabilitation information, sexually transmitted disease information, or information about family planning).				
4. ◆	Verify that you have pulled the correct patient file.				
5. ◆	Locate the documents to be copied.				
6. ★	Review the documents to be copied to verify that they carry the correct patient name and contain the information requested in the authorization to release information and only that information.				
7. ◆	Copy the appropriate documents.				
8. ◆	Send the copies to the requesting agency.				
9. ★	File the release-of-records request in the patient's medical record with a notation of the documents that were copied and sent.				

Name: _____

Date: _____

Document: Enter the appropriate information in the chart below.

Grading

Points Earned	_____		
Points Possible	_____	63	63
Percent Grade (Points Earned/Points Possible)	_____		
PASS:	_____	❏ YES ❏ NO ❏ N/A	❏ YES ❏ NO ❏ N/A

Instructor Sign-Off

Instructor: _____ **Date:** _____

Procedure 5-1:

Use Effective Listening Skills in Patient Interviews

Objective: To use effective listening skills in interviewing the patient correctly within the time limit set by the instructor

Supplies: Patient history form and pen

Affective Behaviors: Affective behaviors provide a professional approach to a skill that enhances the patient encounter. These behaviors may also display sensitivity to a patient's rights and enhance communication. Pay close attention to these skills, which will be in **_bold, italicized_** font.

Notes to the Student

_____

_____

_____

_____

_____

_____

Skills Assessment Requirements

Read and familiarize yourself with the procedure; complete the minimum practice requirements. Document each MPR using proper charting technique. Complete each procedure within a reasonable amount of time, with a minimum of 85 percent accuracy.

Name: _____

Date: _____

POINT VALUE ✦ = 3–6 points ⋆ = 7–9 points		PRACTICE TRIAL	GRADED TRIAL #1	GRADED TRIAL #2	NOTES
1. ✦	**Smile, and introduce** yourself to the patient.				
2. ⋆	Identify the patient by verifying the patient's birth date.				
3. ⋆	Verify that you have the correct patient chart.				
4. ✦	Maintain a professional persona.				
5. ✦	**Maintain eye contact with the patient.**				
6. ✦	Ask the patient open-ended questions.				
7. ✦	Do not interrupt the patient.				
8. ✦	Paraphrase the patient's statements to verify comprehension.				
9. ✦	**Watch for the patient's nonverbal communication.**				
10. ✦	**Summarize the patient's statements, and conclude the interview.**				
11. ⋆	Document appropriate information in the patient's file.				

Name: _____

Date: _____

Document: Enter the appropriate information in the chart below.

Grading

Points Earned	_____		
Points Possible	_____	75	75
Percent Grade (Points Earned/Points Possible)	_____		
PASS:	_____	❏ YES ❏ NO ❏ N/A	❏ YES ❏ NO ❏ N/A

Instructor Sign-Off

Instructor: _____   **Date:** _____

Procedure 5-2:

Communicate with the Hearing-Impaired Patient

Objective: Communicate with a hearing-impaired patient correctly within the time limit set by the instructor.

Supplies: Patient's file and pen

Affective Behaviors: Affective behaviors provide a professional approach to a skill that enhances the patient encounter. These behaviors may also display sensitivity to a patient's rights and enhance communication. Pay close attention to these skills, which will be in **_bold, italicized_** font.

Notes to the Student

_____

_____

_____

_____

_____

_____

Skills Assessment Requirements

Read and familiarize yourself with the procedure; complete the minimum practice requirements. Document each MPR using proper charting technique. Complete each procedure within a reasonable amount of time, with a minimum of 85 percent accuracy.

Name: _____

Date: _____

POINT VALUE ✦ = 3–6 points ⋆ = 7–9 points		PRACTICE TRIAL	GRADED TRIAL # 1	GRADED TRIAL # 2	NOTES
1. ✦	Alert the patient that you are ready to take him to the examination room by entering the reception area, touching the patient's arm to get his attention, and motioning to follow.				
2. ✦	If the patient has an interpreter, also have the interpreter enter the examination room.				
3. ⋆	**When speaking, look directly at the patient and speak slowly.**				
4. ⋆	When the patient can read lips, verify understanding through patient questioning. **When comprehension is lacking, write instructions for the patient.**				
5. ✦	When asking a patient to change into a gown, ask the patient to flip a switch or crack the door open when ready. People with hearing impairments cannot hear a knock to announce the physician's arrival.				
6. ⋆	At the end of the patient's visit, chart all communications, including verification of the patient's understanding.				

Document: Enter the appropriate information in the chart below.

Grading

Points Earned	_____		
Points Possible	_____	42	42
Percent Grade (Points Earned/Points Possible)	_____		
PASS:	_____	❏ YES ❏ NO ❏ N/A	❏ YES ❏ NO ❏ N/A

Instructor Sign-Off

Instructor: _____   **Date:** _____

Procedure 5-3:

Communicate with a Sight-Impaired Patient

Objective: Communicate with a sight-impaired patient correctly within the time limit set by the instructor.

Supplies: Patient's file and pen

Affective Behaviors: Affective behaviors provide a professional approach to a skill that enhances the patient encounter. These behaviors may also display sensitivity to a patient's rights and enhance communication. Pay close attention to these skills, which will be in **_bold, italicized_** font.

Notes to the Student

_____

_____

_____

_____

_____

_____

Skills Assessment Requirements

Read and familiarize yourself with the procedure; complete the minimum practice requirements. Document each MPR using proper charting technique. Complete each procedure within a reasonable amount of time, with a minimum of 85 percent accuracy.

POINT VALUE ✦ = 3–6 points ⋆ = 7–9 points		PRACTICE TRIAL	GRADED TRIAL #1	GRADED TRIAL #2	NOTES
1. ✦	Alert the patient that you are ready to visit the examination room by entering the reception area, touching the patient's arm, and offering your arm for the patient to hold.				
2. ✦	Ensure that any service animal accompanies the patient to the examination room.				
3. ⋆	Alert the patient to any steps, doorways, ramps, or slopes along the way.				
4. ✦	Take the patient to a private area, outside of other patients' views or hearing ranges.				
5. ✦	Place the patient's hand on the chair or table where sitting is desired. Ensure that the patient is comfortable by asking "Do you feel comfortable?"				
6. ✦	Arrange for any service animal to sit directly next to the patient.				
7. ✦	Ask the patient the questions on the history form, and write down the answers. Ensure the patient's responses are clearly understood and verify information obtained.				
8. ⋆	At the end of the patient's visit, chart all communications, including how the patient's understanding was verified.				
9. ⋆	Sign and date the patient history form and note that the history form was completed for the patient due to sight impairment.				

Name: _____

Date: _____

Document: Enter the appropriate information in the chart below.

Grading

Points Earned	_____		
Points Possible	_____	63	63
Percent Grade (Points Earned/Points Possible)	_____		
PASS:	_____	❏ YES ❏ NO ❏ N/A	❏ YES ❏ NO ❏ N/A

Instructor Sign-Off

Instructor: _____ **Date:** _____

Procedure 5-4:

Communicate with Patients via an Interpreter

Objective: Communicate with a patient via an interpreter correctly within the time limit set by the instructor.

Supplies: Patient's file and pen

Affective Behaviors: Affective behaviors provide a professional approach to a skill that enhances the patient encounter. These behaviors may also display sensitivity to a patient's rights and enhance communication. Pay close attention to these skills, which will be in **_bold, italicized_** font.

Notes to the Student

_____

_____

_____

_____

_____

_____

Skills Assessment Requirements

Read and familiarize yourself with the procedure; complete the minimum practice requirements. Document each MPR using proper charting technique. Complete each procedure within a reasonable amount of time, with a minimum of 85 percent accuracy.

Name: _____

Date: _____

POINT VALUE ✦ = 3–6 points ⋆ = 7–9 points		PRACTICE TRIAL	GRADED TRIAL # 1	GRADED TRIAL # 2	NOTES
1. ✦	When the patient arrives in the office with an interpreter, obtain the name of the interpreter and verify the spelling.				
2. ⋆	**Obtain the interpreter's contact information for the patient's medical record.** If the interpreter has a business card, attach it to the patient's file.				
3. ✦	Communicate with the patient directly; **do not speak directly to the interpreter.**				
4. ✦	When any of the interpreter's comments are unclear, **ask for clarification. Ask the patient if her or she has any questions prior to leaving the room.**				
5. ⋆	Document all essential parts of the interview in the patient's chart.				

Name: _____

Date: _____

Document: Enter the appropriate information in the chart below.

Grading

Points Earned	_____		
Points Possible	_____	36	36
Percent Grade (Points Earned/Points Possible)	_____		
PASS:	_____	❏ YES ❏ NO ❏ N/A	❏ YES ❏ NO ❏ N/A

Instructor Sign-Off

Instructor: _____ Date: _____

Name: _____

Date: _____

Procedure 5-5:

Identify Community Resources

Objective: To identify community resources correctly within the time limit set by the instructor.

Supplies: A computer with Internet access, written pamphlets and brochures, telephone directories

Notes to the Student

_____

_____

_____

_____

_____

_____

Skills Assessment Requirements

Read and familiarize yourself with the procedure; complete the minimum practice requirements. Document each MPR using proper charting technique. Complete each procedure within a reasonable amount of time, with a minimum of 85 percent accuracy.

POINT VALUE	PRACTICE TRIAL	GRADED TRIAL #1	GRADED TRIAL #2	NOTES
✦ = 3–6 points ★ = 7–9 points				
1. ★ Locate the name, address, telephone number and Web site address for each of the following need categories in your community: • Homeless services • HIV/AIDS resources • Disability services • Domestic violence services • Public assistance • Housing authority/services • Ombudsman services • Foster care for children • Foster care for adults • Senior services • Legal aid • Rape victim services • Crime victim services • Culturally specific services (Native American, military, etc.) • Medical assistant services (Medicaid, etc.)				
2. ✦ Identify at least one to three resources for each category.				
3. ★ Create a written document to give to patients.				

Document: Enter the appropriate information in the chart below.

Grading

Points Earned	————		
Points Possible	————	24	24
Percent Grade (Points Earned/Points Possible)	————		
PASS:	————	❏ YES ❏ NO ❏ N/A	❏ YES ❏ NO ❏ N/A

Instructor Sign-Off

Instructor: _____   **Date:** _____

Name: _____

Date: _____

Procedure 5-6:

Prepare a Patient's Specialist Referral

Objective: Prepare a referral for a patient to see a specialist correctly within the time limit set by the instructor.

Supplies: Telephone, blue or black ink pen, patient's file, referral form to a specialist

Affective Behaviors: Affective behaviors provide a professional approach to a skill that enhances the patient encounter. These behaviors may also display sensitivity to a patient's rights and enhance communication. Pay close attention to these skills, which will be in **_bold, italicized_** font.

Notes to the Student

_____

_____

_____

_____

_____

_____

Skills Assessment Requirements

Read and familiarize yourself with the procedure; complete the minimum practice requirements. Document each MPR using proper charting technique. Complete each procedure within a reasonable amount of time, with a minimum of 85 percent accuracy.

POINT VALUE ✦ = 3–6 points ⋆ = 7–9 points	PRACTICE TRIAL	GRADED TRIAL # 1	GRADED TRIAL # 2	NOTES
1. ⋆ **Verify the patient file is correct.**				
2. ✦ Verify the referral form for the specialist is correct.				
3. ✦ Verify the doctor's instructions (e.g., What does the doctor want the patient to be seen for? How soon does the patient need to be seen?).				
4. ✦ **Choose a private location, out of the hearing range of other patients, to discuss the referral with the patient.**				
5. ✦ If the pending referral is not an emergency and the patient is in the clinic, ask the patient for a convenient time of day to see the specialist.				
6. ✦ Call the specialist's office, and ask to speak to the person who handles the schedule.				
7. ✦ Provide personal identification and the name of the referring doctor or clinic.				
8. ✦ State the reason for the call.				
9. ✦ Give patient information as requested by the specialist's office. **Only provide the required patient information.**				
10. ✦ Set an appointment date and time. If the patient is in the clinic, verify the date and time.				
11. ✦ Document the appointment's date and time on the referral form. If the patient is in the clinic, give the patient the referral form. Choose to mail the referral form when there is time before the appointment.				
12. ⋆ Document the call's results in the patient's chart.				

Name: _____

Date: _____

Document: Enter the appropriate information in the chart below.

Grading

Points Earned	_____		
Points Possible	_____	78	78
Percent Grade (Points Earned/Points Possible)	_____		
PASS:	_____	❏ YES ❏ NO ❏ N/A	❏ YES ❏ NO ❏ N/A

Instructor Sign-Off

Instructor: _____ **Date:** _____

Procedure 6-1:

Use the Internet to Find Patient Education Materials

Objective: Use the Internet to find patient education materials correctly within the time limit set by the instructor.

Supplies: Computer and printer, patient chart, blue or black pen

Affective Behaviors: Affective behaviors provide a professional approach to a skill that enhances the patient encounter. These behaviors may also display sensitivity to a patient's rights and enhance communication. Pay close attention to these skills, which will be in **_bold, italicized_** font.

Notes to the Student

_____

_____

_____

_____

_____

_____

Skills Assessment Requirements

Read and familiarize yourself with the procedure; complete the minimum practice requirements. Document each MPR using proper charting technique. Complete each procedure within a reasonable amount of time, with a minimum of 85 percent accuracy.

Name: _____

Date: _____

POINT VALUE ✦ = 3–6 points ★ = 7–9 points		PRACTICE TRIAL	GRADED TRIAL # 1	GRADED TRIAL # 2	NOTES
1. ✦	Using the computer, **locate reputable Web sites for desired materials.**				
2. ✦	Print copies of materials.				
3. ★	Show materials to the physician for approval.				
4. ✦	Give/mail the materials to the patient.				
5. ✦	Explain the materials to the patient as needed.				
6. ✦	Place a copy of the materials in the patient's file.				
7. ★	Document how the materials were given to the patient and any verbal education provided with the materials.				

Name: _____

Date: _____

Document: Enter the appropriate information in the chart below.

Grading

Points Earned	_____		
Points Possible	_____	48	48
Percent Grade (Points Earned/Points Possible)	_____		
PASS:	_____	❏ YES ❏ NO ❏ N/A	❏ YES ❏ NO ❏ N/A

Instructor Sign-Off

Instructor: _____   **Date:** _____

Procedure 8-1:

Compose a Business Letter

Objective: Compose a business letter correctly within the time limit set by the instructor.

Supplies: Computer with word-processing software, information for the letter

Affective Behaviors: Affective behaviors provide a professional approach to a skill that enhances the patient encounter. These behaviors may also display sensitivity to a patient's rights and enhance communication. Pay close attention to these skills, which will be in **bold, *italicized*** font.

Notes to the Student

_____

_____

_____

_____

_____

_____

Skills Assessment Requirements

Read and familiarize yourself with the procedure; complete the minimum practice requirements. Document each MPR using proper charting technique. Complete each procedure within a reasonable amount of time, with a minimum of 85 percent accuracy.

Name: _____

Date: _____

POINT VALUE ✦ = 3–6 points ⋆ = 7–9 points		PRACTICE TRIAL	GRADED TRIAL # 1	GRADED TRIAL # 2	NOTES
1. ✦	Determine the recipient and content of the letter.				
2. ✦	Using the word-processing software, type the date of the letter.				
3. ✦	Type the recipient of the letter.				
4. ✦	Type the subject line.				
5. ✦	Type the greeting of the letter.				
6. ✦	Type the body of the letter. **Consider the recipient's level of understanding when communicating.**				
7. ✦	Type the salutation.				
8. ✦	Indicate enclosures, if any.				
9. ✦	Indicate if a copy of the letter will be sent to another party.				
10. ✦	Enter the initials of the letter's author, followed by your initials as the typist.				
11. ⋆	Perform complete electronic spelling and grammar checks.				
12. ✦	Print the letter.				
13. ⋆	**On paper, perform manual spelling and grammar checks.**				
14. ⋆	Give the letter to the physician for a signature.				
15. ✦	Address an envelope.				
16. ✦	Send the letter.				

Document: Enter the appropriate information in the chart below.

Grading

Points Earned	_____		
Points Possible	_____	105	105
Percent Grade (Points Earned/Points Possible)	_____		
PASS:	_____	❏ YES ❏ NO ❏ N/A	❏ YES ❏ NO ❏ N/A

Instructor Sign-Off

Instructor: _____   **Date:** _____

Procedure 8-2:

Prepare a Document for Photocopying

Objective: Prepare a document for photocopying correctly within the time limit set by the instructor.

Supplies: Photocopier, document to be copied, envelope, patient medical record

Notes to the Student

_____

_____

_____

_____

_____

_____

Skills Assessment Requirements

Read and familiarize yourself with the procedure; complete the minimum practice requirements. Document each MPR using proper charting technique. Complete each procedure within a reasonable amount of time, with a minimum of 85 percent accuracy.

Name: _____

Date: _____

POINT VALUE ✦ = 3–6 points * = 7–9 points		PRACTICE TRIAL	GRADED TRIAL # 1	GRADED TRIAL # 2	NOTES
1. ✦	Turn the photocopy machine on and allow for time to warm up.				
2. ✦	Place the document to be copied face down on the glass surface of the photocopier, following the diagram on the photocopier.				
3. ✦	Indicate the number of copies needed by entering the number in the appropriate place on the photocopier.				
4. ✦	Press the "copy" button on the photocopier.				
5. *	Once the copy has been made, remove the original.				
6. ✦	Place the original document into an envelope to be mailed to the patient.				
7. *	Place the photocopy of the document into the patient's file.				

Name: _____

Date: _____

Document: Enter the appropriate information in the chart below.

Grading

Points Earned	_____		
Points Possible	_____	48	48
Percent Grade (Points Earned/Points Possible)	_____		
PASS:	_____	❏ YES ❏ NO ❏ N/A	❏ YES ❏ NO ❏ N/A

Instructor Sign-Off

Instructor: _____   **Date:** _____

Procedure 8-3:

Send a Letter to a Patient Regarding a Missed Appointment

Objective: Send a letter to a patient regarding a missed appointment correctly within the time limit set by the instructor.

Supplies: Computer with word-processing software, patient's medical record

Affective Behaviors: Affective behaviors provide a professional approach to a skill that enhances the patient encounter. These behaviors may also display sensitivity to a patient's rights and enhance communication. Pay close attention to these skills, which will be in ***bold, italicized*** font.

Notes to the Student

_____

_____

_____

_____

_____

_____

Skills Assessment Requirements

Read and familiarize yourself with the procedure; complete the minimum practice requirements. Document each MPR using proper charting technique. Complete each procedure within a reasonable amount of time, with a minimum of 85 percent accuracy.

Name: _____

Date: _____

POINT VALUE ✦ = 3–6 points * = 7–9 points	PRACTICE TRIAL	GRADED TRIAL # 1	GRADED TRIAL # 2	NOTES
1. ✦ Using the word-processing software, type the date at the top of the letter.				
2. ✦ Type the patient's name and mailing address.				
3. ✦ For the subject line, type "RE: Missed Appointment."				
4. ✦ In the body of the letter, describe the appointment that was missed, including its date. **Maintain politeness in the tone of the letter.**				
5. * Per the physician's instructions or office policy, list the reasons the patient should call to reschedule the missed appointment.				
6. * Copy the letter for the patient's file.				
7. ✦ Obtain the signature of the letter's author (you or the physician).				
8. ✦ Send the patient the original letter.				

Name: _____

Date: _____

Document: Enter the appropriate information in the chart below.

Grading

Points Earned	_____		
Points Possible	_____	54	54
Percent Grade (Points Earned/Points Possible)	_____		
PASS:	_____	❏ YES ❏ NO ❏ N/A	❏ YES ❏ NO ❏ N/A

Instructor Sign-Off

Instructor: _____   **Date:** _____

Procedure 8-4:

Proofread Written Documents

Objective: Proofread a written document correctly within the time limit set by the instructor.

Supplies: Computer document to be proofread, computer with word-processing software

Notes to the Student

_____

_____

_____

_____

_____

_____

Skills Assessment Requirements

Read and familiarize yourself with the procedure; complete the minimum practice requirements. Document each MPR using proper charting technique. Complete each procedure within a reasonable amount of time, with a minimum of 85 percent accuracy.

Name: _____

Date: _____

POINT VALUE ✦ = 3–6 points ⋆ = 7–9 points		PRACTICE TRIAL	GRADED TRIAL # 1	GRADED TRIAL # 2	NOTES
1. ✦	Open the document using the word-processing software.				
2. ✦	Use the word processor's spelling and grammar checking functions.				
3. ✦	Save any changes.				
4. ⋆	Starting at the top, read the entire document to verify that all spelling, punctuation, and grammatical errors were corrected.				
5. ✦	Save any changes and print the document.				
6. ⋆	Review the entire document to verify that all spelling, punctuation, and grammatical errors were corrected.				
7. ✦	If changes were made, reprint the document.				
8. ✦	Give the document to the physician for signature.				

Name: _____

Date: _____

Document: Enter the appropriate information in the chart below.

Grading

Points Earned	_____		
Points Possible	_____	54	54
Percent Grade (Points Earned/Points Possible)	_____		
PASS:	_____	❑ YES ❑ NO ❑ N/A	❑ YES ❑ NO ❑ N/A

Instructor Sign-Off

Instructor: _____ **Date:** _____

Name: _____

Date: _____

Procedure 8-5:

Fold Documents for Window Envelopes

Objective: Fold a document for use with a window envelope correctly within the time limit set by the instructor.

Supplies: Document to be mailed, window envelope

Notes to the Student

_____

_____

_____

_____

_____

_____

Skills Assessment Requirements

Read and familiarize yourself with the procedure; complete the minimum practice requirements. Document each MPR using proper charting technique. Complete each procedure within a reasonable amount of time, with a minimum of 85 percent accuracy.

Name: _____

Date: _____

POINT VALUE ✦ = 3–6 points ⋆ = 7–9 points		PRACTICE TRIAL	GRADED TRIAL # 1	GRADED TRIAL # 2	NOTES
1. ✦	Locate the mailing address on the document.				
2. ✦	Compare the location of the mailing address to the location of the window on the envelope.				
3. ⋆	Fold the document such that the mailing address will be viewable through the envelope's window once the document has been inserted in the envelope.				
4. ✦	Insert the document in the envelope.				
5. ⋆	Verify that the address is viewable through the window.				
6. ✦	Seal the envelope.				

Document: Enter the appropriate information in the chart below.

Grading

Points Earned	_____		
Points Possible	_____	42	42
Percent Grade (Points Earned/Points Possible)	_____		
PASS:	_____	❏ YES ❏ NO ❏ N/A	❏ YES ❏ NO ❏ N/A

Instructor Sign-Off

Instructor: _____ Date: _____

Name: _____

Date: _____

Procedure 8-6:

Open and Sort Mail

Objective: Open and sort the office mail correctly within the time limit set by the instructor.

Supplies: A stack of incoming mail, including payments from insurance companies and patients, advertisements, drug samples, magazines, professional journals, bills for office services, a letter to the physician marked "Personal and Confidential," and consultation reports from other physicians, date stamp, letter opener

Affective Behaviors: Affective behaviors provide a professional approach to a skill that enhances the patient encounter. These behaviors may also display sensitivity to a patient's rights and enhance communication. Pay close attention to these skills, which will be in ***bold, italicized*** font.

Notes to the Student

_____

_____

_____

_____

_____

_____

Skills Assessment Requirements

Read and familiarize yourself with the procedure; complete the minimum practice requirements. Document each MPR using proper charting technique. Complete each procedure within a reasonable amount of time, with a minimum of 85 percent accuracy.

Name: _____

Date: _____

POINT VALUE ✦ = 3–6 points ⋆ = 7–9 points		PRACTICE TRIAL	GRADED TRIAL # 1	GRADED TRIAL # 2	NOTES
1. ✦	Using a date stamp, stamp the date on each received item.				
2. ⋆	***Remember: Information contained in the mail may be regarding patient care, and patient privacy must be respected.*** Sort the mail into the appropriate files according to the following: • Physician—correspondence from other physicians, hospitals, or laboratories, as well as any professional journals • Office manager—bills for office services, drug samples, advertisements for supplies or services • Receptionist—magazines • Billing office—payments from patients or insurance companies, correspondence from insurance companies				
3. ✦	Open each piece of mail, except for the piece marked "Personal and Confidential."				
4. ✦	Distribute the mail appropriately. Leave the mail piece marked "Personal and Confidential" on the physician's desk.				

Name: _____

Date: _____

Document: Enter the appropriate information in the chart below.

Grading

Points Earned	_____		
Points Possible	_____	27	27
Percent Grade (Points Earned/Points Possible)	_____		
PASS:	_____	❏ YES ❏ NO ❏ N/A	❏ YES ❏ NO ❏ N/A

Instructor Sign-Off

Instructor: _____ **Date:** _____

Procedure 8-7:

Annotate Written Correspondence

Objective: Annotate a written correspondence correctly within the time limit set by the instructor.

Supplies: Written correspondence, highlighter pen, letter opener

Notes to the Student

_____

_____

_____

_____

_____

_____

Skills Assessment Requirements

Read and familiarize yourself with the procedure; complete the minimum practice requirements. Document each MPR using proper charting technique. Complete each procedure within a reasonable amount of time, with a minimum of 85 percent accuracy.

Name: _____

Date: _____

POINT VALUE ✦ = 3–6 points ⋆ = 7–9 points		**PRACTICE TRIAL**	**GRADED TRIAL #1**	**GRADED TRIAL #2**	**NOTES**
1. ✦	Open the envelope with the document to be annotated.				
2. ✦	Read the document once in its entirety.				
3. ⋆	Using the highlighter pen, review the document again, highlighting such pertinent information as: • Patient's name • Findings of any examination or laboratory work • Dates for followup appointments • Diagnosis				
4. ⋆	Read the document a third time to ensure all pertinent information has been noted.				
5. ✦	Place the annotated document on the physician's desk for review.				

Document: Enter the appropriate information in the chart below.

Grading

Points Earned	_____		
Points Possible	_____	42	42
Percent Grade (Points Earned/Points Possible)	_____		
PASS:	_____	❏ YES ❏ NO ❏ N/A	❏ YES ❏ NO ❏ N/A

Instructor Sign-Off

Instructor: _____ **Date:** _____

Procedure 9-1:

Answer the Telephone

Objective: Answer the medical office telephone correctly within the time limit set by the instructor.

Supplies: Pen, paper, and telephone

Affective Behaviors: Affective behaviors provide a professional approach to a skill that enhances the patient encounter. These behaviors may also display sensitivity to a patient's rights and enhance communication. Pay close attention to these skills, which will be in **_bold, italicized_** font.

Notes to the Student

_____

_____

_____

_____

_____

_____

Skills Assessment Requirements

Read and familiarize yourself with the procedure; complete the minimum practice requirements. Document each MPR using proper charting technique. Complete each procedure within a reasonable amount of time, with a minimum of 85 percent accuracy.

Name: _____

Date: _____

POINT VALUE ✦ = 3–6 points ⋆ = 7–9 points		PRACTICE TRIAL	GRADED TRIAL #1	GRADED TRIAL #2	NOTES
1. ⋆	**Smile** as you answer the telephone; **answer it between the second and third ring** and state the office's name, followed by your name.				
2. ✦	If the caller fails to provide a personal name, ask for it.				
3. ✦	Determine the reason for the call.				
4. ✦	If the caller is having a medical emergency, ask if someone can come to the phone to speak about it. If not, motion a coworker to dial for emergency services, while keeping the patient on the line.				
5. ✦	If the patient is calling to speak with another member of the health care team, transfer the call to that person when available.				
6. ⋆	When a requested party is unavailable, record a message. Include the name of the caller, the date and time of the call, the telephone number where the caller can be reached, the reason for the call, and the name of the person the caller wishes to reach.				
7. ✦	When taking a message, inform the caller when the call will be returned.				
8. ✦	Clarify information (e.g., appointment time) as appropriate.				
9. ✦	**End the call by asking "Is there anything else I can do for you?" and then by saying "Thank you and have a nice day."** Allow the caller to hang up before hanging up.				
10. ✦	Route any message to the proper staff member.				
11. ⋆	Chart any health-care-related information into the patient's chart as appropriate.				

Name: _____

Date: _____

Document: Enter the appropriate information in the chart below.

Grading

Points Earned	_____		
Points Possible	_____	75	75
Percent Grade (Points Earned/Points Possible)	_____		
PASS:	_____	❑ YES ❑ NO ❑ N/A	❑ YES ❑ NO ❑ N/A

Instructor Sign-Off

Instructor: _____ **Date:** _____

Procedure 9-2:

Take a Telephone Message

Objective: Take a message correctly within the time limit set by the instructor.

Supplies: Telephone, pen, message pad

Affective Behaviors: Affective behaviors provide a professional approach to a skill that enhances the patient encounter. These behaviors may also display sensitivity to a patient's rights and enhance communication. Pay close attention to these skills, which will be in ***bold, italicized*** font.

Notes to the Student

_____

_____

_____

_____

_____

_____

Skills Assessment Requirements

Read and familiarize yourself with the procedure; complete the minimum practice requirements. Document each MPR using proper charting technique. Complete each procedure within a reasonable amount of time, with a minimum of 85 percent accuracy.

Name: _____

Date: _____

POINT VALUE ✦ = 3–6 points ⋆ = 7–9 points		PRACTICE TRIAL	GRADED TRIAL # 1	GRADED TRIAL # 2	NOTES
1. ⋆	**Smile and answer the telephone call by the second or third ring.**				
2. ✦	Once the caller identifies the desired party, reach for the message pad.				
3. ✦	Ask for the caller's full name, verify the spelling, and document it on the pad.				
4. ✦	Verify the name of the party the caller is trying to reach, and document it on the pad.				
5. ✦	Ask for the reason for the call, and document it on the pad.				
6. ✦	Ask for the caller's telephone number, including area code, and document it on the pad.				
7. ✦	**Repeat the telephone number to the caller to verify it was documented correctly.**				
8. ✦	Write the date and time of the call on the pad.				
9. ✦	Write your name or initials on the pad.				
10. ✦	**Tell the caller when to expect a return call.**				
11. ⋆	**Ask if there is anything you can do for the caller, say thank you, and then good-by. Allow the caller to hang up before hanging up.**				
12. ✦	Give the message to its intended recipient.				

Document: Enter the appropriate information in the chart below.

Grading

Points Earned	_____		
Points Possible	_____	78	78
Percent Grade (Points Earned/Points Possible)	_____		
PASS:	_____	❏ YES ❏ NO ❏ N/A	❏ YES ❏ NO ❏ N/A

Instructor Sign-Off

Instructor: _____ **Date:** _____

Name: _____

Date: _____

Procedure 9-3:

Call a Pharmacy with a Prescription Order

Objective: Call a pharmacy with a new or refill prescription order within the time limit set by the instructor.

Supplies: Telephone, patient's chart, pen, prescription information, pharmacy telephone number

Affective Behaviors: Affective behaviors provide a professional approach to a skill that enhances the patient encounter. These behaviors may also display sensitivity to a patient's rights and enhance communication. Pay close attention to these skills, which will be in *bold, italicized* font.

Notes to the Student

_____

_____

_____

_____

_____

_____

Skills Assessment Requirements

Read and familiarize yourself with the procedure; complete the minimum practice requirements. Document each MPR using proper charting technique. Complete each procedure within a reasonable amount of time, with a minimum of 85 percent accuracy.

POINT VALUE ✦ = 3–6 points ★ = 7–9 points		PRACTICE TRIAL	GRADED TRIAL #1	GRADED TRIAL #2	NOTES
1. ✦	Carefully read the prescription the physician has ordered.				
2. ★	**Ask the physician any questions about the prescription.**				
3. ✦	Call the pharmacy where the patient would like the prescription filled.				
4. ✦	Give the pharmacist the patient's name, and **verify the name's spelling.**				
5. ✦	Give the pharmacist the patient's birth date.				
6. ✦	Give the pharmacist the medication's name, dosage, and directions per the physician.				
7. ★	**Ask the pharmacist to repeat the information for verification,** and inform the pharmacist if the patient is en route to the pharmacy.				
8. ★	Note the prescription, including pharmacy name and telephone number, on the medication record in the patient's medical chart.				

Document: Enter the appropriate information in the chart below.

Grading

Points Earned	_____		
Points Possible	_____	57	57
Percent Grade (Points Earned/Points Possible)	_____		
PASS:	_____	❏ YES ❏ NO ❏ N/A	❏ YES ❏ NO ❏ N/A

Instructor Sign-Off

Instructor: _____ **Date:** _____

Procedure 10-1:

Open the Office

Objective: Open the medical office correctly within the time limit set by the instructor.

Supplies: Checklist of office opening procedures

Affective Behaviors: Affective behaviors provide a professional approach to a skill that enhances the patient encounter. These behaviors may also display sensitivity to a patient's rights and enhance communication. Pay close attention to these skills, which will be in ***bold, italicized*** font.

Notes to the Student

_____

_____

_____

_____

_____

_____

Skills Assessment Requirements

Read and familiarize yourself with the procedure; complete the minimum practice requirements. Document each MPR using proper charting technique. Complete each procedure within a reasonable amount of time, with a minimum of 85 percent accuracy.

POINT VALUE ✦ = 3–6 points ⋆ = 7–9 points		PRACTICE TRIAL	GRADED TRIAL # 1	GRADED TRIAL # 2	NOTES
1. ⋆	**Arrive in the office at least 15 minutes before the first patient appointment.**				
2. ✦	Turn off the office alarm system.				
3. ✦	Turn on all appropriate lights and equipment.				
4. ✦	Retrieve messages from the office answering system, and return telephone calls as appropriate.				
5. ✦	Verify that all patient charts needed for the morning were pulled the previous night and that all needed information is attached to those charts.				
6. ✦	Check the office for **safety and cleanliness issues.** For example, be sure all garbage cans are empty.				
7. ✦	When the office is ready, unlock the door for patients to enter.				

Document: Enter the appropriate information in the chart below.

Grading

Points Earned	_____		
Points Possible	_____	45	45
Percent Grade (Points Earned/Points Possible)	_____		
PASS:	_____	❏ YES ❏ NO ❏ N/A	❏ YES ❏ NO ❏ N/A

Instructor Sign-Off

Instructor: _____ **Date:** _____

Procedure 10-2:

Greet and Register Patients

Objective: Correctly greet and register patients.

Supplies: Patient history form, pen, clipboard

Affective Behaviors: Affective behaviors provide a professional approach to a skill that enhances the patient encounter. These behaviors may also display sensitivity to a patient's rights and enhance communication. Pay close attention to these skills, which will be in ***bold, italicized*** font.

Notes to the Student

_____

_____

_____

_____

_____

_____

Skills Assessment Requirements

Read and familiarize yourself with the procedure; complete the minimum practice requirements. Document each MPR using proper charting technique. Complete each procedure within a reasonable amount of time, with a minimum of 85 percent accuracy.

Name: _____

Date: _____

POINT VALUE ✦ = 3–6 points ⋆ = 7–9 points		PRACTICE TRIAL	GRADED TRIAL # 1	GRADED TRIAL # 2	NOTES
1. ⋆	As the patient arrives in at the front desk, look up and **make eye contact right away.** If you are on the telephone, **make a motion to the patient with your index finger to indicate that you will be with the patient in one moment.** If you are not on the telephone, **smile and ask the patient for his or her name.**				
2. ✦	Once you have obtained the patient's name, check the appointment schedule to verify the patient is there at the right time and to verify the type of appointment the patient is scheduled to have.				
3. ✦	If the patient is new to the office, give him or her the appropriate new patient forms to fill out on a clipboard, along with a pen.				
4. ✦	Ask the patient to take a seat in the reception area and provide the patient with an approximate amount of time that he or she can expect to wait before being taken back to see the provider.				
5. ✦	Alert the clinical medical assistant of the patient's arrival.				

Name: _____

Date: _____

Document: Enter the appropriate information in the chart below.

Grading

Points Earned	_____		
Points Possible	_____	36	36
Percent Grade (Points Earned/Points Possible)	_____		
PASS:	_____	❏ YES ❏ NO ❏ N/A	❏ YES ❏ NO ❏ N/A

Instructor Sign-Off

Instructor: _____ **Date:** _____

Procedure 10-3:

Collect Payments at the Front Desk

Objective: Correctly collect payments at the front desk.

Supplies: Pen, cash receipt book. credit card machine, check endorsement stamp

Affective Behaviors: Affective behaviors provide a professional approach to a skill that enhances the patient encounter. These behaviors may also display sensitivity to a patient's rights and enhance communication. Pay close attention to these skills, which will be in **_bold, italicized_** font.

Notes to the Student

_____

_____

_____

_____

_____

_____

Skills Assessment Requirements

Read and familiarize yourself with the procedure; complete the minimum practice requirements. Document each MPR using proper charting technique. Complete each procedure within a reasonable amount of time, with a minimum of 85 percent accuracy.

Name: _____

Date: _____

POINT VALUE ✦ = 3–6 points ✶ = 7–9 points		PRACTICE TRIAL	GRADED TRIAL # 1	GRADED TRIAL # 2	NOTES
1. ✶	As the patient arrives at the front desk, check the computer or chart to verify the patient's copayment amount.				
2. ✦	After registering the patient, let the patient know the amount of the expected payment.				
3. ✦	Ask the patient if he or she would prefer to make the payment via cash, check, or credit card. **If the patient does not have the copayment, approach the matter in a sensitive manner while politely explaining the office policy regarding payment at time of service.**				
4. ✦	If the patient pays via cash, write a receipt from the cash receipt book.				
5. ✦	If the patient pays via check, endorse the check with the bank endorsement stamp. Ask the patient if he or she would like a written receipt. If so, write a receipt from the cash receipt book.				
6. ✦	If the patient pays via credit card, process the credit card on the credit card machine, have the patient sign the slip, and provide the patient with their portion as the receipt.				

Document: Enter the appropriate information in the chart below.

Grading

Points Earned	_____		
Points Possible	_____	39	39
Percent Grade (Points Earned/Points Possible)	_____		
PASS:	_____	❏ YES ❏ NO ❏ N/A	❏ YES ❏ NO ❏ N/A

Instructor Sign-Off

Instructor: _____   **Date:** _____

Procedure 10-4:

Close the Office

Objective: Close the medical office correctly within the time limit set by the instructor.

Supplies: Checklist of office closing procedures

Affective Behaviors: Affective behaviors provide a professional approach to a skill that enhances the patient encounter. These behaviors may also display sensitivity to a patient's rights and enhance communication. Pay close attention to these skills, which will be in **_bold, italicized_** font.

Notes to the Student

_____

_____

_____

_____

_____

_____

Skills Assessment Requirements

Read and familiarize yourself with the procedure; complete the minimum practice requirements. Document each MPR using proper charting technique. Complete each procedure within a reasonable amount of time, with a minimum of 85 percent accuracy.

Name: _____

Date: _____

POINT VALUE ✦ = 3–6 points ⋆ = 7–9 points	PRACTICE TRIAL	GRADED TRIAL #1	GRADED TRIAL #2	NOTES
1. ✦ Ensure all patients have exited the office. Check treatment rooms and restrooms.				
2. ✦ Verify that all the day's patient files have been routed to the appropriate areas (e.g., billing, physician, clinical medical assistant).				
3. ✦ Pull all files for patients scheduled for the following morning.				
4. ⋆ Confirm that all information needed for the morning's patients (e.g., lab reports or consultations) is available. **Take time to locate information that is not readily available.**				
5. ✦ Attach needed information to patient files.				
6. ✦ Call to confirm any patient appointments made prior to a couple of days. **Be certain to follow HIPAA guidelines regarding patient privacy.**				
7. ⋆ Forward the telephones over to the answering system.				
8. ✦ Turn off all appropriate equipment and lights.				
9. ⋆ Activate the alarm and lock the doors while leaving the building.				

Document: Enter the appropriate information in the chart below.

Grading

Points Earned	_____		
Points Possible	_____	63	63
Percent Grade (Points Earned/Points Possible)	_____		
PASS:	_____	❏ YES ❏ NO ❏ N/A	❏ YES ❏ NO ❏ N/A

Instructor Sign-Off

Instructor: _____   **Date:** _____

Procedure 11-1:

Establish an Appointment Matrix

Objective: Correctly establish an appointment matrix.

Supplies: Pen, appointment book

Notes to the Student

_____

_____

_____

_____

_____

_____

Skills Assessment Requirements

Read and familiarize yourself with the procedure; complete the minimum practice requirements. Document each MPR using proper charting technique. Complete each procedure within a reasonable amount of time, with a minimum of 85 percent accuracy.

Name: _____

Date: _____

POINT VALUE ✦ = 3–6 points ⋆ = 7–9 points		PRACTICE TRIAL	GRADED TRIAL # 1	GRADED TRIAL # 2	NOTES
1. ✦	Determine the amount of time the providers want patients to have for each appointment type.				
2. ⋆	Within the appointment book, block out the time when the providers will be out of the office for lunch or other appointments.				
3. ⋆	Highlight or create blocks of time in the appointment book for appointments the provider specifies as those he would only like a limited number of, such as physical exams.				
4. ✦	Go over the created appointment matrix with the providers to determine where any adjustments need to be made.				

Name: _____

Date: _____

Document: Enter the appropriate information in the chart below.

Grading

Points Earned	_____		
Points Possible	_____	30	30
Percent Grade (Points Earned/Points Possible)	_____		
PASS:	_____	❏ YES ❏ NO ❏ N/A	❏ YES ❏ NO ❏ N/A

Instructor Sign-Off

Instructor: _____ **Date:** _____

Procedure 11-2:

Schedule a New Patient

Objective: Correctly schedule a new patient that calls the medical office.

Supplies: Telephone, blue or black pen, paper, appointment book

Affective Behaviors: Affective behaviors provide a professional approach to a skill that enhances the patient encounter. These behaviors may also display sensitivity to a patient's rights and enhance communication. Pay close attention to these skills, which will be in *bold, italicized* font.

Notes to the Student

_____

_____

_____

_____

_____

_____

Skills Assessment Requirements

Read and familiarize yourself with the procedure; complete the minimum practice requirements. Document each MPR using proper charting technique. Complete each procedure within a reasonable amount of time, with a minimum of 85 percent accuracy.

Name: _____

Date: _____

POINT VALUE ✦ = 3–6 points ★ = 7–9 points		PRACTICE TRIAL	GRADED TRIAL # 1	GRADED TRIAL # 2	NOTES
1. ✦	Using a **professional, friendly voice, answer the telephone by the second ring.**				
2. ✦	State the office name followed by your name.				
3. ✦	When the caller does not self-identify as a new patient, ask the caller if he or she has been in to the office previously.				
4. ✦	Ask the patient to spell his or her first and last names.				
5. ✦	Write the patient's full name on the paper.				
6. ✦	Ask the patient for work and home telephone numbers, and home address.				
7. ✦	Ask the patient how he or she was referred to the office.				
8. ✦	Ask the patient to identify the type of health insurance that he or she will be using.				
9. ★	Confirm that your physician participates in the patient's health care plan.				
10. ✦	If the physician does not participate in the patient's health plan, advise the patient that he or she may fail to receive preferred benefits or may need to pay in full for their services.				
11. ✦	Ask the patient to state the condition prompting the visit.				
12. ✦	Ask the patient to define the length of the condition.				

Name: _____

Date: _____

		PRACTICE TRIAL	GRADED TRIAL # 1	GRADED TRIAL # 2	NOTES
13. ✦	Offer the patient appointment times to see the physician.				
14. ⋆	Schedule the patient.				
15. ✦	If mailing paperwork to the patient to complete before the appointment, direct the patient to complete the paperwork before the visit.				
16. ✦	If the patient will need to complete the paperwork at the first visit, direct him or her to arrive 15 minutes before the appointment's scheduled start time.				
17. ✦	Document the patient's information in the manual or electronic appointment schedule.				
18. ✦	Ask the patient if directions are needed.				
19. ✦	Give the patient any needed parking information.				
20. ⋆	Confirm the appointment date and time with the patient. **Thank the patient for calling and ask if there is anything else you can do for him or her.**				
21. ✦	**Allow the patient to hang up the telephone before hanging up yourself.**				

Name: _____

Date: _____

Document: Enter the appropriate information in the chart below.

Grading

Points Earned	_____		
Points Possible	_____	135	135
Percent Grade (Points Earned/Points Possible)	_____		
PASS:	_____	❏ YES ❏ NO ❏ N/A	❏ YES ❏ NO ❏ N/A

Instructor Sign-Off

Instructor: _____ Date: _____

Name: _____

Date: _____

Procedure 11-3:

Schedule an Established Patient Appointment

Objective: Schedule a patient appointment correctly within the time limit set by the instructor.

Supplies: Appointment schedule, blue or black pen, patient's chart

Affective Behaviors: Affective behaviors provide a professional approach to a skill that enhances the patient encounter. These behaviors may also display sensitivity to a patient's rights and enhance communication. Pay close attention to these skills, which will be in **bold, *italicized*** font.

Notes to the Student

_____

_____

_____

_____

_____

_____

Skills Assessment Requirements

Read and familiarize yourself with the procedure; complete the minimum practice requirements. Document each MPR using proper charting technique. Complete each procedure within a reasonable amount of time, with a minimum of 85 percent accuracy.

Name: _____

Date: _____

POINT VALUE ✦ = 3–6 points * = 7–9 points		PRACTICE TRIAL	GRADED TRIAL #1	GRADED TRIAL #2	NOTES
1. *	**_Using a professional, friendly voice, smile and answer the telephone by the second ring._**				
2. ✦	Locate the chart of the patient to be scheduled.				
3. ✦	Determine the type of appointment that is needed.				
4. ✦	Determine the patient's schedule.				
5. ✦	Determine the physician's schedule.				
6. ✦	Enter the patient in the appointment schedule. Restate the appointment date and time to the patient.				
7. *	Remind the patient to bring any needed items to the appointment or to follow any procedures (e.g., fasting before the visit). If the patient is in the office, provide a written reminder card. If the patient called on the phone, **_thank the patient for calling and ask if there is anything else you can do for him or her._**				

Name: _____

Date: _____

Document: Enter the correct information in the chart below.

Grading

Points Earned	_____		
Points Possible	_____	48	48
Percent Grade (Points Earned/Points Possible)	_____		
PASS:	_____	❏ YES ❏ NO ❏ N/A	❏ YES ❏ NO ❏ N/A

Instructor Sign-Off

Instructor: _____ Date: _____

Procedure 11-4:

Use Patient Reminder Cards

Objective: Correctly use patient reminder cards.

Supplies: Pen, appointment book, appointment reminder cards

Affective Behaviors: Affective behaviors provide a professional approach to a skill that enhances the patient encounter. These behaviors may also display sensitivity to a patient's rights and enhance communication. Pay close attention to these skills, which will be in **_bold, italicized_** font.

Notes to the Student

_____

_____

_____

_____

_____

_____

Skills Assessment Requirements

Read and familiarize yourself with the procedure; complete the minimum practice requirements. Document each MPR using proper charting technique. Complete each procedure within a reasonable amount of time, with a minimum of 85 percent accuracy.

Name: _____

Date: _____

POINT VALUE ✦ = 3–6 points * = 7–9 points		PRACTICE TRIAL	GRADED TRIAL # 1	GRADED TRIAL # 2	NOTES
1. ✦	As the patient arrives at the reception desk, look at the fee slip to verify when the provider wants the patient to return for an appointment.				
2. ✦	Ask the patient if there is a day or time that works best for their schedule for the appointment.				
3. ✦	Check the appointment book to find an appointment time that fits with the patient's schedule.				
4. ✦	After verifying that the appointment will work with the patient's schedule, write or type the appointment into the appointment schedule.				
5. *	Write the patient's appointment on a reminder card and give the card to the patient. **Thank the patient for visiting the office and bid the patient a good day.**				

Name: _____

Date: _____

Document: Enter the appropriate information in the chart below.

Grading

Points Earned	_____		
Points Possible	_____	33	33
Percent Grade (Points Earned/Points Possible)	_____		
PASS:	_____	❏ YES ❏ NO ❏ N/A	❏ YES ❏ NO ❏ N/A

Instructor Sign-Off

Instructor: _____ **Date:** _____

Name: _____

Date: _____

Procedure 11-5:

Reschedule a Missed Patient Appointment

Objective: Reschedule a missed patient appointment correctly within the time limit set by the instructor.

Supplies: Appointment schedule, blue or black pen, patient's chart

Affective Behaviors: Affective behaviors provide a professional approach to a skill that enhances the patient encounter. These behaviors may also display sensitivity to a patient's rights and enhance communication. Pay close attention to these skills, which will be in **bold, *italicized*** font.

Notes to the Student

_____

_____

_____

_____

_____

_____

Skills Assessment Requirements

Read and familiarize yourself with the procedure; complete the minimum practice requirements. Document each MPR using proper charting technique. Complete each procedure within a reasonable amount of time, with a minimum of 85 percent accuracy.

POINT VALUE ✦ = 3–6 points ⋆ = 7–9 points		PRACTICE TRIAL	GRADED TRIAL # 1	GRADED TRIAL # 2	NOTES
1. ✦	**Fifteen minutes after the patient's appointment time, call the patient's home telephone number.**				
2. ⋆	If the patient answers: • Point out the missed appointment time and **politely ask for an appropriate time to reschedule.** • If the patient reschedules the appointment, document the new appointment in the appointment book as well as the patient's chart. Also chart that the patient missed the originally scheduled appointment. • If the patient does not wish to reschedule, **politely state that you will inform the physician.** Chart the missed appointment and refusal to reschedule in the patient's chart, and give the chart to the physician.				
3. ⋆	If the patient fails to answer: • Leave a message on voice mail or with the person who answers. **Be certain not to disclose confidential patient information.** • In the patient's chart, document the missed appointment and the message.				

Name: _____

Date: _____

Document: Enter the correct information in the chart below.

Grading

Points Earned	_____		
Points Possible	_____	24	24
Percent Grade (Points Earned/Points Possible)	_____		
PASS:	_____	❏ YES ❏ NO ❏ N/A	❏ YES ❏ NO ❏ N/A

Instructor Sign-Off

Instructor: _____ Date: _____

Procedure 11-6:

Manage the Physician's Professional Schedule and Travel

Objective: Manage physician's professional schedule for travel correctly within the time limit set by the instructor.

Supplies: A list of the physician's travel needs, including dates and times of the meeting or seminar, place of the seminar, and physician preference for airline and hotel arrangements, telephone, paper and a pen

Notes to the Student

_____

_____
_____
_____
_____
_____
_____

Skills Assessment Requirements

Read and familiarize yourself with the procedure; complete the minimum practice requirements. Document each MPR using proper charting technique. Complete each procedure within a reasonable amount of time, with a minimum of 85 percent accuracy.

Name: _____

Date: _____

POINT VALUE ✦ = 3–6 points ⋆ = 7–9 points		PRACTICE TRIAL	GRADED TRIAL # 1	GRADED TRIAL # 2	NOTES
1. ✦	Call the physician's preferred airline and book the appropriate flight.				
2. ⋆	Make a note of the date, time, airline, and flight number for both departure time and arrival time for both the outgoing flight and the return flight.				
3. ✦	Call the physician's preferred hotel and book the appropriate room.				
4. ⋆	Make a note of the confirmation number for the hotel room.				
5. ✦	Arrange for any necessary transportation to or from the hotel and airport.				
6. ✦	Create a list of all arrangements made and give the list to the physician.				
7. ✦	Give a copy of the list of arrangements to the office manager and to the receptionist.				
8. ⋆	Verify the receptionist has blocked out the dates the physician will be away, if applicable.				

Document: Enter the correct information in the chart below.

Grading

Points Earned	_____		
Points Possible	_____	57	57
Percent Grade (Points Earned/Points Possible)	_____		
PASS:	_____	❏ YES ❏ NO ❏ N/A	❏ YES ❏ NO ❏ N/A

Instructor Sign-Off

Instructor: _____   **Date:** _____

Procedure 11-7:

Schedule a Hospital Procedure

Objective: Schedule a hospital procedure correctly within the time limit set by the instructor.

Supplies: Patient's chart, hospital/surgery scheduling form, scheduling guidelines, calendar, telephone, notepad, pen

Affective Behaviors: Affective behaviors provide a professional approach to a skill that enhances the patient encounter. These behaviors may also display sensitivity to a patient's rights and enhance communication. Pay close attention to these skills, which will be in *bold, italicized* font.

Notes to the Student

_____

_____

_____

_____

_____

_____

Skills Assessment Requirements

Read and familiarize yourself with the procedure; complete the minimum practice requirements. Document each MPR using proper charting technique. Complete each procedure within a reasonable amount of time, with a minimum of 85 percent accuracy.

POINT VALUE ✦ = 3–6 points ★ = 7–9 points	PRACTICE TRIAL	GRADED TRIAL # 1	GRADED TRIAL # 2	NOTES
1. ✦ Obtain information from the physician or clinical medical assistant about the needed surgery or procedure and the desired hospital.				
2. ✦ Call the patient's insurance carrier to obtain preauthorization for the procedure.				
3. ★ Document the preauthorization number in the patient's chart.				
4. ✦ If the patient is in the clinic, ask what date or time would be most convenient for the procedure. If the patient is not in the clinic, call the patient to determine scheduling needs.				
5. ✦ Call the hospital to communicate the procedure the physician has planned, the time needed for the procedure, and the date preferred for the procedure.				
6. ★ Provide the hospital staff the patient's information, including name, birth date, address, telephone number, insurance information, and preauthorization number. Also relay all pertinent information, such as allergies or disabilities. **Only provide the hospital with the necessary patient information.**				
7. ✦ After agreeing on a date and time, give the information to the patient and enter it in the physician's appointment schedule.				

		PRACTICE TRIAL	GRADED TRIAL # 1	GRADED TRIAL # 2	NOTES
8. ✦	Advise the patient that the hospital will likely call to provide instructions and verify the check-in date and time.				
9. ✦	Schedule the patient for a post-operative appointment in the physician's office, if needed.				
10. ⋆	Chart all information in the patient's medical record, and give the chart to the physician for review.				

Document: Enter the correct information in the chart below.

Grading

Points Earned	_____		
Points Possible	_____	69	69
Percent Grade (Points Earned/Points Possible)	_____		
PASS:	_____	❏ YES ❏ NO ❏ N/A	❏ YES ❏ NO ❏ N/A

Instructor Sign-Off

Instructor: _____ **Date:** _____

Procedure 11-8:

Schedule an Inpatient Admission

Objective: Schedule an inpatient admission correctly within the time limit set by the instructor.

Supplies: Patient's chart, inpatient scheduling guidelines, calendar, telephone, notepad, pen

Affective Behaviors: Affective behaviors provide a professional approach to a skill that enhances the patient encounter. These behaviors may also display sensitivity to a patient's rights and enhance communication. Pay close attention to these skills, which will be in ***bold, italicized*** font.

Notes to the Student

_____

_____

_____

_____

_____

_____

Skills Assessment Requirements

Read and familiarize yourself with the procedure; complete the minimum practice requirements. Document each MPR using proper charting technique. Complete each procedure within a reasonable amount of time, with a minimum of 85 percent accuracy.

POINT VALUE ✦ = 3–6 points ⋆ = 7–9 points		PRACTICE TRIAL	GRADED TRIAL #1	GRADED TRIAL #2	NOTES
1. ✦	Call the patient's insurance carrier to obtain preauthorization for the procedure, the needed followup, and the allowable number of hospital days. ***Thank the insurance representative for their assistance.***				
2. ⋆	Document the preauthorization number in the patient's chart.				
3. ⋆	Call the hospital admissions office with the patient's name, physician's name, and reason for admission.				
4. ✦	Let the admissions office know when the physician would like the patient to be admitted.				
5. ✦	Give the admissions office the patient's contact information, birth date, insurance information, and preauthorization number.				
6. ✦	Instruct the patient when to arrive at the hospital and where to go once there.				
7. ✦	Give the patient any specifics on what to bring (or not) to the hospital. ***Ask the patient if he or she has any questions that need to be answered.***				
8. ⋆	Chart all information in the patient's medical record, and give the chart to the physician for review.				

Name: _____

Date: _____

Document: Enter the correct information in the chart below.

Grading

Points Earned	_____		
Points Possible	_____	57	57
Percent Grade (Points Earned/Points Possible)	_____		
PASS:	_____	❏ YES ❏ NO ❏ N/A	❏ YES ❏ NO ❏ N/A

Instructor Sign-Off

Instructor: _____ **Date:** _____

Procedure 12-1:

Preparing the Medical Chart

Objective: Prepare a patient medical chart correctly within the time limit set by the instructor.

Supplies: Medical chart, metal file clips, medication record sheet, progress notes record, color-coded alphabet stickers, file label, two-hole punch, patient's name

Notes to the Student

_____

_____

_____

_____

_____

_____

_____

Skills Assessment Requirements

Read and familiarize yourself with the procedure; complete the minimum practice requirements. Document each MPR using proper charting technique. Complete each procedure within a reasonable amount of time, with a minimum of 85 percent accuracy.

Name: _____

Date: _____

POINT VALUE ✦ = 3–6 points ⋆ = 7–9 points		PRACTICE TRIAL	GRADED TRIAL # 1	GRADED TRIAL # 2	NOTES
1. ✦	Print the patient's name on a file label, with the last name followed by first name and middle initial. For example, print "Smith, John R." on the file label.				
2. ⋆	Verify the spelling of the patient's name.				
3. ✦	Using the color-coded alphabet stickers, place the first two letters of the patient's last name on the file near the file label. In the preceding example, "SM" stickers would appear near the file label.				
4. ✦	One space after the stickers in the preceding step, place a color-coded alphabet sticker for the first letter of the patient's first name. Building on the preceding example for John R. Smith, the file stickers would read "SM [space] J."				
5. ✦	Add metal file clips to both sides of the file.				
6. ✦	Using the two-hole punch, punch holes in the top of the documents to be filed in the patient's chart. Punch such documents as the patient's history form, the Health Insurance Portability and Accountability Act (HIPAA) notification form, and the patient's consent to be examined.				
7. ✦	Place the medication record sheet on one side of the chart.				

Name: _____

Date: _____

		PRACTICE TRIAL	GRADED TRIAL # 1	GRADED TRIAL # 2	NOTES
8. ✦	Place the progress report sheet on the other side of the chart.				
9. ⋆	On the front of the chart in red ink, note any of the patient's known allergies. When the patient has no known allergies, write "NKA" (i.e., no known allergies) on the front of the chart.				

Name: _____

Date: _____

Document: Enter the correct information in the chart below.

Grading

Points Earned	_____		
Points Possible	_____	60	60
Percent Grade (Points Earned/Points Possible)	_____		
PASS:	_____	❏ YES ❏ NO ❏ N/A	❏ YES ❏ NO ❏ N/A

Instructor Sign-Off

Instructor: _____ **Date:** _____

Procedure 12-2:

Charting Patient Telephone Calls

Objective: Chart a patient telephone call correctly within the time limit set by the instructor.

Supplies: Notepad and pen, patient's chart

Affective Behaviors: Affective behaviors provide a professional approach to a skill that enhances the patient encounter. These behaviors may also display sensitivity to a patient's rights and enhance communication. Pay close attention to these skills, which will be in ***bold, italicized*** font.

Notes to the Student

_____

_____

_____

_____

_____

_____

Skills Assessment Requirements

Read and familiarize yourself with the procedure; complete the minimum practice requirements. Document each MPR using proper charting technique. Complete each procedure within a reasonable amount of time, with a minimum of 85 percent accuracy.

Name: _____

Date: _____

POINT VALUE ✦ = 3–6 points ⋆ = 7–9 points		PRACTICE TRIAL	GRADED TRIAL # 1	GRADED TRIAL # 2	NOTES
1. ✦	While answering an incoming patient call, determine if the call is medically relevant to the patient's care in the office.				
2. ✦	When the call is medically relevant to the patient's care, note the call's time and date, the patient's complete name, and the nature of the message.				
3. ✦	When the call ends, pull the patient's chart.				
4. ✦	In the progress notes section of the patient's chart, note the current date and time.				
5. ⋆	Write the medically relevant portion of the call in the patient's medical record, using quotation marks to indicate any direct quotes from the patient.				
6. ✦	**Sign your name and credentials at the end of the chart entry.**				
7. ⋆	When the call requires the physician's attention, leave the chart on the physician's desk.				
8. ✦	When the call does not require the physician's attention, file the chart.				
9. ⋆	After transferring all relevant information to the chart, **shred any notes from the call that contain personal patient information.**				

Name: _____

Date: _____

Document: Enter the correct information in the chart below.

Grading

Points Earned	_____		
Points Possible	_____	63	63
Percent Grade (Points Earned/Points Possible)	_____		
PASS:	_____	❏ YES ❏ NO ❏ N/A	❏ YES ❏ NO ❏ N/A

Instructor Sign-Off

Instructor: _____ **Date:** _____

Name: _____

Date: _____

Procedure 12-3:

File Documents Using the Alphabetical Filing System

Objective: Correctly file documents using the alphabetical filing system.

Supplies: Patient medical records, color-coded alphabetical file letter stickers

Notes to the Student

_____

_____

_____

_____

_____

_____

Skills Assessment Requirements

Read and familiarize yourself with the procedure; complete the minimum practice requirements. Document each MPR using proper charting technique. Complete each procedure within a reasonable amount of time, with a minimum of 85 percent accuracy.

Name: _____

Date: _____

POINT VALUE ✦ = 3–6 points ⋆ = 7–9 points		PRACTICE TRIAL	GRADED TRIAL # 1	GRADED TRIAL # 2	NOTES
1. ✦	Using the color-coded alphabetical file letter stickers, apply stickers to each medical record using the patient's first two letters from the last name.				
2. ⋆	Arrange the medical records into the alphabetical order by last name.				
3. ⋆	File the medical records accurately into the filing cabinet.				

Name: _____

Date: _____

Document: Enter the appropriate information in the chart below.

Grading

Points Earned	_____		
Points Possible	_____	24	24
Percent Grade (Points Earned/Points Possible)	_____		
PASS:	_____	❏ YES ❏ NO ❏ N/A	❏ YES ❏ NO ❏ N/A

Instructor Sign-Off

Instructor: _____   **Date:** _____

Procedure 12-4:

File Manually Using a Subject Filing System

Objective: Correctly file manually using a subject filing system.

Supplies: Documents to be filed by subject, alphabetic card file, index card listing subjects

Notes to the Student

_____

_____

_____

_____

_____

_____

Skills Assessment Requirements

Read and familiarize yourself with the procedure; complete the minimum practice requirements. Document each MPR using proper charting technique. Complete each procedure within a reasonable amount of time, with a minimum of 85 percent accuracy.

Name: _____

Date: _____

POINT VALUE ✦ = 3–6 points ⋆ = 7–9 points		PRACTICE TRIAL	GRADED TRIAL # 1	GRADED TRIAL # 2	NOTES
1. ⋆	Organize the documents by subject matter.				
2. ✦	Match the subject of the document to the appropriate category on the index cards.				
3. ✦	Underline the subject title on the document.				
4. ⋆	File the document under the appropriate category.				
5. ✦	If the document fits into more than one category, create an index card as a cross-reference, listing the name of the document and the category under which it is filed.				

Name: _____

Date: _____

Document: Enter the appropriate information in the chart below.

Grading

Points Earned	_____		
Points Possible	_____	36	36
Percent Grade (Points Earned/Points Possible)	_____		
PASS:	_____	❑ YES ❑ NO ❑ N/A	❑ YES ❑ NO ❑ N/A

Instructor Sign-Off

Instructor: _____ **Date:** _____

Name: _____

Date: _____

Procedure 12-5:

Filing Documents in Patient Medical Records

Objective: File documents into a patient's medical record correctly within the time limit set by the instructor.

Supplies: Patient medical record, documents to be filed, two-hole punch

Notes to the Student

_____

_____

_____

_____

_____

_____

Skills Assessment Requirements

Read and familiarize yourself with the procedure; complete the minimum practice requirements. Document each MPR using proper charting technique. Complete each procedure within a reasonable amount of time, with a minimum of 85 percent accuracy.

POINT VALUE ✦ = 3–6 points ⋆ = 7–9 points		PRACTICE TRIAL	GRADED TRIAL # 1	GRADED TRIAL # 2	NOTES
1. ✦	Using the two-hole punch, punch holes in the top of each document to be filed.				
2. ⋆	Verify that the physician has viewed any report to be filed (e.g., laboratory or pathology report) by locating the physician's initials on the report.				
3. ⋆	Verify that the patient file matches the name on the documents to be filed.				
4. ✦	Using the metal clips in the file, place the documents in the patient medical record with the most recent documents on top.				
5. ✦	Fasten the metal clips.				

Name: _____

Date: _____

Document: Enter the correct information in the chart below.

Grading

Points Earned	_____		
Points Possible	_____	36	36
Percent Grade (Points Earned/Points Possible)	_____		
PASS:	_____	❏ YES ❏ NO ❏ N/A	❏ YES ❏ NO ❏ N/A

Instructor Sign-Off

Instructor: _____ Date: _____

Procedure 12-6:

Use the Numeric System to File the Medical Record

Objective: Correctly use the numeric system to file medical records.

Supplies: Patient medical records, color-coded numeric file stickers

Notes to the Student

_____

_____

_____

_____

_____

_____

Skills Assessment Requirements

Read and familiarize yourself with the procedure; complete the minimum practice requirements. Document each MPR using proper charting technique. Complete each procedure within a reasonable amount of time, with a minimum of 85 percent accuracy.

Name: _____

Date: _____

POINT VALUE ✦ = 3–6 points ⋆ = 7–9 points		PRACTICE TRIAL	GRADED TRIAL # 1	GRADED TRIAL # 2	NOTES
1. ✦	Using the color-coded numeric file stickers, attach the first two numbers of the patient's medical record.				
2. ✦	After verifying that the patient's numeric identification number is accurately recorded on a master sheet kept away from the patient's files, organize the records in numerical order.				
3. ⋆	File the medical records in numerical order into the medical records filing system.				

Document: Enter the appropriate information in the chart below.

Grading

Points Earned	_____		
Points Possible	_____	21	21
Percent Grade (Points Earned/Points Possible)	_____		
PASS:	_____	❏ YES ❏ NO ❏ N/A	❏ YES ❏ NO ❏ N/A

Instructor Sign-Off

Instructor: _____   **Date:** _____

Procedure 12-7:

Correcting Errors in the Patient Medical Record

Objective: Correct an error in the patient medical record correctly within the time limit set by the instructor.

Supplies: Patient medical record, blue or black ink pen

Notes to the Student

_____

_____

_____

_____

_____

_____

Skills Assessment Requirements

Read and familiarize yourself with the procedure; complete the minimum practice requirements. Document each MPR using proper charting technique. Complete each procedure within a reasonable amount of time, with a minimum of 85 percent accuracy.

Name: _____

Date: _____

POINT VALUE ✦ = 3–6 points ⋆ = 7–9 points		PRACTICE TRIAL	GRADED TRIAL #1	GRADED TRIAL #2	NOTES
1. ✦	Locate the error in the patient's medical record.				
2. ✦	Draw a straight line through the error.				
3. ⋆	Initial and place the date above the line.				
4. ⋆	When the corrected entry will fit above the line, write the correction there. Include the date of the new entry and your initials. When the corrected entry will not fit above the line, add a new entry to the progress notes with the day's date and the word "ADDENDUM" in all capitals. Include the date of the addendum, enter the corrected entry, and initial the entry.				

Document: Enter the correct information in the chart below.

Grading

Points Earned	_____		
Points Possible	_____	30	30
Percent Grade (Points Earned/Points Possible)	_____		
PASS:	_____	❏ YES ❏ NO ❏ N/A	❏ YES ❏ NO ❏ N/A

Instructor Sign-Off

Instructor: _____ **Date:** _____

Name: _____

Date: _____

Procedure 13-1:

Correct an Electronic Medical Record

Objective: Correctly correct an electronic medical record.

Supplies: Computer with electronic patient medical record

Notes to the Student

_____

_____

_____

_____

_____

_____

_____

Skills Assessment Requirements

Read and familiarize yourself with the procedure; complete the minimum practice requirements. Document each MPR using proper charting technique. Complete each procedure within a reasonable amount of time, with a minimum of 85 percent accuracy.

Name: _____

Date: _____

POINT VALUE ✦ = 3–6 points ⋆ = 7–9 points		PRACTICE TRIAL	GRADED TRIAL # 1	GRADED TRIAL # 2	NOTES
1. ✦	Identify the correct patient electronic medical record where the error was made.				
2. ✦	Locate the error within the record.				
3. ⋆	Using the rules associated with the software you are using, make the appropriate correction within the medical record.				
4. ⋆	Sign off on the changes as necessary, according to the steps required within the software program.				
5. ✦	Verify the change made is correct before closing the patient's electronic medical record.				

Name: _____

Date: _____

Document: Enter the appropriate information in the chart below.

Grading

Points Earned	_____		
Points Possible	_____	36	36
Percent Grade (Points Earned/Points Possible)	_____		
PASS:	_____	❏ YES ❏ NO ❏ N/A	❏ YES ❏ NO ❏ N/A

Instructor Sign-Off

Instructor: _____ **Date:** _____

Procedure 14-1:

Use Computer Software to Maintain Office Systems

Objective: Utilize computer software to maintain office systems correctly within the time limit set by the instructor.

Supplies: Computer with spreadsheet software, list of equipment to enter into the computer.

Affective Behaviors: Affective behaviors provide a professional approach to a skill that enhances the patient encounter. These behaviors may also display sensitivity to a patient's rights and enhance communication. Pay close attention to these skills, which will be in **bold, _italicized_** font.

Notes to the Student

_____

_____

_____

_____

_____

_____

Skills Assessment Requirements

Read and familiarize yourself with the procedure; complete the minimum practice requirements. Document each MPR using proper charting technique. Complete each procedure within a reasonable amount of time, with a minimum of 85 percent accuracy.

POINT VALUE ✦ = 3–6 points ⋆ = 7–9 points		PRACTICE TRIAL	GRADED TRIAL #1	GRADED TRIAL #2	NOTES
1. ✦	Launch the spreadsheet software.				
2. ✦	Using the list of equipment, enter each piece of equipment onto a separate line on the spreadsheet.				
3. ✦	Enter the date each piece of equipment was purchased or leased by the medical office.				
4. ⋆	Enter the name of the man-ufacturer that supplied the piece of equipment.				
5. ✦	Enter the type of maintenance the piece of equipment needs on a regular basis.				
6. ✦	Enter information about the needed maintenance, such as the name of the company that performs the repairs, and the schedule for which the equip-ment must be maintained. **Enter as much information as possible as to maintain time efficiency at the time of repairs and maintenance.**				

Name: _____

Date: _____

Document: Enter the appropriate information in the chart below.

Grading

Points Earned	_____		
Points Possible	_____	39	39
Percent Grade (Points Earned/Points Possible)	_____		
PASS:	_____	❏ YES ❏ NO ❏ N/A	❏ YES ❏ NO ❏ N/A

Instructor Sign-Off

Instructor: _____ **Date:** _____

Procedure 14-2:

Using an Internet Search Engine

Objective: Use the computer to search for a topic via an Internet search engine correctly within the time limit set by the instructor.

Supplies: A computer with Internet access

Notes to the Student

_____

_____

_____

_____

_____

_____

Skills Assessment Requirements

Read and familiarize yourself with the procedure; complete the minimum practice requirements. Document each MPR using proper charting technique. Complete each procedure within a reasonable amount of time, with a minimum of 85 percent accuracy.

Name: _____

Date: _____

POINT VALUE ✦ = 3–6 points ⋆ = 7–9 points		PRACTICE TRIAL	GRADED TRIAL #1	GRADED TRIAL #2	NOTES
1. ✦	Turn on the computer.				
2. ✦	Launch an Internet browser.				
3. ✦	Visit the uniform resource locator (URL) of the search engine.				
4. ✦	Enter the search keywords.				
5. ✦	Visit retrieved Web sites to obtain the desired information.				
6. ✦	To refine the search, enter more or different key words.				

Document: Enter the appropriate information in the chart below.

Grading

Points Earned	_____		
Points Possible	_____	36	36
Percent Grade (Points Earned/Points Possible)	_____		
PASS:	_____	❏ YES ❏ NO ❏ N/A	❏ YES ❏ NO ❏ N/A

Instructor Sign-Off

Instructor: _____   **Date:** _____

Procedure 14-3:

Verify Preferred Provider Status of an Insurance Company Web Site

Objective: Verify a provider's preferred status on an insurance company Web site within the time limit set by the instructor.

Supplies: Computer with Internet connection, insurance company's URL, name of target physician

Notes to the Student

_____

_____

_____

_____

_____

_____

Skills Assessment Requirements

Read and familiarize yourself with the procedure; complete the minimum practice requirements. Document each MPR using proper charting technique. Complete each procedure within a reasonable amount of time, with a minimum of 85 percent accuracy.

Name: _____

Date: _____

POINT VALUE ✦ = 3–6 points ⋆ = 7–9 points		PRACTICE TRIAL	GRADED TRIAL # 1	GRADED TRIAL # 2	NOTES
1. ✦	Using the computer, launch an Internet browser.				
2. ✦	Enter the URL of the insurance company.				
3. ✦	Navigate to the provider page or section.				
4. ✦	In the search field, enter the provider's name and/or location.				
5. ✦	Verify if the physician is preferred with the target insurance company.				

Name: _____

Date: _____

Document: Enter the appropriate information in the chart below.

Grading

Points Earned	_____		
Points Possible	_____	30	30
Percent Grade (Points Earned/Points Possible)	_____		
PASS:	_____	❑ YES ❑ NO ❑ N/A	❑ YES ❑ NO ❑ N/A

Instructor Sign-Off

Instructor: _____ **Date:** _____

Procedure 15-1:

Taking Inventory of Administrative Equipment

Objective: Perform an inventory of administrative equipment correctly within the time limit set by the instructor.

Supplies: Paper, pen, computer with word-processing or spreadsheet software

Affective Behaviors: Affective behaviors provide a professional approach to a skill that enhances the patient encounter. These behaviors may also display sensitivity to a patient's rights and enhance communication. Pay close attention to these skills, which will be in **_bold, italicized_** font.

Notes to the Student

_____

_____

_____

_____

_____

_____

Skills Assessment Requirements

Read and familiarize yourself with the procedure; complete the minimum practice requirements. Document each MPR using proper charting technique. Complete each procedure within a reasonable amount of time, with a minimum of 85 percent accuracy.

Name: _____

Date: _____

POINT VALUE ✦ = 3–6 points ⋆ = 7–9 points		PRACTICE TRIAL	GRADED TRIAL #1	GRADED TRIAL #2	NOTES
1. ✦	Locate all administrative equipment in the medical office.				
2. ⋆	List each piece of equipment with manufacturer name, serial number, and date of purchase, when known.				
3. ✦	Include information about the company maintaining the equipment.				
4. ✦	Include information about the supplies needed to maintain the equipment, including where those supplies are purchased.				
5. ✦	Using word-processing or spreadsheet software, create an inventory sheet of all equipment information. ***The inventory sheet should be easy to read and should contain succinct information on all items, ensuring time efficacy.***				
6. ✦	Update the inventory sheet as needed when new equipment is purchased or older equipment is replaced.				

Name: _____

Date: _____

Document: Enter the appropriate information in the chart below.

Grading

Points Earned	_____		
Points Possible	_____	39	39
Percent Grade (Points Earned/Points Possible)	_____		
PASS:	_____	❏ YES ❏ NO ❏ N/A	❏ YES ❏ NO ❏ N/A

Instructor Sign-Off

Instructor: _____ **Date:** _____

Procedure 15-2:

Perform Routine Maintenance of a Computer Printer

Objective: Perform routine maintenance of a computer printer correctly within the time limit set by the instructor.

Supplies: Paper, pen, computer printer, maintenance logbook

Notes to the Student

_____

_____

_____

_____

_____

Skills Assessment Requirements

Read and familiarize yourself with the procedure; complete the minimum practice requirements. Document each MPR using proper charting technique. Complete each procedure within a reasonable amount of time, with a minimum of 85 percent accuracy.

POINT VALUE ✦ = 3–6 points ⋆ = 7–9 points		PRACTICE TRIAL	GRADED TRIAL #1	GRADED TRIAL #2	NOTES
1. ✦	Review the maintenance log-book for the computer printer.				
2. ✦	Following the manufacturer's directions, open the printer cover and remove the toner cartridge.				
3. ✦	Using the manufacturer-provided cleaning tool, clean any dust and spilled toner from within the printer.				
4. ✦	Replace the cleaning tool and the toner cartridge.				
5. ✦	Close the printer cover.				
6. ⋆	In the maintenance logbook, enter information about the maintenance, including the date and your signature.				

Name: _____

Date: _____

Document: Enter the appropriate information in the chart below.

Grading

Points Earned	_____		
Points Possible	_____	39	39
Percent Grade (Points Earned/Points Possible)	_____		
PASS:	_____	❏ YES ❏ NO ❏ N/A	❏ YES ❏ NO ❏ N/A

Instructor Sign-Off

Instructor: _____   Date: _____

Name: _____

Date: _____

Procedure 15-3:

Fax a Document

Objective: Fax a document using a fax machine correctly within the time limit set by the instructor.

Supplies: Document to be faxed, HIPAA-compliant fax cover sheet, pen, fax machine

Affective Behaviors: Affective behaviors provide a professional approach to a skill that enhances the patient encounter. These behaviors may also display sensitivity to a patient's rights and enhance communication. Pay close attention to these skills, which will be in ***bold, italicized*** font.

Notes to the Student

_____

_____

_____

_____

_____

_____

Skills Assessment Requirements

Read and familiarize yourself with the procedure; complete the minimum practice requirements. Document each MPR using proper charting technique. Complete each procedure within a reasonable amount of time, with a minimum of 85 percent accuracy.

Name: _____

Date: _____

POINT VALUE ✦ = 3–6 points ⋆ = 7–9 points		PRACTICE TRIAL	GRADED TRIAL # 1	GRADED TRIAL # 2	NOTES
1. ✦	Complete the **HIPAA fax cover sheet** with personal name, phone number, and clinic contact information.				
2. ✦	Fill in the name and fax number of the fax recipient.				
3. ✦	List the number of pages in the fax, including the cover sheet.				
4. ✦	Properly orient the fax cover sheet and document to be faxed in the fax machine.				
5. ✦	Dial the target fax number. **Prior to hitting the "send" button, double check that the fax number has been accurately entered.**				
6. ⋆	When the fax has fully transmitted, remove the documents and file them with the fax confirmation sheet to the patient's file.				

Name: _____

Date: _____

Document: Enter the appropriate information in the chart below.

Grading

Points Earned	_____		
Points Possible	_____	39	39
Percent Grade (Points Earned/Points Possible)	_____		
PASS:	_____	❏ YES ❏ NO ❏ N/A	❏ YES ❏ NO ❏ N/A

Instructor Sign-Off

Instructor: _____ **Date:** _____

Name: _____

Date: _____

Procedure 15-4:

Prepare a Purchase Order

Objective: Prepare a purchase order correctly within the time limit set by the instructor.

Supplies: List of needed supplies, purchase order form, pen, fax machine or telephone

Notes to the Student

_____

_____

_____

_____

_____

_____

Skills Assessment Requirements

Read and familiarize yourself with the procedure; complete the minimum practice requirements. Document each MPR using proper charting technique. Complete each procedure within a reasonable amount of time, with a minimum of 85 percent accuracy.

Name: _____

Date: _____

POINT VALUE ✦ = 3–6 points * = 7–9 points	PRACTICE TRIAL	GRADED TRIAL #1	GRADED TRIAL #2	NOTES
1. ✦ Review the list of needed supplies, grouping them according to the vendor they will be ordered from.				
2. ✦ Fill in the name and fax number of the company the supplies are to be ordered from.				
3. * List each supply individually on the purchase order, taking care to note the quantity needed of each and the part number associated with each item.				
4. ✦ If the physician's signature is required, obtain his or her signature. If it is not required, sign and date the form with your own signature.				
5. * If the purchase order can be faxed to the supplier, fax the document and make a note of the date and time the fax went through. **or** If the purchase order cannot be faxed to the supplier, call the supplier and place the order over the telephone. Document the name of the person you spoke to and the date and time of the call.				
6. ✦ File the purchase order in a folder for pending orders.				

Name: _____

Date: _____

Document: Enter the appropriate information in the chart below.

Grading

Points Earned	_____		
Points Possible	_____	42	42
Percent Grade (Points Earned/Points Possible)	_____		
PASS:	_____	❏ YES ❏ NO ❏ N/A	❏ YES ❏ NO ❏ N/A

Instructor Sign-Off

Instructor: _____ Date: _____

Name: _____

Date: _____

Procedure 15-5:

Receive a Supply Shipment

Objective: Receive a supply shipment correctly within the time limit set by the instructor.

Supplies: Box of supplies, packing slip, supply inventory log book, pen

Notes to the Student

_____

_____

_____

_____

_____

_____

Skills Assessment Requirements

Read and familiarize yourself with the procedure; complete the minimum practice requirements. Document each MPR using proper charting technique. Complete each procedure within a reasonable amount of time, with a minimum of 85 percent accuracy.

Name: _____

Date: _____

POINT VALUE ✦ = 3–6 points ✱ = 7–9 points		PRACTICE TRIAL	GRADED TRIAL # 1	GRADED TRIAL # 2	NOTES
1. ✦	Open the box of supplies, and locate the packing slip.				
2. ✦	Remove each item from the box, checking it on the packing slip.				
3. ✦	On the packing slip, circle any missing supplies.				
4. ✦	Put the supplies away, newer ones behind older ones.				
5. ✦	Note in the supply log that the supplies have been received.				
6. ✱	When any supplies on the packing slip are absent from the shipment, notify the supplier.				
7. ✦	When any supplies on the packing slip are on back order, retain the slip until the back-ordered supplies arrive.				
8. ✱	When the packing slip also serves as an invoice, route it to the accounts payable department.				
9. ✦	Discard packing materials appropriately.				

Name: _____

Date: _____

Document: Enter the appropriate information in the chart below.

Grading

Points Earned	_____		
Points Possible	_____	60	60
Percent Grade (Points Earned/Points Possible)	_____		
PASS:	_____	❏ YES ❏ NO ❏ N/A	❏ YES ❏ NO ❏ N/A

Instructor Sign-Off

Instructor: _____ **Date:** _____

Procedure 16-1:

Create an Office Brochure

Objective: Create an office brochure correctly within the time limit set by the instructor.

Supplies: Computer with word-processing software, list of information the physician would like in an office brochure

Affective Behaviors: Affective behaviors provide a professional approach to a skill that enhances the patient encounter. These behaviors may also display sensitivity to a patient's rights and enhance communication. Pay close attention to these skills, which will be in **bold, *italicized*** font.

Notes to the Student

_____

_____

_____

_____

_____

_____

Skills Assessment Requirements

Read and familiarize yourself with the procedure; complete the minimum practice requirements. Document each MPR using proper charting technique. Complete each procedure within a reasonable amount of time, with a minimum of 85 percent accuracy.

Name: _____

Date: _____

POINT VALUE ✦ = 3–6 points ⋆ = 7–9 points		PRACTICE TRIAL	GRADED TRIAL # 1	GRADED TRIAL # 2	NOTES
1. ✦	Gather information on the brochure's subject.				
2. ✦	Launch the word-processing software.				
3. ✦	Create a title for the brochure, such as "Living with Diabetes."				
4. ✦	**Add information to the brochure in an easy-to-read format. Use simple terms rather than medical terminology.**				
5. ✦	Add information regarding where the patient can look for further resources, such as Web sites.				
6. ✦	Include the office's name, address, and telephone number.				
7. ⋆	Check for typographical and grammatical errors.				
8. ⋆	Print the brochure, and **give it to the physician for review before making copies for patients.**				

Document: Enter the appropriate information in the chart below.

Grading

Points Earned	_____		
Points Possible	_____	54	54
Percent Grade (Points Earned/Points Possible)	_____		
PASS:	_____	❏ YES ❏ NO ❏ N/A	❏ YES ❏ NO ❏ N/A

Instructor Sign-Off

Instructor: _____ **Date:** _____

Name: _____

Date: _____

Procedure 16-2:

Create a Clinical Procedure for the Procedure Manual

Objective: Correctly create a clinical procedure for an office procedure manual.

Supplies: Computer with word processing software

Affective Behaviors: Affective behaviors provide a professional approach to a skill that enhances the patient encounter. These behaviors may also display sensitivity to a patient's rights and enhance communication. Pay close attention to these skills, which will be in **_bold, italicized_** font.

Notes to the Student

_____

_____

_____

_____

_____

_____

Skills Assessment Requirements

Read and familiarize yourself with the procedure; complete the minimum practice requirements. Document each MPR using proper charting technique. Complete each procedure within a reasonable amount of time, with a minimum of 85 percent accuracy.

POINT VALUE ✦ = 3–6 points ⋆ = 7–9 points		PRACTICE TRIAL	GRADED TRIAL # 1	GRADED TRIAL # 2	NOTES
1. ✦	Determine the type of clinical procedure for which you need to create a written description.				
2. ✦	Gather the information on how this clinical procedure should be performed.				
3. ✦	Title the procedure (e.g., "Collecting a Urine Sample").				
4. ✦	Describe the policy's purpose (e.g. "Purpose: To describe the method for collecting a urine sample from a patient"). **Ensure that each step fits well within the scope of practice and is succinct and time efficient.**				
5. ⋆	List each step in the procedure.				
6. ⋆	Print the procedure, and give it to the office manager for approval.				
7. ✦	Once approved, place the procedure in the clinical portion of the office procedure manual.				

Name: _____

Date: _____

Document: Enter the appropriate information in the chart below.

Grading

Points Earned	_____		
Points Possible	_____	48	48
Percent Grade (Points Earned/Points Possible)	_____		
PASS:	_____	❏ YES ❏ NO ❏ N/A	❏ YES ❏ NO ❏ N/A

Instructor Sign-Off

Instructor: _____ **Date:** _____

Procedure 16-3:

Create an Administrative Procedure for the Procedure Manual

Objective: Create a procedure for an office procedure manual correctly within the time limit set by the instructor.

Supplies: Computer with word-processing software

Affective Behaviors: Affective behaviors provide a professional approach to a skill that enhances the patient encounter. These behaviors may also display sensitivity to a patient's rights and enhance communication. Pay close attention to these skills, which will be in **_bold, italicized_** font.

Notes to the Student

_____

_____

_____

_____

_____

_____

Skills Assessment Requirements

Read and familiarize yourself with the procedure; complete the minimum practice requirements. Document each MPR using proper charting technique. Complete each procedure within a reasonable amount of time, with a minimum of 85 percent accuracy.

Name: _____

Date: _____

POINT VALUE

✦ = 3–6 points

⋆ = 7–9 points

		PRACTICE TRIAL	GRADED TRIAL # 1	GRADED TRIAL # 2	NOTES
1. ✦	Determine the type of procedure to be created.				
2. ✦	Gather the information on how this procedure is to be per-formed.				
3. ✦	Title the procedure (e.g., "Policy: Sorting Incoming Mail"), and determine if it will be listed under administrative, clinical, infection control, personnel, or quality improvement and risk management.				
4. ✦	Describe the policy's purpose (e.g., "Purpose: To describe the method of routing incoming mail to appropriate staff").				
5. ✦	List each step in the procedure. **Ensure that each step fits well within the scope of practice and is succinct and time efficient.**				
6. ⋆	Print the procedure, and give it to the office manager for approval.				
7. ✦	Once approved, place the procedure in the office pro-cedure manual.				

Name: _____

Date: _____

Document: Enter the appropriate information in the chart below.

Grading

Points Earned	_____		
Points Possible	_____	45	45
Percent Grade (Points Earned/Points Possible)	_____		
PASS:	_____	❏ YES ❏ NO ❏ N/A	❏ YES ❏ NO ❏ N/A

Instructor Sign-Off

Instructor: _____ **Date:** _____

Procedure 17-1:

Calculate Deductible, Coinsurance, and Allowable Amounts

Objective: Calculate deductible, coinsurance, and allowable amounts correctly within the time limit set by the instructor.

Supplies: Pen, paper, insurance verification form, patient's insurance identification card

Affective Behaviors: Affective behaviors provide a professional approach to a skill that enhances the patient encounter. These behaviors may also display sensitivity to a patient's rights and enhance communication. Pay close attention to these skills, which will be in **bold, *italicized*** font.

Notes to the Student

_____

_____

_____

_____

_____

_____

Skills Assessment Requirements

Read and familiarize yourself with the procedure; complete the minimum practice requirements. Document each MPR using proper charting technique. Complete each procedure within a reasonable amount of time, with a minimum of 85 percent accuracy.

Name: _____

Date: _____

POINT VALUE ✦ = 3–6 points ⋆ = 7–9 points		PRACTICE TRIAL	GRADED TRIAL # 1	GRADED TRIAL # 2	NOTES
1. ✦	After the patient's insurance coverage has been verified, locate the information on the verification form regarding any deductible and coinsurance amount.				
2. ✦	***Inform the patient of the deductible amount that will need to be paid at the beginning of the calendar or fiscal year.***				
3. ✦	***Explain to the patient that the amount charged for any particular procedure in the medical office will likely be reduced to a lower amount (called the allowed amount) when processed by the insurance carrier.***				
4. ⋆	• Imagine the patient has a $100 yearly deductible and a 10% copayment. The patient has had an examination, with a charge of $95.00, an X-ray with a charge of $75.00, and laboratory work with a charge of $102.00. • Imagine the insurance carrier in this situation allows $72.00 for the examination, $51.00 for the X-ray, and $80.00 for the laboratory work. Calculate the patient's amount owed by adding the allowed figures to come to a total of allowed charges.				
5. ✦	Subtract the $100.00 deductible from the total of the allowed charges.				
6. ✦	Multiply 20% by the remaining allowed amount to determine the patient's coinsurance.				
7. ✦	Add the $100.00 deductible to the 20% coinsurance amount to determine the amount the patient will need to pay for the visit.				
8. ⋆	***Explain the figures to the patient and collect the fees.***				

Name: _____

Date: _____

Document: Enter the appropriate information in the chart below.

Grading

Points Earned	_____		
Points Possible	_____	54	54
Percent Grade (Points Earned/Points Possible)	_____		
PASS:	_____	❏ YES ❏ NO ❏ N/A	❏ YES ❏ NO ❏ N/A

Instructor Sign-Off

Instructor: _____ **Date:** _____

Procedure 17-2:

Verify a Patient's Insurance Eligibility

Objective: Verify a patient's insurance eligibility correctly within the time limit set by the instructor.

Supplies: Insurance identification card, patient's registration form, telephone, paper, and a pen

Affective Behaviors: Affective behaviors provide a professional approach to a skill that enhances the patient encounter. These behaviors may also display sensitivity to a patient's rights and enhance communication. Pay close attention to these skills, which will be in ***bold, italicized*** font.

Notes to the Student

_____

_____

_____

_____

_____

_____

Skills Assessment Requirements

Read and familiarize yourself with the procedure; complete the minimum practice requirements. Document each MPR using proper charting technique. Complete each procedure within a reasonable amount of time, with a minimum of 85 percent accuracy.

Name: _____

Date: _____

POINT VALUE ✦ = 3–6 points ⋆ = 7–9 points		PRACTICE TRIAL	GRADED TRIAL #1	GRADED TRIAL #2	NOTES
1. ✦	Looking at the patient's registration form, locate the patient's birth and the patient's relationship to the insured.				
2. ✦	Looking at the patient's insurance identification card, locate the name of the insured, the insured member identification number, and the telephone number of the insurance company.				
3. ✦	Call the insurance company at the provider customer service telephone number listed on the insurance identification card.				
4. ⋆	***When the customer service representative answers the call, state your name and the reason for the telephone call in a warm and friendly voice. Write down the name of the customer service representative, and the date and time of the call.***				
5. ✦	Verify spelling of policyholder's name and birthdate.				
6. ✦	Verify patient's name and birthdate.				
7. ⋆	Verify the coverage for type of service to be rendered, including frequency or number of visits.				
8. ✦	Verify when preauthorization is needed.				
9. ⋆	Verify patient's financial responsibility for deductible, copayment, or coinsurance amounts.				
10. ⋆	Verify coordination of benefits rules if more than one policy covers the patient.				
11. ✦	Verify provider's participating or nonparticipating status.				

Name: _____

Date: _____

Document: Enter the appropriate information in the chart below.

Grading

Points Earned	_____		
Points Possible	_____	78	78
Percent Grade (Points Earned/Points Possible)	_____		
PASS:	_____	❏ YES ❏ NO ❏ N/A	❏ YES ❏ NO ❏ N/A

Instructor Sign-Off

Instructor: _____ Date: _____

Procedure 17-3:

Obtain a Managed Care Referral

Objective: Obtain a managed care referral for a patient correctly within the time limit set by the instructor.

Supplies: Telephone, patient's medical chart, name and telephone number of patient's primary care provider

Affective Behaviors: Affective behaviors provide a professional approach to a skill that enhances the patient encounter. These behaviors may also display sensitivity to a patient's rights and enhance communication. Pay close attention to these skills, which will be in **_bold, italicized_** font.

Notes to the Student

_____

_____

_____

_____

_____

_____

_____

Skills Assessment Requirements

Read and familiarize yourself with the procedure; complete the minimum practice requirements. Document each MPR using proper charting technique. Complete each procedure within a reasonable amount of time, with a minimum of 85 percent accuracy.

Name: _____

Date: _____

POINT VALUE ✦ = 3–6 points ⋆ = 7–9 points		PRACTICE TRIAL	GRADED TRIAL # 1	GRADED TRIAL # 2	NOTES
1. ✦	Call the patient's primary care provider's office, and ask for the person in charge of referrals.				
2. ✦	**Warmly greet the representative, state your name and give the referral assistant the patient's information, including name and birth date.**				
3. ✦	Inform the referral assistant of the need for a referral to the physician, including the reason for the patient's visit in the medical office.				
4. ✦	Ask the referral assistant if any information from the patient's file is needed to process the referral.				
5. ✦	Ask the referral assistant when to expect the referral. If needed, provide the office fax number for information transmittal. **Thank the referral assistant for their guidance and bid the assistant a good day.**				
6. ⋆	Document in the patient's file the content of the telephone call.				
7. ✦	Notify the physician and the patient of the content of the telephone call.				

Document: Enter the appropriate information in the chart below.

Grading

Points Earned	_____		
Points Possible	_____	45	45
Percent Grade (Points Earned/Points Possible)	_____		
PASS:	_____	❏ YES ❏ NO ❏ N/A	❏ YES ❏ NO ❏ N/A

Instructor Sign-Off

Instructor: _____ **Date:** _____

Name: _____

Date: _____

Procedure 17-4:

Obtain Authorization from an Insurance Company

Objective: Obtain an authorization from an insurance carrier for a procedure correctly within the time limit set by the instructor.

Supplies: Patient insurance information (i.e., I.D. number, birth date of the insured, name and telephone number for provider customer service at the insurance company), paper and pen, description of the procedure the doctor has prescribed, including current procedural terminology (CPT) code, patient's diagnosis pertaining to the needed procedure, location where procedure is to be performed (e.g., office, outpatient surgery, inpatient hospitalization), date by which the procedure must be performed

Affective Behaviors: Affective behaviors provide a professional approach to a skill that enhances the patient encounter. These behaviors may also display sensitivity to a patient's rights and enhance communication. Pay close attention to these skills, which will be in **_bold, italicized_** font.

Notes to the Student

_____

_____

_____

_____

_____

_____

Skills Assessment Requirements

Read and familiarize yourself with the procedure; complete the minimum practice requirements. Document each MPR using proper charting technique. Complete each procedure within a reasonable amount of time, with a minimum of 85 percent accuracy.

POINT VALUE ✦ = 3–6 points ★ = 7–9 points	PRACTICE TRIAL	GRADED TRIAL #1	GRADED TRIAL #2	NOTES
1. ★ Write down the date and time of the call, the name of the insurance company, and the name of the insurance company representative on the phone.				
2. ✦ **Warmly greet the insurance company representative and state your name and your office's/physician's name.**				
3. ✦ Give the insurance company representative the name of the patient, the name of the insured, and the insured's I.D. number.				
4. ✦ Let the representative know what the procedure is your doctor has prescribed for the patient and the date by which the procedure must be performed.				
5. ✦ Provide the representative any other requested information (e.g., procedure code, diagnosis code, and place where the procedure is to be performed).				
6. ★ Write down the authorization number the representative provides.				
7. ★ Ask the representative if any supporting documentation (e.g., chart notes, operative report, laboratory report, or pathology report) will be needed with the CMS-1500 billing form. If so, write down the required documentation. **Thank the representative and end the call.**				
8. ★ Keep all preceding information in the patient's file for reference in case the claim is not paid by the insurance carrier.				

Name: _____

Date: _____

Document: Enter the appropriate information in the chart below.

Grading

Points Earned	_____		
Points Possible	_____	60	60
Percent Grade (Points Earned/Points Possible)	_____		
PASS:	_____	❏ YES ❏ NO ❏ N/A	❏ YES ❏ NO ❏ N/A

Instructor Sign-Off

Instructor: _____ **Date:** _____

Procedure 17-5:

Abstract Data to Complete a Paper CMS-1500 Claim Form

Objective: Abstract data from the medical record to complete a CMS-1500 form.

Supplies: Klaus Davies patient registration form, insurance I.D. card, encounter form, Capital City Medical fee schedule, instructions on completing the CMS-1500 claim form, blank CMS-1500 form, ink pen, and calculator

Notes to the Student

_____

_____

_____

_____

_____

_____

_____

Skills Assessment Requirements

Read and familiarize yourself with the procedure; complete the minimum practice requirements. Document each MPR using proper charting technique. Complete each procedure within a reasonable amount of time, with a minimum of 85 percent accuracy.

POINT VALUE ◆ = 3–6 points ⋆ = 7–9 points		**PRACTICE TRIAL**	**GRADED TRIAL # 1**	**GRADED TRIAL # 2**	**NOTES**
1. ◆	Enter the insurance company name and mailing address in the carrier area.				
2. ◆	Check the correct box in FL 1.				
3. ◆	Enter the insured's I.D. number in FL 1a.				
4. ◆	Enter the patient's name in FL 2.				
5. ◆	Complete FL 3.				
6. ◆	Complete FL 4.				
7. ◆	Enter the patient's address and phone in FL 5. Note there are three lines of information to complete.				
8. ◆	Complete FL 6.				
9. ◆	Leave FL 7 blank.				
10. ◆	Complete FL 8 for marital status and employment status.				
11. ◆	Leave FL 9a to 9d blank.				
12. ◆	Complete FL 10a, 10b, and 10c.				
13. ◆	Leave FL 10d blank.				
14. ◆	Enter the group's number in FL 11.				
15. ◆	Leave FL 11a blank.				
16. ◆	Enter the employer in FL 11a.				
17. ◆	Enter the insurance plan name in FL 11c.				
18. ◆	Mark NO in FL 11d.				
19. ◆	Enter "SOF" in FL 12.				
20. ◆	Enter "SOF" in FL 13.				
21. ◆	Leave FL 14 to 19 blank.				
22. ◆	Mark NO in FL 20.				
23. ⋆	Enter the first diagnosis code in FL 21, line 1.				

		PRACTICE TRIAL	GRADED TRIAL # 1	GRADED TRIAL # 2	NOTES
24. ★	Enter the second diagnosis code in FL 21, line 2.				
25. ✦	Leave FL 22 to FL 23 blank.				
26. ✦	In FL 24a, line 1, enter the date of service in both the FROM and TO fields.				
27. ✦	Enter the code number for place of service in FL 24b.				
28. ✦	Leave FL 24c blank.				
29. ★	Enter the first CPT code in FL 24d.				
30. ★	In FL 24e enter "12" to designate that both diagnosis 1 and 2 relate to this.				
31. ★	Look on the encounter form to find the description for CPT code 99231. Then look on the fee schedule to find the fee for this service and enter it FL 24f.				
32. ✦	Enter 1 for units in FL 24g.				
33. ✦	Leave FL 24h and FL 24i blank.				
34. ✦	Enter the physician's NPI number on the unshaded portion of 24j. You will find this on the encounter form.				
35. ✦	Repeat these steps for lines 2 through 6. In FL 24e be certain you designate the correct diagnosis reference for each service, as some lines will be only "1" or only "2."				
36. ✦	When all services are completed, enter the EIN in FL 25 and mark X in the appropriate box. You will find this on the patient registration.				

		PRACTICE TRIAL	GRADED TRIAL # 1	GRADED TRIAL # 2	NOTES
37. ◆	Enter the patient's account number in FL 26. You will find this on the patient registration form.				
38. ◆	Leave FL 27 blank.				
39. ◆	Add up the total charges in column 24f. Write the total in FL 28.				
40. ◆	Leave FL 29 and FL 30 blank.				
41. ◆	Enter the physician's signature, credentials, and date in FL 31. Be certain to stay within the lines of the box.				
42. ◆	Enter the name and address of the clinic in FL 32.				
43. ◆	Enter the clinic's group NPI number in FL 32a. You will find this on the patient registration form.				
44. ◆	Leave FL 32b blank.				
45. ◆	In FL 33, enter the clinic's phone number in the top right corner.				
46. ◆	Enter the clinic's name and address in FL 33.				
47. ◆	Enter the clinic's NPI number in FL 33a.				
48. ◆	Leave FL 33b blank.				
49. ⋆	Proofread your work. Check all spelling and numbers against your source documents.				
50. ◆	Check your claim against the sample CMS-1500 form in Figure 17-26.				

Name: _____

Date: _____

Document: Enter the appropriate information in the chart below.

Grading

Points Earned	_____		
Points Possible	_____	318	318
Percent Grade (Points Earned/Points Possible)	_____		
PASS:	_____	❏ YES ❏ NO ❏ N/A	❏ YES ❏ NO ❏ N/A

Instructor Sign-Off

Instructor: _____   **Date:** _____

Name: _____

Date: _____

Procedure 17-6:

Complete a Computerized Insurance Claim Form

Objective: Complete an insurance claim form correctly within the time limit set by the instructor.

Supplies: Computer with medical billing software, patient medical chart, fee slip for patient's visit

Notes to the Student

_____

_____

_____

_____

_____

_____

Skills Assessment Requirements

Read and familiarize yourself with the procedure; complete the minimum practice requirements. Document each MPR using proper charting technique. Complete each procedure within a reasonable amount of time, with a minimum of 85 percent accuracy.

POINT VALUE ✦ = 3–6 points ⋆ = 7–9 points	PRACTICE TRIAL	GRADED TRIAL # 1	GRADED TRIAL # 2	NOTES
1. ✦ Enter the patient's account ledger in the computer billing software.				
2. ⋆ Verify that the fee slip is for the patient with the account opened on the computer.				
3. ✦ Enter the charges and coding as appropriate.				
4. ✦ Complete the patient insurance information field.				
5. ✦ Enter the patient's information, including address, telephone number, and birth date.				
6. ✦ Enter the insured's information, including address, telephone number, and birth date.				
7. ✦ Enter the patient's relationship to the insured.				
8. ✦ Enter the insured's identification and group number.				
9. ✦ Check the appropriate box to indicate the patient has authorized the release of information to the insurance company.				
10. ✦ Check the appropriate box to indicate the patient has assigned the benefits (payment) to the provider.				
11. ✦ Check the appropriate boxes to indicate if the visit was related to an accident. If the visit was due to an accident, enter the accident's date.				
12. ✦ Enter any information regarding a referring physician, if applicable.				

	PRACTICE TRIAL	GRADED TRIAL # 1	GRADED TRIAL # 2	NOTES
13. ✦ Enter any information regarding the patient's need for hospitalization for these charges, if applicable.				
14. ✦ Enter the treating provider's name, address, telephone number, national provider identification (NPI) number, and Internal Revenue Service (IRS) tax identification number.				
15. ✦ Enter information regarding the facility where the services were performed if not performed in the provider's office.				
16. ✦ Check the appropriate box to indicate the provider accepts assignment.				
17. ★ Print the patient's insurance claim form. Review the form for accuracy and completeness.				
18. ✦ Send the claim to the insurance company.				

Name: _____

Date: _____

Document: Enter the appropriate information in the chart below.

Grading

Points Earned	_____		
Points Possible	_____	114	114
Percent Grade (Points Earned/Points Possible)	_____		
PASS:	_____	❏ YES ❏ NO ❏ N/A	❏ YES ❏ NO ❏ N/A

Instructor Sign-Off

Instructor: _____ **Date:** _____

Name: _____

Date: _____

Procedure 17-7:

Handle a Denied Insurance Claim

Objective: Handle a denied insurance claim correctly within the time limit set by the instructor.

Supplies: Patient insurance information, paper and pen, copy of the explanation of benefits (EOB) received, description of the procedure the doctor has performed, including CPT code, patient's diagnosis pertaining to the procedure performed, location where procedure was performed, date the procedure was performed, any documentation of the service having been preauthorized by the office

Affective Behaviors: Affective behaviors provide a professional approach to a skill that enhances the patient encounter. These behaviors may also display sensitivity to a patient's rights and enhance communication. Pay close attention to these skills, which will be in **_bold, italicized_** font.

Notes to the Student

_____

_____

_____

_____

_____

_____

Skills Assessment Requirements

Read and familiarize yourself with the procedure; complete the minimum practice requirements. Document each MPR using proper charting technique. Complete each procedure within a reasonable amount of time, with a minimum of 85 percent accuracy.

Name: _____

Date: _____

	POINT VALUE ✦ = 3–6 points ⋆ = 7–9 points	PRACTICE TRIAL	GRADED TRIAL # 1	GRADED TRIAL # 2	NOTES
1. ✦	Organize all materials.				
2. ✦	Call the insurance company's provider customer service phone number as listed on the patient's insurance identification card.				
3. ⋆	***Write down the date and time of the telephone call, the number called, and the name of the customer service telephone representative on the phone.***				
4. ✦	***Warmly greet and self-identify to the customer service representative,*** and provide the patient's identification number and date of service.				
5. ✦	If the service was preauthorized, give that information to the customer service representative.				
6. ⋆	Ask the customer service representative why the procedure was not paid as anticipated.				
7. ✦	If there was an error in processing the service for payment, ask the customer service representative if any other information is needed to process the claim correctly. Ask the customer service representative when the office can expect payment for the procedure.				
8. ⋆	If the customer service representative says the claim was correctly processed, request the reason for the denial.				
9. ✦	If the reason for the denial was lack of supporting documentation, ask the customer service representative if faxing the information is a solution. If the answer is yes, get the customer service representative's direct fax line and fax the needed documentation.				

		PRACTICE TRIAL	GRADED TRIAL # 1	GRADED TRIAL # 2	NOTES
10. ★	If the reason for the denial requires an appeal be filed, ask the customer service representative to explain the insurance company's process for appeals.				
11. ★	Write down any pertinent information, such as where to mail the appeal and what information the appeal should contain.				
12. ✦	Call the patient with the findings and get the patient involved as needed. *Take the time to ensure that the patient understands the outcome.*				

Name: _____

Date: _____

Document: Enter the appropriate information in the chart below.

Grading

Points Earned	_____		
Points Possible	_____	87	87
Percent Grade (Points Earned/Points Possible)	_____		
PASS:	_____	❏ YES ❏ NO ❏ N/A	❏ YES ❏ NO ❏ N/A

Instructor Sign-Off

Instructor: _____   **Date:** _____

Name: _____

Date: _____

Procedure 18-1:

Perform Diagnostic Coding

Objective: Perform diagnostic coding correctly within the time limit set by the instructor.

Supplies: Patient's medical chart, current ICD-9-CM coding book, superbill with doctor's written diagnosis

Affective Behaviors: Affective behaviors provide a professional approach to a skill that enhances the patient encounter. These behaviors may also display sensitivity to a patient's rights and enhance communication. Pay close attention to these skills, which will be in **_bold, italicized_** font.

Notes to the Student

_____

_____

_____

_____

_____

_____

Skills Assessment Requirements

Read and familiarize yourself with the procedure; complete the minimum practice requirements. Document each MPR using proper charting technique. Complete each procedure within a reasonable amount of time, with a minimum of 85 percent accuracy.

Name: _____

Date: _____

POINT VALUE ✦ = 3–6 points ✶ = 7–9 points	PRACTICE TRIAL	GRADED TRIAL #1	GRADED TRIAL #2	NOTES
1. ✦ Locate the patient's diagnostic code(s) on the superbill or in the chart notes.				
2. ✶ Verify that the diagnostic code(s) on the superbill also appear in the patient's chart in the form of a patient complaint (subjective finding) or a test finding (objective finding).				
3. ✦ Using Volume II (the Alphabetic Index) of the ICD-9-CM coding book, find the diagnostic code(s).				
4. ✦ Using Volume I (the Tabular Index), confirm that the written description matches the chart notes. If in doubt, check with the physician.				
5. ✦ Read and defer to the conventions in the Tabular List.				
6. ✶ Assign the code for each diagnostic, primary diagnosis first. **Code to the highest level of specificity to ensure the highest reimbursement allowed.**				

Name: _____

Date: _____

Document: Enter the appropriate information in the chart below.

Grading

Points Earned	_____		
Points Possible	_____	42	42
Percent Grade (Points Earned/Points Possible)	_____		
PASS:	_____	❏ YES ❏ NO ❏ N/A	❏ YES ❏ NO ❏ N/A

Instructor Sign-Off

Instructor: _____ Date: _____

Procedure 19-1:

Code for a Procedure

Objective: Assign a Procedure code correctly within the time limit set by the instructor.

Supplies: CPT-4 coding book, superbill/encounter form, patient's chart

Affective Behaviors: Affective behaviors provide a professional approach to a skill that enhances the patient encounter. These behaviors may also display sensitivity to a patient's rights and enhance communication. Pay close attention to these skills, which will be in **_bold, italicized_** font.

Notes to the Student

_____

_____

_____

_____

_____

_____

Skills Assessment Requirements

Read and familiarize yourself with the procedure; complete the minimum practice requirements. Document each MPR using proper charting technique. Complete each procedure within a reasonable amount of time, with a minimum of 85 percent accuracy.

Name: _____

Date: _____

POINT VALUE ✦ = 3–6 points ⋆ = 7–9 points		PRACTICE TRIAL	GRADED TRIAL # 1	GRADED TRIAL # 2	NOTES
1. ✦	On the superbill, locate the procedure code the physician has circled.				
2. ✦	Identify the primary and secondary services or procedures performed, as stated in the medical record.				
3. ✦	Locate the main term in the alphabetic index.				
4. ⋆	Review any modifying terms or instructional notes associated with the main term.				
5. ✦	Identify the tentative codes associated with the most appropriate modifying terms.				
6. ✦	Locate the tentative codes in the tabular index.				
7. ⋆	Interpret the conventions used in the tabular index.				
8. ⋆	***Select the code with the highest level of specificity to ensure the highest reimbursement allowed.***				
9. ✦	Review the code for appropriate billing, add-on codes, and quantity.				
10. ⋆	Determine if modifiers are required.				
11. ⋆	Verify the final code against documentation.				
12. ✦	Assign the code.				

Name: _____

Date: _____

Document: Enter the appropriate information in the chart below.

Grading

Points Earned	_____		
Points Possible	_____	87	87
Percent Grade (Points Earned/Points Possible)	_____		
PASS:	_____	❏ YES ❏ NO ❏ N/A	❏ YES ❏ NO ❏ N/A

Instructor Sign-Off

Instructor: _____   **Date:** _____

Name: _____

Date: _____

Procedure 20-1:

Post an Entry on a Day Sheet

Objective: Post an entry on a day sheet correctly within the time allowed by the instructor.

Supplies: Pegboard, day sheet, patient ledger card, superbill, blue or black ink pen, calculator

Notes to the Student

_____

_____

_____

_____

_____

_____

Skills Assessment Requirements

Read and familiarize yourself with the procedure; complete the minimum practice requirements. Document each MPR using proper charting technique. Complete each procedure within a reasonable amount of time, with a minimum of 85 percent accuracy.

POINT VALUE ✦ = 3–6 points ★ = 7–9 points	PRACTICE TRIAL	GRADED TRIAL #1	GRADED TRIAL #2	NOTES
1. ✦ Place the patient's ledger card on the day sheet.				
2. ✦ Place the patient's superbill on top of the ledger card.				
3. ★ Pressing hard enough to impact all copies, enter the date, procedures, charges, and any payment in the appropriate boxes.				
4. ✦ In the appropriate box, enter the new balance.				
5. ✦ Verify that the entry appears on all copies.				
6. ✦ File the patient's ledger card.				

Document: Enter the appropriate information in the chart below.

Grading

Points Earned	_____		
Points Possible	_____	39	39
Percent Grade (Points Earned/Points Possible)	_____		
PASS:	_____	❏ YES ❏ NO ❏ N/A	❏ YES ❏ NO ❏ N/A

Instructor Sign-Off

Instructor: _____ Date: _____

Procedure 20-2:

Prepare an Accounts Receivable Trial Balance

Objective: Correctly prepare an accounts receivable trial balance.

Supplies: Patient accounts in computerized or paper ledger format, computer (if using a computerized billing system), fee slips for services rendered to the patients for the day, calculator, pegboard system (if using a manual billing system), pen

Notes to the Student

_____

_____

_____

_____

_____

_____

Skills Assessment Requirements

Read and familiarize yourself with the procedure; complete the minimum practice requirements. Document each MPR using proper charting technique. Complete each procedure within a reasonable amount of time, with a minimum of 85 percent accuracy.

POINT VALUE ✦ = 3–6 points ⋆ = 7–9 points		PRACTICE TRIAL	GRADED TRIAL # 1	GRADED TRIAL # 2	NOTES
1. ⋆	Calculate the total of the charges on the fee slips for the day.				
2. ⋆	Using the computer or the manual ledger card system, calculate the total of the charges posted to patient accounts for the day.				
3. ✦	Compare the total of the charges from the fee slips to the total of the charges in the computer or on the manual ledger card system.				
4. ✦	If the balances do not match, calculate the totals a second time to verify you added them correctly.				
5. ✦	If the balances continue to differ, go through the fee slips to see where the error in entry has occurred.				
6. ✦	Correct the entry error and calculate the totals again.				
7. ✦	If the balances continue to differ, go through the above steps until they match.				

Document: Enter the appropriate information in the chart below.

Grading

Points Earned	_____		
Points Possible	_____	48	48
Percent Grade Points Earned/Points Possible)	_____		
PASS:	_____	❏ YES ❏ NO ❏ N/A	❏ YES ❏ NO ❏ N/A

Instructor Sign-Off

Instructor: _____   **Date:** _____

Procedure 20-3:

Explain Professional Fees to a Patient

Objective: Explain the physician's professional fees to a patient correctly within the time limit set by the instructor.

Supplies: Patient medical record, copy of office fee schedule, blue or black pen, payment contract

Affective Behaviors: Affective behaviors provide a professional approach to a skill that enhances the patient encounter. These behaviors may also display sensitivity to a patient's rights and enhance communication. Pay close attention to these skills, which will be in **bold, *italicized*** font.

Notes to the Student

_____

_____

_____

_____

_____

_____

Skills Assessment Requirements

Read and familiarize yourself with the procedure; complete the minimum practice requirements. Document each MPR using proper charting technique. Complete each procedure within a reasonable amount of time, with a minimum of 85 percent accuracy.

Name: _____

Date: _____

POINT VALUE ✦ = 3–6 points ⋆ = 7–9 points		PRACTICE TRIAL	GRADED TRIAL #1	GRADED TRIAL #2	NOTES
1. ✦	**Find a private location** to sit with the patient.				
2. ✦	Explain to the patient the procedure the physician has prescribed.				
3. ✦	Explain to the patient the fee for the procedure.				
4. ✦	Explain to the patient any insurance coverage for the fee.				
5. ✦	**With a professional tone, explain to the patient the payment amount and deadline. Try to remain sensitive to the patient's financial situation.**				
6. ✦	Secure an agreement from the patient about the payment date.				
7. ✦	Enter the payment agreement and arrangements on the payment contract. **Ask the patient if he or she has any questions prior to signing the contract.**				
8. ⋆	On the payment contract, obtain the patient's signature and sign as the witness.				
9. ✦	Answer any questions the patient may have about the fee or the procedure.				
10. ⋆	Place the payment agreement in the patient's financial record.				

Name: _____

Date: _____

Document: Enter the appropriate information in the chart below.

Grading

Points Earned	_____		
Points Possible	_____	66	66
Percent Grade (Points Earned/Points Possible)	_____		
PASS:	_____	❏ YES ❏ NO ❏ N/A	❏ YES ❏ NO ❏ N/A

Instructor Sign-Off

Instructor: _____ **Date:** _____

Procedure 20-4:

Calling a Patient Regarding an Overdue Account

Objective: Call a patient regarding an overdue account correctly within the time limit set by the instructor.

Supplies: Telephone, patient's ledger information, blue or black pen

Affective Behaviors: Affective behaviors provide a professional approach to a skill that enhances the patient encounter. These behaviors may also display sensitivity to a patient's rights and enhance communication. Pay close attention to these skills, which will be in **_bold, italicized_** font.

Notes to the Student

_____

_____

_____

_____

_____

_____

Skills Assessment Requirements

Read and familiarize yourself with the procedure; complete the minimum practice requirements. Document each MPR using proper charting technique. Complete each procedure within a reasonable amount of time, with a minimum of 85 percent accuracy.

Name: _____

Date: _____

POINT VALUE ✦ = 3–6 points ★ = 7–9 points		PRACTICE TRIAL	GRADED TRIAL #1	GRADED TRIAL #2	NOTES
1. ✦	Dial the patient's home telephone number.				

2. ★	If you reach the patient, ***using a professional and non-confrontational voice:***
	  a. Identify yourself and the name of your clinic and state the reason for the call.
	  b. Ask the patient when payment on the out-standing bill will be made.
	  c. If the patient agrees to pay via credit card, take the credit card information over the telephone, verify the amount to be charged, and mail the patient a receipt.
	  d. If the patient agrees to mail payment to the office, secure a date by which the payment is to be received and note the date in the patient's billing ledger.
	  e. If the patient expresses an inability to make a payment at this time, secure a date by which the patient expects to be able to make a payment and note the date in the patient's billing ledger.
	Express thanks to the patient for assisting in resolving the matter.				

3. ✦	If unable to reach the patient, leave a message that dis-closes no personal infor-mation about the patient's care in the office.				
4. ★	Note the message in the patient's billing ledger.				

Document: Enter the appropriate information in the chart below.

Grading

Points Earned	_____		
Points Possible	_____	30	30
Percent Grade (Points Earned/Points Possible)	_____		
PASS:	_____	❏ YES ❏ NO ❏ N/A	❏ YES ❏ NO ❏ N/A

Instructor Sign-Off

Instructor: _____ Date: _____

Procedure 20-5:

Send a Patient Billing Statement

Objective: Send a patient billing statement correctly within the time limit set by the instructor.

Supplies: Computer with medical billing software, printer (computerized billing), patient ledger card (manual billing), copy machine (manual billing)

Notes to the Student

_____

_____

_____

_____

_____

_____

Skills Assessment Requirements

Read and familiarize yourself with the procedure; complete the minimum practice requirements. Document each MPR using proper charting technique. Complete each procedure within a reasonable amount of time, with a minimum of 85 percent accuracy.

Name: _____

Date: _____

POINT VALUE ✦ = 3–6 points ⋆ = 7–9 points		PRACTICE TRIAL	GRADED TRIAL #1	GRADED TRIAL #2	NOTES
1.	Manual billing:				
✦	Make a photocopy of the patient's ledger card.				
✦	Make a notation on the ledger card of the date and write "Bill to Patient" on the ledger.				
⋆	Verify that the information on the ledger is correct, including that the balance has been correctly totaled.				
✦	Place the copy of the ledger card in an envelope.				
✦	Stamp the envelope, and place it in the mail.				
2.	Computerized billing:				
⋆	Within the billing software, follow the appropriate steps to print a patient billing statement.				
✦	Once printed, verify the information on the bill is correct.				
✦	Place the copy of the ledger card into an envelope.				
✦	Stamp the envelope and place it in the mail.				

Name: _____

Date: _____

Document: Enter the appropriate information in the chart below.

Grading

Points Earned	_____		
Points Possible	_____	60	60
Percent Grade (Points Earned/Points Possible)	_____		
PASS:	_____	❏ YES ❏ NO ❏ N/A	❏ YES ❏ NO ❏ N/A

Instructor Sign-Off

Instructor: _____   **Date:** _____

Name: _____

Date: _____

Procedure 20-6:

Post a Nonsufficient Funds Check

Objective: Post an NSF check correctly within the time limit set by the instructor.

Supplies: Check returned due to NSF. For manual billing: patient billing ledger, day sheet, blue or black pen. For computerized billing: computer with medical billing software

Notes to the Student

_____

_____

_____

_____

_____

_____

Skills Assessment Requirements

Read and familiarize yourself with the procedure; complete the minimum practice requirements. Document each MPR using proper charting technique. Complete each procedure within a reasonable amount of time, with a minimum of 85 percent accuracy.

POINT VALUE ✦ = 3–6 points ⋆ = 7–9 points		PRACTICE TRIAL	GRADED TRIAL # 1	GRADED TRIAL # 2	NOTES
1. ✦	Verify that you have the correct patient ledger.				
	When billing manually:				
2. ⋆	Place the patient's ledger on the day sheet.				
	On the ledger card, write the NSF check and any applicable fees.				
	Calculate the new total on the account.				
	When billing via computer:				
3. ⋆	Enter the NSF check and any fees on the patient's ledger.				
4. ✦	Notify the patient via phone that the check was returned. Indicate any corresponding fees.				
5. ✦	Secure a date by which to secure a replacement payment.				
6. ⋆	In the patient's financial record or ledger, note the outcome of the conversation.				

Name: _____

Date: _____

Document: Enter the appropriate information in the chart below.

Grading

Points Earned	_____		
Points Possible	_____	45	45
Percent Grade (Points Earned/Points Possible)	_____		
PASS:	_____	❏ YES ❏ NO ❏ N/A	❏ YES ❏ NO ❏ N/A

Instructor Sign-Off

Instructor: _____ **Date:** _____

Name: _____

Date: _____

Procedure 20-7:

Post an Adjustment to a Patient Account

Objective: Post an adjustment to a patient account correctly within the time limit set by the instructor.

Supplies: For manual billing: patient's ledger, day sheet, blue or black pen, calculator. For computerized billing: medical billing software

Notes to the Student

_____

_____

_____

_____

_____

_____

Skills Assessment Requirements

Read and familiarize yourself with the procedure; complete the minimum practice requirements. Document each MPR using proper charting technique. Complete each procedure within a reasonable amount of time, with a minimum of 85 percent accuracy.

POINT VALUE ✦ = 3–6 points ★ = 7–9 points		PRACTICE TRIAL	GRADED TRIAL # 1	GRADED TRIAL # 2	NOTES
1. ★	**When billing manually:**				
	Place the patient's billing ledger on the day sheet.				
	Pressing hard enough to impact all layers of paper, enter the type of adjustment on the ledger card.				
	Add or subtract adjustments as appropriate.				
	Calculate the new balance.				
	Enter the new balance on the ledger card.				
2. ★	**When billing via computer:**				
	Locate the correct patient ledger in the computer.				
	Enter the adjustment as a debit or a credit.				
3. ★	In the patient's financial record, note the reason for the adjustment.				

Name: _____

Date: _____

Document: Enter the appropriate information in the chart below.

Grading

Points Earned	_____		
Points Possible	_____	27	27
Percent Grade (Points Earned/Points Possible)	_____		
PASS:	_____	❏ YES ❏ NO ❏ N/A	❏ YES ❏ NO ❏ N/A

Instructor Sign-Off

Instructor: _____ **Date:** _____

Name: _____

Date: _____

Procedure 20-8:

Post a Collection Agency Payment

Objective: Post a collection agency payment correctly within the time limit set by the instructor.

Supplies: For a manual posting system: day sheet, ledger card, pegboard, calculator, blue or black pen, collection agency payment. For a computerized posting system: calculator, computer, collection agency payment

Notes to the Student

_____

_____

_____

_____

_____

_____

Skills Assessment Requirements

Read and familiarize yourself with the procedure; complete the minimum practice requirements. Document each MPR using proper charting technique. Complete each procedure within a reasonable amount of time, with a minimum of 85 percent accuracy.

Name: _____

Date: _____

POINT VALUE ✦ = 3–6 points ★ = 7–9 points		PRACTICE TRIAL	GRADED TRIAL # 1	GRADED TRIAL # 2	NOTES
	When billing manually:				
1. ✦	Verify which patient account will receive the payment.				
2. ✦	Align the patient's ledger card with the next line on the day sheet.				
3. ★	In the appropriate columns, enter the patient's name, previous balance, payment date, payment amount, and name of the collection agency.				
4. ✦	In the checks column of the day sheet's deposit section, enter the payment amount.				
5. ✦	Subtract the payment from the previous patient balance.				
6. ✦	Record the new balance on the patient's ledger card.				
7. ★	When an adjustment is to be made to the account due to collection agency fee, record the amount in brackets [ ] in the adjustment column of the ledger card and enter as the description "collection agency fee."				
8. ✦	Subtract the amount of the adjustment from the previous patient balance, and record the new balance on the patient's ledger card.				
	When using a computerized system:				
9. ✦	Find the patient's account in the computer.				

Name: _____

Date: _____

		PRACTICE TRIAL	GRADED TRIAL # 1	GRADED TRIAL # 2	NOTES
10. ✦	Verify the patient account is correct.				
11. ⭑	Post the payment, choosing "collection payment" as the payment source.				
12. ✦	If applicable, enter any adjustment due to collection agency fee.				
13. ✦	Verify the payment amount and adjustment.				
14. ⭑	Save all changes.				

Name: _____

Date: _____

Document: Enter the appropriate information in the chart below.

Grading

Points Earned	_____		
Points Possible	_____	84	84
Percent Grade (Points Earned/Points Possible)	_____		
PASS:	_____	❑ YES ❑ NO ❑ N/A	❑ YES ❑ NO ❑ N/A

Instructor Sign-Off

Instructor: _____ Date: _____

Procedure 20-9:

Process a Patient Refund

Objective: Process a refund to a patient correctly within the time limit set by the instructor.

Supplies: For a manual posting system: day sheet, patient ledger card, calculator, blue or black pen. For a computerized posting system: computer with medical billing software

Notes to the Student

_____

_____

_____

_____

_____

_____

Skills Assessment Requirements

Read and familiarize yourself with the procedure; complete the minimum practice requirements. Document each MPR using proper charting technique. Complete each procedure within a reasonable amount of time, with a minimum of 85 percent accuracy.

Name: _____

Date: _____

POINT VALUE ✦ = 3–6 points ★ = 7–9 points		PRACTICE TRIAL	GRADED TRIAL # 1	GRADED TRIAL # 2	NOTES
	When billing manually:				
1. ✦	Place the patient's ledger card on the day sheet.				
2. ✦	Pressing hard enough to impact all copies, enter "Patient Refund" on the line.				
3. ✦	Enter the dollar amount of the refund being sent to the patient.				
4. ✦	Add the refund amount to the patient's balance.				
5. ✦	Enter the new balance in the proper box.				
	When billing via computer:				
6. ✦	Locate the proper patient ledger in the billing software.				
7. ✦	Enter the refund amount.				
8. ✦	Choose the adjustment code for "Refund to Patient."				
9. ★	Obtain a refund check from the physician or office manager.				
10. ✦	Send the refund check to the patient.				
11. ★	In the patient ledger, note the party receiving the refund and the number of the refund check.				
12. ★	Post the payment, choosing "Collection Payment" as the payment source.				
13. ✦	If applicable, enter any adjustment due to collection agency fee.				
14. ✦	Verify the payment amount and adjustment.				
15. ★	Save all changes.				

Name: _____

Date: _____

Document: Enter the appropriate information in the chart below.

Grading

Points Earned	_____		
Points Possible	_____	72	72
Percent Grade (Points Earned/Points Possible)	_____		
PASS:	_____	❑ YES ❑ NO ❑ N/A	❑ YES ❑ NO ❑ N/A

Instructor Sign-Off

Instructor: _____ **Date:** _____

Procedure 20-10:

Process an Insurance Company Overpayment

Objective: Process a refund to an insurance company correctly within the time limit set by the instructor.

Supplies: For manual billing: patient ledger card, day sheet, blue or black pen, copies of insurance companies' explanations of benefits. For computerized billing: computer with medical billing software, copies of insurance companies' explanations of benefits

Notes to the Student

_____

_____

_____

_____

_____

_____

Skills Assessment Requirements

Read and familiarize yourself with the procedure; complete the minimum practice requirements. Document each MPR using proper charting technique. Complete each procedure within a reasonable amount of time, with a minimum of 85 percent accuracy.

POINT VALUE ✦ = 3–6 points ⋆ = 7–9 points	PRACTICE TRIAL	GRADED TRIAL #1	GRADED TRIAL #2	NOTES
1. ✦ Using the insurance companies' explanations of benefits, determine which company is the patient's primary insurance carrier and which is secondary.				
When billing manually:				
2. ✦ Place the patient's ledger card on the day sheet.				
3. ✦ Pressing hard enough to impact all copies, enter the refund amount and write "Refund to insurance company."				
4. ✦ Enter the new balance.				
When billing via computer:				
5. ✦ Find the appropriate patient ledger in the computer.				
6. ✦ Using the appropriate code, enter the refund to the insurance company.				
7. ⋆ Obtain a refund check from the physician or office manager.				
8. ⋆ Send a note to the insurance company explaining the reason for the refund, as well as copies of the primary and secondary insurance companies' explanations of benefits.				

Name: _____

Date: _____

Document: Enter the appropriate information in the chart below.

Grading

Points Earned	_____		
Points Possible	_____	54	54
Percent Grade (Points Earned/Points Possible)	_____		
PASS:	_____	❏ YES ❏ NO ❏ N/A	❏ YES ❏ NO ❏ N/A

Instructor Sign-Off

Instructor: _____   Date: _____

Procedure 21-1:

Create a New Employee Record

Objective: Create a new employee record correctly within the time limit set by the instructor.

Supplies: Pen, paper, employee file, copy machine

Notes to the Student

_____

_____

_____

_____

_____

_____

Skills Assessment Requirements

Read and familiarize yourself with the procedure; complete the minimum practice requirements. Document each MPR using proper charting technique. Complete each procedure within a reasonable amount of time, with a minimum of 85 percent accuracy.

Name: _____

Date: _____

POINT VALUE ✦ = 3–6 points ⋆ = 7–9 points		PRACTICE TRIAL	GRADED TRIAL #1	GRADED TRIAL #2	NOTES
1. ✦	Ask the new employee to bring the following items with them on their first day of employment: • Picture identification or other proof of ability to work in the United States. • Social Security card • Copies of any certification or professional licenses				
2. ⋆	Photocopy any documents the employee has brought for the employee record.				
3. ✦	Give the employee a W-4 IRS form to complete to indicate the number of exemptions to be claimed.				
4. ✦	Place the employee's resume and application into the employee record.				
5. ✦	Give the employee an I-9 form to complete to verify citizenship.				

Document: Enter the appropriate information in the chart below.

Grading

Points Earned	_____		
Points Possible	_____	33	33
Percent Grade (Points Earned/Points Possible)	_____		
PASS:	_____	❏ YES ❏ NO ❏ N/A	❏ YES ❏ NO ❏ N/A

Instructor Sign-Off

Instructor: _____ **Date:** _____

Procedure 21-2:

Calculate an Employee's Payroll

Objective: Calculate the amount of an employee's payroll correctly within the time limit set by the instructor.

Supplies: Calculator, employee's W-4 form, IRS Circular E list of federal tax deduction amounts, record of number of hours the employee worked, employee's payroll record

Affective Behaviors: Affective behaviors provide a professional approach to a skill that enhances the patient encounter. These behaviors may also display sensitivity to a patient's rights and enhance communication. Pay close attention to these skills, which will be in **_bold, italicized_** font.

Notes to the Student

_____

_____

_____

_____

_____

_____

Skills Assessment Requirements

Read and familiarize yourself with the procedure; complete the minimum practice requirements. Document each MPR using proper charting technique. Complete each procedure within a reasonable amount of time, with a minimum of 85 percent accuracy.

POINT VALUE ✦ = 3–6 points ⋆ = 7–9 points		PRACTICE TRIAL	GRADED TRIAL # 1	GRADED TRIAL # 2	NOTES
1. ⋆	Calculate the number of hours the employee worked during the payroll period.				
2. ✦	For an hourly employee, calculate the employee's gross wage by multiplying the number of hours worked in the payroll period by the employee's hourly wage. ***Keep in mind that the employee's wage is confidential and should never be discussed with anyone other than the employee.***				
3. ✦	If the employee worked any overtime hours, first multiply the employee's hourly wage by 1.5 and then multiply that amount by the employee's overtime hours.				
4. ✦	Consult the employee's W-4 form to determine filing status (i.e., married or single) and the number of deductions.				
5. ✦	Consult the IRS Circular E form to determine the amount to be withheld from the employee's gross wages.				
6. ⋆	Deduct the federal withholding tax from the Circular E form from the employee's gross payroll.				
7. ✦	Multiply the employee's gross payroll amount by 6.2 percent to determine the FICA (Social Security) to withhold from the employee's payroll.				
8. ✦	Multiply the employee's gross payroll amount by 1.45 percent to determine the Medicare tax to withhold from the employee's payroll.				

		PRACTICE TRIAL	GRADED TRIAL # 1	GRADED TRIAL # 2	NOTES
9. ★	Consult the employee's file to determine any other deductions (e.g., health insurance or retirement contributions) to withhold from the employee's payroll.				
10. ◆	Determine the net payroll by subtracting all deductions from the gross payroll.				

Name: _____

Date: _____

Document: Enter the appropriate information in the chart below.

Grading

Points Earned	_____		
Points Possible	_____	69	69
Percent Grade (Points Earned/Points Possible)	_____		
PASS:	_____	❏ YES ❏ NO ❏ N/A	❏ YES ❏ NO ❏ N/A

Instructor Sign-Off

Instructor: _____ **Date:** _____

Procedure 21-3:

Write Checks to Pay Bills

Objective: Write checks in payment of office bills correctly within the time limit set by the instructor.

Supplies: Office checkbook register, bills to be paid, blue or black pen, calculator

Notes to the Student

_____

_____

_____

_____

_____

_____

Skills Assessment Requirements

Read and familiarize yourself with the procedure; complete the minimum practice requirements. Document each MPR using proper charting technique. Complete each procedure within a reasonable amount of time, with a minimum of 85 percent accuracy.

POINT VALUE ✦ = 3–6 points ⋆ = 7–9 points	PRACTICE TRIAL	GRADED TRIAL # 1	GRADED TRIAL # 2	NOTES
1. ✦ Verify the bill is accurate and that the supplies or services were received.				
2. ✦ Determine if the company offers a discount if the bill is paid by a certain date. If so, pay the bill by the discount due date to obtain the discount.				
3. ⋆ Complete the check, providing the date, name of the vendor or supplier, and check amount.				
4. ✦ On the invoice, write the date, check number, and payment amount.				
5. ✦ File the invoice.				
6. ⋆ Give the check to the physician or office manager for signature.				
7. ✦ In the checkbook register, note the payment category.				

Name: _____

Date: _____

Document: Enter the appropriate information in the chart below.

Grading

Points Earned	_____		
Points Possible	_____	48	48
Percent Grade (Points Earned/Points Possible)	_____		
PASS:	_____	❏ YES ❏ NO ❏ N/A	❏ YES ❏ NO ❏ N/A

Instructor Sign-Off

Instructor: _____   **Date:** _____

Procedure 21-4:

Pay an Office Supply Invoice

Objective: Pay an office supply invoice correctly within the time limit set by the instructor.

Supplies: Office supply invoice, office checkbook and checkbook register, blue or black pen, calculator

Notes to the Student

_____

_____

_____

_____

_____

_____

Skills Assessment Requirements

Read and familiarize yourself with the procedure; complete the minimum practice requirements. Document each MPR using proper charting technique. Complete each procedure within a reasonable amount of time, with a minimum of 85 percent accuracy.

Name: _____

Date: _____

Name: _____

Date: _____

Document: Enter the appropriate information in the chart below.

Grading

Points Earned	_____		
Points Possible	_____	42	42
Percent Grade (Points Earned/Points Possible)	_____		
PASS:	_____	❏ YES ❏ NO ❏ N/A	❏ YES ❏ NO ❏ N/A

Instructor Sign-Off

Instructor: _____ Date: _____

Procedure 21-5:

Complete a Deposit Slip

Objective: Fill out a deposit slip correctly within the time limit set by the instructor.

Supplies: Calculator, deposit slip, printout from the electronic or manual billing system showing amount received for the day, pen, and endorsement stamp

Affective Behaviors: Affective behaviors provide a professional approach to a skill that enhances the patient encounter. These behaviors may also display sensitivity to a patient's rights and enhance communication. Pay close attention to these skills, which will be in ***bold, italicized*** font.

Notes to the Student

_____

_____

_____

_____

_____

_____

Skills Assessment Requirements

Read and familiarize yourself with the procedure; complete the minimum practice requirements. Document each MPR using proper charting technique. Complete each procedure within a reasonable amount of time, with a minimum of 85 percent accuracy.

POINT VALUE ✦ = 3–6 points ⋆ = 7–9 points		PRACTICE TRIAL	GRADED TRIAL # 1	GRADED TRIAL # 2	NOTES
1. ✦	**Perform this task out of view of patients, such as in a back office.** Check to see that all checks have been properly endorsed.				
2. ✦	Total all cash receipts.				
3. ✦	On the line marked "cash" on the deposit slip, list the cash receipt total.				
4. ✦	On the deposit slip, list each check individually by bank routing number or name of the patient or insurance company.				
5. ✦	Total the checks.				
6. ✦	On the appropriate line of the deposit slip, list the check total.				
7. ⋆	Total the checks and cash.				
8. ✦	On the appropriate line of the deposit slip, list the checks and cash total. **Doublecheck calculations for errors.**				
9. ✦	Attach the deposit slip, cash, and checks via paperclip.				
10. ✦	Place the paperclipped deposit in an envelope.				
11. ✦	Take the deposit to the bank.				
12. ✦	Secure a receipt.				
13. ✦	Return to the office.				
14. ⋆	Using the receipt, record the deposit amount in the clinic checkbook register.				

Document: Enter the appropriate information in the chart below.

Grading

Points Earned	_____		
Points Possible	_____	90	90
Percent Grade (Points Earned/Points Possible)	_____		
PASS:	_____	❏ YES ❏ NO ❏ N/A	❏ YES ❏ NO ❏ N/A

Instructor Sign-Off

Instructor: _____ **Date:** _____

Procedure 21-6:

Account for Petty Cash

Objective: Balance the petty cash fund correctly within the time limit set by the instructor.

Supplies: Petty cash record, receipts for petty cash purchases, blue or black pen, calculator

Affective Behaviors: Affective behaviors provide a professional approach to a skill that enhances the patient encounter. These behaviors may also display sensitivity to a patient's rights and enhance communication. Pay close attention to these skills, which will be in **_bold, italicized_** font.

Notes to the Student

_____

_____

_____

_____

_____

Skills Assessment Requirements

Read and familiarize yourself with the procedure; complete the minimum practice requirements. Document each MPR using proper charting technique. Complete each procedure within a reasonable amount of time, with a minimum of 85 percent accuracy.

POINT VALUE ✦ = 3–6 points ★ = 7–9 points		PRACTICE TRIAL	GRADED TRIAL # 1	GRADED TRIAL # 2	NOTES
1. ★	**Perform this task out of view of patients, such as in a back office.** Verify that all petty cash expenditures have been listed on the petty cash record and that each has a receipt.				
2. ✦	Subtract all expenditures from the petty cash balance.				
3. ✦	Enter the new balance on the petty cash record.				
4. ✦	Count the money in petty cash.				
5. ✦	Verify that the petty cash amount matches the resulting amount in Step 2.				
6. ✦	If the amounts do not match, verify all subtraction was done accurately and that all receipts were entered in the petty cash record.				
7. ★	Once the account balances, obtain a check for the total expenditures from the physician or office manager.				
8. ✦	Cash the check at the bank.				
9. ✦	Enter the money in the petty cash record.				

Name: _____

Date: _____

Document: Enter the appropriate information in the chart below.

Grading

Points Earned	_____		
Points Possible	_____	60	60
Percent Grade (Points Earned/Points Possible)	_____		
PASS:	_____	❏ YES ❏ NO ❏ N/A	❏ YES ❏ NO ❏ N/A

Instructor Sign-Off

Instructor: _____   **Date:** _____

Name: _____

Date: _____

Procedure 21-7:

Reconcile a Bank Statement

Objective: Balance the clinic bank statement correctly within the time limit set by the instructor.

Supplies: Bank statement, checkbook register, calculator, blue or black pen

Notes to the Student

_____

_____

_____

_____

_____

_____

Skills Assessment Requirements

Read and familiarize yourself with the procedure; complete the minimum practice requirements. Document each MPR using proper charting technique. Complete each procedure within a reasonable amount of time, with a minimum of 85 percent accuracy.

POINT VALUE ✦ = 3–6 points ⋆ = 7–9 points		PRACTICE TRIAL	GRADED TRIAL #1	GRADED TRIAL #2	NOTES
1. ⋆	Comparing the bank statement to the checkbook register, make a check mark next to each check processed by the bank.				
2. ✦	Write the ending balance on the bank statement.				
3. ✦	Add any deposits made since the bank statement was printed.				
4. ✦	Subtract any checks not yet processed when the bank statement was printed.				
5. ✦	Add any interest awarded by the bank.				
6. ✦	Subtract any bank service fees taken by the bank.				
7. ⋆	If the resulting balance fails to match that in the checkbook register balance, verify that Steps 1 through 6 were performed correctly.				
8. ✦	If the balances still do not match, check for addition or subtraction errors in the checkbook register.				

Name: _____

Date: _____

Document: Enter the appropriate information in the chart below.

Grading

Points Earned	_____		
Points Possible	_____	54	54
Percent Grade (Points Earned/Points Possible)	_____		
PASS:	_____	❏ YES ❏ NO ❏ N/A	❏ YES ❏ NO ❏ N/A

Instructor Sign-Off

Instructor: _____ **Date:** _____

Procedure 22-1:

Direct a Staff Meeting

Objective: Direct a staff meeting correctly within the time limit set by the instructor.

Supplies: Blue or black pen, paper, clock or watch to keep time, staff meeting agenda

Affective Behaviors: Affective behaviors provide a professional approach to a skill that enhances the patient encounter. These behaviors may also display sensitivity to a patient's rights and enhance communication. Pay close attention to these skills, which will be in ***bold, italicized*** font.

Notes to the Student

_____

_____

_____

_____

_____

_____

Skills Assessment Requirements

Read and familiarize yourself with the procedure; complete the minimum practice requirements. Document each MPR using proper charting technique. Complete each procedure within a reasonable amount of time, with a minimum of 85 percent accuracy.

Name: _____

Date: _____

POINT VALUE ✦ = 3–6 points ⋆ = 7–9 points		PRACTICE TRIAL	GRADED TRIAL # 1	GRADED TRIAL # 2	NOTES
1. ✦	Before the staff meeting, create an agenda of the meeting's discussion topics.				
2. ⋆	**Provide a copy of the meeting's agenda to each member of staff,** prior to its start.				
3. ✦	**Start the meeting on time.**				
4. ✦	Note staff in attendance and staff who are absent.				
5. ✦	Discuss the agenda items one at a time, being mindful of the time.				
6. ⋆	**Considering time management, when non-agenda items arise, determine if they should be included in this meeting or moved to the next.**				
7. ✦	Address any issues or concerns that arise.				
8. ✦	**End the meeting at the prearranged time.**				

Name: _____

Date: _____

Document: Enter the correct information in the chart below.

Grading

Points Earned	_____		
Points Possible	_____	54	54
Percent Grade (Points Earned/Points Possible)	_____		
PASS:	_____	❏ YES ❏ NO ❏ N/A	❏ YES ❏ NO ❏ N/A

Instructor Sign-Off

Instructor: _____   **Date:** _____

Name: _____

Date: _____

Procedure 22-2:

Write a Job Description

Objective: Write a job description correctly within the time limit set by the instructor.

Supplies: Computer with word-processing software, list of skills needed for the position, list of duties required for the position

Affective Behaviors: Affective behaviors provide a professional approach to a skill that enhances the patient encounter. These behaviors may also display sensitivity to a patient's rights and enhance communication. Pay close attention to these skills, which will be in **_bold, italicized_** font.

Notes to the Student

_____

_____

_____

_____

_____

_____

Skills Assessment Requirements

Read and familiarize yourself with the procedure; complete the minimum practice requirements. Document each MPR using proper charting technique. Complete each procedure within a reasonable amount of time, with a minimum of 85 percent accuracy.

POINT VALUE ✦ = 3–6 points ⋆ = 7–9 points		PRACTICE TRIAL	GRADED TRIAL #1	GRADED TRIAL #2	NOTES
1. ✦	Create a title for the job position.				
2. ✦	List the name of the supervisor for the position.				
3. ⋆	Create a summary description of the position's duties. **Be sure that the duties fall within the scope of practice for the given job title.**				
4. ✦	List the hours required of the position.				
5. ✦	List the location of the position, when it varies.				
6. ⋆	**List any employment requirements (e.g., certification, malpractice insurance).**				
7. ⋆	**List any physical requirements for the position (e.g., lifting, excessive sitting, or standing).**				
8. ✦	Describe the evaluation process for the position.				
9. ✦	Review the job description for accuracy, as well as with the physician if needed.				

Name: _____

Date: _____

Document: Enter the correct information in the chart below.

Grading

Points Earned	_____		
Points Possible	_____	63	63
Percent Grade (Points Earned/Points Possible)	_____		
PASS:	_____	❏ YES ❏ NO ❏ N/A	❏ YES ❏ NO ❏ N/A

Instructor Sign-Off

Instructor: _____ **Date:** _____

Procedure 22-3:

Conduct an Interview

Objective: Conduct an interview correctly within the time limit set by the instructor.

Supplies: Pen, notebook, applicant's resume

Affective Behaviors: Affective behaviors provide a professional approach to a skill that enhances the patient encounter. These behaviors may also display sensitivity to a patient's rights and enhance communication. Pay close attention to these skills, which will be in ***bold, italicized*** font.

Notes to the Student

_____

_____

_____

_____

_____

_____

Skills Assessment Requirements

Read and familiarize yourself with the procedure; complete the minimum practice requirements. Document each MPR using proper charting technique. Complete each procedure within a reasonable amount of time, with a minimum of 85 percent accuracy.

Name: _____

Date: _____

POINT VALUE ✦ = 3–6 points ⋆ = 7–9 points		PRACTICE TRIAL	GRADED TRIAL # 1	GRADED TRIAL # 2	NOTES
1. ✦	Before meeting the applicant, read the resume.				
2. ✦	Highlight any areas of concern or interest on the resume.				
3. ✦	Highlight resume items that apply to the position being filled.				
4. ✦	**Greet the applicant while making direct eye contact, and state your name.**				
5. ✦	**Use a firm handshake to shake hands with the applicant and lead the applicant to a private room.**				
6. ✦	Show the applicant where to sit for the interview.				
7. ✦	Ask the applicant about the potential to perform the job.				
8. ⋆	Review any areas of concern highlighted on the resume.				
9. ⋆	Review the job description				
10. ✦	Verify the applicant's ability to perform the required tasks.				
11. ✦	Ask the applicant if he or she has any questions about the office or physicians.				
12. ✦	**Provide a decision date for the position.**				
13. ✦	**Thank the applicant, and escort the applicant out of the office.**				

Name: _____

Date: _____

Document: Enter the correct information in the chart below.

Grading

Points Earned	_____		
Points Possible	_____	84	84
Percent Grade (Points Earned/Points Possible)	_____		
PASS:	_____	❏ YES ❏ NO ❏ N/A	❏ YES ❏ NO ❏ N/A

Instructor Sign-Off

Instructor: _____ **Date:** _____

Procedure 22-4:

Call Employee References

Objective: Call for an employee reference correctly within the time limit set by the instructor.

Supplies: Telephone, employee resume, pen

Affective Behaviors: Affective behaviors provide a professional approach to a skill that enhances the patient encounter. These behaviors may also display sensitivity to a patient's rights and enhance communication. Pay close attention to these skills, which will be in ***bold, italicized*** font.

Notes to the Student

_____

_____

_____

_____

_____

_____

Skills Assessment Requirements

Read and familiarize yourself with the procedure; complete the minimum practice requirements. Document each MPR using proper charting technique. Complete each procedure within a reasonable amount of time, with a minimum of 85 percent accuracy.

Name: _____

Date: _____

POINT VALUE ✦ = 3–6 points ⋆ = 7–9 points		PRACTICE TRIAL	GRADED TRIAL # 1	GRADED TRIAL # 2	NOTES
1. ✦	Call the applicant's previous employer.				
2. ✦	Ask to speak with the office manager or supervisor.				
3. ⋆	**In a friendly voice self-identify, and give the reason for the call.**				
4. ✦	Ask the previous employer open-ended questions about the employee.				
5. ✦	Ask the previous employer if the employee would be eligible for rehire.				
6. ⋆	Ask specifics as to the employee's job duties and job performance.				
7. ⋆	Ask the previous employer for any other relevant information.				
8. ✦	Note all of the previous employers' statements.				
9. ✦	**Thank the previous employer and end the phone call in a kind manner.**				

Name: _____

Date: _____

Document: Enter the correct information in the chart below.

Grading

Points Earned	_____		
Points Possible	_____	63	63
Percent Grade (Points Earned/Points Possible)	_____		
PASS:	_____	❏ YES ❏ NO ❏ N/A	❏ YES ❏ NO ❏ N/A

Instructor Sign-Off

Instructor: _____ Date: _____

Procedure 22-5:

Perform an Employee Evaluation

Objective: Perform an employee evaluation correctly within the time limit set by the instructor.

Supplies: Employee evaluation form, pen

Affective Behaviors: Affective behaviors provide a professional approach to a skill that enhances the patient encounter. These behaviors may also display sensitivity to a patient's rights and enhance communication. Pay close attention to these skills, which will be in **_bold, italicized_** font.

Notes to the Student

_____

_____

_____

_____

_____

_____

Skills Assessment Requirements

Read and familiarize yourself with the procedure; complete the minimum practice requirements. Document each MPR using proper charting technique. Complete each procedure within a reasonable amount of time, with a minimum of 85 percent accuracy.

POINT VALUE ✦ = 3–6 points ⋆ = 7–9 points		PRACTICE TRIAL	GRADED TRIAL # 1	GRADED TRIAL # 2	NOTES
1. ⋆	Before the evaluation meeting, ask the employee to complete a self-evaluation form on job performance. Be sure to include job performance goals for the next year.				
2. ✦	Meet with the employee *at a prearranged time and in a private room.*				
3. ✦	Compare the employee's self-evaluation form with your evaluation.				
4. ✦	Address any discrepancies between the two evaluations.				
5. ✦	*Address any areas of concern in performance or behavior while maintaining a professional persona.*				
6. ✦	Review the last evaluation's goals, and discuss progress toward those goals.				
7. ✦	Review the goals set for the next evaluation, and set timelines as needed.				
8. ✦	Discuss any pay raise associated with employee's performance.				
9. ⋆	Have the employee sign the employee evaluation.				
10. ✦	Place the evaluation in the employee's personnel file.				
11. ✦	*Raise any concerns about the performance evaluation with the physician.*				

Name: _____

Date: _____

Document: Enter the correct information in the chart below.

Grading

Points Earned	_____		
Points Possible	_____	72	72
Percent Grade (Points Earned/Points Possible)	_____		
PASS:	_____	❏ YES ❏ NO ❏ N/A	❏ YES ❏ NO ❏ N/A

Instructor Sign-Off

Instructor: _____ **Date:** _____

Procedure 22-6:

Discipline an Employee

Objective: Discipline an employee correctly within the time limit set by the instructor.

Supplies: Pen and paper

Affective Behaviors: Affective behaviors provide a professional approach to a skill that enhances the patient encounter. These behaviors may also display sensitivity to a patient's rights and enhance communication. Pay close attention to these skills, which will be in ***bold, italicized*** font.

Notes to the Student

_____

_____

_____

_____

_____

_____

Skills Assessment Requirements

Read and familiarize yourself with the procedure; complete the minimum practice requirements. Document each MPR using proper charting technique. Complete each procedure within a reasonable amount of time, with a minimum of 85 percent accuracy.

Name: _____

Date: _____

POINT VALUE ✦ = 3–6 points ⋆ = 7–9 points		PRACTICE TRIAL	GRADED TRIAL #1	GRADED TRIAL #2	NOTES
1. ⋆	**Verify all facts before meeting with the employee.**				
2. ✦	Write a disciplinary notice that contains the reason for the discipline and the action to be taken by the office and/or by the employee as a result.				
3. ✦	Request a meeting with the employee.				
4. ✦	**Hold the employee meeting in a private room.**				
5. ✦	Let the employee know the reason for the meeting.				
6. ✦	Discuss the disciplinary action being levied on the employee. **This should be done in a calm voice.**				
7. ✦	Discuss your expectations of the employee.				
8. ✦	Discuss the outcome if the employee's behavior does not change. **It is important not to threaten, but rather state the facts of the situation.**				
9. ⋆	Ask the employee to sign the disciplinary statement.				
10. ⋆	If the employee refuses to sign the statement, make a note on the statement of "Contents reviewed with employee. Employee refused to sign." Sign your signature and date the document.				

Name: _____

Date: _____

		PRACTICE TRIAL	GRADED TRIAL # 1	GRADED TRIAL # 2	NOTES
11. ✦	Place the statement in the employee's personnel record.				
12. ✦	Agree to a future date on which you will meet with the employee to discuss progress.				
13. ★	***Inform the physician of the meeting's outcome.***				

Name: _____

Date: _____

Document: Enter the correct information in the chart below.

Grading

Points Earned	_____		
Points Possible	_____	90	90
Percent Grade (Points Earned/Points Possible)	_____		
PASS:	_____	❏ YES ❏ NO ❏ N/A	❏ YES ❏ NO ❏ N/A

Instructor Sign-Off

Instructor: _____ **Date:** _____

Procedure 22-7:

Terminate an Employee

Objective: Terminate an employee correctly within the time limit set by the instructor.

Supplies: Pen and paper

Affective Behaviors: Affective behaviors provide a professional approach to a skill that enhances the patient encounter. These behaviors may also display sensitivity to a patient's rights and enhance communication. Pay close attention to these skills, which will be in **_bold, italicized_** font.

Notes to the Student

_____

_____

_____

_____

_____

_____

Skills Assessment Requirements

Read and familiarize yourself with the procedure; complete the minimum practice requirements. Document each MPR using proper charting technique. Complete each procedure within a reasonable amount of time, with a minimum of 85 percent accuracy.

Document: Enter the correct information in the chart below.

Grading

Points Earned	_____		
Points Possible	_____	30	30
Percent Grade (Points Earned/Points Possible)	_____		
PASS:	_____	❏ YES ❏ NO ❏ N/A	❏ YES ❏ NO ❏ N/A

Instructor Sign-Off

Instructor: _____ **Date:** _____

Procedure 23-2:

Developing an Exposure Control Plan

Objective: Develop an exposure control plan within the time limit set by the instructor.

Supplies: List of personal protective equipment within the office, training manual

Affective Behaviors: Affective behaviors provide a professional approach to a skill that enhances the patient encounter. These behaviors may also display sensitivity to a patient's rights and enhance communication. Pay close attention to these skills, which will be in **_bold, italicized_** font.

Notes to the Student

_____

_____

_____

_____

_____

_____

Skills Assessment Requirements

Read and familiarize yourself with the procedure; complete the minimum practice requirements. Document each MPR using proper charting technique. Complete each procedure within a reasonable amount of time, with a minimum of 85 percent accuracy.

POINT VALUE ✦ = 3–6 points ⋆ = 7–9 points		PRACTICE TRIAL	GRADED TRIAL #1	GRADED TRIAL #2	NOTES
1. ✦	List each piece of personal protective equipment in the office.				
2. ✦	List the situations when each piece of equipment should/must be used.				
3. ⋆	**Hold an in-office training session to review each item and to discuss its use. Discuss the use in terms understood by all in the office.**				
4. ✦	Demonstrate each item's use.				
5. ✦	**Discuss how the office can reduce or eliminate exposures in the office.**				
6. ✦	**Discuss the steps the employees should take in the event of exposure.**				
7. ⋆	Document everything discussed at the meeting, and **distribute copies to all staff.**				

Document: Enter the correct information in the chart below.

Grading

Points Earned	_____		
Points Possible	_____	48	48
Percent Grade (Points Earned/Points Possible)	_____		
PASS:	_____	❏ YES ❏ NO ❏ N/A	❏ YES ❏ NO ❏ N/A

Instructor Sign-Off

Instructor: _____   **Date:** _____

Procedure 24-1:

Complete a History Form

Objective: The student will be able to complete a patient history form.

Supplies: Chart, file folder for chart, patient history form, black or blue ink pen

Affective Behaviors: Affective behaviors provide a professional approach to a skill that enhances the patient encounter. These behaviors may also display sensitivity to a patient's rights and enhance communication. Pay close attention to these skills, which will be in **bold, *italicized*** font.

Notes to the Student

_____

_____

_____

_____

_____

_____

Skills Assessment Requirements

Read and familiarize yourself with the procedure; complete the minimum practice requirements. Document each MPR using proper charting technique. Complete each procedure within a reasonable amount of time, with a minimum of 85 percent accuracy.

Name: _____

Date: _____

POINT VALUE ✦ = 3–6 points ⭑ = 7–9 points		PRACTICE TRIAL	GRADED TRIAL # 1	GRADED TRIAL # 2	NOTES
1. ⭑	*Greet the patient in a formal or age-appropriate manner. Introduce yourself by stating your name and indicating that you are a medical assistant.*				
2. ✦	Explain the health history form. Explain to the patient or parent that additional information beyond the original questions is always important and can be added.				
3. ✦	Observe patient's body language and *respond appropriately or tactfully to encourage open sharing of medical information.*				
4. ✦	The order of interview for the patient history form follows the order of the form unless office policy dictates otherwise.				
5. ✦	Instruct the patient to fill in the patient identification section. Review it to *make sure the information is complete.*				

		PRACTICE TRIAL	GRADED TRIAL # 1	GRADED TRIAL # 2	NOTES
6. ∗	Use open-ended questions to obtain details of the patient's CC, or present illness, such as: • How long have the symptoms been occurring? • Where do the symptoms occur? • What activity brings on the symptoms or makes the symptoms worse? • Do the symptoms occur suddenly or gradually? • What activity helps the symptom(s) disappear or lessen? • When symptoms occur, how long do they last?				
7. ✦	Proceed through the questions about past medical history, family medical history, and social/occupational history as presented on the patient history form.				

Name: _____

Date: _____

Document: Enter the appropriate information in the chart below.

Grading

Points Earned	_____		
Points Possible	_____	48	48
Percent Grade (Points Earned/Points Possible)	_____		
PASS:	_____	❏ YES ❏ NO ❏ N/A	❏ YES ❏ NO ❏ N/A

Instructor Sign-Off

Instructor: _____ Date: _____

Procedure 24-2:

Document a Clinical Visit and Procedure

Objective: The student should be able accurately to document a clinical visit or procedure.

Supplies: Patient chart, narrative or progress note forms to be added to the chart, black or blue ink pen

Affective Behaviors: Affective behaviors provide a professional approach to a skill that enhances the patient encounter. These behaviors may also display sensitivity to a patient's rights and enhance communication. Pay close attention to these skills, which will be in **_bold, italicized_** font.

Notes to the Student

_____

_____

_____

_____

_____

_____

Skills Assessment Requirements

Read and familiarize yourself with the procedure; complete the minimum practice requirements. Document each MPR using proper charting technique. Complete each procedure within a reasonable amount of time, with a minimum of 85 percent accuracy.

Name: _____

Date: _____

POINT VALUE ✦ = 3–6 points ⋆ = 7–9 points		**PRACTICE TRIAL**	**GRADED TRIAL # 1**	**GRADED TRIAL # 2**	**NOTES**
1. ⋆	Verify that the chart is the correct chart for the patient being seen.				
2. ✦	If notes are insufficient for documentation, add the appropriate form.				
3. ✦	With narrative charting or SOAP charting, avoid leaving blank areas.				
4. ✦	**Write the date and time in the left-hand column of the notes.**				
5. ✦	**Continue writing in the charting format used by the medical office.**				
6. ⋆	**Document immediately after performance of procedures.**				
7. ✦	Use only standard, accepted abbreviations and describe clinical observations during performance of the procedure.				
8. ✦	**Document only facts. DO NOT make diagnoses or judgmental statements.**				
9. ⋆	**Sign your name and add your title at the end of the documentation.**				

Document: Enter the appropriate information in the chart below.

Grading

Points Earned	_____		
Points Possible	_____	63	63
Percent Grade (Points Earned/Points Possible)	_____		
PASS:	_____	❑ YES ❑ NO ❑ N/A	❑ YES ❑ NO ❑ N/A

Instructor Sign-Off

Instructor: _____ **Date:** _____

Name: _____

Date: _____

Procedure 25-1:

Hand Washing

Objective: The student, using the supplies and equipment listed below, will demonstrate how to wash hands following medically aseptic technique.

Supplies: Soap (bar or pump), paper towels, waste container, nail brush or cuticle stick

Notes to the Student

_____

_____

_____

_____

_____

_____

Skills Assessment Requirements

Read and familiarize yourself with the procedure; complete the minimum practice requirements. Document each MPR using proper charting technique. Complete each procedure within a reasonable amount of time, with a minimum of 85 percent accuracy.

POINT VALUE ✦ = 3–6 points ⋆ = 7–9 points	PRACTICE TRIAL	GRADED TRIAL # 1	GRADED TRIAL # 2	NOTES
1. ⋆ Remove and secure most jewelry. Wedding bands and professional watches are allowed. Push the watch higher than your wrist. Avoid touching the contaminated sink front with your uniform.				
2. ✦ With a paper towel, turn on the water and adjust to a warm temperature. The water should run continuously until you have finished the procedure. Discard the paper towel.				
3. ✦ With your hands and fingers lower than your elbows, wet your wrists and hands.				
4. ⋆ Apply soap and scrub lather over the hands and fingers, between the fingers, under and around the nails, and rinse. Apply soap and lather to the wrists and forearms. The purpose of this washing order is to wash the dirtiest areas first. A circular motion and friction rubbing will loosen dirt and microorganisms. If you are using bar soap, rinse it before returning it to the soap dish.				
5. ✦ Use the cuticle stick or nail brush to clean your nails. If you are wearing a wedding band, scrub around it with the nail brush.				
6. ✦ Rinse off the lather, keeping your hands in a downward position. Avoid splashing and touching the sink or faucets.				
7. ✦ Dry your hands with a paper towel and discard it.				
8. ✦ Turn off the faucet with another paper towel and discard it; using a new paper towel prevents the contamination of clean hands.				

Name: _____

Date: _____

Document: Enter the appropriate information in the chart below.

Grading

Points Earned	_____		
Points Possible	_____	54	54
Percent Grade (Points Earned/Points Possible)	_____		
PASS:	_____	❑ YES ❑ NO ❑ N/A	❑ YES ❑ NO ❑ N/A

Instructor Sign-Off

Instructor: _____ **Date:** _____

Procedure 25-2:

Nonsterile Gloving

Objective: The student, using the supplies and equipment listed below, will demonstrate the application, removal, and disposal of nonsterile gloves following medically aseptic technique.

Supplies: Nonsterile gloves, waste receptacle

Notes to the Student

_____

_____

_____

_____

_____

_____

Skills Assessment Requirements

Read and familiarize yourself with the procedure; complete the minimum practice requirements. Document each MPR using proper charting technique. Complete each procedure within a reasonable amount of time, with a minimum of 85 percent accuracy.

Name: _____

Date: _____

POINT VALUE ✦ = 3–6 points ⋆ = 7–9 points		PRACTICE TRIAL	GRADED TRIAL # 1	GRADED TRIAL # 2	NOTES
1. ✦	Wash and dry your hands.				
2. ⋆	Choose gloves of the right size. They should not be so loose that they fall off during a procedure. If they are too tight, they may tear and new gloves will have to be applied.				
3. ✦	Take one glove from the box and pull it on over your hand to the wrist.				
4. ✦	Take a second glove and pull it on to the wrist				
5. ✦	Adjust the gloves so that the wrists are covered.				
6. ✦	To remove the first glove, grasp the outside of the glove at the wrist with the other gloved hand and pull down. This motion will keep the contaminated surface inside and is called the "glove touch glove." Discard the first glove immediately.				
7. ✦	With your ungloved hand, reach inside the second glove. Grasp the inside of the glove and pull it down and off. This second glove removal also keeps the contaminated surface on the inside and is called "ungloved hand touch hand inside before removing." Discard the second glove immediately.				
8. ✦	Wash and dry your hands.				

Document: Enter the appropriate information in the chart below.

Grading

Points Earned	_____		
Points Possible	_____	51	51
Percent Grade (Points Earned/Points Possible)	_____		
PASS:	_____	❏ YES ❏ NO ❏ N/A	❏ YES ❏ NO ❏ N/A

Instructor Sign-Off

Instructor: _____ **Date:** _____

Procedure 26-1:

Sanitization

Objective: The student, using the supplies and equipment listed below, will demonstrate performance of manually cleaning and sanitizing of instruments.

Supplies: Contaminated instruments, basin for soaking instruments, examination gloves, utility gloves, neutral low-suds detergent, scrubbing brush, paper towel, cotton towel

Notes to the Student

_____

_____

_____

_____

_____

_____

Skills Assessment Requirements

Read and familiarize yourself with the procedure; complete the minimum practice requirements. Document each MPR using proper charting technique. Complete each procedure within a reasonable amount of time, with a minimum of 85 percent accuracy.

POINT VALUE ✦ = 3–6 points ⋆ = 7–9 points	PRACTICE TRIAL	GRADED TRIAL # 1	GRADED TRIAL # 2	NOTES
1. ⋆ With examination and utility gloves on your hands, place the contaminated instruments in an empty basin, cover it with a cotton towel, and transport it to the cleaning area. Remove the towel and add disinfectant or water with detergent to the basin. After the patient is discharged, clean, disinfect, and supply the room for the next patient.				
2. ✦ In the instrument cleaning area, drain off the disinfectant or detergent and remove the instruments. Carefully wipe away blood and/or any tissue **debris.** Hold the instruments by their finger openings when possible.				
3. ✦ Place the instruments in a basin with the recommended amount of cleaning agent and water.				
4. ✦ Cleaning one instrument at a time, use a soft brush on all serrated and smooth edges, grooves, and opened hinges.				
5. ✦ Rinse all the instruments with hot water.				
6. ✦ Dry each instrument with a paper towel and allow to air-dry completely on a cotton towel. Lubricate the hinges with a water-based lubricant.				
7. ⋆ Follow the manufacturer's directions for disposing of cleaning solution. *Do not reuse.*				

Name: _____

Date: _____

		PRACTICE TRIAL	GRADED TRIAL # 1	GRADED TRIAL # 2	NOTES
8. ✦	Remove the gloves and wash your hands.				
9. ✦	Inspect each instrument for defects and proper function. Package the instruments as needed to ready for sterilization.				
	Ultrasonic Cleansing:				
10. ⋆	With examination and utility gloves on your hands, prepare the cleaning solution for the ultrasonic cleaner as directed by the manufacturer. Observe all MSDS safety and accidental spill precautions.				
11. ✦	Place instruments made of different metals in separate ultrasonic cleaning loads.				
12. ✦	Place the instruments in the ultrasonic cleaner with their hinges open and sharp edges not touching other instruments. Make sure that all the instruments are covered with the ultrasonic cleaning solution. Turn on the ultrasonic cleaner.				
13. ⋆	When the recommended cleaning time has passed, remove the instruments and rinse each one with hot tap water.				
14. ✦	Dry each instrument with a paper towel and allow to air dry completely on a cotton towel. Lubricate the hinges with a water-based lubricant.				

		PRACTICE TRIAL	GRADED TRIAL # 1	GRADED TRIAL # 2	NOTES
15. ✦	Follow the manufacturer's directions for changing the cleaning solution.				
16. ✦	Remove the gloves and wash your hands.				
17. ✦	Inspect each instrument for defects and proper function. Package the instruments as needed to ready for sterilization.				

Document: Enter the appropriate information in the chart below.

Grading

Points Earned	_____		
Points Possible	_____	114	114
Percent Grade (Points Earned/Points Possible)	_____		
PASS:	_____	❑ YES ❑ NO ❑ N/A	❑ YES ❑ NO ❑ N/A

Instructor Sign-Off

Name: _____

Date: _____

Procedure 26-2:

Disinfection

Objective: The student, using the supplies and equipment listed below, will demonstrate how to perform the steps of disinfection correctly and safely.

Supplies: Contaminated articles, MSDS, disposable gloves, utility gloves, chemical disinfectant, soaking container, paper towels, cotton towel

Affective Behaviors: Affective behaviors provide a professional approach to a skill that enhances the patient encounter. These behaviors may also display sensitivity to a patient's rights and enhance communication. Pay close attention to these skills, which will be in **_bold, italicized_** font.

Notes to the Student

_____

_____

_____

_____

_____

_____

Skills Assessment Requirements

Read and familiarize yourself with the procedure; complete the minimum practice requirements. Document each MPR using proper charting technique. Complete each procedure within a reasonable amount of time, with a minimum of 85 percent accuracy.

POINT VALUE ✦ = 3–6 points ⋆ = 7–9 points		PRACTICE TRIAL	GRADED TRIAL #1	GRADED TRIAL #2	NOTES
1. ⋆	**Review the MSDS, noting potential hazards, how to clean accidental spills, and whether PPE should be worn.**				
2. ✦	Apply disposable gloves to place the contaminated items into the basin. Then apply an additional layer of utility gloves.				
3. ✦	Complete the sanitizing steps in Procedure 8-1. Remember to cover the basin of contaminated instruments with a cloth towel when you move them to the cleaning area.				
4. ⋆	Check the expiration date of the disinfectant and follow the manufacturer's directions for mixing and use.				
5. ✦	With gloves on, completely immerse the contaminated articles in the container of disinfectant. Cover the container and soak the instruments for the length of time recommended by the manufacturer.				
6. ✦	Remove and rinse each instrument thoroughly. Dry the instruments with paper towels.				
7. ✦	Place the disinfected instruments on muslin or into sterilizing packets for the autoclave.				

Document: Enter the appropriate information in the chart below.

Grading

Points Earned	_____		
Points Possible	_____	48	48
Percent Grade (Points Earned/Points Possible)	_____		
PASS:	_____	❏ YES ❏ NO ❏ N/A	❏ YES ❏ NO ❏ N/A

Instructor Sign-Off

Instructor: _____ **Date:** _____

Procedure 26-3:

Wrapping Surgical Instruments for Autoclave Sterilization

Objective: The student, using the supplies and equipment listed below, will demonstrate how to package and wrap instruments and supplies to be placed in the autoclave correctly.

Supplies: Dry wrapping paper, muslin cloth, or sealable bags, sanitized and disinfected items to be sterilized, sterilization indicators for interior and exterior of packages, marker pen

Notes to the Student

_____

_____

_____

_____

_____

_____

Skills Assessment Requirements

Read and familiarize yourself with the procedure; complete the minimum practice requirements. Document each MPR using proper charting technique. Complete each procedure within a reasonable amount of time, with a minimum of 85 percent accuracy.

Name: _____

Date: _____

POINT VALUE ✦ = 3–6 points ⋆ = 7–9 points		PRACTICE TRIAL	GRADED TRIAL # 1	GRADED TRIAL # 2	NOTES
1. ✦	Place the sanitized items to be sterilized in the center of the dry wrapping paper, muslin, or sealable bag. Place an indicator tape inside the package. The sealable bag may need to be sealed if it is not manufacturer-prepared.				
2. ⋆	For cloth or paper packaging, fold up one corner to cover the items. Double-back a small fold to use as a pull-corner for unwrapping. Do the same fold and double-back fold for the right side and left side. Fold the last side once toward the center and tuck the corner under before applying sterilization indicator tape.				
3. ✦	Use the marker to label the tape with the date, contents, and preparer's initials.				

Name: _____

Date: _____

Document: Enter the appropriate information in the chart below.

Grading

Points Earned	_____		
Points Possible	_____	21	21
Percent Grade (Points Earned/Points Possible)	_____		
PASS:	_____	❏ YES ❏ NO ❏ N/A	❏ YES ❏ NO ❏ N/A

Instructor Sign-Off

Instructor: _____ **Date:** _____

Name: _____

Date: _____

Procedure 26-4:

Loading and Operating an Autoclave

Objective: The student, using the supplies and equipment listed below, will demonstrate loading and operating an autoclave correctly and safely to ensure complete sterilization.

Supplies: Wrapped or unwrapped sanitized and disinfected instruments, distilled water, heat-resistant gloves, manual or automatic autoclave, manufacturer's instruction manual, sterile transfer forceps, storage containers or shelf areas

Notes to the Student

_____

_____

_____

_____

_____

_____

Skills Assessment Requirements

Read and familiarize yourself with the procedure; complete the minimum practice requirements. Document each MPR using proper charting technique. Complete each procedure within a reasonable amount of time, with a minimum of 85 percent accuracy.

POINT VALUE ✦ = 3–6 points ⋆ = 7–9 points	PRACTICE TRIAL	GRADED TRIAL # 1	GRADED TRIAL # 2	NOTES
1. ✦ Wash your hands and assemble materials.				
2. ✦ Check the level of distilled water in the autoclave reservoir and fill as necessary.				
3. ⋆ Load the autoclave, asking yourself the following questions: • Are the autoclave trays 1 inch apart? • Are small packs 1 to 3 inches apart? • Are any of the packs touching the inside of the autoclave chamber? • Are glassware and jars on their sides? • Are dressings and sterilization pouches in a vertical position, on their sides? • Are any materials leaning against plastic items? • For a mixed load of porous and nonporous materials, are materials such as dressings on the top shelf and instruments on the lower shelf?				
4. ✦ Close and latch the door. Turn on the autoclave.				
5. ✦ Sterilization time starts when the correct pressure and temperature have been reached.				
6. ✦ After steam pressure has been manually or automatically released, open the autoclave door slightly to allows the load to dry. Larger packs with dressings may take 45 to 60 minutes to dry.				

	PRACTICE TRIAL	GRADED TRIAL # 1	GRADED TRIAL # 2	NOTES
7. ✦ Wearing heat-resistant gloves, remove the dry packages. Inspect for holes, tears, and indicator tape color change. Use the sterile transfer forceps to remove single instruments or items to a clean container. Place sterile items toward the back of the stock so that the oldest dated materials are used first. Avoid storing in cool areas that may cause condensation, make the materials damp, and require additional wrapping and sterilizing.				
8. ✦ Remove the gloves and wash your hands.				
9. ★ Record the date, autoclave load contents, and use of sterilization indicators and quality controls in the sterilization control log.				

Name: _____

Date: _____

Document: Enter the appropriate information in the chart below.

Grading

Points Earned	_____		
Points Possible	_____	60	60
Percent Grade (Points Earned/Points Possible)	_____		
PASS:	_____	❏ YES ❏ NO ❏ N/A	❏ YES ❏ NO ❏ N/A

Instructor Sign-Off

Instructor: _____ Date: _____

Procedure 26-5:

Pour Sterile Solution onto a Sterile Field

Objective: Correctly pour a sterile solution onto a sterile field.

Supplies: Bottle of sterile solution, sterile stainless steel bowl or container, sterile field, and a waste container

Affective Behaviors: Affective behaviors provide a professional approach to a skill that enhances the patient encounter. These behaviors may also display sensitivity to a patient's rights and enhance communication. Pay close attention to these skills, which will be in **_bold, italicized_** font.

Notes to the Student

_____

_____

_____

_____

_____

_____

Skills Assessment Requirements

Read and familiarize yourself with the procedure; complete the minimum practice requirements. Document each MPR using proper charting technique. Complete each procedure within a reasonable amount of time, with a minimum of 85 percent accuracy.

POINT VALUE ✦ = 3–6 points ⋆ = 7–9 points	PRACTICE TRIAL	GRADED TRIAL # 1	GRADED TRIAL # 2	NOTES
1. ✦ Wash your hands.				
2. ✦ Gather your supplies.				
3. ⋆ **Read the label to ensure that you have the correct solution.**				
4. ✦ Check the expiration date on the solution.				
5. ✦ Place the palm of your hand over the label to avoid staining the label (Figure 26-16).				
6. ⋆ Remove the cap by touching only the outside and place the cap on a flat surface with the open end up.				
7. ✦ Pour a small amount of the solution into a waste container to rinse the lip of the bottle.				
8. ⋆ Without splashing the solution, pour the proper amount of solution into the sterile container located on the sterile field.				
9. ⋆ Replace the cap on the container without contaminating it.				
10. ⋆ **Check the label for a final time to ensure that you have poured the correct solution.**				

Document: Enter the appropriate information in the chart below.

Grading

Points Earned	_____		
Points Possible	_____	75	75
Percent Grade (Points Earned/Points Possible)	_____		
PASS:	_____	❏ YES ❏ NO ❏ N/A	❏ YES ❏ NO ❏ N/A

Instructor Sign-Off

Instructor: _____ **Date:** _____

Procedure 26-6:

Opening a Sterile Surgical Pack to Create a Sterile Field

Objective: The student, using the supplies and equipment listed below, will demonstrate how to use sterile technique to open a sterile surgical pack for a sterile field.

Supplies: Mayo stand, sterile packet(s), sterile transfer forceps, sterile gloves, sterile towels or drapes, waste container

Notes to the Student

_____

_____

_____

_____

_____

_____

Skills Assessment Requirements

Read and familiarize yourself with the procedure; complete the minimum practice requirements. Document each MPR using proper charting technique. Complete each procedure within a reasonable amount of time, with a minimum of 85 percent accuracy.

POINT VALUE ✦ = 3–6 points ⋆ = 7–9 points		PRACTICE TRIAL	GRADED TRIAL # 1	GRADED TRIAL # 2	NOTES
1. ✦	Wash your hands and assemble the equipment.				
2. ✦	Adjust the height of the Mayo stand to a comfortable working position.				
3. ✦	Position the sterile surgical pack on the Mayo stand so that the top flap will open away from you.				
4. ✦	Remove the sterilization indicator tape from the pack, note whether or not the appropriate color change occurred to indicate sterility, and discard.				
5. ✦	Pull the top flap away from you and down to hang over the edge of the Mayo stand. Pull each of the side flaps away from the packet and over the edge.				
6. ⋆	Without reaching over the sterile field, bring the last flap toward you and down to hang over the edge. Do not touch your body to any part of the sterile field while opening the pack or at any time during a sterile procedure.				

Name: _____

Date: _____

		PRACTICE TRIAL	GRADED TRIAL # 1	GRADED TRIAL # 2	NOTES
7. *	The inside of the pack is now the sterile field. To move items on the sterile field, use sterile transfer forceps. • To add items to a sterile field, open other packages without touching the inner side of the package or contents, then dump the contents on the sterile field without crossing or touching it. • To open the inner package of another sterile pack during the procedure, a person with clean hands may open the outer package so that a person with sterile gloves may take the inner packet of instruments and supplies.				
8. ◆	Cover the tray with sterile towels or drape until ready to use. This is done by opening a pack of sterile gloves and a pack of sterile drapes or towels, then putting on the sterile gloves to unfold the drape or towel over the sterile field. Some sterile packets come with material for draping the sterile field.				

Document: Enter the appropriate information in the chart below.

Grading

Points Earned	_____		
Points Possible	_____	54	54
Percent Grade (Points Earned/Points Possible)	_____		
PASS:	_____	❏ YES ❏ NO ❏ N/A	❏ YES ❏ NO ❏ N/A

Instructor Sign-Off

Instructor: _____   **Date:** _____

Name: _____

Date: _____

Procedure 26-7:

Using Sterile Transfer Forceps

Objective: The student, using the supplies and equipment listed below, will demonstrate how to move sterile instruments and supplies within a sterile field, onto a sterile field, or into a sterile gloved hand without contaminating.

Supplies: Transfer forceps, sterile tray set upon a Mayo stand, forceps, container two-thirds full of Cidex or other sterilant, sterile 4 × 4 gauze package, instrument or supply pack for use with sterile transfer forceps

Notes to the Student

_____

_____

_____

_____

_____

_____

Skills Assessment Requirements

Read and familiarize yourself with the procedure; complete the minimum practice requirements. Document each MPR using proper charting technique. Complete each procedure within a reasonable amount of time, with a minimum of 85 percent accuracy.

POINT VALUE ✦ = 3–6 points ⋆ = 7–9 points		PRACTICE TRIAL	GRADED TRIAL #1	GRADED TRIAL #2	NOTES
1. ✦	Open the 4 × 4 gauze package using sterile technique and lay it on the countertop or Mayo stand.				
2. ✦	Grasp the forceps handles, keeping the tips together. Remove the forceps vertically from the container without touching the sides.				
3. ⋆	Touch the forceps tips to the gauze 4 × 4 to dry them. Do not allow the forceps to touch the sterile field. Holding them vertically, pick up and move an item from the open pack to the sterile field. To move a sterile item on the sterile field, keep the forceps vertical, pick up the item, and lift it to the desired location without touching the sterile field.				
4. ✦	Place the transfer forceps back into the standing container without touching the sides.				

Name: _____

Date: _____

Document: Enter the appropriate information in the chart below.

Grading

Points Earned	_____		
Points Possible	_____	27	27
Percent Grade (Points Earned/Points Possible)	_____		
PASS:	_____	❑ YES ❑ NO ❑ N/A	❑ YES ❑ NO ❑ N/A

Instructor Sign-Off

Instructor: _____ **Date:** _____

Name: _____

Date: _____

Procedure 26-8:

Performing a Sterile Scrub (Surgical Hand Washing)

Objective: The student, using the supplies and equipment listed below, will demonstrate how to perform surgical hand washing using sterile technique correctly.

Supplies: Germicidal liquid soap in dispenser, large wall clock, sink with hand, knee, or foot on/off controls, sterile towel packet, sterile scrub sponge, orangewood stick or nail file

Notes to the Student

_____

_____

_____

_____

_____

_____

Skills Assessment Requirements

Read and familiarize yourself with the procedure; complete the minimum practice requirements. Document each MPR using proper charting technique. Complete each procedure within a reasonable amount of time, with a minimum of 85 percent accuracy.

Name: _____

Date: _____

		PRACTICE TRIAL	GRADED TRIAL #1	GRADED TRIAL #2	NOTES
POINT VALUE ✦ = 3–6 points ⋆ = 7–9 points					
1. ✦	Without touching the inside, open the sterile towel packet some distance from potential water spray.				
2. ✦	Remove all jewelry from your hands and wrists. Use an orangewood stick or nail file to remove dirt from under your fingernails.				
3. ✦	Turn on the water with hand, knee, or foot controls and adjust the temperature. Wet your arm from the fingertips to the elbows.				
4. ⋆	Apply liquid soap to your hands and lower arms. For 5 minutes, use a circular motion to create lather, starting from the fingertips and working toward the elbows. Be sure to wash between the fingers and under the fingernails.				
5. ⋆	Rinse the lather from your arm, beginning at the fingertips and proceeding to the elbows. Keep hands above your elbows.				
6. ✦	Repeat the process, applying liquid soap to your hands and lower arms. Scrub from the fingertips to the elbows with the sponge for 3 minutes.				
7. ✦	Rinse thoroughly and leave the water running. Use a sterile towel to dry your hands.				
8. ⋆	Use the towel to turn off a hand-controlled faucet or, if necessary, use your elbow. Otherwise, release the foot pedal or move the knee control to turn off the water.				

Document: Enter the appropriate information in the chart below.

Grading

Points Earned	_____		
Points Possible	_____	57	57
Percent Grade (Points Earned/Points Possible)	_____		
PASS:	_____	❏ YES ❏ NO ❏ N/A	❏ YES ❏ NO ❏ N/A

Instructor Sign-Off

Instructor: _____ **Date:** _____

Procedure 26-9:

Glove While Wearing a Sterile Gown

Objective: Correctly apply sterile gloves while wearing a sterile gown.

Supplies: Sterile gloves, opened on a sterile field, and a sterile gown, mask, goggles, and hair cover

Notes to the Student

_____

_____

_____

_____

_____

_____

Skills Assessment Requirements

Read and familiarize yourself with the procedure; complete the minimum practice requirements. Document each MPR using proper charting technique. Complete each procedure within a reasonable amount of time, with a minimum of 85 percent accuracy.

POINT VALUE ✦ = 3–6 points ✶ = 7–9 points	PRACTICE TRIAL	GRADED TRIAL #1	GRADED TRIAL #2	NOTES
1. ✦ A sterile glove package should be opened up and placed on a sterile field.				
2. ✶ Using your dominant hand, and keeping it within the cuff of the left sleeve, pick up the glove, from the inner wrap of the glove package, by grasping the folded cuff with your thumb and forefinger.				
3. ✦ Place the glove in the palm of your nondominant hand, with glove fingers pointing to the elbows.				
4. ✦ With both hands, pinch the rolled edges of the glove and stretch the glove up and over the gown cuff.				
5. ✦ Pull the glove over your hand as you push through the gown cuff. Remember that the bare hand will only touch the inside of the glove. Gently slide your fingers in the glove.				
6. ✶ Unroll the glove cuff so that it covers the stockinette sleeve cuff.				
7. ✦ With your nondominant hand gloved, place your fingers under the cuff of the second glove.				
8. ✦ Pull the glove over your hand as you push through the gown cuff.				
9. ✦ Adjust the cuffs and make sure that each gown cuff is secured and covered completely by the cuff of the glove. Lastly, adjust the fingers of the glove as necessary so that they fit snugly.				

Document: Enter the appropriate information in the chart below.

Grading

Points Earned	_____		
Points Possible	_____	53	53
Percent Grade (Points Earned/Points Possible)	_____		
PASS:	_____	❏ YES ❏ NO ❏ N/A	❏ YES ❏ NO ❏ N/A

Instructor Sign-Off

Instructor: _____ **Date:** _____

Name: _____

Date: _____

Procedure 26-10:

Sterile Gloving and Glove Removal

Objective: The student, using the supplies and equipment listed below, will demonstrate how to apply gloves using sterile technique correctly.

Supplies: Sterile glove pack in correct size

Notes to the Student

_____

_____

_____

_____

_____

_____

Skills Assessment Requirements

Read and familiarize yourself with the procedure; complete the minimum practice requirements. Document each MPR using proper charting technique. Complete each procedure within a reasonable amount of time, with a minimum of 85 percent accuracy.

POINT VALUE ✦ = 3–6 points ⋆ = 7–9 points		PRACTICE TRIAL	GRADED TRIAL # 1	GRADED TRIAL # 2	NOTES
1. ✦	Open the pack of sterile gloves, touching only the outside of the pack. Touching only the outside of the inner packet, turn the cuff end toward you.				
2. ⋆	Open the inner packet by pulling each edge to the side. The gloves will be lying on the sterile field created by opening the inner pack. *Do not* touch the inside of the inner pack.				
3. ✦	Perform a sterile scrub.				
4. ⋆	The following directions are for a right-handed person. Perform the opposite actions if you are left handed. With the thumb and fingers of the left hand, grasp only the folded-back cuff area (skin to skin: your skin touches what is to be the inside of the glove). While dangling the glove with the left hand, carefully slide the right hand in. *Do not* touch the outside of the glove with your ungloved hand. Keep your hands above your waist and in front of you.				
5. ⋆	To don the second sterile glove, slide the fingers of your gloved hand under the cuff (sterile to sterile: the outside of the gloved hand is sterile against the sterile outside of the second glove). With the second glove "hooked" by the fingers of your gloved hand, slide your second hand into the glove. Continue to keep your hands above your waist and in front of you.				

		PRACTICE TRIAL	GRADED TRIAL # 1	GRADED TRIAL # 2	NOTES
6. ✦	Adjust the finger and thumb fit of the gloves (sterile to sterile).				
7. ✦	To remove the gloves, use the fingers of one gloved hand to grasp the other glove at the wrist. Pull the glove over itself and hold it in the palm of the gloved hand. Slide the fingers of the of the ungloved hand under the cuff of the remaining glove, grasp the inside, and pull it down over the glove and off the hand.				
8. ✦	Discard the gloves in a bio-hazard waste receptacle.				

Name: _____

Date: _____

Document: Enter the appropriate information in the chart below.

Grading

Points Earned	_____		
Points Possible	_____	57	57
Percent Grade (Points Earned/Points Possible)	_____		
PASS:	_____	❏ YES ❏ NO ❏ N/A	❏ YES ❏ NO ❏ N/A

Instructor Sign-Off

Instructor: _____   **Date:** _____

Procedure 27-1:

Demonstrate Safety Measures to Prepare, Administer, and Document Medication

Objective: Correctly and safely prepare, administer, and document medication.

Supplies: Written medication order, including name of patient, drug name, strength, dose, and route of medication, *Physician's Drug Reference* (PDR) or drug package insert, container of ordered medication, correct supplies for administering the drug, and patient chart

Affective Behaviors: Affective behaviors provide a professional approach to a skill that enhances the patient encounter. These behaviors may also display sensitivity to a patient's rights and enhance communication. Pay close attention to these skills, which will be in ***bold, italicized*** font.

Notes to the Student

_____

_____

_____

_____

_____

_____

Skills Assessment Requirements

Read and familiarize yourself with the procedure; complete the minimum practice requirements. Document each MPR using proper charting technique. Complete each procedure within a reasonable amount of time, with a minimum of 85 percent accuracy.

POINT VALUE ✦ = 3–6 points ⋆ = 7–9 points		PRACTICE TRIAL	GRADED TRIAL # 1	GRADED TRIAL # 2	NOTES
1. ⋆	Read the medication order and clarify the medication order with the physician, if needed.				
2. ✦	If unfamiliar with the drug, refer to the PDR or the package insert to determine the medication's function, usual dose, side effects, and any pertinent precautions or contraindications. **Follow the "six rights" to prevent errors.**				
3. ⋆	Based upon the information on the medication order and the medication on hand, calculate the dosage to match the medication order. Confirm the answer with the physician if you have any questions.				
4. ✦	Wash your hands.				
5. ✦	Dispense the medication in a well lit, quiet, low traffic area.				
6. ⋆	Perform the three checks to prevent errors: a. **Compare the written label with the label on the medication container or vial when you remove it from storage, check the expiration date and properly dispose of any expired medication.** b. **Compare the written order with the label on the medication container before dispensing or drawing up medication. Ensure that the strength on the label matches the medication order or that you dispense the correctly calculated dose.** c. **Compare the written order and the label on the medication container or vial before returning it to storage or discarding.**				

Name: _____

Date: _____

		PRACTICE TRIAL	GRADED TRIAL # 1	GRADED TRIAL # 2	NOTES
7. ✦	If at any time you have any doubts about the function of the medication, the dosage, or route of medication, or the possibility of an allergic reaction, *immediately* consult the physician.				
8. *	**Greet and identify the patient and escort him or her to the treatment area. Verify allergy information in the chart and ask the patient if they have any allergies.**				
9. ✦	Wash your hands and put on gloves.				
10. *	Administer the medication according to the medication order and **follow the "six rights" to prevent errors and ensure Occupational Safety and Health Administration (OSHA) precautions.**				
11. ✦	Provide patient education on the function of the drug administered, typical side effects, and dosage and storage information, if applicable. Refer to the physician if additional information is needed.				
12. *	Document the procedure. Include the date, time, medication, route, and amount administered. **Sign the entry with your name and credentials.** Follow the office policy for recording expiration date and lot number.				

Name: _____

Date: _____

Document: Enter the appropriate information in the chart below.

Grading

Points Earned	_____		
Points Possible	_____	90	90
Percent Grade (Points Earned/Points Possible)	_____		
PASS:	_____	❑ YES ❑ NO ❑ N/A	❑ YES ❑ NO ❑ N/A

Instructor Sign-Off

Instructor: _____   **Date:** _____

Procedure 27-2:

Demonstrate the Preparation of a Prescription for the Physician's Signature

Objective: The student should be able to prepare a prescription for the physician's signature.

Supplies: Physician's order for medication, patient chart, ink pen, computer if Rx is typed, blank prescription

Affective Behaviors: Affective behaviors provide a professional approach to a skill that enhances the patient encounter. These behaviors may also display sensitivity to a patient's rights and enhance communication. Pay close attention to these skills, which will be in ***bold, italicized*** font.

Notes to the Student

_____

_____

_____

_____

_____

_____

Skills Assessment Requirements

Read and familiarize yourself with the procedure; complete the minimum practice requirements. Document each MPR using proper charting technique. Complete each procedure within a reasonable amount of time, with a minimum of 85 percent accuracy.

POINT VALUE ✦ = 3–6 points ⋆ = 7–9 points		PRACTICE TRIAL	GRADED TRIAL # 1	GRADED TRIAL # 2	NOTES
1. ✦	Gather the equipment.				
2. ✦	Obtain the prescription information (name, dose, amount, frequency, refills) from the physician.				
3. ✦	**Correctly and legibly write out the prescription according to the information received from the physician.**				
4. ⋆	Document the procedure. Include the date, time, medication, strength, dose, frequency, and refills allowed. **Sign the entry with your name and credentials.** Some offices will want a photocopy of the written Rx.				

Name: _____

Date: _____

Document: Enter the appropriate information in the chart below.

Grading

Points Earned	_____		
Points Possible	_____	27	27
Percent Grade (Points Earned/Points Possible)	_____		
PASS:	_____	❏ YES ❏ NO ❏ N/A	❏ YES ❏ NO ❏ N/A

Instructor Sign-Off

Instructor: _____ Date: _____

Name: _____

Date: _____

Procedure 27-3:

Demonstrate Withdrawing Medication from an Ampule

Objective: The student, using the supplies and equipment listed below, will demonstrate how to withdraw medication from an ampule correctly.

Supplies: Sterile filter needle/syringe set, ampule of medication, sterile gauze 2 × 4s or 4 × 4s, alcohol wipes, gloves, sharps container, patient chart

Affective Behaviors: Affective behaviors provide a professional approach to a skill that enhances the patient encounter. These behaviors may also display sensitivity to a patient's rights and enhance communication. Pay close attention to these skills, which will be in **_bold, italicized_** font.

Notes to the Student

_____

_____

_____

_____

_____

_____

Skills Assessment Requirements

Read and familiarize yourself with the procedure; complete the minimum practice requirements. Document each MPR using proper charting technique. Complete each procedure within a reasonable amount of time, with a minimum of 85 percent accuracy.

POINT VALUE ✦ = 3–6 points ∗ = 7–9 points		PRACTICE TRIAL	GRADED TRIAL # 1	GRADED TRIAL # 2	NOTES
1. ✦	Wash your hands and gather equipment.				
2. ✦	**Check to make sure the medication matches the physician's order.** Calculate the dosage, if necessary. Look up information relating to the medication's function, usual doses, and side effects. Check for patient allergies.				
3. ✦	Check the medication label a second time against the physician's order.				
4. ∗	**Identify the patient, introduce yourself, and escort the patient to the treatment area.**				
5. ✦	Put on your gloves.				
6. ✦	Dislodge any medication that may be trapped in the ampule neck by holding the ampule by the neck and quickly flicking your wrist in a downward motion.				
7. ✦	Disinfect the ampule with an alcohol swab and check the label again for correct medication and dosage.				
8. ✦	Completely wrap the neck of the ampule with the sterile cotton gauze and snap off the top by pulling it toward you. Discard the top in a sharps container.				
9. ✦	With a filtered needle, withdraw the necessary medication amount. You can withdraw the medication with the ampule either inverted or not.				

	PRACTICE TRIAL	GRADED TRIAL # 1	GRADED TRIAL # 2	NOTES
10. * Change needles and discard the filtered needle into a sharps container.				
11. * Identify the patient.				
12. ✦ Administer the medication according to the physician's orders.				
13. ✦ Discard the used needle into the sharps container.				
14. ✦ Remove the gloves and wash your hands.				
15. * Document the procedure. Include date, time, site, medication, route, and amount administered. **Sign the entry with your name and credentials.** Follow office policy for recording the expiration date and lot number.				

Name: _____

Date: _____

Document: Enter the appropriate information in the chart below.

Grading

Points Earned	_____		
Points Possible	_____	102	102
Percent Grade (Points Earned/Points Possible)	_____		
PASS:	_____	❏ YES ❏ NO ❏ N/A	❏ YES ❏ NO ❏ N/A

Instructor Sign-Off

Instructor: _____ **Date:** _____

Procedure 27-4:

Demonstrate Withdrawing Medication from a Vial

Objective: The student, using the supplies and equipment listed below, will demonstrate accurately withdrawing a medication for injection from a vial.

Supplies: Vial of medication, bandage strip(s), sharps container, patient chart

Affective Behaviors: Affective behaviors provide a professional approach to a skill that enhances the patient encounter. These behaviors may also display sensitivity to a patient's rights and enhance communication. Pay close attention to these skills, which will be in ***bold, italicized*** font.

Notes to the Student

_____

_____

_____

_____

_____

_____

Skills Assessment Requirements

Read and familiarize yourself with the procedure; complete the minimum practice requirements. Document each MPR using proper charting technique. Complete each procedure within a reasonable amount of time, with a minimum of 85 percent accuracy.

Name: _____

Date: _____

POINT VALUE ✦ = 3–6 points ★ = 7–9 points		PRACTICE TRIAL	GRADED TRIAL # 1	GRADED TRIAL # 2	NOTES
1. ✦	Wash your hands and gather equipment.				
2. ★	Select the correct-size needle to withdraw the medication. Viscous medications require a larger needle gauge.				
3. ★	Check the vial label against the physician's medication order.				
4. ✦	Remove the plastic cap from the vial if necessary. If the vial has already been used, wipe the rubber stopper with an alcohol wipe.				
5. ✦	Inject air into the vial in an amount equal to the medication being removed.				
6. ✦	Place the vial on a firm surface and insert the needle through the rubber stopper.				
7. ✦	Inject air into the vial.				
8. ✦	Invert the vial with the needle tip under the surface of the medication to avoid getting air into the syringe.				
9. ✦	Pull back the plunger to withdraw the necessary amount of medication.				
10. ✦	If air bubbles are present, tap firmly on the syringe to release the bubbles and re-inject them into the vial.				
11. ✦	Check the level of medication in the vial and withdraw more if needed.				
12. ✦	Withdraw the needle from the vial and replace the cap.				

Name: _____

Date: _____

		PRACTICE TRIAL	GRADED TRIAL #1	GRADED TRIAL #2	NOTES
13. ✦	Remove the needle and discard it in a sharps container.				
14. ✦	Replace the needle with a sharp, sterile needle of appropriate size.				
15. ✦	Inject the medication at the appropriate site.				
16. ★	Document the procedure. Include the date, time, medication, site, route, and amount administered. **Sign the entry with your name and credentials.** Follow office policy for recording the medication expiration date and lot number.				

Document: Enter the appropriate information in the chart below.

Grading

Points Earned	_____		
Points Possible	_____	105	105
Percent Grade (Points Earned/Points Possible)	_____		
PASS:	_____	❏ YES ❏ NO ❏ N/A	❏ YES ❏ NO ❏ N/A

Instructor Sign-Off

Instructor: _____ **Date:** _____

Name: _____

Date: _____

Procedure 27-5:

Demonstrate the Reconstitution of a Powdered Drug for Injection Administration

Objective: The student, using the supplies and equipment listed below, will demonstrate accurate reconstitution of a powdered medication for injection

Supplies: Gloves, alcohol wipes, two appropriate-size syringes with needles, vial of medication, sterile water, sharps container, fine-tip permanent marker, and patient's chart

Affective Behaviors: Affective behaviors provide a professional approach to a skill that enhances the patient encounter. These behaviors may also display sensitivity to a patient's rights and enhance communication. Pay close attention to these skills, which will be in ***bold, italicized*** font.

Notes to the Student

_____

_____

_____

_____

_____

_____

Skills Assessment Requirements

Read and familiarize yourself with the procedure; complete the minimum practice requirements. Document each MPR using proper charting technique. Complete each procedure within a reasonable amount of time, with a minimum of 85 percent accuracy.

Name: _____

Date: _____

POINT VALUE ✦ = 3–6 points ⋆ = 7–9 points		PRACTICE TRIAL	GRADED TRIAL # 1	GRADED TRIAL # 2	NOTES
1. ✦	Wash your hands and gather the equipment.				
2. ⋆	**Check to make sure the medication matches the physician's order.** Calculate the dosage if necessary. Look up information relating to the function of the medication, usual dosage, and side effects.				
3. ✦	Check the medication label again against the physician's order to make sure it is the right medication.				
4. ✦	Remove the protective tops from the diluent (sterile water) and medication and wipe both with alcohol.				
5. ✦	Insert one needle into the diluent, making certain to inject an amount of air equal to the amount of solution you are removing. Withdraw the necessary amount of diluent.				
6. ✦	Inject the diluent into the powdered medication vial.				
7. ✦	Discard the used needle in the sharps container.				
8. ✦	Roll the vial containing the diluent and powder between your palms. It may take several minutes to mix the solution thoroughly. Avoid shaking the vial.				

		PRACTICE TRIAL	GRADED TRIAL # 1	GRADED TRIAL # 2	NOTES
9. *	*If the medication will not be used immediately, label the vial with the date and time prepared, your initials, and the expiration date/time.*				
10. ✦	With the second needle, draw up the correct amount of prepared medication to give to the patient.				
11. *	Document the procedure. Include the date, time, medication, site, route, amount administered. *Sign the entry with your name and credentials.* Follow office policy for recording the medication expiration date and lot number.				

Name: _____

Date: _____

Document: Enter the appropriate information in the chart below.

Grading

Points Earned	_____		
Points Possible	_____	75	75
Percent Grade (Points Earned/Points Possible)	_____		
PASS:	_____	❏ YES ❏ NO ❏ N/A	❏ YES ❏ NO ❏ N/A

Instructor Sign-Off

Instructor: _____ **Date:** _____

Procedure 27-6:

Demonstrate the Administration of Medication during Infusion Therapy

Objective: The student, using the supplies and equipment listed below, will demonstrate correct administration of medication through an intermittent infusion device.

Supplies: Three syringes with needles, medication to be administered, normal saline (0.9%) 4 mL, alcohol wipes, gloves, sharps container, patient chart

Affective Behaviors: Affective behaviors provide a professional approach to a skill that enhances the patient encounter. These behaviors may also display sensitivity to a patient's rights and enhance communication. Pay close attention to these skills, which will be in **_bold, italicized_** font.

Notes to the Student

_____

_____

_____

_____

_____

_____

Skills Assessment Requirements

Read and familiarize yourself with the procedure; complete the minimum practice requirements. Document each MPR using proper charting technique. Complete each procedure within a reasonable amount of time, with a minimum of 85 percent accuracy.

POINT VALUE ✦ = 3–6 points ⋆ = 7–9 points	PRACTICE TRIAL	GRADED TRIAL #1	GRADED TRIAL #2	NOTES
1. ✦ Wash your hands and gather the equipment. **Greet and identify the patient, and introduce yourself.**				
2. ⋆ **Check to make sure the medication matches the physician's order.** Calculate the dosage, if necessary. Look up information relating to the medication's function, usual doses, and side effects. Check for patient allergies.				
3. ⋆ Check medication compatibility with the infusion product being used.				
4. ✦ Put on gloves.				
5. ✦ Disinfect the cannula port with the alcohol wipe.				
6. ⋆ Verify that the cannula and vein are freely open, with no blockages.				
7. ✦ With the first of the three syringes, slowly inject 2 mL of the normal saline into the cannula port.				
8. ✦ With the second syringe, administer the medication as prescribed by the physician into the cannula port.				
9. ✦ With the final syringe, inject 2 mL of normal saline into the cannula port.				

		PRACTICE TRIAL	GRADED TRIAL # 1	GRADED TRIAL # 2	NOTES
10. ✦	Remove the gloves and wash your hands.				
11. ⋆	Document the procedure. Include date, time, site, medication, route, and amount administered. **Sign the entry with your name and credentials.**				
12. ✦	Follow office policy for recording the expiration date and lot number.				

Document: Enter the appropriate information in the chart below.

Grading

Points Earned	_____		
Points Possible	_____	84	84
Percent Grade (Points Earned/Points Possible)	_____		
PASS:	_____	❏ YES ❏ NO ❏ N/A	❏ YES ❏ NO ❏ N/A

Instructor Sign-Off

Instructor: _____ **Date:** _____

Name: _____

Date: _____

Procedure 27-7:

Demonstrate the Preparation and Administration of Oral Medication

Objective: The student, using the supplies and equipment listed below, will demonstrate preparation and administration of oral medication.

Supplies: Vial of medication, gloves, patient chart

Affective Behaviors: Affective behaviors provide a professional approach to a skill that enhances the patient encounter. These behaviors may also display sensitivity to a patient's rights and enhance communication. Pay close attention to these skills, which will be in **_bold, italicized_** font.

Notes to the Student

_____

_____

_____

_____

_____

_____

Skills Assessment Requirements

Read and familiarize yourself with the procedure; complete the minimum practice requirements. Document each MPR using proper charting technique. Complete each procedure within a reasonable amount of time, with a minimum of 85 percent accuracy.

POINT VALUE ✦ = 3–6 points ∗ = 7–9 points		PRACTICE TRIAL	GRADED TRIAL #1	GRADED TRIAL #2	NOTES
1. ✦	Wash your hands and gather equipment. ***Greet and identify the patient, and introduce yourself to the patient.***				
2. ✦	Put on gloves.				
3. ∗	***Check to make sure the medication matches the physician's order.*** Calculate the dosage, if necessary. Look up information relating to the medication's function, usual doses, and side effects.				
4. ✦	Check for patient allergies.				
5. ✦	Check the medication label a second time against the physician's order.				
6. ∗	Identify the patient and escort him or her to the treatment area.				
7. ✦	Pour the correct amount of medication.				
8. ∗	*For pills, capsules, and tablets:* Pour the correct amount from the container directly into a medicine cup. *For liquids and suspensions:* If the ingredients are not evenly mixed, shake the bottle gently but thoroughly. Allow time for any bubbles to disappear. When pouring, hold the medication bottle with your palm over the label and hold the medicine cup at eye level.				

		PRACTICE TRIAL	GRADED TRIAL # 1	GRADED TRIAL # 2	NOTES
9. ✦	Check a third time to match the medication against the physician's order.				
10. ✦	If at any time you have doubts about the function of the medication, the dosage or route of administration, or the possibility of an allergic reaction, immediately consult the physician.				
11. ✦	Give the medicine cup to the patient. Have drinking water available for pills, capsules, and tablets, as well as for liquids or suspensions, if necessary.				
12. ✦	Observe as the patient takes the medication to ensure that it is swallowed completely, without difficulty.				
13. ✦	Dispose of the used medication cup and preparation supplies. Wash your hands and return the multiple-use medication bottle to the storage shelf.				
14. ★	Document the procedure. Include date, time, site, medication, route, and amount administered. **Sign the entry with your name and credentials.** Follow office policy for recording the expiration date and lot number.				

Name: _____

Date: _____

Document: Enter the appropriate information in the chart below.

Grading

Points Earned	_____		
Points Possible	_____	96	96
Percent Grade (Points Earned/Points Possible)	_____		
PASS:	_____	❑ YES ❑ NO ❑ N/A	❑ YES ❑ NO ❑ N/A

Instructor Sign-Off

Instructor: _____   **Date:** _____

Procedure 27-8:

Demonstrate the Administration of a Subcutaneous Injection

Objective: The student, using the supplies and equipment listed below, will demonstrate correct administration of a subcutaneous injection.

Supplies: Gloves, alcohol wipes, syringe with needle, vial or ampule of medication, bandage strip(s), sharps container, patient chart

Affective Behaviors: Affective behaviors provide a professional approach to a skill that enhances the patient encounter. These behaviors may also display sensitivity to a patient's rights and enhance communication. Pay close attention to these skills, which will be in **_bold, italicized_** font.

Notes to the Student

_____

_____

_____

_____

_____

_____

Skills Assessment Requirements

Read and familiarize yourself with the procedure; complete the minimum practice requirements. Document each MPR using proper charting technique. Complete each procedure within a reasonable amount of time, with a minimum of 85 percent accuracy.

POINT VALUE ✦ = 3–6 points ✶ = 7–9 points		PRACTICE TRIAL	GRADED TRIAL #1	GRADED TRIAL #2	NOTES
1. ✦	Wash your hands and gather the equipment.				
2. ✶	**Check to make sure the medication matches the physician's order.** Calculate dosage if necessary. Look up information relating to the function of the medication, usual dosage, and side effects.				
3. ✦	Check the medication label again against the physician's order to make sure it is the right medication.				
4. ✶	**Greet and identify the patient, introduce yourself, and escort patient to treatment area.**				
5. ✦	Select the subcutaneous site. Put on gloves. Loosen the cap of the needle so that you can drop it on the counter just before you withdraw medication from the ampule or vial. Cleanse the skin site with an alcohol wipe and allow it to thoroughly air dry.				
6. ✦	Withdraw the correct amount of medication. If necessary, cover the needle by the slide cap method. Otherwise, if the patient is nearby, do not recap the needle.				
7. ✦	Check a third time to match the medication against the physician's order.				

		PRACTICE TRIAL	GRADED TRIAL # 1	GRADED TRIAL # 2	NOTES
8. ✦	If you have any doubts, consult the physician immediately before administering the medication.				
9. ✦	Lightly stretch the skin immediately surrounding the injection site with your nondominant hand.				
10. ✶	Quickly insert the needle at a 45-degree angle. Hold the barrel of the syringe with your nondominant hand and pull (aspirate) the plunger with your dominant hand. If no blood appears in the syringe barrel, move your nondominant hand to the skin position and hold the syringe with your dominant hand. Push the plunger down with your index finger.				
11. ✦	Withdraw the needle and blot the area gently with an alcohol wipe. Discard the syringe into the sharps container. Apply a bandage strip to protect the patient's clothing.				
12. ✦	Remove the gloves and wash your hands.				
13. ✶	Document the procedure. Include the date, time, medication, site, route, and amount administered. ***Sign the entry with your name and credentials.*** Follow office policy for recording the medication expiration date and lot number.				

Name: _____

Date: _____

Document: Enter the appropriate information in the chart below.

Grading

Points Earned	_____		
Points Possible	_____	90	90
Percent Grade (Points Earned/Points Possible)	_____		
PASS:	_____	❏ YES ❏ NO ❏ N/A	❏ YES ❏ NO ❏ N/A

Instructor Sign-Off

Instructor: _____ Date: _____

Procedure 27-9:

Demonstrate the Administration of an Intramuscular Injection to Adults and Children

Objective: The student, using the supplies and equipment listed below, will demonstrate correct administration of an intramuscular injection to an adult or child.

Supplies: Gloves, alcohol wipes, syringe with needle, vial or ampule of medication, bandage strips, sharps container, patient chart

Affective Behaviors: Affective behaviors provide a professional approach to a skill that enhances the patient encounter. These behaviors may also display sensitivity to a patient's rights and enhance communication. Pay close attention to these skills, which will be in ***bold, italicized*** font.

Notes to the Student

_____

_____

_____

_____

_____

_____

Skills Assessment Requirements

Read and familiarize yourself with the procedure; complete the minimum practice requirements. Document each MPR using proper charting technique. Complete each procedure within a reasonable amount of time, with a minimum of 85 percent accuracy.

POINT VALUE ✦ = 3–6 points ⋆ = 7–9 points		PRACTICE TRIAL	GRADED TRIAL #1	GRADED TRIAL #2	NOTES
1. ✦	Wash your hands and gather the equipment.				
2. ⋆	**Check to make sure the medication matches the physician's order.** Calculate dosage if necessary. Look up information relating to the function of the medication, usual dosage, and side effects.				
3. ✦	Check the medication label again against the physician's order to make sure it is the right medication.				
4. ⋆	**Greet and identify the patient, identify yourself, and escort the patient to treatment area. Ask parents to identify the child patient.**				
5. ✦	Select the intramuscular site. Put on gloves. Loosen the cap of the needle so that you can drop it on the counter just before you withdraw medication from the ampule or vial. Cleanse the skin site with an alcohol wipe and allow it to thoroughly air dry.				
6. ✦	Follow the procedure for withdrawing medication from a vial or ampule. Withdraw the correct amount. If necessary, cover the needle by the slide cap method. Otherwise, do not recap the needle.				

Name: _____

Date: _____

		PRACTICE TRIAL	GRADED TRIAL # 1	GRADED TRIAL # 2	NOTES
7. ✦	Check a third time to match the medication against the physician's order.				
8. ✦	If you have any doubts, consult the physician immediately before administering the medication.				
9. ✦	Grasp the skin immediately surrounding the injection site with your nondominant hand. For a small child, ask another clinical staff person to hold the child, then grasp the upper outer quadrant area of the vastus lateralis muscle.				
10. ⋆	Quickly but lightly thrust the needle at a 90-degree (perpendicular) angle. Hold the barrel of the syringe with your nondominant hand and with your dominant hand pull (aspirate) the plunger. If no blood appears in the syringe barrel, move your nondominant hand to the skin position and hold the syringe with your dominant hand. Push the plunger down with your index finger.				
11. ✦	Withdraw the needle and apply pressure with an alcohol wipe. Massage the muscle unless contraindicated. Discard the syringe into the sharps container. Apply a bandage strip to protect the patient's clothing.				

Name: _____

Date: _____

		PRACTICE TRIAL	GRADED TRIAL # 1	GRADED TRIAL # 2	NOTES
12. ✦	Remove the gloves and wash your hands.				
13. ✶	Document the procedure. Include the date, time, medication, site, route, and amount administered. **Sign the entry with your name and credentials.** Follow office policy for recording the medication expiration date and lot number.				

Name: _____

Date: _____

Document: Enter the appropriate information in the chart below.

Grading

Points Earned	_____		
Points Possible	_____	90	90
Percent Grade (Points Earned/Points Possible)	_____		
PASS:	_____	❏ YES ❏ NO ❏ N/A	❏ YES ❏ NO ❏ N/A

Instructor Sign-Off

Instructor: _____ Date: _____

Procedure 27-10:

Demonstrate the Administration of a Z-Track Injection

Objective: The student, using the supplies and equipment listed below, will demonstrate correctly how to administer a Z-track injection.

Supplies: Gloves, alcohol wipes, tuberculin syringe with needle, vial of medication, bandage strips, sharps container, patient chart

Affective Behaviors: Affective behaviors provide a professional approach to a skill that enhances the patient encounter. These behaviors may also display sensitivity to a patient's rights and enhance communication. Pay close attention to these skills, which will be in ***bold, italicized*** font.

Notes to the Student

_____

_____

_____

_____

_____

_____

Skills Assessment Requirements

Read and familiarize yourself with the procedure; complete the minimum practice requirements. Document each MPR using proper charting technique. Complete each procedure within a reasonable amount of time, with a minimum of 85 percent accuracy.

POINT VALUE ✦ = 3–6 points ⋆ = 7–9 points		PRACTICE TRIAL	GRADED TRIAL #1	GRADED TRIAL #2	NOTES
1. ✦	Wash your hands and gather the equipment.				
2. ⋆	**Greet and identify the patient, identify yourself, and escort patient to the treatment area.**				
3. ✦	Select the appropriate intramuscular site. Put on the gloves.				
4. ✦	Cleanse the skin with an alcohol wipe and allow to thoroughly air dry.				
5. ✦	Cleanse the top of the medication vial with an alcohol wipe and allow to air dry. Withdraw the correct dosage from the vial and hold the syringe in your dominant hand.				
6. ✦	With your nondominant hand, pull the skin laterally toward the side opposite the site.				
7. ⋆	Quickly but lightly thrust the needle into the site at a 90-degree (perpendicular) angle. While still holding the skin away from the needle site, inject the medication and wait for 10 seconds.				
8. ⋆	After 10 seconds, quickly withdraw the needle and allow the skin to track back over the original injection site.				

		PRACTICE TRIAL	GRADED TRIAL # 1	GRADED TRIAL # 2	NOTES
9. ✦	Blot the area gently with an alcohol wipe. Discard the syringe into the sharps container. Apply a bandage strip to protect the patient's clothing.				
10. ⋆	Do not massage the injection site. Document the procedure. Include the date, time, medication, site, route, and amount administered. **Sign the entry with your name and credentials.** Follow office policy for recording the medication expiration date and lot number.				

Name: _____

Date: _____

Document: Enter the appropriate information in the chart below.

Grading

Points Earned	_____		
Points Possible	_____	72	72
Percent Grade (Points Earned/Points Possible)	_____		
PASS:	_____	❑ YES ❑ NO ❑ N/A	❑ YES ❑ NO ❑ N/A

Instructor Sign-Off

Instructor: _____   Date: _____

Name: _____

Date: _____

Procedure 28-1:

Obtain an Oral Temperature with an Electronic Digital Thermometer

Objective: The student, using the supplies and equipment listed below, will demonstrate correctly measuring oral temperature with a digital electronic thermometer.

Supplies: Electronic digital thermometer, thermometer probe covers, watch with second hand (for pulse and respiration count), examination gloves

Affective Behaviors: Affective behaviors provide a professional approach to a skill that enhances the patient encounter. These behaviors may also display sensitivity to a patient's rights and enhance communication. Pay close attention to these skills, which will be in **bold, *italicized*** font.

Notes to the Student

_____

_____

_____

_____

_____

_____

Skills Assessment Requirements

Read and familiarize yourself with the procedure; complete the minimum practice requirements. Document each MPR using proper charting technique. Complete each procedure within a reasonable amount of time, with a minimum of 85 percent accuracy.

POINT VALUE ✦ = 3–6 points * = 7–9 points		PRACTICE TRIAL	GRADED TRIAL #1	GRADED TRIAL #2	NOTES
1. *	**Greet and identify the patient, identify yourself and escort patient to the examination room, and offer a place to sit on a chair or the examination table.**				
2. ✦	Wash your hands and apply gloves.				
3. *	Ask the patient if he or she has had hot or cold drinks or food, or smoked a cigarette within the last 10 minutes. If so, wait 10 minutes. If not, proceed with taking the oral temperature.				
4. ✦	Remove the electronic thermometer from its charge base and place a cover on the probe.				
5. ✦	Place the probe under the tongue near the frenulum linguae. Instruct the patient to close the mouth around the thermometer.				
6. ✦	Explain to the patient that the thermometer will need to stay in place until the beep sounds. You may count pulse and respirations now (see procedures 7-6 through 7-8) or after the temperature is taken.				
7. ✦	When the beep sounds, remove the thermometer from the patient's mouth, note the temperature, and discard the probe cover in a waste receptacle.				
8. ✦	Remove the gloves and wash your hands. Return the thermometer to its charge base. **Ask the patient if he or she has any questions prior to leaving the examination room.**				
9. *	**Record the temperature in the appropriate place on the chart. Sign the entry with your name and credentials.** Return the thermometer to its designated storage location.				

Document: Enter the appropriate information in the chart below.

Grading

Points Earned	_____		
Points Possible	_____	63	63
Percent Grade (Points Earned/Points Possible)	_____		
PASS:	_____	❑ YES ❑ NO ❑ N/A	❑ YES ❑ NO ❑ N/A

Instructor Sign-Off

Instructor: _____   **Date:** _____

Procedure 28-2:

Obtain an Axillary Temperature with an Electronic Digital Thermometer

Objective: The student, using the supplies and equipment listed below, will demonstrate accurately measuring an axillary temperature with a digital electronic thermometer.

Supplies: Digital electronic thermometer, thermometer probe cover, watch with second hand (for pulse and respiration count), examination gloves

Affective Behaviors: Affective behaviors provide a professional approach to a skill that enhances the patient encounter. These behaviors may also display sensitivity to a patient's rights and enhance communication. Pay close attention to these skills, which will be in **bold, *italicized*** font.

Notes to the Student

_____

_____

_____

_____

_____

_____

Skills Assessment Requirements

Read and familiarize yourself with the procedure; complete the minimum practice requirements. Document each MPR using proper charting technique. Complete each procedure within a reasonable amount of time, with a minimum of 85 percent accuracy.

POINT VALUE ✦ = 3–6 points ⋆ = 7–9 points	PRACTICE TRIAL	GRADED TRIAL #1	GRADED TRIAL #2	NOTES
1. ⋆ **Greet and identify the patient, identify yourself and escort the patient to the examination room, and offer a place to sit on a chair or the examination table.** Have the patient either unbutton or take off his or her shirt to allow access to the axilla.				
2. ✦ Wash your hands and apply gloves.				
3. ⋆ Observe the axillary area for dryness or diaphoresis. Pat the area dry with a washcloth or towel if it is diaphoretic.				
4. ✦ Remove the electronic thermometer from its charge base and place a cover on the probe.				
5. ✦ Ask the patient to raise an arm. Place the thermometer in direct contact with the skin of the axilla and have the patient lower the arm against the side of the chest.				
6. ✦ Explain that the thermometer will need to stay in place until the beep sounds. You may count pulse and respirations now or after the temperature is taken.				
7. ✦ When the beep sounds, remove the thermometer and discard the probe cover in a waste receptacle.				

		PRACTICE TRIAL	GRADED TRIAL # 1	GRADED TRIAL # 2	NOTES
8. ✦	Remove the gloves and wash your hands. ***Ask the patient if he or she has any questions prior to leaving the examination room.*** Return the thermometer to its charge base.				
9. ⋆	Record the temperature (Figure 10-7), pulse, and respirations in the appropriate place on the chart. Write "A" after the temperature to indicate that the axillary route was used. ***Sign the entry with your name and credentials.***				
10. ✦	Return the thermometer to its designated storage location.				

Name: _____

Date: _____

Document: Enter the appropriate information in the chart below.

Grading

Points Earned	_____		
Points Possible	_____	69	69
Percent Grade (Points Earned/Points Possible)	_____		
PASS:	_____	❏ YES ❏ NO ❏ N/A	❏ YES ❏ NO ❏ N/A

Instructor Sign-Off

Instructor: _____ Date: _____

Name: _____

Date: _____

Procedure 28-3:

Obtain a Rectal Temperature with an Electronic Digital Thermometer

Objective: The student, using the supplies and equipment listed below, will demonstrate accurately measuring a rectal temperature with a digital thermometer.

Supplies: Digital electronic thermometer (rectal) and probe covers, lubricant, tissue, examination gloves

Affective Behaviors: Affective behaviors provide a professional approach to a skill that enhances the patient encounter. These behaviors may also display sensitivity to a patient's rights and enhance communication. Pay close attention to these skills, which will be in **_bold, italicized_** font.

Notes to the Student

_____

_____

_____

_____

_____

_____

Skills Assessment Requirements

Read and familiarize yourself with the procedure; complete the minimum practice requirements. Document each MPR using proper charting technique. Complete each procedure within a reasonable amount of time, with a minimum of 85 percent accuracy.

Name: _____

Date: _____

POINT VALUE ✦ = 3–6 points * = 7–9 points	PRACTICE TRIAL	GRADED TRIAL # 1	GRADED TRIAL # 2	NOTES
1. * **Greet and identify the patient, identify yourself and escort the patient to the examination room.** Assist the patient in removing clothing from the waist down. Keeping the patient draped, assist him or her into a left side-lying position (Sims' position) on the examination table. **Drape for exposure of the buttocks only. Try to ease the patient if he or she seems apprehensive.**				
2. ✦ Wash your hands and apply gloves.				
3. ✦ Remove the electronic thermometer from its charge base and place a cover on the probe.				
4. ✦ Place a small amount of lubricant on a tissue next to the patient. Dip the tip of the probe cover in the lubricant.				
5. * **Inform the patient of procedure before you insert the rectal probe.** For an adult, insert the lubricated probe cover approximately 1 1/2 inches into the anus. For an infant, insert it 1/4 to 1/2 inch, and for a child, 1/2 to 1 inch.				
6. ✦ Hold the thermometer in place until it beeps. Remove the thermometer and discard the probe cover in a waste receptacle.				
7. ✦ Remove the gloves and wash your hands. Return the thermometer to its charge base.				
8. * Record the temperature in the appropriate place on the chart. Write an "R" after the measurement to indicate the rectal route. **Sign the entry with your name and credentials.**				
9. ✦ Return the thermometer to its designated storage location.				

Name: _____

Date: _____

Document: Enter the appropriate information in the chart below.

Grading

Points Earned	_____		
Points Possible	_____	63	63
Percent Grade (Points Earned/Points Possible)	_____		
PASS:	_____	❑ YES ❑ NO ❑ N/A	❑ YES ❑ NO ❑ N/A

Instructor Sign-Off

Instructor: _____ Date: _____

Name: _____

Date: _____

Procedure 28-4:

Obtain an Aural Temperature with a Tympanic Thermometer

Objective: The student, using the supplies and equipment listed below, will demonstrate accurately taking an aural temperature according to the patient's age.

Supplies: Tympanic thermometer, probe cover, and examination gloves

Affective Behaviors: Affective behaviors provide a professional approach to a skill that enhances the patient encounter. These behaviors may also display sensitivity to a patient's rights and enhance communication. Pay close attention to these skills, which will be in **_bold, italicized_** font.

Notes to the Student

_____

_____

_____

_____

_____

_____

Skills Assessment Requirements

Read and familiarize yourself with the procedure; complete the minimum practice requirements. Document each MPR using proper charting technique. Complete each procedure within a reasonable amount of time, with a minimum of 85 percent accuracy.

POINT VALUE ◆ = 3–6 points * = 7–9 points	PRACTICE TRIAL	GRADED TRIAL # 1	GRADED TRIAL # 2	NOTES
1. *	**Greet and identify the patient, identify yourself and escort the patient to the examination room, and offer a place to sit on a chair or the examination table.** If the patient is a child, encourage the parent to sit and hold the child.			
2. ◆	Wash your hands and apply gloves.			
3. ◆	**Explain the basic procedure to the patient or parent. Assess whether the patient has had an aural temperature taken before. Depending on the patient's age and previous experience or knowledge of the procedure, you may need to assure him or her that the procedure is painless or demonstrate on the parent before taking a child's temperature.**			
4. ◆	Remove the tympanic thermometer from its charge base and place a cover on the probe.			
5. *	For an adult, pull the outer ear in an upward direction. For a child or infant, pull the outer ear in a downward direction.			
6. ◆	With your hand insert the probe-covered earpiece of the thermometer into the ear canal and press the scan button to obtain the temperature reading.			

	PRACTICE TRIAL	GRADED TRIAL # 1	GRADED TRIAL # 2	NOTES
7. ✦ When the thermometer beeps, withdraw it from the patient's ear and pop the probe cover into the waste receptacle. Read the temperature reading in the thermometer's display window.				
8. ✦ Remove the gloves and wash your hands. Return the thermometer to its charge base. **Prior to leaving the examination room, ask the patient if he or she has any questions.**				
9. ★ Record the temperature on the patient's chart, followed by a "T" to indicate tympanic temperature. **Sign the entry with your name and credentials.**				
10. ✦ Return the tympanic thermometer to its designated storage location.				

Document: Enter the appropriate information in the chart below.

Grading

Points Earned	_____		
Points Possible	_____	69	69
Percent Grade (Points Earned/Points Possible)	_____		
PASS:	_____	❏ YES ❏ NO ❏ N/A	❏ YES ❏ NO ❏ N/A

Instructor Sign-Off

Instructor: _____ **Date:** _____

Procedure 28-5:

Obtain a Dermal Temperature with a Disposable Thermometer

Objective: The student, using the supplies and equipment listed below, will demonstrate accurately measuring a dermal temperature with a disposable thermometer.

Supplies: Disposable dermal strips; clean, dry washcloth; examination gloves

Notes to the Student

_____

_____

_____

_____

_____

_____

Skills Assessment Requirements

Read and familiarize yourself with the procedure; complete the minimum practice requirements. Document each MPR using proper charting technique. Complete each procedure within a reasonable amount of time, with a minimum of 85 percent accuracy.

Name: _____

Date: _____

POINT VALUE ✦ = 3–6 points * = 7–9 points		PRACTICE TRIAL	GRADED TRIAL # 1	GRADED TRIAL # 2	NOTES
1. *	**Greet and identify the patient, identify yourself and escort the patient to the examination room,** and offer a place to sit on a chair or the examination table.				
2. ✦	Wash your hands and apply gloves.				
3. ✦	Observe the forehead for dryness or diaphoresis. Pat the area dry with a washcloth if it is diaphoretic.				
4. ✦	Carefully unwrap the dermal strip without touching the chemical dots and place it on the forehead.				
5. *	Leave the strip on the forehead for the length of time recommended by the manufacturer, usually about 15 seconds.				
6. ✦	After noting the temperature of the last color-changed dot, remove and dispose of the dermal thermometer in a waste receptacle.				
7. ✦	Remove the gloves and wash your hands. **Prior to leaving the examination room, ask the patient if he or she has any questions.**				
8. *	Record the temperature on the patient's chart, followed by the word "dermal." **Sign the entry with your name and credentials.**				

Name: _____

Date: _____

Document: Enter the appropriate information in the chart below.

Grading

Points Earned	_____		
Points Possible	_____	57	57
Percent Grade (Points Earned/Points Possible)	_____		
PASS:	_____	❏ YES ❏ NO ❏ N/A	❏ YES ❏ NO ❏ N/A

Instructor Sign-Off

Instructor: _____ **Date:** _____

Name: _____

Date: _____

Procedure 28-6:

Perform a Radial Pulse Count

Objective: The student, using the supplies and equipment listed below, will demonstrate accurately measuring a radial pulse.

Supplies: Watch with second hand

Affective Behaviors: Affective behaviors provide a professional approach to a skill that enhances the patient encounter. These behaviors may also display sensitivity to a patient's rights and enhance communication. Pay close attention to these skills, which will be in **_bold, italicized_** font.

Notes to the Student

_____

_____

_____

_____

_____

_____

Skills Assessment Requirements

Read and familiarize yourself with the procedure; complete the minimum practice requirements. Document each MPR using proper charting technique. Complete each procedure within a reasonable amount of time, with a minimum of 85 percent accuracy.

POINT VALUE ✦ = 3–6 points ✳ = 7–9 points		PRACTICE TRIAL	GRADED TRIAL # 1	GRADED TRIAL # 2	NOTES
1. ✳	The patient has been identified, escorted to the examination room, and offered a place to sit on a chair or the examination table. **Introduce yourself to the patient.**				
2. ✦	Wash your hands (unless you have already done so prior to taking the temperature).				
3. ✦	**Explain the procedure to the patient** (unless you have already done so prior to taking the temperature). Do not mention that you will be counting respirations after taking the pulse.				
4. ✦	Position the patient's arm at about heart level, with the palm facing down. Identify the radial artery with the three middle fingertips by feeling pulsation through the arterial wall.				
5. ✦	Palpate for the pulsation of the radial artery on the inside of the wrist below the thumb. Note the strength and rhythm of the pulse. Do not palpate the pulse with your thumb.				
6. ✳	Looking at your watch, start counting the pulse beats when the second hand is at 3, 6, 9, or 12. Count for one full minute. While still holding the wrist, observe the patient's respiratory efforts and count as instructed in Procedure 10-8.				
7. ✳	Document the rate, strength, and rhythm of the pulse on the chart. **Sign the entry with your name and credentials.**				
8. ✦	Wash your hands. **Prior to leaving the examination room, ask the patient if he or she has any questions.**				

Document: Enter the appropriate information in the chart below.

Grading

Points Earned	_____		
Points Possible	_____	57	57
Percent Grade (Points Earned/Points Possible)	_____		
PASS:	_____	❏ YES ❏ NO ❏ N/A	❏ YES ❏ NO ❏ N/A

Instructor Sign-Off

Instructor: _____   **Date:** _____

Name: _____

Date: _____

Procedure 28-7:

Perform an Apical Pulse Count

Objective: The student, using the supplies and equipment listed below, will demonstrate accurately performing an apical pulse count.

Supplies: Stethoscope, alcohol prep, watch with a second hand

Affective Behaviors: Affective behaviors provide a professional approach to a skill that enhances the patient encounter. These behaviors may also display sensitivity to a patient's rights and enhance communication. Pay close attention to these skills, which will be in **_bold, italicized_** font.

Notes to the Student

_____
_____
_____
_____
_____
_____

Skills Assessment Requirements

Read and familiarize yourself with the procedure; complete the minimum practice requirements. Document each MPR using proper charting technique. Complete each procedure within a reasonable amount of time, with a minimum of 85 percent accuracy.

POINT VALUE ✦ = 3–6 points ⋆ = 7–9 points		PRACTICE TRIAL	GRADED TRIAL # 1	GRADED TRIAL # 2	NOTES
1. ⋆	The patient has already been identified, and you have washed your hands to obtain vital signs. **Introduce yourself to the patient.**				
2. ✦	**Explain the procedure to the patient.** Do not mention that you will be counting respirations after you have noted the apical pulse.				
3. ✦	Wipe the stethoscope earpieces with the alcohol prep. With the earpieces pointed toward the nose, place the stethoscope earpieces in your ears. Place the bell or diaphragm on the patient's chest in the area of the apex of the heart.				
4. ✦	Begin counting heartbeats (each "lub-dub" counts as one heartbeat) when the second hand of the watch is at 3, 6, 9, or 12.				
5. ✦	Count for one full minute. Note the quality and regularity of the heartbeat.				
6. ⋆	Chart the rate, rhythm, and any other pertinent information. **Sign the entry with your name and credentials.** If the radial pulse is also documented, write "RP" before the radial pulse rate and "AP" before the apical pulse rate. **Prior to leaving the examination room, ask the patient if he or she has any questions.**				

Name: _____

Date: _____

Document: Enter the appropriate information in the chart below.

Grading

Points Earned	_____		
Points Possible	_____	42	42
Percent Grade (Points Earned/Points Possible)	_____		
PASS:	_____	❏ YES ❏ NO ❏ N/A	❏ YES ❏ NO ❏ N/A

Instructor Sign-Off

Instructor: _____ Date: _____

Procedure 28-8:

Perform a Respiration Count

Objective: The student, using the supplies and equipment listed below, will demonstrate accurately performing a respiratory count without the patient being aware that the MA is doing this count.

Supplies: Watch with second hand

Affective Behaviors: Affective behaviors provide a professional approach to a skill that enhances the patient encounter. These behaviors may also display sensitivity to a patient's rights and enhance communication. Pay close attention to these skills, which will be in ***bold, italicized*** font.

Notes to the Student

_____

_____

_____

_____

_____

_____

Skills Assessment Requirements

Read and familiarize yourself with the procedure; complete the minimum practice requirements. Document each MPR using proper charting technique. Complete each procedure within a reasonable amount of time, with a minimum of 85 percent accuracy.

Name: _____

Date: _____

POINT VALUE ✦ = 3–6 points ⋆ = 7–9 points		PRACTICE TRIAL	GRADED TRIAL # 1	GRADED TRIAL # 2	NOTES
1. ⋆	This procedure is a continuation of the radial or apical pulse count. The patient has been identified and you have washed your hands.				
2. ✦	After counting the radial or apical pulse and mentally noting the rate, continue holding the patient's wrist or holding the stethoscope chestpiece in place.				
3. ✦	Watch the patient's chest rise (inspiration) and fall (expiration) and count the respiratory cycles for 30 seconds. Observe the regularity and depth of the respirations. Make a mental note of the respiratory rate.				
4. ⋆	Multiply the 30-second count by two and record that figure as the respiratory rate. Record the pulse as well. Add any appropriate comments about the regularity or depth of the respirations on the chart. **Sign the entry with your name and credentials. Prior to leaving the examination room, ask the patient if he or she has any questions.**				

Name: _____

Date: _____

Document: Enter the appropriate information in the chart below.

Grading

Points Earned	_____		
Points Possible	_____	30	30
Percent Grade (Points Earned/Points Possible)	_____		
PASS:	_____	❏ YES ❏ NO ❏ N/A	❏ YES ❏ NO ❏ N/A

Instructor Sign-Off

Instructor: _____ **Date:** _____

Procedure 28-9:

Perform a Blood Pressure Measurement

Objective: The student, using the supplies and equipment listed below, will demonstrate obtaining an accurate blood pressure reading.

Supplies: Stethoscope, 70% isopropyl alcohol wipes, sphygmomanometer (aneroid or mercury)

Affective Behaviors: Affective behaviors provide a professional approach to a skill that enhances the patient encounter. These behaviors may also display sensitivity to a patient's rights and enhance communication. Pay close attention to these skills, which will be in **_bold, italicized_** font.

Notes to the Student

_____

_____

_____

_____

_____

_____

Skills Assessment Requirements

Read and familiarize yourself with the procedure; complete the minimum practice requirements. Document each MPR using proper charting technique. Complete each procedure within a reasonable amount of time, with a minimum of 85 percent accuracy.

Name: _____

Date: _____

POINT VALUE ✦ = 3–6 points ⋆ = 7–9 points		PRACTICE TRIAL	GRADED TRIAL # 1	GRADED TRIAL # 2	NOTES
1. ✦	Wash your hands and assemble the equipment. Squeeze the bladder of the sphygmomanometer cuff to make sure it is completely deflated.				
2. ⋆	***Greet and identify the patient and escort to a central area or patient examination room. Introduce yourself to the patient.*** Have the patient sit either on a chair or on the examination table. Explain the procedure to the patient.				
3. ✦	Cleanse the earpieces, diaphragm, and bell of the stethoscope with the alcohol wipes.				
4. ✦	Expose the patient's upper arm and ask the patient to extend the arm with the palm facing upward. You may have to assist the patient in rolling up the sleeve.				
5. ✦	Place the sphygmomanometer cuff around the patient's upper arm and secure it snugly, centering over the brachial artery.				
6. ✦	Palpate the brachial pulse.				
7. ✦	Hold the arm with the attached sphygmomanometer at heart level.				
8. ✦	Place the sphygmomanometer gauge where you can monitor it easily or ask the patient to hold it.				

		PRACTICE TRIAL	GRADED TRIAL # 1	GRADED TRIAL # 2	NOTES
9. ✦	Place the stethoscope earpieces in your ears. Place the diaphragm of the stethoscope over the location where you felt the brachial pulse. Hold the bell of the stethoscope in place with the thumb of your nondominant hand while supporting the elbow with your fingers.				
10. ✦	With your dominant hand, close the thumbscrew on the hand bulb by turning it clockwise. Quickly and evenly pump the bulb to inflate the cuff.				
11. ✦	Slowly turn the thumbscrew counterclockwise, releasing air at approximately 2–3 mm per second.				
12. *	Listen and mentally note when you hear the first pulsation. Slowly continue to release air until the pulsation sounds cease, and make a mental note of that reading.				
13. ✦	Quickly release the rest of the air, deflating the cuff. Remove the cuff.				
14. ✦	If it is necessary to check the blood pressure reading because of an error in the procedure or an abnormally high or low reading, wait one minute before retaking the blood pressure on the same arm.				

		PRACTICE TRIAL	GRADED TRIAL # 1	GRADED TRIAL # 2	NOTES
15. ✦	Clean the earpieces and diaphragm with 70% ethyl alcohol. Return the sphyg-momanometer and stetho-scope to their usual storage place.				
16. ✦	Wash your hands.				
17. ＊	After recording the date and time, document the first pulsation sounds as systolic and the last sounds as diastolic readings. Write the systolic over diastolic readings in fraction format. **Sign the entry with your name and credentials.** If the blood pressure was taken with the patient standing or lying down, specify the position in the chart. **If the patient asks for the reading and office policy allows it, you may inform the patient of the reading. Prior to leaving the examination room, ask the patient if he or she has any questions.**				

Name: _____

Date: _____

Document: Enter the appropriate information in the chart below.

Grading

Points Earned	_____		
Points Possible	_____	111	111
Percent Grade (Points Earned/Points Possible)	_____		
PASS:	_____	❑ YES ❑ NO ❑ N/A	❑ YES ❑ NO ❑ N/A

Instructor Sign-Off

Instructor: _____ **Date:** _____

Procedure 28-10:

Obtain Weight and Height Measurements

Objective: The student, using the supplies and equipment listed below, will demonstrate accurately obtaining height and weight measurements.

Supplies: Upright balance scales with height bar, paper towel

Affective Behaviors: Affective behaviors provide a professional approach to a skill that enhances the patient encounter. These behaviors may also display sensitivity to a patient's rights and enhance communication. Pay close attention to these skills, which will be in ***bold, italicized*** font.

Notes to the Student

_____

_____

_____

_____

_____

_____

Skills Assessment Requirements

Read and familiarize yourself with the procedure; complete the minimum practice requirements. Document each MPR using proper charting technique. Complete each procedure within a reasonable amount of time, with a minimum of 85 percent accuracy.

Name: _____

Date: _____

POINT VALUE ✦ = 3–6 points ⭑ = 7–9 points	PRACTICE TRIAL	GRADED TRIAL #1	GRADED TRIAL #2	NOTES
1. ⭑ **Greet and identify the patient, introduce yourself to the patient, and escort him or her to the examination room.**				
2. ✦ Wash your hands.				
3. ✦ **Explain the procedure to the patient. Explain that most personal items may be left in the room, although a female patient may want to take her purse. Escort the patient to the scales.**				
4. ⭑ Balance the scales to read zero.				
5. ✦ Instruct the patient to step on the scales. You may need to place a paper towel on the scale for patients who wish to remove their shoes. **Assist the patient onto the scales and provide support as needed.**				
6. ✦ Instruct the patient to stand still. Move the weights until the scale balances.				
7. ⭑ Note the weight and return the balance weights to zero. **Do not state the patient's weight out loud, unless directly asked by the patient. If asked, state the weight in a discreet manner.**				
8. ✦ **Ask the patient to step off the scales, assisting as necessary.**				

		PRACTICE TRIAL	GRADED TRIAL # 1	GRADED TRIAL # 2	NOTES
9. ✦	Help the patient to step on the scales backwards so that his or her back is against the scale. Ask the patient to stand erect, eyes looking ahead.				
10. *	Raise the height bar in a collapsed position above the patient's head. Extend the bar and slowly bring it down until it touches the top of the patient's head. Note the height.				
11. ✦	Raise the entire height bar up over the patient's head, collapse it, and return it to its original position.				
12. ✦	**Ask the patient to step off the scales, assisting as necessary.**				
13. *	Record the height and weight on the patient's chart. **Sign the entry with your name and credentials. Prior to leaving the examination room, ask the patient if he or she has any questions.**				

Name: _____

Date: _____

Document: Enter the appropriate information in the chart below.

Grading

Points Earned	_____		
Points Possible	_____	93	93
Percent Grade (Points Earned/Points Possible)	_____		
PASS:	_____	❏ YES ❏ NO ❏ N/A	❏ YES ❏ NO ❏ N/A

Instructor Sign-Off

Instructor: _____ **Date:** _____

Name: _____

Date: _____

Procedure 28-11:

Demonstrate Patient Positions Used in a Medical Examination

Objective: The student, using the supplies and equipment listed below, will demonstrate correctly assisting the patient into the sitting, supine, Sims', prone, dorsal recumbent, and lithotomy positions.

Supplies: Patient gown, pants, and drapes; examination table paper

Affective Behaviors: Affective behaviors provide a professional approach to a skill that enhances the patient encounter. These behaviors may also display sensitivity to a patient's rights and enhance communication. Pay close attention to these skills, which will be in **_bold, italicized_** font.

Notes to the Student

_____

_____

_____

_____

_____

_____

Skills Assessment Requirements

Read and familiarize yourself with the procedure; complete the minimum practice requirements. Document each MPR using proper charting technique. Complete each procedure within a reasonable amount of time, with a minimum of 85 percent accuracy.

POINT VALUE ✦ = 3–6 points ✱ = 7–9 points		PRACTICE TRIAL	GRADED TRIAL # 1	GRADED TRIAL # 2	NOTES
1. ✱	**Greet and identify the patient, introduce yourself and escort him or her to the examination room.**				
2. ✦	Wash your hands.				
3. ✦	**Explain the procedure to the patient.** Ask the patient to completely undress and to put on a patient gown. For a breast examination, instruct the patient to tie the gown in the front.				
4. ✦	Instruct the patient to sit on the examination table, assisting as necessary. **Cover the patient with the drape.**				
5. ✦	Assist the patient into the supine position.				
6. ✦	Assist the patient into Sim's position.				
7. ✦	Assist the patient into the prone position.				
8. ✦	Assist the patient back into the supine position, then into the dorsal recumbent position.				
9. ✦	Assist the patient into the lithotomy position.				
10. ✦	Assist the patient in returning to the sitting position and stepping off the examination table. **Prior to leaving the examination room, ask the patient if he or she has any questions.**				

		PRACTICE TRIAL	GRADED TRIAL # 1	GRADED TRIAL # 2	NOTES
11. *	After the examination has been completed and the physician has discussed the procedure with the patient, clean the examination room. Remove the used paper from the examination table and replace it with clean paper for the next patient.				
12. *	Wash your hands and complete documentation in the patient's chart. **Sign the entry with your name and credentials.**				

Name: _____

Date: _____

Document: Enter the appropriate information in the chart below.

Grading

Points Earned	_____		
Points Possible	_____	81	81
Percent Grade (Points Earned/Points Possible)	_____		
PASS:	_____	❏ YES ❏ NO ❏ N/A	❏ YES ❏ NO ❏ N/A

Instructor Sign-Off

Instructor: _____ Date: _____

Name: _____

Date: _____

Procedure 28-12:

Prepare the Patient for Medical Examination and Assist the Physician

Objective: The student, using the supplies and equipment listed below, will assist the physician with the physical examination.

Supplies: Examination table with clean covering (sheet) and stirrups if pelvic examination is to be performed, patient gown and appropriate drapes, pillow with disposable cover, scales with height rod, Snellen chart and color vision charts, disposable gloves, lubricant and tissues, emesis basin, alcohol swabs, laryngeal mirror, nasal and ear speculums, ophthalmoscope and otoscope, pen light, reflex hammer, sphygmomanometer and stethoscope, tape measure, thermometer, tongue depressors, tuning fork, urine specimen container, gooseneck lamp.

Affective Behaviors: Affective behaviors provide a professional approach to a skill that enhances the patient encounter. These behaviors may also display sensitivity to a patient's rights and enhance communication. Pay close attention to these skills, which will be in **_bold, italicized_** font.

Notes to the Student

_____

_____

_____

_____

_____

_____

Skills Assessment Requirements

Read and familiarize yourself with the procedure; complete the minimum practice requirements. Document each MPR using proper charting technique. Complete each procedure within a reasonable amount of time, with a minimum of 85 percent accuracy.

POINT VALUE ✦ = 3–6 points ⋆ = 7–9 points		PRACTICE TRIAL	GRADED TRIAL #1	GRADED TRIAL #2	NOTES
1. ⋆	Equip each examination room with the necessary supplies, equipment, and instruments. Ensure that instruments are in working order and the room temperature is comfortable.				
2. ⋆	**Greet and identify the patient, introduce yourself and escort him or her to the examination room.**				
3. ✦	Wash your hands.				
4. ✦	Obtain the patient's weight and height, **usually in a semiprivate but central location in the clinical area.**				
5. ✦	Obtain vital signs and pain assessment.				
6. ✦	Instruct the patient to remove necessary clothing and to put on the gown or cover. **Offer to assist the patient if necessary and explain where to place removed clothing.**				
7. ✦	Instruct the patient to sit on the examination table and provide a drape.				
8. ✦	Obtain the patient history through interview and review of the complete forms.				
9. ✦	Gather the instruments the physician will need. **Prior to leaving the examination room, ask the patient if he or she has any questions.**				

Competency Check-Offs **943**

	PRACTICE TRIAL	GRADED TRIAL # 1	GRADED TRIAL # 2	NOTES
10. ✦ Notify the physician that the patient is ready.				
11. ★ *When the physician is ready, assist with positioning the patient and the physical examination. Drape and adjust the drape to ensure modesty. Be prepared to gather additional supplies and assist the physician with any instruments or supplies necessary for the examination.*				
12. ✦ Upon completion of the examination, *assist the patient from the examination table.*				
13. ★ Prepare specimens for examination and/or transport by labeling and completing appropriate forms.				
14. ✦ Remove soiled instruments and equipment to the dirty utility room for cleaning.				
15. ✦ Clean the room and dispose of any waste. Wash your hands.				
16. ✦ Prepare the room for the next patient.				

Document: Enter the appropriate information in the chart below.

Grading

Points Earned	_____		
Points Possible	_____	108	108
Percent Grade (Points Earned/Points Possible)	_____		
PASS:	_____	❏ YES ❏ NO ❏ N/A	❏ YES ❏ NO ❏ N/A

Instructor Sign-Off

Instructor: _____ **Date:** _____

Name: _____

Date: _____

Procedure 29-1:

Prepare the Skin for a Surgical Procedure

Objective: The student, using the supplies and equipment listed below, will demonstrate how to prepare the patient's skin for a surgical procedure with a surgical scrub and shave.

Supplies: Shave prep kit, including razor, sterile basin pack, antiseptic germicidal soap, sterile 4 × 4s, sterile applicators, sterile sponge forceps, Mayo stand or side tray, sterile water or saline, waste receptacle, hazardous waste container, plastic bags for disposal of contaminated material, sterile gloves, sterile towels, sterile drapes, antiseptic

Affective Behaviors: Affective behaviors provide a professional approach to a skill that enhances the patient encounter. These behaviors may also display sensitivity to a patient's rights and enhance communication. Pay close attention to these skills, which will be in **_bold, italicized_** font.

Notes to the Student

_____

_____

_____

_____

_____

_____

Skills Assessment Requirements

Read and familiarize yourself with the procedure; complete the minimum practice requirements. Document each MPR using proper charting technique. Complete each procedure within a reasonable amount of time, with a minimum of 85 percent accuracy.

POINT VALUE ✦ = 3–6 points ★ = 7–9 points		PRACTICE TRIAL	GRADED TRIAL # 1	GRADED TRIAL # 2	NOTES
1. ✦	Wash your hands thoroughly. Gather equipment and supplies.				
2. ★	***Greet and identify the patient, introduce yourself and guide him or her to the treatment area. Explain the entire procedure to the patient.***				
3. ✦	Instruct the patient to void if necessary.				
4. ✦	Have the patient remove appropriate clothing and wear a patient gown until it is time for positioning and draping.				
5. ★	Unwrap the outer wraps of all packs. Unwrap the basin pack. Following correct technique for pouring liquids in a sterile field, pour germicidal soap into one basin, sterile water or saline into the second basin, and germicidal solution into the third basin.				
6. ✦	Wash your hands and apply sterile gloves. Position the patient and remove the gown as necessary. ***Explain the following steps to the patient, as necessary.***				
7. ✦	You may need to shave the area before it is surgically scrubbed. If so, apply soap solution to the area.				
8. ✦	Remove the razor from the shave prep pack that has been placed outside the sterile field.				
9. ✦	Pull the skin gently taut at the surgical site. Shave in the direction of hair growth.				

		PRACTICE TRIAL	GRADED TRIAL # 1	GRADED TRIAL # 2	NOTES
10. ✦	Rinse the skin with sterile saline or water in an outward circular motion, then pat the area dry.				
11. ✦	Wash your hands and put on sterile gloves.				
12. ✦	Apply soapy solution to the patient's skin in a circular motion with a sterile sponge, starting at the center of the surgical site and moving outward. During the application the circles should not overlap each other or repeat over the same area.				
13. ✦	Cleanse the skin by continuing from the center of the circle making your way to the outer rim. During the application the circles should not overlap each other or repeat over the same area.				
14. ✦	Rinse the area in the same circular manner with new sterile sponges.				
15. ✦	Allow area to air dry.				
16. ✦	Apply germicidal solution in concentric circles with a sterile sponge or cotton-tipped applicators.				
17. ✦	After allowing the prep area to completely air dry, drape 3 to 5 inches above and below the surgical site with sterile towels.				
18. ✦	Drape the prepared surgical site with a sterile towel. If the patient must be left unattended at any time after the surgical scrub, another medical assistant or scrub float will need to cover the prepped area with a sterile towel.				

		PRACTICE TRIAL	GRADED TRIAL #1	GRADED TRIAL #2	NOTES
19. ⋆	If the physician did not participate in the patient prep or setting up the surgical tray, alert him or her that the patient has been prepped. ***Prior to leaving the examination room, ask the patient if he or she has any questions.***				
20. ⋆	Document the scrub procedure with patient education notes. ***Sign the entry with your name and credentials.***				

Name: _____

Date: _____

Document: Enter the appropriate information in the chart below.

Grading

Points Earned	_____		
Points Possible	_____	132	132
Percent Grade (Points Earned/Points Possible)	_____		
PASS:	_____	❏ YES ❏ NO ❏ N/A	❏ YES ❏ NO ❏ N/A

Instructor Sign-Off

Instructor: _____ Date: _____

Procedure 29-2:

Set Up a Surgical Tray and Assist the Physician with Minor Surgical Procedures

Objective: The student, using the supplies and equipment listed below, will demonstrate how to assist the physician with minor surgery by preparing for the procedure, anticipating physician needs, and providing or reinforcing instruction to the patient or significant other(s).

Supplies: Sterile surgical pack, including two pairs of sterile gloves, towel pack, 4 × 4 sponge pack, sterile drapes, needle pack and suture materials, sterile instrument pack, sterile syringe pack, two sterile surgical basins, and sterile specimen containers, Mayo stand and/or a surgical instrument table, transfer forceps and holder, waste container lined with plastic bag, sharps disposal container, biohazard waste container, local anesthetic, and alcohol preps

Affective Behaviors: Affective behaviors provide a professional approach to a skill that enhances the patient encounter. These behaviors may also display sensitivity to a patient's rights and enhance communication. Pay close attention to these skills, which will be in **bold, *italicized*** font.

Notes to the Student

_____

_____

_____

_____

_____

_____

Skills Assessment Requirements

Read and familiarize yourself with the procedure; complete the minimum practice requirements. Document each MPR using proper charting technique. Complete each procedure within a reasonable amount of time, with a minimum of 85 percent accuracy.

Name: _____

Date: _____

POINT VALUE ✦ = 3–6 points ⋆ = 7–9 points		PRACTICE TRIAL	GRADED TRIAL # 1	GRADED TRIAL # 2	NOTES
1. ✦	Determine scrub and float assistant staffing needs for the procedure.				
2. ✦	Wash your hands.				
3. ✦	Sanitize and disinfect a Mayo instrument stand by using a 4 × 4 gauze square that has been soaked in 70% isopropyl alcohol. Starting from the middle of the tray, use a circular motion to cleanse the entire tray, including the rim.				
4. ✦	If your place of employment uses sterile disposable drapes, place the package on a counter and carefully peel back the top layer to expose the fan-folded drape. Grasping only the corner of the drape with your thumb and forefinger, raise it quickly to a height that allows it to carefully unfold, *without* touching the counter top, or any portion of your body. If your place of employment uses sterile towels, they will be folded in the same manner and placed inside towel canisters. Sterile towels will be removed the same way.				
5. ✦	With the drape held firmly with the thumb and forefinger of one hand well above waist level, take your other hand and pinch the opposite corner of the drape between your thumb and forefinger. Both corners along the shortest side of the drape are now firmly held.				

		PRACTICE TRIAL	GRADED TRIAL # 1	GRADED TRIAL # 2	NOTES
6. ✦	With the drape held above waist level, carefully reach over the Mayo stand and pull the drape toward you as you lay it on the stand. It is critical that the bottom edge of the drape not touch the stand as you are reaching across. The drape must also not swing and touch any portion of your body at any time.				
7. ✦	At this point in the procedure the tray is now considered sterile. It must not be left unattended, reached over, or touched. If the sterile drape needs to be adjusted, you may reach under and use the draping portions to make minor adjustments.				
8. ✦	Gather the appropriate supplies needed for the procedure. If you gather items that are wrapped twice you must apply them in a sterile manner.				
9. ✦	Position the package in your nondominant hand with the flap facing up. The package should look like an envelope, with the envelope opening on top and toward your fingertips. You may adjust the package as needed at this point, as this outer wrapping is not sterile and neither is your hand.				
10. ✦	Pull open the top flap by gently grasping it with your other hand and pulling it up and underneath, ticking it into the fingers of the nondominant hand.				

		PRACTICE TRIAL	GRADED TRIAL # 1	GRADED TRIAL # 2	NOTES
11. ✦	Follow the same procedure, pulling the right flap to the right and the left flap to the left, without crossing over your nondominant hand. Rationale: This method allows the inner package to remain sterile while it is being exposed for removal. Gathering the loose ends into your fingers prevents them from being dragged across the sterile field or folding back onto the sterile package before it is placed on the tray.				
12. ✦	Carefully apply the package to the sterile field by holding it well above the tray and letting it carefully fall onto the tray.				
13. ✦	Items that have been sterilized in plastic pouches must also be applied in a sterile manner.				
14. ✦	Carefully peel apart the package and allow the instrument to fall onto the sterile field.				
15. ✦	Do not allow the package to touch the sterile field and do not allow the instruments to slide or bounce as they land on the tray.				

	PRACTICE TRIAL	GRADED TRIAL #1	GRADED TRIAL #2	NOTES
16. ★ Once all items have been applied to the sterile field, you may wash your hands using a surgical scrub and apply sterile gloves. With sterile gloves on, you may open the previously applied sterile package and verify its contents. You may also arrange the items on the tray according to physician preference. *Note:* If you drop your hands below your waist or touch any item outside of the sterile area you are once again contaminated. You must also pay very close attention to your clothes, as scrubs that are worn too loosely will fall forward and contaminate the sterile tray. Once you have verified that all items are present and arranged according to physician preference you must cover the sterile tray. To cover the sterile tray follow the instructions for setup, but instead of crossing over the field and pulling the drape to you, you must hold the drape in front of you at a level so that the top towel and bottom towel are even and carefully lay it over the tray.				
17. ★ ***Greet and identify the patient, introduce yourself and guide him or her to the treatment area. Explain the entire procedure to the patient.***				
18. ✦ Instruct the patient to void if necessary. Provide draping or a gown for the patient as required for the procedure. Sometimes patients disrobe and gown in another room before entering the treatment area.				
19. ✦ Assist the patient onto the examination table.				
20. ★ Perform a skin prep as described in procedure 8-1.				

		PRACTICE TRIAL	GRADED TRIAL # 1	GRADED TRIAL # 2	NOTES
21. ✦	Assist the physician in scrubbing, gowning, and gloving as needed.				
22. ✦	The physician may want you to open the packet of sterile gloves for him or her and place the packet where it can be easily accessed at the start of the procedure. (Depending on the duties of the scrub assistant during the procedure, you may be designated to scrub, and to gown, mask, and glove.)				
23. ✦	When the physician is ready to proceed, he or she may remove the drapes from the tray setups without contaminating the trays or the sterile field. If you are directed to do this, grasp the towel or drape at the distal corners (away from the center). Lift the towel toward you without reaching over the tray and unprotected sterile field.				
24. ✦	In anticipation of soiled dressings, place a bag or container to the side for the physician to discard them into. *Note:* You may fulfill the role of scrub assistant or circulating assistant, depending on the procedure and the needs of the physician.				
25. ∗	**Observe closely and anticipate the physician's needs.** If a specimen container is needed, hold it to receive a specimen.				
26. ✦	In most cases the physician will prefer to apply the first sterile dressing but occasionally may direct the scrub to do it. You will reinforce or anchor the dressing.				

		PRACTICE TRIAL	GRADED TRIAL # 1	GRADED TRIAL # 2	NOTES
27. ✦	When the procedure has been completed, collect all soiled instruments in a basin and remove them from the patient's view. Dispose of soiled dressings in biohazard containers.				
28. ✦	Remove your gloves and discard. Wash your hands.				
29. ⋆	If specimen containers have been contaminated, use clean gloves to place and tighten lids on them. Label and bag specimens before transporting or sending them to the lab.				
30. ⋆	Obtain and chart vital signs following office policy and document your recovery observations, including mental status, changes in drainage and size of drainage on dressings, and ability to ambulate and urinate. (Observation requirements may vary according to the medical office specialty.) **Sign the entry with your name and credentials.**				
31. ✦	Review your observations with the physician. When the physician determines discharge readiness, he or she discusses care instructions with the patient and significant other(s).				
32. ⋆	Give the patient a printed copy of the physician's discharge instructions, and **review and reinforce them with the patient. Before the patient leaves the facility, help with any additional paperwork, such as followup appointments. Clarify any questions as necessary.**				
33. ✦	Assist or transport the patient to significant others or, in some cases, to the car.				

		PRACTICE TRIAL	GRADED TRIAL # 1	GRADED TRIAL # 2	NOTES
34. ★	Chart the results of patient instruction immediately. ***Sign the entry with your name and credentials.***				
35. ✦	Don appropriate PPE to clean and sanitize the room for the next patient.				
36. ✦	Wash your hands.				

Document: Enter the appropriate information in the chart below.

Grading

Points Earned	_____		
Points Possible	_____	240	240
Percent Grade (Points Earned/Points Possible)	_____		
PASS:	_____	❏ YES ❏ NO ❏ N/A	❏ YES ❏ NO ❏ N/A

Instructor Sign-Off

Instructor: _____   **Date:** _____

Name: _____

Date: _____

Procedure 29-3:

Assist the Physician with Suturing

Objective: The student, using the supplies and equipment listed below, will demonstrate sterile technique when assisting with suture repair of an incision.

Supplies: Sterile packs, including patient drapes, towels, and 4 × 4s, scalpels with blades or blades (size according to physician's preference), suture and needle pack (according to physician's preference), sterile suture pack, including scalpel handle, thumb forceps, needle holder, scissors, hemostats, Mayo stand and side stand or table, anesthetic (usually local), sterile transfer forceps and holder, sterile basins, sterile saline or water, sterile gloves, needle and syringe pack, waste container, with plastic bag liner, biohazard waste container, sharps container

Affective Behaviors: Affective behaviors provide a professional approach to a skill that enhances the patient encounter. These behaviors may also display sensitivity to a patient's rights and enhance communication. Pay close attention to these skills, which will be in **_bold, italicized_** font.

Notes to the Student

_____

_____

_____

_____

_____

_____

Skills Assessment Requirements

Read and familiarize yourself with the procedure; complete the minimum practice requirements. Document each MPR using proper charting technique. Complete each procedure within a reasonable amount of time, with a minimum of 85 percent accuracy.

Name: _____

Date: _____

POINT VALUE ✦ = 3–6 points ⋆ = 7–9 points		PRACTICE TRIAL	GRADED TRIAL # 1	GRADED TRIAL # 2	NOTES
1. ✦	Wash your hands.				
2. ⋆	**Greet and identify the patient, introduce yourself and guide him or her to the treatment area. Explain the entire procedure to the patient.**				
3. ✦	Position the patient on the exam table so that the area to be sutured is exposed.				
4. ✦	Drape to cover the patient's clothing. Follow the guidelines for prepping the skin and draping it for minor surgery.				
5. ⋆	Perform a 5-minute sterile scrub.				
6. ✦	Put on sterile gloves.				
7. ✦	Take a position standing opposite the physician.				
8. ✦	Place two sterile sponges near the wound site.				
9. ✦	Have additional sponges ready as needed.				
10. ⋆	Pass instruments to the physician as requested, with a firm "snap" into the palm of the physician's hand.				
11. ⋆	Prepare a scalpel handle with blade according to the physician's preference. Pass the scalpel to the physician when necessary.				
12. ✦	Sponge the area as necessary and as directed by the physician.				
13. ✦	Pass other instruments, such as toothed forceps, as necessary.				

		PRACTICE TRIAL	GRADED TRIAL # 1	GRADED TRIAL # 2	NOTES
14. ★	Place the needle in the needle holder. Pass the needle holder, needle, and suture to the physician, keeping the suture material within the sterile field.				
15. ✦	Keep a hold on the distal end of the suture until the physician sees it and takes it.				
16. ✦	With suture scissors, cut sutures as directed by the physician 1/8 to 1/4 inch above the knot.				
17. ✦	Sponge the closed wound during suturing and discard the soiled sponges.				
18. ✦	Place used instruments in a disinfectant-filled instrument basin immediately.				
19. ✦	Add unused sterile instruments to the disinfectant at the same time, or use another disinfectant-filled instrument basin.				
20. ✦	Remove the gloves and discard. Wash your hands.				
21. ✦	Apply dressings as instructed by the physician.				
22. ✦	**Help the patient into a comfortable position.** Monitor vital signs according to office procedures.				
23. ★	**Provide the patient with both oral and written postoperative instructions, including the date and time of the followup appointment. Clarify any questions as necessary.**				
24. ✦	Make sure the patient is stable for discharge.				

	PRACTICE TRIAL	GRADED TRIAL # 1	GRADED TRIAL # 2	NOTES
25. ★ Complete requisitions for specimens. Transport them to the laboratory or secure them for courier transport to the laboratory.				
26. ✦ Clean, sanitize, and sterilize the instruments. Inspect them for residual tissue or body fluids and remove any you discover.				
27. ✦ Clean and sanitize the room for the next patient.				
28. ✦ Wash your hands.				

Document: Enter the appropriate information in the chart below.

Grading

Points Earned	_____		
Points Possible	_____	189	189
Percent Grade (Points Earned/Points Possible)	_____		
PASS:	_____	❏ YES ❏ NO ❏ N/A	❏ YES ❏ NO ❏ N/A

Instructor Sign-Off

Instructor: _____ Date: _____

Name: _____

Date: _____

Procedure 29-4:

Assist the Physician with Suture or Staple Removal

Objective: The student should be able to assist the physician with suture or staple removal.

Supplies: Suture removal kit, including suture scissors, thumb forceps, and sterile 4 × 4 gauze, or staple removal kit, including staple remover and sterile 4 × 4 gauze; antiseptic swabs; sterile 4 × 4 gauze, gloves, surgical tape, biohazard waste container, sharps container, if necessary

Affective Behaviors: Affective behaviors provide a professional approach to a skill that enhances the patient encounter. These behaviors may also display sensitivity to a patient's rights and enhance communication. Pay close attention to these skills, which will be in **bold, _italicized_** font.

Notes to the Student

_____

_____

_____

_____

_____

_____

Skills Assessment Requirements

Read and familiarize yourself with the procedure; complete the minimum practice requirements. Document each MPR using proper charting technique. Complete each procedure within a reasonable amount of time, with a minimum of 85 percent accuracy.

POINT VALUE ✦ = 3–6 points ⋆ = 7–9 points		PRACTICE TRIAL	GRADED TRIAL # 1	GRADED TRIAL # 2	NOTES
1. ✦	Wash your hands.				
2. ⋆	**Greet and identify the patient, introduce yourself and guide him or her to the treatment area. Explain the entire procedure to the patient.**				
3. ✦	**Describe the sensation of pulling or tugging normally felt as the sutures or staples are removed.**				
4. ✦	Apply gloves.				
5. ✦	Remove any dressing present. Moisten adhered dressing with sterile saline or hydrogen peroxide before removal, if necessary.				
6. ✦	Grasp the edge of the dressing and lift it halfway to the point of the suture line. Then lift the other edge in the same manner. Once the dressing is free of the suture area, it can be disposed of in a biohazard container.				
7. ✦	Cleanse the suture or staple area and surrounding skin.				
8. ✦	Open the sterile suture or staple removal kit.				
9. ✦	Wash your hands and put on sterile gloves.				
	For sutures: **Explain the following steps to the patient, as necessary.**				
10. ⋆	With the thumb forceps, grasp the suture knot. Gently lift the knot upward.				

		PRACTICE TRIAL	GRADED TRIAL #1	GRADED TRIAL #2	NOTES
11. ★	With your other hand, slip the notched edge of the suture scissors under the suture as close to the skin as possible. Close the scissors to cut the suture.				
12. ★	Gently pull on the knot and pull the unexposed suture through the skin. Place it on the 4 × 4 gauze.				
13. ✦	Continue until all the sutures are removed. Check the patient chart for total number of sutures applied to verify that all sutures have been removed. If the count is inconsistent you must report this to the physician for further instructions.				
14. ✦	Cleanse the skin with an antiseptic swab.				
15. ✦	Allow the skin to air dry and apply adhesive skin closures or dressing as the physician directs. **Prior to leaving the examination room, ask the patient if he or she has any questions.**				
	For staples: Explain the following steps to the patient, as necessary.				
16. ★	Slide the bottom jaw of the staple remover under the staple.				
17. ★	Squeeze the staple remover handles together. The staple will bend slightly into a "V" shape.				
18. ★	Carefully lift the staple from the skin. Place it on the 4 × 4 gauze.				

Name: _____

Date: _____

		PRACTICE TRIAL	GRADED TRIAL #1	GRADED TRIAL #2	NOTES
19. ✦	Continue the process until all the staples are removed.				
20. ✦	Cleanse the skin with antiseptic swab.				
21. ✦	Allow the skin to air dry and apply adhesive skin closures or dressing as the physician directs. *Prior to leaving the examination room, ask the patient if he or she has any questions.*				
	Cleanup for both procedures:				
22. ✦	Dispose of contaminated materials in a biohazard or sharps container as appropriate.				
23. ✦	Remove the gloves and discard.				
24. ✦	Wash your hands.				
25. ★	Document the procedure. *Sign the entry with your name and credentials.*				

Document: Enter the appropriate information in the chart below.

Grading

Points Earned	_____		
Points Possible	_____	174	174
Percent Grade (Points Earned/Points Possible)	_____		
PASS:	_____	❑ YES ❑ NO ❑ N/A	❑ YES ❑ NO ❑ N/A

Instructor Sign-Off

Instructor: _____ **Date:** _____

Procedure 29-5:

Change a Sterile Dressing

Objective: The student, using the supplies and equipment listed below, will demonstrate a sterile dressing change.

Supplies: Prepackaged dressing pack, including sterile gauze or sponges, sterile thumb forceps, sterile dressings, adhesive tape (or tape most appropriate for skin condition and dressing function); Mayo stand and side tray; antiseptic solution; sterile transfer forceps; sterile gloves; scissors; sterile basins; thumb forceps; disposable gloves; waste container with plastic bag liner, biohazard waste container

Affective Behaviors: Affective behaviors provide a professional approach to a skill that enhances the patient encounter. These behaviors may also display sensitivity to a patient's rights and enhance communication. Pay close attention to these skills, which will be in **_bold, italicized_** font.

Notes to the Student

_____

_____

_____

_____

_____

_____

Skills Assessment Requirements

Read and familiarize yourself with the procedure; complete the minimum practice requirements. Document each MPR using proper charting technique. Complete each procedure within a reasonable amount of time, with a minimum of 85 percent accuracy.

Name: _____

Date: _____

POINT VALUE ✦ = 3–6 points ★ = 7–9 points	PRACTICE TRIAL	GRADED TRIAL #1	GRADED TRIAL #2	NOTES
1. ★ **Greet and identify the patient, introduce yourself and guide him or her to the treatment area. Explain the entire procedure to the patient.**				
2. ✦ Wash your hands.				
3. ✦ Assemble the equipment on the Mayo stand or side table, using aseptic technique. Arrange the supplies and equipment.				
4. ✦ Apply nonsterile gloves and remove the dressing by pulling it in the direction of the wound.				
5. ✦ Place the removed dressing into a biohazard bag, without touching the outside of the bag. Be careful not to pass it over your sterile tray.				
6. ★ Arrange the supplies and equipment. Inspect the patient's wound and make a mental note to later document in the chart. A description of the wound size, shape, and any indication of infection, such as pus or inflammation, should be noted.				
7. ✦ Hold the antiseptic container with your palm covering the label. Pour some of the antiseptic into a sink or waste container. As the solution flows across the edge of the container, the edge will be disinfected. Pour the antiseptic into the sterile basin.				
8. ✦ Wash your hands with a surgical scrub and apply sterile gloves.				

		PRACTICE TRIAL	GRADED TRIAL # 1	GRADED TRIAL # 2	NOTES
9. ✦	Using sterile forceps and sterile cotton balls or sterile gauze pads, depending on the size of the wound, cleanse the wound. Disposable materials can be discarded in biohazard, and reusable items will be cleaned at the end of the procedure.				
10. ⋆	Cleanse the wound by moving from the inside to the outside, wiping from the top of the wound to the bottom, one time. The cotton ball must be changed with each stroke.				
11. ⋆	Apply the sterile dressing to the wound and remove your gloves. Verify that your patient does not have an allergy to adhesives. If any allergy is present, secure the dressing with nonadhesive disposable bandage wrap such as Coban.				
12. ✦	Secure the dressing with adhesive tape. Tape should cover the entire dressing or be wrapped completely around the extremity.				
13. ⋆	***Provide the patient with written and verbal instructions on wound care, signs of infection, and when they should follow up with the physician. Prior to the patient leaving the procedure area, ask if he or she has any questions.***				

Name: _____

Date: _____

		PRACTICE TRIAL	GRADED TRIAL # 1	GRADED TRIAL # 2	NOTES
14. ✦	When the patient has exited the procedure area you may apply nonsterile gloves and clean the room in preparation for the next patient.				
15. ⋆	**Document the procedure and sign the entry with your name and credentials.**				

Document: Enter the appropriate information in the chart below.

Grading

Points Earned	_____		
Points Possible	_____	108	108
Percent Grade (Points Earned/Points Possible)	_____		
PASS:	_____	❏ YES ❏ NO ❏ N/A	❏ YES ❏ NO ❏ N/A

Instructor Sign-Off

Instructor: _____   **Date:** _____

Procedure 30-1:

Check the Accuracy of Glucometer Results
Using Quality Control Methods

Objective: The student, using the supplies and equipment listed below, will demonstrate how to perform quality control testing of the glucometer.

Supplies: Quality control log book, glucometer, quality controls specific to brand of glucometer

Notes to the Student

_____

_____

_____

_____

_____

Skills Assessment Requirements

Read and familiarize yourself with the procedure; complete the minimum practice requirements. Document each MPR using proper charting technique. Complete each procedure within a reasonable amount of time, with a minimum of 85 percent accuracy.

Name: _____

Date: _____

POINT VALUE ✦ = 3–6 points ⋆ = 7–9 points		PRACTICE TRIAL	GRADED TRIAL # 1	GRADED TRIAL # 2	NOTES
1. ✦	Wash your hands and assemble materials.				
2. ⋆	Perform control testing as recommended by the manufacturer and per office policy. a. Check unsealed quality control vials and test strips for open and discard dates and expiration dates. Label the control vials and test strips if you are opening them for the first time. b. If you are changing code strips, calibrate and change the number per manufacturer's instructions.				
3. ✦	Record the test results in a quality control log. If control results are abnormal, report them to the supervisor. Label the glucometer "Repair" and remove it from the clinical area to prevent other staff from using it. Return the glucometer to the clinical area only after the problem has been corrected.				
4. ✦	Dispose of waste materials in the appropriate container.				
5. ✦	Wash your hands and return the glucometer and quality test control equipment to the designated storage area.				

Name: _____

Date: _____

Document: Enter the appropriate information in the chart below.

Grading

Points Earned	_____		
Points Possible	_____	33	33
Percent Grade (Points Earned/Points Possible)	_____		
PASS:	_____	❏ YES ❏ NO ❏ N/A	❏ YES ❏ NO ❏ N/A

Instructor Sign-Off

Instructor: _____ **Date:** _____

Procedure 30-2:

Demonstrate Screening and Followup of Test Results

Objective: The student, using the supplies and equipment listed below, will demonstrate how to screen and follow up on returned laboratory results.

Supplies: Returned laboratory reports, patient chart, blue or black ink pen, telephone

Affective Behaviors: Affective behaviors provide a professional approach to a skill that enhances the patient encounter. These behaviors may also display sensitivity to a patient's rights and enhance communication. Pay close attention to these skills, which will be in **_bold, italicized_** font.

Notes to the Student

_____

_____

_____

_____

_____

_____

Skills Assessment Requirements

Read and familiarize yourself with the procedure; complete the minimum practice requirements. Document each MPR using proper charting technique. Complete each procedure within a reasonable amount of time, with a minimum of 85 percent accuracy.

	POINT VALUE ✦ = 3–6 points ★ = 7–9 points		PRACTICE TRIAL	GRADED TRIAL #1	GRADED TRIAL #2	NOTES
1. ✦	Sort lab reports according to physician.					
2. ✦	Sort the reports according to last name, first name, and initial for each physician.					
3. ✦	Match patient identification numbers in cases where names are similar.					
4. ★	Attach the new reports to the patient chart and place them in a designated area for the physician to read and interpret. The physician will initial each laboratory test that he or she reads.					
5. ★	Call patients with their laboratory results or set up appointments to discuss the results as designated by the physician. *If an answering machine or voicemail is activated, do not include patient information in your message.* Leave a phone number for the patient to return the call.					
6. ✦	Place the laboratory reports in the chart according to office procedure.					
7. ✦	On a tickler file, note the next scheduled date for routinely scheduled laboratory procedures.					
8. ✦	*Work with the patient to schedule the next appointment if the laboratory procedure is weekly or monthly. Prior to hanging up the phone, ask the patient if he or she has any questions.*					

Name: _____

Date: _____

Document: Enter the appropriate information in the chart below.

Grading

Points Earned	_____		
Points Possible	_____	54	54
Percent Grade (Points Earned/Points Possible)	_____		
PASS:	_____	❏ YES ❏ NO ❏ N/A	❏ YES ❏ NO ❏ N/A

Instructor Sign-Off

Instructor: _____ Date: _____

Procedure 31-1:

Demonstrate Using the Microscope

Objective: The student, using the supplies and equipment listed below, will demonstrate how to use the microscope and focus all three objectives.

Supplies: Microscope, lens paper, lens cleaner, prepared slide (with or without cover slip), immersion oil, disposable gloves, tissues

Notes to the Student

_____

_____

_____

_____

_____

_____

Skills Assessment Requirements

Read and familiarize yourself with the procedure; complete the minimum practice requirements. Document each MPR using proper charting technique. Complete each procedure within a reasonable amount of time, with a minimum of 85 percent accuracy.

POINT VALUE ✦ = 3–6 points ★ = 7–9 points	PRACTICE TRIAL	GRADED TRIAL #1	GRADED TRIAL #2	NOTES
1. ✦ Wash your hands and put on disposable gloves.				
2. ✦ Remove the cover from the microscope.				
3. ✦ Check that the microscope is clean and in working order. Replace the light bulb if necessary.				
4. ✦ Turn the light off until you are ready to focus the objectives on the specimen slide.				
5. ✦ Clean the lenses and eyepieces (oculars) with lens paper. Use lens cleaner as necessary, but do *not* oversaturate the glue holding the lens in place.				
6. ✦ Secure the slide on the stage with the slide clips.				
7. ✦ Revolve the low-power objective into place until it is seated or you hear a click.				
8. ✦ Adjust the oculars so that you see only one field rather than separate left and right views.				
9. ✦ Using the coarse adjustment control knob, raise the body tube of the microscope and swivel the 10× objective into place.				
10. ✦ Turn the light on.				
11. ✦ Lower the body tube with the coarse adjustment control knob, to bring the slide into general focus.				

		PRACTICE TRIAL	GRADED TRIAL # 1	GRADED TRIAL # 2	NOTES
12. ✦	With the iris controls, adjust the light to cover the slide. It is not important at this point to achieve clear focus.			₹	
13. ✦	Observing from the side, lower the body tube to bring the objective closer to the slide without touching it.				
14. ✦	Look through the oculars, using the coarse adjustment to bring the specimen into focus. Adjust the iris if you need more light.				
15. ✦	Observing from the side, switch to the high-power objective without touching the slide. The body tube may need to be adjusted during this process.				
16. ✦	When the high-power objective (40×) is in place, adjust the fine focus controls to bring the specimen into clear focus.				
17. ✦	If the slide specimen is dry and does not have a cover slip, apply a drop of oil and turn the oil immersion objective into place. Lower the objective until it is covered with oil.				
18. ✦	After the specimen has been examined, lower the stage.				
19. ✦	Remove the slide specimen and dispose of it in a biohazard waste receptacle.				
20. ✦	Turn off the light.				

Name: _____

Date: _____

		PRACTICE TRIAL	GRADED TRIAL # 1	GRADED TRIAL # 2	NOTES
21. ✦	Clean the lenses with lens cleaner and lens paper. Clean the stage.				
22. ✦	Rotate the objectives to return the low-power objective directly above the stage.				
23. ✦	Cover the microscope.				
24. ✦	Clean the work area.				
25. ✦	Dispose of the gloves and wash your hands.				

Name: _____

Date: _____

Document: Enter the appropriate information in the chart below.

Grading

Points Earned	_____		
Points Possible	_____	150	150
Percent Grade (Points Earned/Points Possible)	_____		
PASS:	_____	❏ YES ❏ NO ❏ N/A	❏ YES ❏ NO ❏ N/A

Instructor Sign-Off

Instructor: _____   **Date:** _____

Procedure 31-2:

Preparing a Specimen Smear for Microbiological Examination

Objective: The student, using the supplies and equipment listed below, will demonstrate how to prepare a slide for microscopic examination.

Supplies: Glass slide (preferably with frosted edge), disposable gloves, sterile distilled water, inoculating loops or specimen swabs, flame source, biohazardous waste container, sharps container

Notes to the Student

_____

_____

_____

_____

_____

_____

Skills Assessment Requirements

Read and familiarize yourself with the procedure; complete the minimum practice requirements. Document each MPR using proper charting technique. Complete each procedure within a reasonable amount of time, with a minimum of 85 percent accuracy.

POINT VALUE ✦ = 3–6 points ⋆ = 7–9 points		PRACTICE TRIAL	GRADED TRIAL # 1	GRADED TRIAL # 2	NOTES
1. ✦	Wash your hands.				
2. ✦	Gather equipment and supplies.				
3. ✦	Wash your hands again and put on disposable gloves.				
4. ⋆	Write the patient information on the frosted edge of the slide.				
5. ✦	Prepare a thin film, or smear, on the slide.				
	For a specimen from a swab:				
6. ✦	Roll and turn the swab across the slide.				
	For a specimen from a petri dish:				
7. ✦	Gather sterile distilled water with a sterile inoculating loop and place it on the slide.				
8. ✦	Use the inoculating loop to gather the microbial specimen, without gathering any culture medium.				
9. ✦	Mix the specimen into the distilled water on the slide.				
10. ✦	Sterilize the loop over the flame.				

Name: _____

Date: _____

		PRACTICE TRIAL	GRADED TRIAL # 1	GRADED TRIAL # 2	NOTES
	For a specimen from a liquid:				
11. ✦	Dip the inside of the sterile inoculating loop in the culture until it appears covered with a film.				
12. ✦	Touch the film to the center of the slide.				
13. ✦	Allow the specimen on the slide to air dry completely.				
14. ✦	Hold and pass the slide through the flame several times. The slide is now ready to stain.				
15. ∗	Clean the work area.				
16. ✦	Dispose of the gloves and wash your hands.				

Name: _____

Date: _____

Document: Enter the appropriate information in the chart below.

Grading

Points Earned	_____		
Points Possible	_____	102	102
Percent Grade (Points Earned/Points Possible)	_____		
PASS:	_____	❏ YES ❏ NO ❏ N/A	❏ YES ❏ NO ❏ N/A

Instructor Sign-Off

Instructor: _____ **Date:** _____

Name: _____

Date: _____

Procedure 31-3:

Prepare a Gram Stain

Objective: The student, using the supplies and equipment listed below, will demonstrate how to prepare a slide for microscopic examination of gram-negative and gram-positive bacteria.

Supplies: Disposable gloves, slide with fixed smear, crystal violet dye, Gram's iodine, alcohol/acetone mixture, safranin dye, wash bottle filled with distilled water, rack and tray for slide staining, forceps, paper towel, biohazardous waste container, sharps container

Notes to the Student

_____

_____

_____

_____

_____

_____

Skills Assessment Requirements

Read and familiarize yourself with the procedure; complete the minimum practice requirements. Document each MPR using proper charting technique. Complete each procedure within a reasonable amount of time, with a minimum of 85 percent accuracy.

POINT VALUE ✦ = 3–6 points ⋆ = 7–9 points	PRACTICE TRIAL	GRADED TRIAL #1	GRADED TRIAL #2	NOTES
1. ✦ Wash your hands.				
2. ✦ Wash your hands again and put on disposable gloves.				
3. ✦ Lay the slide on the slide rack and tray.				
4. ⋆ Pour crystal violet on the slide and allow it to stain for 1 minute.				
5. ✦ Rinse the slide gently with water from the wash bottle.				
6. ✦ Lay the slide on the slide rack and tray.				
7. ⋆ Pour Gram's iodine, also known as mordant, on the slide. Allow it to stain for 2 minutes.				
8. ✦ Lift the slide diagonally with the forceps and rinse gently with water from the wash bottle.				
9. ✦ Maintaining the vertical hold, gently pour the acetone/alcohol decolorizing mixture over the slide. Pour until the runoff is clear (approximately 1 minute).				
10. ✦ Lay the slide on the slide rack and tray.				
11. ⋆ Pour safranin dye on the slide and allow it to stain for 30 seconds.				
12. ✦ Lift the slide angled vertically with the forceps and rinse gently.				
13. ✦ Let the slide air dry vertically, or blot—do not wipe—the stained area with a paper towel.				

		PRACTICE TRIAL	GRADED TRIAL # 1	GRADED TRIAL # 2	NOTES
14. ✦	Mount the slide on the micro-scope for examination.				
15. ✦	Return supplies to storage.				
16. ∗	Clean the work area.				
17. ✦	Dispose of biohazardous waste and sharps in the appropriate containers.				
18. ✦	Dispose of the gloves and wash your hands.				

Name: _____

Date: _____

Document: Enter the appropriate information in the chart below.

Grading

Points Earned	_____		
Points Possible	_____	120	120
Percent Grade (Points Earned/Points Possible)	_____		
PASS:	_____	❏ YES ❏ NO ❏ N/A	❏ YES ❏ NO ❏ N/A

Instructor Sign-Off

Instructor: _____ **Date:** _____

Name: _____

Date: _____

Procedure 31-4:

Instruct a Patient in Collecting a Fecal Specimen for Occult Blood or Culture Testing

Objective: The student, using the supplies and equipment listed below, will demonstrate how to provide verbal and written instruction to the patient.

Supplies: *Fecal occult blood:* patient chart, testing kit, clean and dry mouth container with spatula, patient label and laboratory requisition form, if needed, disposable gloves, black ink pen. *Fecal culture testing:* patient chart, specimen container for transport, spatula, patient label and laboratory requisition form, if needed, disposable gloves, black ink pen. *Fecal culture developing:* disposable gloves, prepared occult blood slides, developing solution, patient chart, waste container

Affective Behaviors: Affective behaviors provide a professional approach to a skill that enhances the patient encounter. These behaviors may also display sensitivity to a patient's rights and enhance communication. Pay close attention to these skills, which will be in **bold, *italicized*** font.

Notes to the Student

_____

_____

_____

_____

_____

_____

Skills Assessment Requirements

Read and familiarize yourself with the procedure; complete the minimum practice requirements. Document each MPR using proper charting technique. Complete each procedure within a reasonable amount of time, with a minimum of 85 percent accuracy.

POINT VALUE ✦ = 3–6 points ⋆ = 7–9 points	PRACTICE TRIAL	GRADED TRIAL #1	GRADED TRIAL #2	NOTES
1. ✦ Wash your hands.				
2. ✦ Gather supplies.				
3. ✦ Check the kit to make sure it has not expired.				
4. ⋆ **Greet and identify the patient, introduce yourself and escort him or her to the examination room.**				
5. ✦ Ask the patient what he or she understands about the reason(s) for the test. **Clarify the information as needed to help the patient understand.**				
6. ✦ Inform the physician if further discussion would benefit the patient.				
7. ⋆ **Provide verbal instructions for fecal occult blood or culture testing.** Reinforce them by giving the patient a written copy of the instructions and the appropriate test kit supplies, lab requisitions, and patient identification labels.				
For **fecal occult blood specimen collection,** instruct the patient as follows:				
8. ✦ Using the spatula provided for each slide, place a thin smear over the first square (labeled A).				
9. ✦ Take a small specimen from a different area and smear it over the second square (labeled B).				
10. ✦ Close the flap covering the slide.				
11. ✦ Allow the slide to air dry.				

		PRACTICE TRIAL	GRADED TRIAL # 1	GRADED TRIAL # 2	NOTES
12. ✦	Repeat these steps for the remaining two slides, according to the physician's order.				
13. ✦	Return the three slides to the medical office as soon as possible. **Ask the patient if he or she has any questions.**				
	For *fecal culture specimen collection*, instruct the patient as follows:				
14. ✦	After collecting the specimen in a clean, dry container, tighten the container lid.				
15. ✦	Transport the specimen immediately or transfer it to a preservative container.				
16. ⋆	Document on the chart the instructions you gave and the patient's understanding. **Sign the entry with your name and credentials.**				
17. ✦	Wash your hands.				
	For *developing the fecal occult blood test*, complete the following steps:				
18. ✦	Wash your hands.				
19. ✦	Gather the supplies.				
20. ⋆	Check the developing solution bottle to ensure that it has not expired.				
21. ✦	Put on disposable gloves.				
22. ✦	Open the back flap of the cardboard slides.				
23. ✦	Apply 2 drops of the developing solution to the guaiac test paper directly over each smear.				

		PRACTICE TRIAL	GRADED TRIAL # 1	GRADED TRIAL # 2	NOTES
24. ★	Read the results within 60 seconds. Any trace of blue on or at the edge of the smear is positive for occult blood.				
25. ★	Perform the quality control procedure to ensure the accuracy and reliability of the test results.				
26. ✦	Dispose the fecal occult blood test in a regular waste container.				
27. ✦	Remove your gloves and sanitize your hands.				
28. ★	Document on the chart the results of the test, including the date and time, the brand name of the test, and the results for each slide. **Sign the entry with your name and credentials.**				

Name: _____

Date: _____

Document: Enter the appropriate information in the chart below.

Grading

Points Earned	_____		
Points Possible	_____	189	189
Percent Grade (Points Earned/Points Possible)	_____		
PASS:	_____	❏ YES ❏ NO ❏ N/A	❏ YES ❏ NO ❏ N/A

Instructor Sign-Off

Instructor: _____ Date: _____

Name: _____

Date: _____

Procedure 31-5:

Perform a Wound or Throat Culture Using Sterile Swabs

Objective: The student, using the supplies and equipment listed below, will perform swab culture collection and prepare it for transport and processing.

Supplies: *Wound*: patient chart, single- or double-swab collection device (one swab for culture inoculation and one for gram stain), setup for anaerobic culture (for nonsuperficial wound, if physician ordered), specimen label, disposable gloves. *Throat*: patient chart, tongue depressor, sterile swab and transport device, specimen label, disposable gloves

Affective Behaviors: Affective behaviors provide a professional approach to a skill that enhances the patient encounter. These behaviors may also display sensitivity to a patient's rights and enhance communication. Pay close attention to these skills, which will be in **bold, *italicized*** font.

Notes to the Student

_____

_____

_____

_____

_____

_____

Skills Assessment Requirements

Read and familiarize yourself with the procedure; complete the minimum practice requirements. Document each MPR using proper charting technique. Complete each procedure within a reasonable amount of time, with a minimum of 85 percent accuracy.

Name: _____

Date: _____

	POINT VALUE ✦ = 3–6 points ✱ = 7–9 points		PRACTICE TRIAL	GRADED TRIAL # 1	GRADED TRIAL # 2	NOTES
1. ✦		Wash your hands.				
2. ✦		Gather supplies.				
3. ✱		**Greet and identify the patient, introduce yourself, then escort him or her to the examination room. Explain the process of specimen collection.**				
4. ✦		Wash your hands again and put on disposable gloves.				
		Wound specimen collection:				
5. ✦		Mentally note the type and amount of drainage; any redness, warmth, or swelling in the surrounding area; any other abnormalities.				
6. ✦		Swab the inside of the wound. Do not swab the surrounding skin area.				
7. ✦		Place the swab in the transport container and medium, if used.				
		Throat culture specimen collection:				
8. ✦		Ask the patient to open the mouth wide and extend the tongue forward.				
9. ✦		Examine the throat and make observe for redness, swelling of throat tissue, amount and type of drainage, or the presence of white patches or pustules.				
10. ✦		Place the tongue depressor firmly on the tongue and press down.				
11. ✦		Swab the posterior pharynx between the tonsillar pillars.				

	PRACTICE TRIAL	GRADED TRIAL # 1	GRADED TRIAL # 2	NOTES
12. ✦ Place the swab in the transport container and medium, if used.				
13. ⋆ Label the container with the patient's name (first and last), date and time of collection, and source of specimen.				
14. ✦ Dispose of any waste materials in the appropriate container(s).				
15. ✦ Remove and dispose of gloves. Wash your hands. **Prior to leaving the examination room, ask the patient if he or she has any questions.**				
16. ✦ Transport the specimen to the testing area.				
17. ⋆ Perform the required charting or laboratory documentation relating to specimen collection. **Sign the entry with your name and credentials.**				

Name: _____

Date: _____

Document: Enter the appropriate information in the chart below.

Grading

Points Earned	_____		
Points Possible	_____	111	111
Percent Grade (Points Earned/Points Possible)	_____		
PASS:	_____	❑ YES ❑ NO ❑ N/A	❑ YES ❑ NO ❑ N/A

Instructor Sign-Off

Instructor: _____ **Date:** _____

Procedure 31-6:

Perform Rapid Group A Strep Testing

Objective: Correctly perform Rapid Group A Strep Testing.

Supplies: Labeled throat specimen, Group A strep kit (controls may be included depending on the kit), personal protective equipment, timer, and a biohazard waste container

Affective Behaviors: Affective behaviors provide a professional approach to a skill that enhances the patient encounter. These behaviors may also display sensitivity to a patient's rights and enhance communication. Pay close attention to these skills, which will be in **_bold, italicized_** font.

Notes to the Student

_____

_____

_____

_____

_____

_____

Skills Assessment Requirements

Read and familiarize yourself with the procedure; complete the minimum practice requirements. Document each MPR using proper charting technique. Complete each procedure within a reasonable amount of time, with a minimum of 85 percent accuracy.

POINT VALUE ✦ = 3–6 points ⋆ = 7–9 points		PRACTICE TRIAL	GRADED TRIAL # 1	GRADED TRIAL # 2	NOTES
1. ✦	Wash your hands and gather supplies.				
2. ⋆	**Verify that the name on the specimen container and the laboratory requisition form are the same.**				
3. ✦	Put on your personal protective equipment.				
4. ⋆	Label one extraction tube with the patient's name, one for the positive control, and one for the negative control.				
5. ✦	Follow the directions for the kit according to the manufacturer's instructions.				
6. ✦	Add the appropriate reagents and drops to each of the extraction tubes.				
7. ✦	Insert the patient's swab into the labeled extraction tube and add the appropriate controls to each of the labeled extraction tubes.				
8. ✦	To ensure accuracy, set the timer for the appropriate time.				
9. ✦	Add the appropriate reagent and drops to each of the extraction tubes.				
10. ⋆	Mix the reagents with the swab and add three drops from the well mixes extraction tube to the sample window of the Strep A test unit. Repeat the procedure for each control.				
11. ✦	Set the timer for the time indicated by the manufacturer.				

		PRACTICE TRIAL	GRADED TRIAL # 1	GRADED TRIAL # 2	NOTES
12. ✦	A positive or negative result appears within 5 minutes. Refer to the direction in the kit to differentiate between a positive or negative result.				
13. ✦	Properly dispose of the equipment and supplies in a biohazard waste container.				
14. ✦	Remove your personal protective equipment and wash your hands.				
15. ⋆	Document the procedure and results in the patient chart. **Sign the entry with your name and credentials.**				
16. ⋆	Sanitize the area.				

Name: _____

Date: _____

Document: Enter the appropriate information in the chart below.

Grading

Points Earned	_____		
Points Possible	_____	111	111
Percent Grade (Points Earned/Points Possible)	_____		
PASS:	_____	❏ YES ❏ NO ❏ N/A	❏ YES ❏ NO ❏ N/A

Instructor Sign-Off

Instructor: _____ Date: _____

Name: _____

Date: _____

Procedure 32-1:

Perform a Butterfly Draw Using a Hand Vein

Objective: The student, using the supplies and equipment listed below, will demonstrate how to obtain a venous blood specimen from the back of the hand using a butterfly system.

Supplies: Gloves, sterile butterfly package, cotton balls, tourniquet, vacutainer or syringe, bandage, Coban, or paper tape, alcohol, sharps container, permanent pen for marking lab sample, patient chart

Affective Behaviors: Affective behaviors provide a professional approach to a skill that enhances the patient encounter. These behaviors may also display sensitivity to a patient's rights and enhance communication. Pay close attention to these skills, which will be in **_bold, italicized_** font.

Notes to the Student

_____

_____

_____

_____

_____

_____

Skills Assessment Requirements

Read and familiarize yourself with the procedure; complete the minimum practice requirements. Document each MPR using proper charting technique. Complete each procedure within a reasonable amount of time, with a minimum of 85 percent accuracy.

Name: _____

Date: _____

POINT VALUE ✦ = 3–6 points ★ = 7–9 points		PRACTICE TRIAL	GRADED TRIAL #1	GRADED TRIAL #2	NOTES
1. ✦	Wash your hands and gather the equipment.				
2. ★	**Greet and identify the patient, introduce yourself and escort him or her to the treatment area.**				
3. ✦	Select the appropriate hand site. Put on gloves. **Explain the procedure to the patient.**				
4. ✦	Cleanse the skin with alcohol.				
5. ✦	Open the sterile butterfly package and stretch the tubing slightly to prevent it from recoiling when you begin the blood draw.				
6. ✦	Apply the tourniquet to the patient's wrist area, proximal to the wrist bone, at least 3 inches above the injection site.				
7. ✦	Have the patient make a fist or hold a stress ball or roll of gauze to slightly elevate the hand.				
8. ★	Enter the vein with the needle. The bevel should face upward, at a 30-degree angle to the skin. Advance the needle into the vein. Some people prefer to pinch the wings upward to hold the needle, while others prefer to hold just one wing from the side. If you enter the vein correctly, you will see blood "flash" into the hub of the needle, occasionally into the tubing. Hand veins have a tendency to "roll," so you may want to do a single-finger or double-finger anchor.				

		PRACTICE TRIAL	GRADED TRIAL # 1	GRADED TRIAL # 2	NOTES
9. ✦	**Single-finger anchor:** With your thumb, pull the skin taut toward the patient's knuckles to hold the vein in place. Do not put excessive pressure on the vein, as it will collapse and be difficult to enter.				
10. ✦	**Double-finger anchor:** Place your thumb below the puncture site and pull the skin toward the knuckles. Place the index finger of the same hand above the puncture site with slight pressure. You will insert the needle between your two fingers, so take great care to avoid an accidental needle stick.				
11. ✦	When blood appears in the tubing, release the tourniquet.				
12. ✱	With the needle secured in the vein, pull back on the plunger to obtain the necessary amount of blood for testing. If you are taking blood from the anetcubital space with a vacutainer, advance the tube onto the collection hub with your other hand, using the wings for support.				
13. ✦	When you have obtained the correct amount of blood, break the suction of the vacutainer by removing the tube. (If you are using a syringe, there is no suction.)				

		PRACTICE TRIAL	GRADED TRIAL # 1	GRADED TRIAL # 2	NOTES
14. ✦	Place a cotton ball or gauze pad over the puncture site without pressure and remove the needle.				
15. ✦	Discard the needle and butterfly collection tubing into a sharps container.				
16. ✦	**Bandage as necessary; ensure that the patient is comfortable and does not have any questions.**				
17. *	Label the blood specimen and fill out the laboratory paperwork.				

Document: Enter the appropriate information in the chart below.

Grading

Points Earned	_____		
Points Possible	_____	114	114
Percent Grade (Points Earned/Points Possible)	_____	.	
PASS:	_____	❏ YES ❏ NO ❏ N/A	❏ YES ❏ NO ❏ N/A

Instructor Sign-Off

Instructor: _____   **Date:** _____

Name: _____

Date: _____

Procedure 32-2:

Demonstrate Venipuncture Using the Evacuation System

Objective: The student should be able to perform a venipuncture using an evacuation system.

Supplies: Phlebotomy tray *or* individual items (antiseptic pads, appropriate vacutainers, holder, and needle), tourniquet, handwritten or preprinted specimen, appropriate labels, disposable gloves, sharps container

Affective Behaviors: Affective behaviors provide a professional approach to a skill that enhances the patient encounter. These behaviors may also display sensitivity to a patient's rights and enhance communication. Pay close attention to these skills, which will be in **bold, *italicized*** font.

Notes to the Student

_____

_____

_____

_____

_____

_____

Skills Assessment Requirements

Read and familiarize yourself with the procedure; complete the minimum practice requirements. Document each MPR using proper charting technique. Complete each procedure within a reasonable amount of time, with a minimum of 85 percent accuracy.

POINT VALUE ✦ = 3–6 points ⋆ = 7–9 points		PRACTICE TRIAL	GRADED TRIAL #1	GRADED TRIAL #2	NOTES
1. ⋆	*Review the physician's order. Verify that the order is legible, includes a diagnosis and other necessary information, and is signed by the physician or by his or her assigned person. If any test order is not legible, or if there is any confusion about which test has been ordered, contact the physician or the office nurse for confirmation. Document on the physician's order the correct tests and the name of the person who confirmed the order.*				
2. ✦	Wash your hands.				
3. ✦	Prepare the laboratory requisition from the physician's order.				
4. ✦	Make sure all routine and special supplies are available for venipuncture and transporting the specimen.				
5. ⋆	*Greet and identify the patient, introduce yourself and escort him or her to the treatment area.*				
6. ✦	Verify that the patient has been properly prepared.				
7. ✦	Position and *reassure the patient.*				
8. ✦	Wash your hands and put on disposable gloves.				

		PRACTICE TRIAL	GRADED TRIAL # 1	GRADED TRIAL # 2	NOTES
9. ✦	Prepare the needle. **For evacuated tubes and holder:** Thread the appropriate needle into the holder until it is secured, using the needle sheath as a wrench.				
10. ✦	**For a syringe:** Insert the needle into the syringe. Move the plunger within the barrel to check movement.				
11. ✦	Apply the tourniquet. Wrap it around the patient's upper arm 3 to 4 inches above the antecubital fossa. Cross the ends of the tourniquet and pull them snugly against the patient's arm. With your thumb and forefinger, hold the tourniquet in place while pulling a loop of one end behind the joined area.				
12. ✦	Select the venipuncture site.				
13. ✦	Ask the patient to make a fist.				
14. ✦	Palpate the antecubital area with your index finger to determine the exact vein location and needle entry site.				
15. ✦	Clean the antecubital area (or other selected site) with an antiseptic wipe, cotton ball soaked in antiseptic, or alcohol wipe. Use a circular motion from the venipuncture site outward.				

Name: _____

Date: _____

		PRACTICE TRIAL	GRADED TRIAL #1	GRADED TRIAL #2	NOTES
16. ✦	Insert the blood collection tube into the holder and onto the needle up to the recessed guideline on the needle holder. Avoid pushing the tube beyond the guideline to prevent loss of vacuum.				
17. ✦	To perform the venipuncture: Make sure the patient's arm (or other venipuncture site) is in a downward position to prevent reflux or "backflow."				
18. ✦	Grasp the patient's arm firmly but gently.				
19. ✦	Draw the patient's skin taut with your thumb to anchor the vein.				
20. *	Line the needle bevel up with the vein. With a single, direct puncture, enter the vein at a 15- to 30-degree angle.				
21. ✦	Hold the needle holder firmly and steadily, and then push the tube forward in the holder until the stopper is punctured with the rear of the needle.				
22. *	As soon as blood is flowing freely, release the tourniquet by pulling on the free end above the loop.				
23. ✦	Ask the patient to release his or her fist. Fill the tubes in the correct order of draw. Invert any tubes containing anticoagulant.				
24. ✦	Remove the last tube from the holder.				

	PRACTICE TRIAL	GRADED TRIAL # 1	GRADED TRIAL # 2	NOTES
25. ✦ Withdraw the needle from the patient's arm.				
26. ✦ Immediately place a clean gauze pad over the site. Apply pressure or instruct the patient to apply pressure.				
27. ✦ Remove the needle from the hub and discard the needle in an approved container. Or, if using a syringe, after filling the tubes in the correct order of draw, discard the syringe in an approved container.				
28. * Label each tube with the patient's first and last name, identification number, date and time of collection, and your initials or identifying code. Or, if preprinted computer labels are available, **initial each label** and attach the labels to the appropriate tubes.				
29. ✦ Bandage as necessary. Instruct the patient to leave the bandage on for at least 15 minutes. **Ensure that the patient is comfortable and does not have any questions.**				
30. ✦ Remove and dispose of your gloves. Wash your hands.				
31. ✦ Evaluate the patient for signs of faintness or color loss. If the patient appears stable, **thank the patient for cooperating and escort him or her back to the waiting room.**				

Document: Enter the appropriate information in the chart below.

Grading

Points Earned	_____		
Points Possible	_____	201	201
Percent Grade (Points Earned/Points Possible)	_____		
PASS:	_____	❏ YES ❏ NO ❏ N/A	❏ YES ❏ NO ❏ N/A

Instructor Sign-Off

Instructor: _____   **Date:** _____

Procedure 32-3:

Demonstrate a Venipuncture Using the Syringe Method

Objective: Correctly demonstrate a venipuncture using the syringe method.

Supplies: Sterile needle (21–22 gauge needle), 10–20 ml syringe and syringe adaptor to transfer to vacutainer tubes, phlebotomy tray or individual items (antiseptic or alcohol pads, appropriate vacutainers, sterile gauze), tourniquet, handwritten or preprinted specimen labels, disposable gloves, sharps container, nonallergic tape or bandage

Affective Behaviors: Affective behaviors provide a professional approach to a skill that enhances the patient encounter. These behaviors may also display sensitivity to a patient's rights and enhance communication. Pay close attention to these skills, which will be in **_bold, italicized_** font.

Notes to the Student

_____

_____

_____

_____

_____

_____

Skills Assessment Requirements

Read and familiarize yourself with the procedure; complete the minimum practice requirements. Document each MPR using proper charting technique. Complete each procedure within a reasonable amount of time, with a minimum of 85 percent accuracy.

POINT VALUE ✦ = 3–6 points ⋆ = 7–9 points	PRACTICE TRIAL	GRADED TRIAL #1	GRADED TRIAL #2	NOTES
1. ⋆ **Review the physician's order. Verify that the order is legible, includes a diagnosis and other necessary information, and is signed by the physician or by his or her assigned person.**				
2. ✦ Wash your hands.				
3. ✦ Prepare the laboratory requisition from the physician's orders.				
4. ⋆ **Greet and identify the patient, introduce yourself and escort him or her to the treatment area.**				
5. ✦ Verify that the patient has been properly prepared.				
6. ✦ Position and reassure the patient.				
7. ✦ Wash your hands and put on the disposable gloves.				
8. ✦ Insert the needle into the syringe. Move the plunger within the barrel to check movement.				
9. ✦ Apply the tourniquet. Wrap it around the patient's upper arm 3-4 inches above the antecubital fossa. Cross the ends of the tourniquet and pull them snugly against the patient's arm. With your thumb and forefinger, hold the tourniquet in place while pulling a loop of one end behind the joined area.				
10. ✦ Select the venipuncture site.				

Name: _____

Date: _____

	PRACTICE TRIAL	GRADED TRIAL #1	GRADED TRIAL #2	NOTES
11. ✦ Ask the patient to make a fist.				
12. ✶ Palpate the antecubital area with your index finger to determine the exact vein location and needle entry site.				
13. ✦ Clean the antecubital area (or other selected site) with an antiseptic or alcohol wipe.				
14. ✦ Allow the site to air dry, or dry it with a clean gauze pad.				
15. ✦ Hold the syringe with your dominant hand. Remove the plastic protective cover from the needle.				
16. ✶ To perform venipuncture: • Make sure the patient's arm is in a downward position to prevent reflux or backflow. • Use your thumb to draw the skin tight to anchor the vein. • Line the needle bevel up with the vein. • With a single direct puncture, enter the vein at a 15- to 30- degree angle. • Observe for a "flash" of blood in the hub of the syringe. • Have the patient release his or her fist.				
17. ✦ Slowly pull back the plunger of the syringe. Be certain that you do not move the needle after entering the vein. Fill the barrel to the needed volume.				

		PRACTICE TRIAL	GRADED TRIAL # 1	GRADED TRIAL # 2	NOTES
18. *	Release the tourniquet when you have obtained the appropriate volume and venipuncture is complete.				
19. ✦	Immediately place a sterile gauze pad over the site and withdraw the needle from the patient's arm.				
20. ✦	Apply pressure or instruct the patient to apply pressure on the puncture site with sterile gauze.				
21. *	Transfer the blood immediately to the required tube(s) using the syringe adaptor. Invert the tubes after the addition of the blood.				
22. ✦	Discard the syringe in an approved container.				
23. *	**Use the preprinted labels or label each tube with the patient's first and last name, identification number (if applicable), date and time of collection, and your initials.**				
24. ✦	Check the venipuncture sight to make sure the bleeding has stopped, and bandage it. Instruct the patient to leave the bandage on for at least 15 minutes. **Ensure that the patient is comfortable and does not have any questions.**				
25. ✦	Remove and dispose of gloves.				

Name: _____

Date: _____

	PRACTICE TRIAL	GRADED TRIAL #1	GRADED TRIAL #2	NOTES
26. ✦ Wash your hands.				
27. ✦ *Evaluate the patient for signs of faintness or color loss.*				
28. * Complete the laboratory requisition, and route the specimen to the proper place.				
29. * Record the procedure in the patient's chart. *Sign the entry with your name and credentials*.				

Document: Enter the appropriate information in the chart below.

Grading

Points Earned	_____		
Points Possible	_____	201	201
Percent Grade (Points Earned/Points Possible)	_____		
PASS:	_____	❏ YES ❏ NO ❏ N/A	❏ YES ❏ NO ❏ N/A

Instructor Sign-Off

Instructor: _____   **Date:** _____

Procedure 32-4:

Perform a Capillary Puncture with Microcollection Tubes

Objective: The student, using the supplies and equipment listed below, will demonstrate a capillary puncture.

Supplies: Phlebotomy tray *or* individual items (antiseptic pads and capillary puncture and collection devices), handwritten or preprinted specimen labels, disposable gloves, sharps container

Affective Behaviors: Affective behaviors provide a professional approach to a skill that enhances the patient encounter. These behaviors may also display sensitivity to a patient's rights and enhance communication. Pay close attention to these skills, which will be in **bold, *italicized*** font.

Notes to the Student

_____

_____

_____

_____

_____

_____

Skills Assessment Requirements

Read and familiarize yourself with the procedure; complete the minimum practice requirements. Document each MPR using proper charting technique. Complete each procedure within a reasonable amount of time, with a minimum of 85 percent accuracy.

Name: _____

Date: _____

POINT VALUE ◆ = 3–6 points ⋆ = 7–9 points		PRACTICE TRIAL	GRADED TRIAL #1	GRADED TRIAL #2	NOTES
1. ⋆	*Review the physician's order and prepare the laboratory requisition.*				
2. ◆	Gather the supplies for capillary puncture and specimen transport.				
3. ◆	Wash your hands.				
4. ⋆	*Greet and identify the patient, ask the parents or guardian of babies or young children for identification information; introduce yourself and escort him or her to the treatment area.*				
5. ◆	Verify that the patient has followed test preparation instructions such as changing the diet or taking special medications and is not allergic to latex.				
6. ◆	Position and **reassure the patient.**				
7. ◆	Select an age-appropriate dermal puncture site where there is no danger of contact with bone. If possible, warm the site with a warming device or a warm, moist cloth (no warmer than 40° C/105° F) for 3 minutes.				
8. ◆	Wash your hands and put on disposable gloves.				
9. ◆	Clean the site with an antiseptic wipe, usually 70% isopropyl alcohol. Allow the area to thoroughly air dry, or dry it with clean gauze.				

		PRACTICE TRIAL	GRADED TRIAL # 1	GRADED TRIAL # 2	NOTES
10. ✦	Choose a puncturing device of the appropriate size. Remove the safety indicator and discard it in the appropriate biohazardous waste container.				
11. ✶	Place the puncturing device firmly on the prepared skin surface, so that the lancet cuts across the grooves of the finger or heel print. Press the safety trigger to release the puncturing lancet.				
12. ✦	For a finger stick, massage gently from the hand to near the puncture site, keeping the hand below elbow level to obtain the required blood sample.				
13. ✶	Wipe away the first drop of blood with clean gauze. The first drop contains tissue fluids and may contaminate the blood sample.				
14. ✦	Follow the correct order of draw for capillary puncture specimens to fill the tubes to the fill line: lavender, the other additive tubes, then red.				
15. ✶	Collect the specimen by holding the scoop of the microcollection tube directly beneath the puncture site. Apply gentle pressure at the puncture site ends, opening the puncture slightly to maximize blood flow. (For a finger stick, apply gentle, intermittent pressure on the entire finger to allow the capillaries to refill with blood and to help ensure continuous blood flow.)				

		PRACTICE TRIAL	GRADED TRIAL # 1	GRADED TRIAL # 2	NOTES
16. ✦	Lightly touch the collection scoop to the underside of the drop of blood so that the blood flows through the scoop and into the collection tube.				
17. ✦	Gently tap each tube containing anticoagulant after the addition of each drop of blood to ensure that the blood falls to the anti-coagulant/blood mixture.				
18. ✦	After filling the tube, invert it back and forth eight to ten times.				
19. ✦	When the blood collection is complete, wipe the site dry and apply pressure with clean gauze until the bleeding stops.				
20. ✦	**Bandage as necessary; ensure that the patient is comfortable and does not have any questions.**				
21. ✦	Dispose of all used sharps and biohazardous waste in the appropriate containers.				
22. *	**Label each tube with the patient's first and last name, identification number, date and time of collection, and your initials or identifying code. Or, if preprinted computer labels are available, initial each label and attach the labels to the appropriate tubes.**				
23. ✦	Remove the disposable gloves and discard appropriately. Wash your hands.				

		PRACTICE TRIAL	GRADED TRIAL # 1	GRADED TRIAL # 2	NOTES
24. ✦	Instruct the patient, or the patient's parent or guardian, to remove the bandage after at least 15 minutes. ***Thank the patient or parent/guardian for cooperating or assisting.***				
25. ✦	Escort the patient to the waiting room for further instructions.				

Name: _____

Date: _____

Document: Enter the appropriate information in the chart below.

Grading

Points Earned	_____		
Points Possible	_____	168	168
Percent Grade (Points Earned/Points Possible)	_____		
PASS:	_____	❏ YES ❏ NO ❏ N/A	❏ YES ❏ NO ❏ N/A

Instructor Sign-Off

Instructor: _____ **Date:** _____

Procedure 32-5:

Perform a WBC and Platelet Count with a Unopette Vial Hemacytometer

Objective: The student should be able to perform a WBC and platelet count with a Unopette vial and hemacytometer.

Supplies: Unopette vial and pipette unit, hemacytometer with Neubauer ruling, petri dish, sterile gauze squares, disposable gloves, sharps container, biohazardous waste container

Notes to the Student

_____

_____

_____

_____

_____

_____

Skills Assessment Requirements

Read and familiarize yourself with the procedure; complete the minimum practice requirements. Document each MPR using proper charting technique. Complete each procedure within a reasonable amount of time, with a minimum of 85 percent accuracy.

Name: _____

Date: _____

POINT VALUE ✦ = 3–6 points ∗ = 7–9 points		PRACTICE TRIAL	GRADED TRIAL #1	GRADED TRIAL #2	NOTES
1. ✦	Wash your hands.				
2. ✦	Gather equipment and supplies.				
3. ✦	Place the Unopette vial on a flat surface. Push the pipette shield through the diaphragm into the neck of the vial.				
4. ✦	Remove the pipette assembly from the vial, then remove the pipette shield.				
5. ∗	Holding the pipette horizontally, touch the tip to the blood sample—venous, mixed EDTA anticoagulated, or capillary. The capillary action filling the pipette will stop when the blood reaches the capillary bore end in the pipette neck.				
6. ✦	Clean any blood from the outside of the pipette, being careful not to remove any blood from the pipette bore.				
7. ∗	Squeeze and maintain a slight pressure on the Unopette vial to force out the air, but not the liquid.				
8. ✦	With your index finger, cover the opening of the pipette overflow chamber. Insert the pipette into the punctured neck opening of the Unopette vial.				
9. ✦	Remove your index finger from the pipette opening. The resulting negative pressure draws blood into the diluent.				
10. ✦	Rinse the capillary pipette bore by gently squeezing the vial two or three times. Thoroughly mix the blood and diluent by swirling the vial.				

Name: _____

Date: _____

		PRACTICE TRIAL	GRADED TRIAL # 1	GRADED TRIAL # 2	NOTES
11. ✦	Leave the vial standing for 10 minutes to hemolyze the red blood cells.				
12. ✦	Invert the vial to thoroughly remix and suspend the cells in the fluid.				
13. ⋆	Convert to a dropper assembly by withdrawing the pipette from the reservoir and reseating it in the reverse position.				
14. ✦	Gently squeeze the sides of the vial and discard the first three or four drops. Fill the chamber of the Neubauer hemacytometer with the diluted blood.				
15. ✦	Place the hemacytometer on moistened paper in a petri dish. Cover the petri dish and leave it standing for 10 minutes so the cells settle.				
16. ⋆	Count and calculate for WBCs and platelets: For WBCs, examine under 40× microscope power with lower light. Count all the white blood cells in the nine large squares of the counting chamber. Count the opposite side in the same manner. Add both sides and divide by two to obtain the average. Calculation formula: average count $\times$ 10/9 $\times$ 100 = WBC/mm^3				

		PRACTICE TRIAL	GRADED TRIAL # 1	GRADED TRIAL # 2	NOTES
17. ★	For platelets, examine under 40× microscope power with lower light. Count all the platelets in center secondary square of the Neubauer ruling of the counting chamber. Count the opposite side in the same manner. Add both sides and divide by two for the average. Calculation formula: average count × 9 × 10/9 × 100 = PLT/mm³				
18. ✦	Dispose of all used sharps and biohazardous waste in the appropriate containers.				
19. ✦	Remove the disposable gloves and discard appropriately. Wash your hands.				

Document: Enter the appropriate information in the chart below.

Grading

Points Earned	_____		
Points Possible	_____	129	129
Percent Grade (Points Earned/Points Possible)	_____		
PASS:	_____	❑ YES ❑ NO ❑ N/A	❑ YES ❑ NO ❑ N/A

Instructor Sign-Off

Instructor: _____ **Date:** _____

Name: _____

Date: _____

Procedure 32-6:

Prepare a Blood Smear for a Differentiated Cell Count

Objective: The student, using the supplies and equipment listed below, will demonstrate how to prepare a blood smear for a differentiated cell count.

Supplies: Materials for venipuncture or capillary puncture, microscope, two glass slides, gauze squares, disposable gloves, sharps container, biohazardous waste container

Affective Behaviors: Affective behaviors provide a professional approach to a skill that enhances the patient encounter. These behaviors may also display sensitivity to a patient's rights and enhance communication. Pay close attention to these skills, which will be in **bold, *italicized*** font.

Notes to the Student

_____

_____

_____

_____

_____

_____

Skills Assessment Requirements

Read and familiarize yourself with the procedure; complete the minimum practice requirements. Document each MPR using proper charting technique. Complete each procedure within a reasonable amount of time, with a minimum of 85 percent accuracy.

POINT VALUE ✦ = 3–6 points ★ = 7–9 points		PRACTICE TRIAL	GRADED TRIAL #1	GRADED TRIAL #2	NOTES
1. ✦	Wash your hands. Gather equipment and supplies.				
2. ✦	Ensure that the microscope is clean and working properly.				
3. ★	**Greet and identify the patient, introduce yourself and escort him or her to the treatment area.**				
4. ✦	Wash your hands and put on disposable gloves.				
5. ★	Obtain a drop of blood by any one of the following methods. Place the blood drop 1/2 to 1 inch from the label end of the slide. *For a capillary puncture:* • Puncture the skin per the capillary puncture method. • Wipe the first drop of blood away with a sterile gauze square. Lightly touch the second drop of blood to a slide. *For a fresh venous specimen:* • After you withdraw the needle from the venipuncture site, immediately touch the drop of blood lightly to a slide. *For a venous specimen from a vacutainer:* • Place a capillary tube in the vacutainer. It will automatically draw the correct amount of blood. • With sterile gauze, wipe away any blood from the outside of the tube, being careful not to remove the blood from the tip. • Lightly touch the drop of blood from the capillary tube to a slide.				

Name: _____

Date: _____

		PRACTICE TRIAL	GRADED TRIAL # 1	GRADED TRIAL # 2	NOTES
6. ✦	Place the second slide lengthwise, in front of and in contact with the drop of blood. Allow the blood to spread along the edge of the slide by capillary action.				
7. ★	At a 30° angle and applying only light pressure, pull the second slide toward the opposite edge of the first slide. After approximately 1 inch and as the specimen is feathering, lift the second slide in a sliding arch away from the first slide.				
8. ✦	Allow the slide to air dry.				
9. ★	Label the slide and place it next to the microscope for examination.				
10. ✦	Follow institutional procedure for the cell count, which is performed by a designated individual.				
11. ✦	Dispose of all used sharps and biohazardous waste in the appropriate containers.				
12. ✦	Remove the disposable gloves and discard appropriately. Wash your hands.				
13. ★	Document the procedure in the chart or log per institutional procedure. **Sign the entry with your name and credentials.**				

Name: _____

Date: _____

Document: Enter the correct information in the chart below.

Grading

Points Earned	_____		
Points Possible	_____	93	93
Percent Grade (Points Earned/Points Possible)	_____		
PASS:	_____	❏ YES ❏ NO ❏ N/A	❏ YES ❏ NO ❏ N/A

Instructor Sign-Off

Instructor: _____ **Date:** _____

Name: _____

Date: _____

Procedure 32-7:

Prepare a Smear Stained with Wright's Stain

Objective: The student, using the supplies and equipment listed below, will demonstrate how to prepare a blood smear stained with Wright's stain.

Supplies: Clean glass slides (more than needed, in case of a break), transfer device, either a pipette or a capillary tube, blood specimen, Wright's stain, disposable gloves

Notes to the Student

_____

_____

_____

_____

_____

_____

Skills Assessment Requirements

Read and familiarize yourself with the procedure; complete the minimum practice requirements. Document each MPR using proper charting technique. Complete each procedure within a reasonable amount of time, with a minimum of 85 percent accuracy.

POINT VALUE ✦ = 3–6 points ⋆ = 7–9 points		PRACTICE TRIAL	GRADED TRIAL # 1	GRADED TRIAL # 2	NOTES
1. ✦	Have all the necessary materials in your laboratory work station.				
2. ✦	Wash your hands and put on the gloves.				
3. ✦	Mix the blood sample. If it has separated, gently swirl it in the tube.				
4. ✦	With a pipette, take a small sample of the blood and drop it on the slide, approximately 1/4 inch from the end of the slide.				
5. ✦	Hold the end of the slide with one hand. With your other hand, place the other slide directly in front of the blood specimen at a 30-degree angle.				
6. ✦	Pull the spreader slide back into the drop of blood, just until contact is made. This will cause the blood to spread out along the edge of the slide in a thin line. You should be pulling the blood back toward the closer end of the slide.				
7. ✦	To avoid air bubbles, push the spreader slide back toward the opposite end of the slide in a quick, smooth motion, being careful to maintain the 30-degree angle.				
8. ✦	Allow the slide to dry.				
9. ✦	When the slide is dry, label the thick end of the smear with a pencil.				
10. ✦	Place the slide on a staining rack with the blood side up. Flood the smear with Wright's stain.				

Name: _____

Date: _____

		PRACTICE TRIAL	GRADED TRIAL # 1	GRADED TRIAL # 2	NOTES
11. ✦	Follow the instructions for the waiting time, generally 1 to 3 minutes.				
12. ✦	Add a buffer in an amount equivalent to the Wright's stain. Mix the stain and buffer and blow gently on the mixture for several minutes until a green, metallic sheen appears.				
13. ✦	Rinse the slide completely with distilled water.				
14. ✦	Allow the excess water to drain off the slide and stand it on end to allow it to dry.				

Name: _____

Date: _____

Document: Enter the appropriate information in the chart below.

Grading

Points Earned	_____		
Points Possible	_____	84	84
Percent Grade (Points Earned/Points Possible)	_____		
PASS:	_____	❏ YES ❏ NO ❏ N/A	❏ YES ❏ NO ❏ N/A

Instructor Sign-Off

Instructor: _____ **Date:** _____

Name: _____

Date: _____

Procedure 32-8:

Perform a Microhematocrit by Capillary Tube

Objective: The student, using the supplies and equipment listed below, will demonstrate how to perform a microhematocrit.

Supplies: Heparinized capillary tubes, microhematocrit centrifuge, microhematocrit reader, tube sealer or sealing clay, gauze squares, disposable gloves, sharps container, biohazardous waste container

Affective Behaviors: Affective behaviors provide a professional approach to a skill that enhances the patient encounter. These behaviors may also display sensitivity to a patient's rights and enhance communication. Pay close attention to these skills, which will be in **bold, italicized** font.

Notes to the Student

_____

_____

_____

_____

_____

_____

Skills Assessment Requirements

Read and familiarize yourself with the procedure; complete the minimum practice requirements. Document each MPR using proper charting technique. Complete each procedure within a reasonable amount of time, with a minimum of 85 percent accuracy.

Name: _____

Date: _____

POINT VALUE ✦ = 3–6 points ⋆ = 7–9 points		PRACTICE TRIAL	GRADED TRIAL # 1	GRADED TRIAL # 2	NOTES
1. ✦	Wash your hands.				
2. ✦	Gather equipment and supplies.				
3. ⋆	**Greet and identify the patient, introduce yourself and escort him or her to the laboratory draw area. Explain the procedure.**				
4. ✦	Wash your hands and put on disposable gloves.				
5. ✦	Perform a capillary puncture or venipuncture.				
6. ✦	Fill a capillary tube with capillary or well mixed anticoagulated blood approximately 3/4 full.				
7. ✦	Wipe excess blood off the outside of the tube.				
8. ✦	Repeat steps 6 and 7. You will use the second tube as a counterbalance weight in the centrifuge or as a second test to confirm the accuracy of the results.				
9. ✦	Holding each capillary tube by its sides, place the blood-filled end in the sealing clay to form a plug. Pull the tube straight up and out of the sealing clay.				
10. ⋆	Place the capillary tubes in the microhematocrit head grooves opposite each other. Make sure the sealed ends of the tubes face away from the center of the centrifuge and are touching the outside rim of the centrifuge head.				

		PRACTICE TRIAL	GRADED TRIAL # 1	GRADED TRIAL # 2	NOTES
11. ✦	Attach and secure the lid of the centrifuge.				
12. ✦	Centrifuge the capillary tubes at 12,000 RPM for the optimum time stated on the instrument, usually 2 to 5 minutes.				
13. ✦	Remove the capillary tubes after the centrifuge has stopped spinning.				
14. ✦	Place one centrifuged capillary tube into the groove on the clear plastic piece of the micro-hematocrit reader with the plug end toward the reader bottom center. The reference line near the top of the groove should be under the separation line in the capillary tube where the clay plug and the RBCs meet.				
15. ✦	Rotate the bottom of the reader plate so that the metal stop on the outer rim makes contact with the left edge of the grooved piece.				
16. ✦	Holding the bottom plate steady, rotate the top plate to align the outer edge of the spiral line with the outer edge of the plasma meniscus.				
17. ✦	Rotate the entire bottom portion of the reader clockwise until the spiral line intersects the line separating the buffy coat and plasma layer.				
18. ⋆	Read the results on the ruled scale where the red line intersects it.				

Name: _____

Date: _____

		PRACTICE TRIAL	GRADED TRIAL #1	GRADED TRIAL #2	NOTES
19. ✦	Dispose of all used sharps and biohazardous waste in the appropriate containers.				
20. ✦	Remove the disposable gloves and discard appropriately. Wash your hands.				
21. ⋆	Document the percentage results on the laboratory requisition or other designated area of the chart. **Sign the entry with your name and credentials.**				

Document: Enter the appropriate information in the chart below.

Grading

Points Earned	_____		
Points Possible	_____	138	138
Percent Grade (Points Earned/Points Possible)	_____		
PASS:	_____	❏ YES ❏ NO ❏ N/A	❏ YES ❏ NO ❏ N/A

Instructor Sign-Off

Instructor: _____ **Date:** _____

Name: _____

Date: _____

Procedure 32-9:

Perform a Hemoglobin Test Using a Hemoglobulinometer

Objective: Correctly perform a hemoglobin test using a hemoglobulinometer.

Supplies: Hemoglobulinometer, applicator sticks, whole blood sample (by capillary puncture), gloves, biohazard waste container, patient record

Affective Behaviors: Affective behaviors provide a professional approach to a skill that enhances the patient encounter. These behaviors may also display sensitivity to a patient's rights and enhance communication. Pay close attention to these skills, which will be in **_bold, italicized_** font.

Notes to the Student

_____

_____

_____

_____

_____

_____

Skills Assessment Requirements

Read and familiarize yourself with the procedure; complete the minimum practice requirements. Document each MPR using proper charting technique. Complete each procedure within a reasonable amount of time, with a minimum of 85 percent accuracy.

Name: _____

Date: _____

POINT VALUE ✦ = 3–6 points ⋆ = 7–9 points		PRACTICE TRIAL	GRADED TRIAL #1	GRADED TRIAL #2	NOTES
1. ✦	Wash your hands and assemble equipment and supplies.				
2. ✦	Put on gloves.				
3. ⋆	Obtain a blood specimen from the patient by capillary puncture following the steps outlined in procedure 32-4.				
4. ⋆	Place well mixed whole blood into the hemoglobulinometer chamber as described by the manufacturer (Figure 32-8).				
5. ✦	Slide the chamber into the hemoglobinometer.				
6. ✦	Remove gloves and discard.				
7. ✦	Wash your hands.				
8. ⋆	Record the hemoglobin level in the patient's record. **Sign the entry with your name and credentials.**				

Name: _____

Date: _____

Document: Enter the appropriate information in the chart below.

Grading

Points Earned	_____		
Points Possible	_____	57	57
Percent Grade (Points Earned/Points Possible)	_____		
PASS:	_____	❏ YES ❏ NO ❏ N/A	❏ YES ❏ NO ❏ N/A

Instructor Sign-Off

Instructor: _____   **Date:** _____

Name: _____

Date: _____

Procedure 32-10:

Perform an ESR Using the Wintrobe Method

Objective: The student, using the supplies and equipment listed below, will demonstrate performing an ESR using the Wintrobe method.

Supplies: Wintrobe tube (calibrated in millimeters), Wintrobe pipette rack, pipette bulb, DTA-anticoagulated patient blood sample, gauze squares, disposable gloves, sharps container, biohazardous waste container

Affective Behaviors: Affective behaviors provide a professional approach to a skill that enhances the patient encounter. These behaviors may also display sensitivity to a patient's rights and enhance communication. Pay close attention to these skills, which will be in **bold, italicized** font.

Notes to the Student

_____

_____

_____

_____

_____

_____

Skills Assessment Requirements

Read and familiarize yourself with the procedure; complete the minimum practice requirements. Document each MPR using proper charting technique. Complete each procedure within a reasonable amount of time, with a minimum of 85 percent accuracy.

POINT VALUE ✦ = 3–6 points ✱ = 7–9 points		PRACTICE TRIAL	GRADED TRIAL # 1	GRADED TRIAL # 2	NOTES
1. ✦	Wash your hands.				
2. ✦	Gather equipment and supplies.				
3. ✱	**Greet and identify the patient, introduce yourself and escort him or her to the laboratory draw area. Explain the procedure.**				
4. ✦	Wash your hands and put on disposable gloves.				
5. ✦	Perform a capillary puncture or venipuncture.				
6. ✦	Mix thoroughly an EDTA-anticoagulated tube of patient blood.				
7. ✦	Attach a disposable pipette bulb to the top of the Wintrobe tube.				
8. ✦	Place the tip of the Wintrobe tube in the blood specimen. With the pipette bulb, draw a blood sample to the 0 mark.				
9. ✦	Place the filled Wintrobe tube in an exactly vertical position in the rack. Set a timer for 60 minutes.				

		PRACTICE TRIAL	GRADED TRIAL # 1	GRADED TRIAL # 2	NOTES
10. ★	At the end of 60 minutes, record the number of mm the red blood cells have fallen. This result is the sed rate in mm/hr.				
11. ✦	Dispose of all used sharps and biohazardous waste in the appropriate containers.				
12. ✦	Remove the disposable gloves and discard appropriately. Wash your hands.				
13. ★	Document the sed rate in mm/hr on the laboratory requisition or other designated area of the chart. **Sign the entry with your name and credentials.**				

Name: _____

Date: _____

Document: Enter the appropriate information in the chart below.

Grading

Points Earned	_____		
Points Possible	_____	87	87
Percent Grade (Points Earned/Points Possible)	_____		
PASS:	_____	❑ YES ❑ NO ❑ N/A	❑ YES ❑ NO ❑ N/A

Instructor Sign-Off

Instructor: _____ Date: _____

Name: _____

Date: _____

Procedure 32-11:

Measure Blood Glucose Using the Accu-Chek™ Glucometer

Objective: The student, using the supplies and equipment listed below, will demonstrate how to measure blood glucose with a glucometer and record patient results.

Supplies: Accu-Chek™ glucometer, Accu-Chek™ test strips, glucose control solutions, puncture device, sterile 2 × 2 gauze, disposable gloves, sharps container, biohazardous waste container

Affective Behaviors: Affective behaviors provide a professional approach to a skill that enhances the patient encounter. These behaviors may also display sensitivity to a patient's rights and enhance communication. Pay close attention to these skills, which will be in **_bold, italicized_** font.

Notes to the Student

_____

_____

_____

_____

_____

_____

Skills Assessment Requirements

Read and familiarize yourself with the procedure; complete the minimum practice requirements. Document each MPR using proper charting technique. Complete each procedure within a reasonable amount of time, with a minimum of 85 percent accuracy.

Name: _____

Date: _____

	POINT VALUE ◆ = 3–6 points ⋆ = 7–9 points	PRACTICE TRIAL	GRADED TRIAL #1	GRADED TRIAL #2	NOTES
1. ◆	Wash your hands.				
2. ◆	Gather equipment and supplies.				
3. ◆	Verify that calibration and quality control have been performed and are acceptable.				
4. ⋆	**Greet and identify the patient, introduce yourself and escort him or her to the laboratory draw area. Explain the procedure.**				
5. ◆	Wash your hands and put on disposable gloves.				
6. ◆	Check the expiration date on the test strip bottle. Obtain a different bottle if the expiration date has passed.				
7. ◆	Turn on the glucometer by pressing the ON button.				
8. ◆	Follow the manufacturer's directions for entering the 3-digit test-strip code in the display if the glucometer code does not match the code on the test strip bottle.				
9. ◆	Enter the patient identification number. (Home glucometers may not require this information.)				
10. ◆	Wait for the indicator that the monitor is ready for a test strip. Within the short time frame specified by the glucometer model, insert one test strip as directed into the monitor.				
11. ◆	Remove the monitor from the charging station.				

		PRACTICE TRIAL	GRADED TRIAL # 1	GRADED TRIAL # 2	NOTES
12. ✦	Obtain a capillary blood specimen from the patient following standard procedure for capillary blood collections. Venous or arterial specimens may also be used.				
13. *	Touch the edge of the test strip to the drop of blood. The blood will be pulled into the strip. Fill the target area of the strip completely.				
14. ✦	The glucose result will appear in the time frame specified by the manufacturer, usually within 30 seconds.				
15. ✦	Remove the test strip and discard in a biohazard container. Dispose of the lancet or blade in the sharps container.				
16. ✦	Return the monitor to the charging/storage unit.				
17. ✦	Remove the disposable gloves and discard appropriately. Wash your hands. **Thank the patient and ask if he or she has any questions.**				
18. *	Document the date, time, finger used, patient's tolerance of the procedure, and results in the designated area of the chart. **Sign the entry with your name and credentials.**				

Name: _____

Date: _____

Document: Enter the appropriate information in the chart below.

Grading

Points Earned	_____		
Points Possible	_____	117	117
Percent Grade (Points Earned/Points Possible)	_____		
PASS:	_____	❏ YES ❏ NO ❏ N/A	❏ YES ❏ NO ❏ N/A

Instructor Sign-Off

Instructor: _____ **Date:** _____

Name: _____

Date: _____

Procedure 32-12:

Determine a Cholesterol Level with the ProAct Testing Device

Objective: The student, using the supplies and equipment listed below, will demonstrate how to measure cholesterol level using a ProAct testing device.

Supplies: ProAct testing device, capillary tube containing lithium heparin, lancet device, 2 × 2 gauze pads, sterile, alcohol pads, disposable gloves, patient's chart

Affective Behaviors: Affective behaviors provide a professional approach to a skill that enhances the patient encounter. These behaviors may also display sensitivity to a patient's rights and enhance communication. Pay close attention to these skills, which will be in **bold, *italicized*** font.

Notes to the Student

_____

_____

_____

_____

_____

_____

Skills Assessment Requirements

Read and familiarize yourself with the procedure; complete the minimum practice requirements. Document each MPR using proper charting technique. Complete each procedure within a reasonable amount of time, with a minimum of 85 percent accuracy.

Name: _____

Date: _____

POINT VALUE ✦ = 3–6 points ⋆ = 7–9 points		PRACTICE TRIAL	GRADED TRIAL # 1	GRADED TRIAL # 2	NOTES
1. ✦	Wash your hands and put on the gloves.				
2. ⋆	*Verify the physician's order and the patient's identity. Introduce yourself and explain the procedure to the patient.*				
3. ✦	Load the lancet device according to the directions.				
4. ✦	Choose a puncture site free of broken skin or bruising.				
5. ✦	Wipe the patient's finger with an alcohol wipe and allow to dry.				
6. ⋆	Puncture the finger and wipe away the first drop of blood that forms with the sterile gauze.				
7. ✦	Hold the capillary tube horizontal to the patient's finger, making sure no air bubbles enter the tube. If air bubbles enter, you must throw away the tube and start over again.				
8. ✦	When the tube has filled, remove it and have the patient put pressure on the puncture site with a sterile gauze square.				
9. ✦	Remove a testing strip from the container and peel away the protective foil. Place the strip on a hard work surface.				
10. ✦	Attach the filled capillary tube to the pipette.				

		PRACTICE TRIAL	GRADED TRIAL #1	GRADED TRIAL #2	NOTES
11. ✦	Without touching the tip of the capillary tube to the testing strip, place one drop in the center of the application zone.				
12. ✶	Allow the blood droplet to soak into the testing mesh for 15 to 20 seconds.				
13. ✦	Place the strip in the ProAct device port. The device will start to count down approximately 160 seconds.				
14. ✦	While the machine is running, clean the test area. Throw the pipette and capillary tube into a sharps container.				
15. ✦	When the LED screen indicates, remove the test strip and observe it for uneven color development. (If the color is uneven, you will need to perform the entire test again.)				
16. ✦	Discard the test strip into a biohazard container.				
17. ✶	*Ask the patient if he or she has any questions. Record the test results as displayed in the patient's chart. Sign the entry with your name and credentials.*				

Document: Enter the appropriate information in the chart below.

Grading

Points Earned	_____		
Points Possible	_____	114	114
Percent Grade (Points Earned/Points Possible)	_____		
PASS:	_____	❏ YES ❏ NO ❏ N/A	❏ YES ❏ NO ❏ N/A

Instructor Sign-Off

Instructor: _____ **Date:** _____

Procedure 32-13:

Perform a Mononucleosis Test

Objective: The student, using the supplies and equipment listed below, will demonstrate how to test for infectious mononucleosis.

Supplies: Mono-Test kit, nonsterile disposable gloves, blood serum or plasma, disposable capillary tube

Affective Behaviors: Affective behaviors provide a professional approach to a skill that enhances the patient encounter. These behaviors may also display sensitivity to a patient's rights and enhance communication. Pay close attention to these skills, which will be in **bold, italicized** font.

Notes to the Student

_____

_____

_____

_____

_____

_____

Skills Assessment Requirements

Read and familiarize yourself with the procedure; complete the minimum practice requirements. Document each MPR using proper charting technique. Complete each procedure within a reasonable amount of time, with a minimum of 85 percent accuracy.

Name: _____

Date: _____

POINT VALUE ✦ = 3–6 points ★ = 7–9 points		PRACTICE TRIAL	GRADED TRIAL # 1	GRADED TRIAL # 2	NOTES
1. ★	Bring all liquid reagents to room temperature. Check the expiration date of all reagents in the kit.				
2. ✦	Wash and dry your hands and put on disposable gloves.				
3. ✦	After obtaining a blood sample from the patient and processing it to separate the serum, fill the capillary tube to the marked line with the serum.				
4. ✦	Using the glass slide and rubber bulb in the kit, place a small drop of the specimen serum in the first of the three circles on the slide.				
5. ✦	Place a single drop of the negative control in the second circle on the slide.				
6. ✦	Place a single drop of the positive control in the third circle.				
7. ✦	Holding the bottle of Mono-Test reagent upright between your palms, gently roll it back and forth, making certain that the reagent RBCs that have settled in the tube are mixed thoroughly.				
8. ✦	Hold the dropper 1 inch above the slide and place one drop of reagent into each of the three circles. Make certain the dropper does not come into contact with the slide and become contaminated.				

		PRACTICE TRIAL	GRADED TRIAL # 1	GRADED TRIAL # 2	NOTES
9. ✦	Using the enclosed stirrers, one for each circle, quickly and thoroughly mix each area and spread it out to the full 1-inch diameter of the circle.				
10. ✦	Observe the slide as you rock it back and forth gently for exactly 2 minutes.				
11. *	Agglutination is a positive test result; no agglutination is negative. Verify the test results by comparing them to the positive and negative controls on the slide.				
12. ✦	Clean the work area, disposing of the test in a biohazard container. Wash your hands.				
13. *	Record the test results. **Sign the entry with your name and credentials.**				

Name: _____

Date: _____

Document: Enter the appropriate information in the chart below.

Grading

Points Earned	_____		
Points Possible	_____	87	87
Percent Grade (Points Earned/Points Possible)	_____		
PASS:	_____	❑ YES ❑ NO ❑ N/A	❑ YES ❑ NO ❑ N/A

Instructor Sign-Off

Instructor: _____ **Date:** _____

Procedure 33-1:

Demonstrate Patient Instruction for a Clean-Catch Urine Specimen

Objective: The student, using the supplies and equipment listed below, will demonstrate how to instruct the patient on obtaining a clean-catch specimen.

Supplies: Sterile specimen container, label, antiseptic wipes, chart, requisition slip if necessary

Affective Behaviors: Affective behaviors provide a professional approach to a skill that enhances the patient encounter. These behaviors may also display sensitivity to a patient's rights and enhance communication. Pay close attention to these skills, which will be in **bold, italicized** font.

Notes to the Student

_____

_____

_____

_____

_____

_____

Skills Assessment Requirements

Read and familiarize yourself with the procedure; complete the minimum practice requirements. Document each MPR using proper charting technique. Complete each procedure within a reasonable amount of time, with a minimum of 85 percent accuracy.

Name: _____

Date: _____

POINT VALUE ✦ = 3–6 points ⋆ = 7–9 points		PRACTICE TRIAL	GRADED TRIAL # 1	GRADED TRIAL # 2	NOTES
1. ✦	Wash your hands. Gather equipment and supplies.				
2. ⋆	**Greet and identify the patient, introduce yourself, and guide the patient to the treatment area.**				
3. ✦	Instruct the patient to wash their hands.				
4. ✦	Open the sterile urine container and place the lid on a flat area with the inside facing up.				
5. ✦	Open the antiseptic wipes and place them on top of their packaging.				
6. ⋆	**If male:** Retract the foreskin, if present. Cleanse the glans penis with the antiseptic wipes with a circular motion from the meatal opening and proceeding outward. Repeat, using all the antiseptic wipes.				
7. ⋆	**If female:** Spread the labia apart with one hand. Wipe from front to back. Use one wipe to cleanse one side, then discard the wipe. Cleanse the other side with a new wipe and discard it. Finally, with a new wipe, cleanse down the middle across the meatus, and discard the wipe.				

		PRACTICE TRIAL	GRADED TRIAL # 1	GRADED TRIAL # 2	NOTES
8. ★	After cleansing, the patient should: • Discard all the used wipes in an appropriate waste container. • Void some urine into the toilet and stop (an uncircumcised male should also bring the foreskin forward) • Restart voiding to half-fill the sterile container. • Finish voiding into the toilet. • Wash the hands. • Put the lid on the container without touching the inside of the lid. • Place it in the designated receiving site. **Before sending the patient into the restroom, have the patient reiterate the instructions and clarify any questions he or she may have.**				
9. ✦	Wash your hands.				
10. ★	Chart your observations of the urine specimen as well as the date, time collected, and tests ordered. **Sign the entry with your name and credentials.**				
11. ✦	If the specimen is to be tested at another laboratory, complete a laboratory requisition slip. Take the specimen to the lab or refrigerator or add preservative.				

Name: _____

Date: _____

Document: Enter the appropriate information in the chart below.

Grading

Points Earned	_____		
Points Possible	_____	81	81
Percent Grade (Points Earned/Points Possible)	_____		
PASS:	_____	❏ YES ❏ NO ❏ N/A	❏ YES ❏ NO ❏ N/A

Instructor Sign-Off

Instructor: _____   Date: _____

Procedure 33-2:

Demonstrate Patient Instruction for Collection of a 24-Hour Specimen

Objective: The student, using the supplies and equipment listed below, will demonstrate being able to instruct the patient to obtain a quality 24-hour specimen for accurate testing, diagnosis, and treatment.

Supplies: 24-hour specimen container, smaller collection container, patient instruction sheet, chart, requisition slip

Affective Behaviors: Affective behaviors provide a professional approach to a skill that enhances the patient encounter. These behaviors may also display sensitivity to a patient's rights and enhance communication. Pay close attention to these skills, which will be in **bold, *italicized*** font.

Notes to the Student

_____

_____

_____

_____

_____

_____

Skills Assessment Requirements

Read and familiarize yourself with the procedure; complete the minimum practice requirements. Document each MPR using proper charting technique. Complete each procedure within a reasonable amount of time, with a minimum of 85 percent accuracy.

Name: _____

Date: _____

POINT VALUE ✦ = 3–6 points ⋆ = 7–9 points		PRACTICE TRIAL	GRADED TRIAL # 1	GRADED TRIAL # 2	NOTES
1. ✦	Wash your hands. Gather equipment and supplies.				
2. ⋆	**Greet and identify the patient, introduce yourself and guide the patient to the treatment area.**				
3. ✦	Instruct the patient to: • Wash the hands.				
4. ✦	• Void into the toilet upon arising and record the time (from this time and for the next 24 hours, all urine will go into the 24-hour collection container).				
5. ⋆	• Void all urine into the smaller collection container to pour into the larger container. • Each time wash, rinse, and air dry the smaller container. • After each specimen is placed in the larger specimen container, screw the lid tightly and put it in the refrigerator or portable cooler.				

		PRACTICE TRIAL	GRADED TRIAL # 1	GRADED TRIAL # 2	
6. ✦	At the end of the 24-hour period, bring the large container to the medical office or laboratory. (The first voided specimen of the second morning is the last specimen to be added to the container, ending the collecting period.) **Ask the patient if he or she has any questions prior to leaving the office and beginning the specimen collection.**				
7. ✦	Ask the patient if any problems occurred during the specimen collection. If too much urine was collected or if some was spilled during collection, tell the patient a new collection must be started.				
8. ✦	Fill out a lab requisition slip for the specimen when it is brought to the office or taken directly to an outside laboratory.				
9. ✶	Chart your observations of the urine specimen, the date, time collected, tests ordered, and any other pertinent information. **Sign and date the entry with your name and credentials.**				

Name: _____

Date: _____

Document: Enter the appropriate information in the chart below.

Grading

Points Earned	_____		
Points Possible	_____	63	63
Percent Grade (Points Earned/Points Possible)	_____		
PASS:	_____	❑ YES ❑ NO ❑ N/A	❑ YES ❑ NO ❑ N/A

Instructor Sign-Off

Instructor: _____ Date: _____

Procedure 33-3:

Perform Catheterization of a Female Patient

Objective: The student, using the supplies and equipment listed below, will demonstrate how to perform catheterization of a female patient.

Supplies: Lighting source, preferably a gooseneck lamp, sterile specimen container, sterile drapes, sterile catheterization kit or straight catheter, sterile K-Y gel or other lubricant, sterilized Mayo stand, sterile gloves, 2 pairs, nonsterile latex gloves, biohazardous waste receptacle, several 2 * 2 sterile gauze squares (minimum of 6), Betadine or other iodine solution, maxipad or pantyliner, patient chart, lab order forms

Affective Behaviors: Affective behaviors provide a professional approach to a skill that enhances the patient encounter. These behaviors may also display sensitivity to a patient's rights and enhance communication. Pay close attention to these skills, which will be in ***bold, italicized*** font.

Notes to the Student

_____

_____

_____

_____

_____

_____

Skills Assessment Requirements

Read and familiarize yourself with the procedure; complete the minimum practice requirements. Document each MPR using proper charting technique. Complete each procedure within a reasonable amount of time, with a minimum of 85 percent accuracy.

POINT VALUE ✦ = 3–6 points ⋆ = 7–9 points		PRACTICE TRIAL	GRADED TRIAL # 1	GRADED TRIAL # 2	NOTES
1. ✦	Gather all needed supplies to bring into the room. Generally, the patient will already be disrobed and covered with a drape. ***Bringing all supplies into the room on one trip avoids opening the door more than once while your patient is in a potentially embarrassing position.***				
2. ✦	***Explain the procedure to the patient and obtain verbal permission to begin touching her.***				
3. ✦	If the patient is not unclothed, explain the correct dorsal recumbent position and draping				
4. ✦	Position the gooseneck lamp to so that it is directed at the genital area, but do not turn it on, as it may heat up quickly and make the patient uncomfortable.				
5. ✦	Wash your hands and put on nonsterile gloves. Open the catheterization kit.				
6. ✦	Ask the patient to keep her knees apart and take slow deep breaths while lifting her hips off the table surface.				
7. ✦	When her hips have cleared the surface, slide a sterile drape beneath her by encircling the corners with your hands. Avoid touching the patient or the table with your hands.				
8. ✦	Open a second sterile drape and place it over the patient's genital area, making sure that the vulvar area is exposed.				

		PRACTICE TRIAL	GRADED TRIAL # 1	GRADED TRIAL # 2	NOTES
9. ✦	Place the insertion portion of the kit on the sterile drape you placed under the patient's hips, between her knees.				
10. ✦	Remove the gloves and wash your hands.				
11. ✦	Following sterile technique, put on sterile gloves.				
12. ✦	Soak the 2 * 2 gauze pads in Betadine or other iodine solution.				
13. ✦	Open the sterile lubricant and place it on the sterile field on the Mayo stand. Open the remaining items, including the sterile container, and place them on the tray.				
14. *	Cleanse the patient with the Betadine-soaked gauze squares. Separate the labia with the thumb and index finger of your nondominant hand. With your other hand, take a gauze square and wipe one side of the labia from top to bottom in one pass. Throw the square away. Take another square, repeat on the other side, and discard. Do not let the hand that is separating the labia touch and thereby contaminate your other hand.				
15. *	With a third gauze square, cleanse the urinary meatus with a circular motion, working from the inside to the outside. Discard the square.				
16. *	With your dominant hand, pick up the catheter, with your thumb and index finger approximately 3 inches from the end to be inserted.				

Name: _____

Date: _____

		PRACTICE TRIAL	GRADED TRIAL # 1	GRADED TRIAL # 2	NOTES
17. ✦	Dip the insertion end of the catheter into the sterile lubricant. Make sure the opposite end of the catheter is in the collection portion of the kit's tray.				
18. ✦	Thread the catheter into the urinary meatus approximately 2 to 3 inches, until urine begins to flow into the collection tray.				
19. *	If you meet resistance when threading the catheter, do not force it in. Resistance can be an indication of a problem. Remove the catheter and notify the physician.				
20. ✦	After a small amount of the urine has flowed into the collection tray, move the end of the catheter into the sterile collection container.				
21. ✦	Measure the urine that has flowed from the bladder. Emptying more than 500 ml at one time may cause the bladder to spasm. If more than 500 ml has been released, clamp the catheter, wait 10 to 15 minutes, and release the remainder of the urine.				
22. ✦	When the bladder is completely empty, gently remove the catheter.				
23. ✦	Secure the collection container's lid in place and prepare the paperwork for laboratory testing.				

		PRACTICE TRIAL	GRADED TRIAL # 1	GRADED TRIAL # 2	NOTES
24. ✦	Remove all supplies and dispose of them in a biohazard container.				
25. ✦	Assist the patient in sitting up and dressing if necessary.				
26. ✦	*Inform the patient that the Betadine used to cleanse the labia may stain her undergarments, and offer her a maxipad or panty-liner to protect her clothing.*				
27. ✶	Document the procedure in the patient's chart. *Sign and date the entry with your name and credentials.*				

Document: Enter the appropriate information in the chart below.

Grading

Points Earned	_____		
Points Possible	_____	177	177
Percent Grade (Points Earned/Points Possible)	_____		
PASS:	_____	❏ YES ❏ NO ❏ N/A	❏ YES ❏ NO ❏ N/A

Instructor Sign-Off

Instructor: _____ **Date:** _____

Name: _____

Date: _____

Procedure 33-4:

Perform Catheterization of a Male Patient

Objective: The student, using the supplies and equipment listed below, will demonstrate how to perform catheterization of a male patient

Supplies: Lighting source, preferably a gooseneck lamp, waterproof underpad, sterile specimen container, sterile catheterization kit or straight catheter, sterile drapes, sterile K-Y gel or other lubricant, sterilized Mayo stand, sterile gloves, 2 pairs, nonsterile latex gloves, biohazardous waste receptacle, several 2 * 2 sterile gauze squares (minimum of 6), Betadine or other iodine solution, fenestrated drape, patient chart, lab order forms

Affective Behaviors: Affective behaviors provide a professional approach to a skill that enhances the patient encounter. These behaviors may also display sensitivity to a patient's rights and enhance communication. Pay close attention to these skills, which will be in **_bold, italicized_** font.

Notes to the Student

_____

_____

_____

_____

_____

_____

Skills Assessment Requirements

Read and familiarize yourself with the procedure; complete the minimum practice requirements. Document each MPR using proper charting technique. Complete each procedure within a reasonable amount of time, with a minimum of 85 percent accuracy.

Name: _____

Date: _____

POINT VALUE ✦ = 3–6 points ⋆ = 7–9 points		PRACTICE TRIAL	GRADED TRIAL #1	GRADED TRIAL #2	NOTES
1. ✦	Wash your hands. Collect all the needed supplies and bring into patient's room.				
2. ✦	**Explain the procedure to the patient and explain that it will be necessary to remove all articles of clothing from the waist down. Obtain permission before touching the patient.**				
3. ✦	Assist the patient, if needed, into the supine position.				
4. ✦	Wash your hands and put on nonsterile gloves.				
5. ✦	Following sterile technique, open the catheterization kit and place the items on the sterile field on the Mayo stand.				
6. ✦	Wrap the corners of the sterile underpad over your hands and place it over the patient's thighs, sliding it under the penis.				
7. ✦	Remove the gloves, wash your hands, and put on sterile gloves.				
8. ✦	Being careful not to touch the patient or the table, place a fenestrated drape over the genital area so that the penis is exposed.				
9. ✦	Soak the 2 ⋆ 2 gauze pads in Betadine and place them on the patient's thighs for easy access.				

		PRACTICE TRIAL	GRADED TRIAL # 1	GRADED TRIAL # 2	NOTES
10. ★	With your nondominant hand grasp the penis below the glans and hold it upright. If the patient is uncircumcised, retract the foreskin to expose the meatus.				
11. ★	With your dominant hand, cleanse the meatus with a gauze square in a circular motion, working from the inside to the outside. Discard the gauze.				
12. ✦	Repeat step 11 a total of three times, using a fresh gauze square each time you cleanse.				
13. ✦	Dip the insertion tip of the catheter into lubricant to cover the 7 or 8 inches that will be inserted into the penis. Place the opposite end of the catheter in the collection tray.				
14. ★	Hold the penis firmly at a straight, upward angle to straighten the urethra for easier insertion.				
15. ✦	Ask the patient to constrict the penis muscles in the same manner as when trying to urinate. While he is doing this, gently thread the catheter into the penis until urine begins to flow, generally 6 to 8 inches.				
16. ★	Never force the catheter. If you meet resistance, discontinue the procedure and notify the physician.				

		PRACTICE TRIAL	GRADED TRIAL # 1	GRADED TRIAL # 2	NOTES
17. ✦	After a small amount of the urine has flowed into the collection tray, move the end of the catheter into the sterile collection container.				
18. ★	Measure the urine that has flowed from the bladder. Emptying more than 500 ml at one time may cause the bladder to spasm. If more than 500 ml has been released, clamp the catheter, wait 10 to 15 minutes, and release the remainder of the urine.				
19. ✦	When the bladder is completely empty, gently remove the catheter.				
20. ✦	Secure the collection container's lid in place and prepare the paperwork for laboratory testing.				
21. ✦	Remove all supplies and dispose of them in a biohazardous container.				
22. ✦	Assist the patient in sitting up and dressing if necessary.				
23. ✦	***Inform the patient that the Betadine used to cleanse the glans may transfer to his undergarments and stain them.***				
24. ★	Document the procedure in the patient's chart. ***Sign and date the entry with your name and credentials.***				

Name: _____

Date: _____

Document: Enter the appropriate information in the chart below.

Grading

Points Earned	_____		
Points Possible	_____	162	162
Percent Grade (Points Earned/Points Possible)	_____		
PASS:	_____	❏ YES ❏ NO ❏ N/A	❏ YES ❏ NO ❏ N/A

Instructor Sign-Off

Instructor: _____   **Date:** _____

Procedure 33-5:

Measure Urine Specific Gravity with a Refractometer

Objective: Correctly measure urine specific gravity with a refractometer.

Supplies: Urine specimen (at room temperature), urinary refractometer, disposable pipette, distilled water (if calibration of refractometer is required), biohazardous waste container, patient chart or laboratory requisition form

Notes to the Student

_____

_____

_____

_____

_____

_____

Skills Assessment Requirements

Read and familiarize yourself with the procedure; complete the minimum practice requirements. Document each MPR using proper charting technique. Complete each procedure within a reasonable amount of time, with a minimum of 85 percent accuracy.

Name: _____

Date: _____

POINT VALUE ✦ = 3–6 points ⋆ = 7–9 points		**PRACTICE TRIAL**	**GRADED TRIAL # 1**	**GRADED TRIAL # 2**	**NOTES**
1. ✦	Wash your hands and gather equipment and supplies.				
2. ✦	Apply gloves and protective clothing and check the specimen container for proper labeling.				
3. ✦	Mix the urine specimen in the urine collection container.				
4. ⋆	Confirm that the refractometer has been calibrated according to the manufacturer's specifications. Record the calibration values in the quality control log.				
5. ✦	Open the hinged lid of the refractometer.				
6. ✦	Draw up a small amount of the specimen into the pipette. Discard the pipette in the biohazard waste container.				
7. ✦	Place one drop of the specimen under the cover and close the lid.				
8. ⋆	Turn on the light or point the device toward a light source. Read the specific gravity value on the scale.				
9. ✦	Discard the urine specimen appropriately.				
10. ✦	Remove the gloves and wash your hands.				
11. ⋆	Record the specific gravity value on the laboratory report form. Sign and date the entry with your name and credentials.				

Name: _____

Date: _____

Document: Enter the appropriate information in the chart below.

Grading

Points Earned	_____		
Points Possible	_____	75	75
Percent Grade (Points Earned/Points Possible)	_____		
PASS:	_____	❏ YES ❏ NO ❏ N/A	❏ YES ❏ NO ❏ N/A

Instructor Sign-Off

Instructor: _____   **Date:** _____

Name: _____

Date: _____

Procedure 33-6:

Perform a Urinalysis with a Chemical Test Strip and Prepare the Specimen for Microscopic Examination

Objective: The student, using the supplies and equipment listed below, will demonstrate how to perform a urinalysis with chemical test strips.

Supplies: Chemical reagent urine test strips, blotting paper, urine container, centrifuge and test tubes, microscope, slide and cover slip, pipette, disposable gloves, biohazardous waste receptacle, urinalysis report form

Affective Behaviors: Affective behaviors provide a professional approach to a skill that enhances the patient encounter. These behaviors may also display sensitivity to a patient's rights and enhance communication. Pay close attention to these skills, which will be in **bold, *italicized*** font.

Notes to the Student

_____

_____

_____

_____

_____

_____

Skills Assessment Requirements

Read and familiarize yourself with the procedure; complete the minimum practice requirements. Document each MPR using proper charting technique. Complete each procedure within a reasonable amount of time, with a minimum of 85 percent accuracy.

Name: _____

Date: _____

POINT VALUE ✦ = 3–6 points ⋆ = 7–9 points	PRACTICE TRIAL	GRADED TRIAL # 1	GRADED TRIAL # 2	NOTES
1. ✦ Wash your hands. Gather equipment and supplies. Check the expiration date on the reagent strip container.				
2. ⋆ ***Greet and identify the patient, introduce yourself, and guide the patient to the treatment area.***				
3. ✦ Provide the patient with a labeled urine container. Instruct the patient on how to obtain the specimen and where to leave it.				
4. ✦ Wash your hands. Put on disposable gloves.				
5. ✦ After the patient leaves the specimen in the designated area, move it to the testing area.				
6. ⋆ Observe and describe the urine's color, quantity, and odor. ***Sign and date the entry with your name and credentials.*** Inform the physician that the specimen is ready for testing.				
7. ✦ Remove one reagent strip and recap the bottle tightly and immediately. Do not touch the test area of the strip. If necessary, place the strip temporarily on a dry paper towel while you open the urine specimen container.				
8. ✦ Dip the test strip briefly in the urine, making sure to cover all testing areas. Pull the strip gently back against the inner edge of the container mouth, then place the length of the strip at a right angle to the blotting paper to remove excess urine.				

		PRACTICE TRIAL	GRADED TRIAL # 1	GRADED TRIAL # 2	NOTES
9. ✦	Hold the reagent test areas of the strip next to, but not touching, the matching areas on the test strip bottle. Note the reaction reading at the time mentioned on the bottle for each square of reagent.				
10. ✦	Dispose of the urine test strip in the biohazardous waste container.				
11. ✶	**Prepare urine for microscopic examination by the physician**: Put approximately 10 cc in a tube on one side of the centrifuge, and on the opposite side an equal amount of liquid in another tube. Run the centrifuge for 5 minutes.				
12. ✦	Pour out most of the liquid (supernatant) from the tube, but keep the sediment.				
13. ✦	Mix the remaining liquid with the sediment and pipette a couple of drops of moistened sediment onto a slide.				
14. ✦	Cover with a cover slip. Position and focus the slide under the lighted microscope.				
15. ✦	Remove the gloves and discard in proper container. Wash your hands.				
16. ✶	Chart the results on the reporting urine lab slip immediately, including the date, time, and urine test strip brand name. Record the color, odor, volume, and cloudiness or sediment.				
17. ✶	On the patient's chart, chart the date and time of specimen collection and procedure performance. **_Sign and date the entry with your name and credentials._**				
18. ✦	Return to the microscope examination area for cleaning and disposal.				

Name: _____

Date: _____

Document: Enter the appropriate information in the chart below.

Grading

Points Earned	_____		
Points Possible	_____	123	123
Percent Grade (Points Earned/Points Possible)	_____		
PASS:	_____	❏ YES ❏ NO ❏ N/A	❏ YES ❏ NO ❏ N/A

Instructor Sign-Off

Instructor: _____ **Date:** _____

Procedure 33-7:

Perform a Multi-Drug Screen Urine Test Using the Instant-View Multi-Drug Screen Test

Objective: Correctly perform a Multi-Drug Screen Test.

Supplies: Instant-View Multi-Drug Screen urine test in a sealed pouch, freshly voided urine sample, timer, biohazardous waste container

Affective Behaviors: Affective behaviors provide a professional approach to a skill that enhances the patient encounter. These behaviors may also display sensitivity to a patient's rights and enhance communication. Pay close attention to these skills, which will be in **bold, *italicized*** font.

Notes to the Student

_____

_____

_____

_____

_____

_____

Skills Assessment Requirements

Read and familiarize yourself with the procedure; complete the minimum practice requirements. Document each MPR using proper charting technique. Complete each procedure within a reasonable amount of time, with a minimum of 85 percent accuracy.

Name: _____

Date: _____

POINT VALUE ✦ = 3–6 points ⋆ = 7–9 points		PRACTICE TRIAL	GRADED TRIAL # 1	GRADED TRIAL # 2	NOTES
1. ✦	Wash your hands and put on your gloves and PPE.				
2. ⋆	Assemble the equipment and urine specimen. Ensure that the test kit has not expired. Expired test kits should be discarded immediately.				
3. ✦	Determine the urine temperature within 4 minutes of voiding. The temperature should be between 90° and 100° F.				
4. ⋆	Remove the cap from the device from the foil pouch and label it with the patient's identification information.				
5. ✦	Remove the cap from the urine specimen cup and dip the device into the specimen for 10 seconds. The surface of the urine must be above the sample well and below the arrowheads in the window.				
6. ✦	Recap the urine specimen.				
7. ✦	Set the timer for 4–7 minutes. Do not read the results after 7 minutes.				
8. ⋆	Interpret the results according to the manufacturer's guidelines.				
9. ✦	Discard all biohazardous waste in the appropriate container.				
10. ✦	Remove your gloves and mask.				
11. ✦	Wash your hands.				
12. ⋆	Record the results in the patient's chart. **Sign and date the entry with your name and credentials.**				

Name: _____

Date: _____

Document: Enter the appropriate information in the chart below.

Grading

Points Earned	_____		
Points Possible	_____	84	84
Percent Grade (Points Earned/Points Possible)	_____		
PASS:	_____	❏ YES ❏ NO ❏ N/A	❏ YES ❏ NO ❏ N/A

Instructor Sign-Off

Instructor: _____ **Date:** _____

Procedure 33-8:

Demonstrate Patient Instruction for Testicular Self-Examination

Objective: The student, using the supplies and equipment listed below, will demonstrate how to instruct the patient on performing a testicular self-examination.

Supplies: None

Affective Behaviors: Affective behaviors provide a professional approach to a skill that enhances the patient encounter. These behaviors may also display sensitivity to a patient's rights and enhance communication. Pay close attention to these skills, which will be in **bold, italicized** font.

Notes to the Student

_____

_____

_____

_____

_____

_____

Skills Assessment Requirements

Read and familiarize yourself with the procedure; complete the minimum practice requirements. Document each MPR using proper charting technique. Complete each procedure within a reasonable amount of time, with a minimum of 85 percent accuracy.

Name: _____

Date: _____

POINT VALUE ✦ = 3–6 points ⋆ = 7–9 points		PRACTICE TRIAL	GRADED TRIAL # 1	GRADED TRIAL # 2	NOTES
1. ✦	Wash your hands.				
2. ⋆	**Greet and identify the patient, introduce yourself and guide him to the treatment area.**				
3. ✦	**Consider the sensitivity of the issue at hand.** Instruct the patient to: • Take a warm bath or shower to relax the scrotum. • In the clinical setting, the patient should take several deep breaths.				
4. ✦	Observe the contour of the scrotum. If one testicle is slightly larger or lies somewhat lower than the other, this is considered normal.				
5. ✦	Elevate the right leg to the level of a toilet, chair, or bed to expose the right testicle.				
6. ✦	With the left hand, lightly support the right testicle. With the right hand, palpate the right testicle for hardness, lumps, or anything unusual.				
7. ✦	Reverse the process by elevating the left leg to examine the left testicle. Support the left testicle with the right hand and, with the left hand, palpate the left testicle.				
8. ✦	If the patient finds any abnormalities or has any questions, he should contact the physician. **Ask the patient if he has any questions prior to leaving the examination room.**				
9. ⋆	Document patient education in the patient's chart. **Sign and date the entry with your name and credentials.**				

Document: Enter the appropriate information in the chart below.

Grading

Points Earned	_____		
Points Possible	_____	60	60
Percent Grade (Points Earned/Points Possible)	_____		
PASS:	_____	❏ YES ❏ NO ❏ N/A	❏ YES ❏ NO ❏ N/A

Instructor Sign-Off

Instructor: _____ **Date:** _____

Procedure 34-1:

General Procedure for X-Ray Examination

Objective: The student, using the supplies and equipment listed below, will demonstrate how to X-ray a patient.

Supplies: Physician's order, patient chart, dosimeter badge, X-ray film, X-ray film holder, X-ray machine, processing machine, lead aprons for MA and patient, paper drapes as needed

Affective Behaviors: Affective behaviors provide a professional approach to a skill that enhances the patient encounter. These behaviors may also display sensitivity to a patient's rights and enhance communication. Pay close attention to these skills, which will be in **_bold, italicized_** font.

Notes to the Student

_____

_____

_____

_____

_____

_____

Skills Assessment Requirements

Read and familiarize yourself with the procedure; complete the minimum practice requirements. Document each MPR using proper charting technique. Complete each procedure within a reasonable amount of time, with a minimum of 85 percent accuracy.

POINT VALUE ✦ = 3–6 points ⋆ = 7–9 points		PRACTICE TRIAL	GRADED TRIAL # 1	GRADED TRIAL # 2	NOTES
1. ⋆	**Greet the patient and verify the patient's identity. Verify the physician's order.**				
2. ✦	Check the X-ray equipment.				
3. ✦	**Explain the procedure to the patient.**				
4. ✦	Instruct the patient to remove the appropriate clothing for the X-ray. Provide paper drapes for modesty. For chest and neck X-rays, the patient should remove all jewelry and large hair bands, which may obstruct the view of the structures.				
5. ✦	Position the patient according to the X-ray view(s) required.				
6. ✦	Set the controls with the X-ray tube and cassette at the proper distance.				
7. ✦	If necessary, ask the patient to take a deep breath and hold it.				
8. ⋆	Stand behind the lead wall or shield to take the X-ray. Instruct the patient to adjust to a comfortable position while you develop the X-rays and have them reviewed. The patient should not dress or leave the X-ray suite until the physician has indicated that the X-rays are satisfactory.				
9. ✦	**With the physician's approval, assist the patient in dressing, if necessary.**				
10. ✦	Label the X-ray and X-ray sleeve according to office procedure.				
11. ⋆	Document the procedure in the patient's chart. **Sign and date the entry with your name and credentials.**				

Name: _____

Date: _____

Document: Enter the appropriate information in the chart below.

Grading

Points Earned	_____		
Points Possible	_____	75	75
Percent Grade (Points Earned/Points Possible)	_____		
PASS:	_____	❏ YES ❏ NO ❏ N/A	❏ YES ❏ NO ❏ N/A

Instructor Sign-Off

Instructor: _____ **Date:** _____

Procedure 34-2:

File and Loan Radiographic Records

Objective: The student, using the supplies and equipment listed below, will demonstrate how to file and loan X-rays.

Supplies: X-ray films, consent form, larger envelope or film jacket, labels

Notes to the Student

_____

_____

_____

_____

_____

_____

Skills Assessment Requirements

Read and familiarize yourself with the procedure; complete the minimum practice requirements. Document each MPR using proper charting technique. Complete each procedure within a reasonable amount of time, with a minimum of 85 percent accuracy.

Name: _____

Date: _____

POINT VALUE ✦ = 3–6 points ⋆ = 7–9 points		PRACTICE TRIAL	GRADED TRIAL # 1	GRADED TRIAL # 2	NOTES
1. ✦	Place the films in a large film envelope labeled with the patient's name, DOB, date of procedure, and physician's name. The films will be taken to a radiologist to be read.				
2. ✦	If the films are to be taken by the patient to another facility or physician, note the destination and receiving physician's name on the patient record.				
3. ✦	Record the transfer of all films in a log or file, along with the time, date, patient's name, destination, and receiving physician.				
4. ⋆	Obtain the patient's signed consent for any films the patient takes from the ownership facility to another physician or diagnostic center.				

Name: _____

Date: _____

Document: Enter the appropriate information in the chart below.

Grading

Points Earned	_____		
Points Possible	_____	27	27
Percent Grade (Points Earned/Points Possible)	_____		
PASS:	_____	❏ YES ❏ NO ❏ N/A	❏ YES ❏ NO ❏ N/A

Instructor Sign-Off

Instructor: _____   **Date:** _____

Name: _____

Date: _____

Procedure 35-1:

Perform an Electrocardiogram

Objective: The student, using the supplies and equipment listed below, will demonstrate how to perform a 12-lead ECG.

Supplies: Electrocardiograph with wires, electrodes, and ECG paper, patient gown and drape as necessary for privacy and warmth, alcohol pads, supplies for shaving if needed

Affective Behaviors: Affective behaviors provide a professional approach to a skill that enhances the patient encounter. These behaviors may also display sensitivity to a patient's rights and enhance communication. Pay close attention to these skills, which will be in **_bold, italicized_** font.

Notes to the Student

_____

_____

_____

_____

_____

_____

Skills Assessment Requirements

Read and familiarize yourself with the procedure; complete the minimum practice requirements. Document each MPR using proper charting technique. Complete each procedure within a reasonable amount of time, with a minimum of 85 percent accuracy.

Name: _____

Date: _____

POINT VALUE ✦ = 3–6 points ✱ = 7–9 points		PRACTICE TRIAL	GRADED TRIAL # 1	GRADED TRIAL # 2	NOTES
1. ✦	Wash your hands. Assemble the equipment and supplies.				
2. ✱	**Greet and identify the patient, introduce yourself and escort him or her to the patient examination room.**				
3. ✦	**Explain the procedure to relieve the patient's apprehension.**				
4. ✦	Ask the patient to disrobe from the waist up. Assist the patient into a gown, with the opening in front. **Assure the patient that his or her privacy will be respected.**				
5. ✦	Help the patient recline on the examination table or bed where the procedure will be performed.				
6. ✦	**Cover the patient with the drape, leaving the arms and legs exposed.** You may need to raise pant legs to expose the calves of the lower legs.				
7. ✦	Cleanse the skin with alcohol pads where the electrodes will be applied. If chest hair will interfere with contact between the electrodes and the skin, remove the hair with soap and/or shaving cream and a disposable razor.				
8. ✱	Apply the electrodes in the correct positions, making sure the wires do not touch the cart or examination table and that they follow the normal contours of the body. The power cord should not cross under the examination table or bed.				

		PRACTICE TRIAL	GRADED TRIAL #1	GRADED TRIAL #2	NOTES
9. ✦	Explain to the patient that the electrocardiograph is a sensitive machine and that he or she must remain as still as possible during the procedure. **Ask the patient if there are any questions prior to beginning.**				
10. ⋆	Calibrate the electrocardiograph and run the ECG. Mark the leads if necessary.				
11. ✦	When the ECG is complete, remove the electrodes and cleanse any residual conduction gel from the patient's skin.				
12. ✦	**Assist the patient in dressing. Discard the gown, if it is disposable; otherwise place it in a laundry hamper.**				
13. ✦	Cleanse the equipment. Sanitize the leads by wiping them with antiseptic solution, then store them in the appropriate compartment of the electrocardiograph cart. Replace any necessary supplies. Wash your hands.				
14. ⋆	Label the electrocardiograph paper with the patient's name, DOB, and the date and time. Document the patient's tolerance of the procedure. **Sign and date the entry with your name and credentials.**				
15. ✦	Per physician preference, instruct the patient to wait to discuss the test with the physician or make a followup appointment.				

Name: _____

Date: _____

Document: Enter the appropriate information in the chart below.

Grading

Points Earned	_____		
Points Possible	_____	102	102
Percent Grade (Points Earned/Points Possible)	_____		
PASS:	_____	❏ YES ❏ NO ❏ N/A	❏ YES ❏ NO ❏ N/A

Instructor Sign-Off

Instructor: _____ **Date:** _____

Procedure 35-2:

Applying a Holter Monitor

Objective: The student, using the supplies and equipment listed below, will demonstrate the application of a holter monitor.

Supplies: Medical order for the Holter monitor, Holter monitor, ECG electrodes, ECG recording cassette, fresh batteries (or recharged batteries), patient gown and drape as necessary for privacy and warmth, supplies for shaving if needed, alcohol pads, 4 × 4 gauze pad, liquid abrasive, adhesive tape, patient diary, patient chart, gloves

Affective Behaviors: Affective behaviors provide a professional approach to a skill that enhances the patient encounter. These behaviors may also display sensitivity to a patient's rights and enhance communication. Pay close attention to these skills, which will be in **bold, italicized** font.

Notes to the Student

_____

_____

_____

_____

_____

_____

Skills Assessment Requirements

Read and familiarize yourself with the procedure; complete the minimum practice requirements. Document each MPR using proper charting technique. Complete each procedure within a reasonable amount of time, with a minimum of 85 percent accuracy.

Name: _____

Date: _____

POINT VALUE ✦ = 3–6 points ⋆ = 7–9 points		PRACTICE TRIAL	GRADED TRIAL #1	GRADED TRIAL #2	NOTES
1. ✦	Run a test of the equipment to make sure it is functioning properly and that the batteries are fresh.				
2. ⋆	*With the patient sitting on the exam table, explain the procedure while showing the patient the equipment.*				
3. ✦	Instruct the patient to remove all clothing from the waist up. If the exam room is cool, offer the patient a blanket.				
4. ✦	Because the electrodes of the Holter monitor must be in constant contact with the skin, you may have to shave the electrode sites. *If so, explain the reason for shaving before you begin.*				
5. ✦	Wash your hands and put on gloves.				
6. ✦	Cleanse the skin with alcohol wipes to remove all lotions, cologne or perfume, and body oil.				
7. ✦	Moisten a 4 × 4 gauze with liquid abrasive and abrade the skin at the electrode sites until it is slightly red, to ensure the electrodes adhere.				
8. ✦	Take the electrodes from their packaging and remove the adhesive covering from each one.				
9. ✦	Check for moist gel on each electrode and apply the adhesive side to the skin site, using circular pressure from the center outward.				

Name: _____

Date: _____

		PRACTICE TRIAL	GRADED TRIAL # 1	GRADED TRIAL # 2	NOTES
10. ✦	Attach the lead wires to the electrodes and tape a loop to the electrode wires to the skin.				
11. ✦	Cover each electrode site with nonallergenic tape, which will remain in place over the next 24 hours.				
12. ✦	Verify the correct electrode placement by connecting the electrodes to the ECG machine and obtaining a test strip.				
13. ✦	Help the patient to dress, if necessary, being careful not to disturb any leads.				
14. ⋆	Test the Holter monitor by placing a cassette into it and making certain it runs smoothly. Plug the electrode cable into the recorder, and note the starting time in the patient diary and patient chart.				
15. ✦	Make an appointment for 24 hours later to review the monitor and remove the electrodes. **Ask the patient if he or she has any questions prior to leaving the examination room.**				
16. ⋆	Document the procedure in the patient's chart. **Sign and date the entry with your name and credentials.**				

Name: _____

Date: _____

Document: Enter the appropriate information in the chart below.

Grading

Points Earned	_____		
Points Possible	_____	105	105
Percent Grade (Points Earned/Points Possible)	_____		
PASS:	_____	❏ YES ❏ NO ❏ N/A	❏ YES ❏ NO ❏ N/A

Instructor Sign-Off

Instructor: _____ **Date:** _____

Name: _____

Date: _____

Procedure 36-1:

Demonstrate Performance of Spirometry

Objective: The student, using the supplies and equipment listed below, will demonstrate how to assist the patient in the performance of spirometry testing.

Supplies: Spirometer, disposable mouthpiece and tubing, nose clip, chart, forms and lab slips for documentation and testing

Affective Behaviors: Affective behaviors provide a professional approach to a skill that enhances the patient encounter. These behaviors may also display sensitivity to a patient's rights and enhance communication. Pay close attention to these skills, which will be in **bold, *italicized*** font.

Notes to the Student

_____

_____

_____

_____

_____

_____

Skills Assessment Requirements

Read and familiarize yourself with the procedure; complete the minimum practice requirements. Document each MPR using proper charting technique. Complete each procedure within a reasonable amount of time, with a minimum of 85 percent accuracy.

Name: _____

Date: _____

POINT VALUE ✦ = 3–6 points ⋆ = 7–9 points		PRACTICE TRIAL	GRADED TRIAL # 1	GRADED TRIAL # 2	NOTES
1. ✦	Wash your hands. Gather equipment and supplies.				
2. ⋆	**Greet and identify the patient, introduce yourself and guide the patient to the treatment area.**				
3. ✦	Record the patient's history and main complaint. **Explain the entire procedure. Ask the patient if he or she has any questions prior to beginning.**				
4. ✦	If the patient is chewing gum, ask him or her to dispose of it (to prevent choking during the test). If a female patient is wearing lipstick, ask her to remove it to create a tight seal.				
5. ✦	Ask the patient to place the mouthpiece in his or her mouth and to close the lips tightly around the mouthpiece to make a good seal.				
6. ✦	Place the nose clips on the patient's nose, sealing the nostrils closed.				
7. ⋆	Ask the patient to inhale as deeply as he or she possibly can and hold the breath for a short time. Then tell the patient to blow the air out into the mouthpiece as hard and as fast as possible—until he or she cannot blow out any more air.				
8. ✦	Repeat this procedure two more times, **giving the patient a few minutes in between.**				

		PRACTICE TRIAL	GRADED TRIAL #1	GRADED TRIAL #2	NOTES
9. ✦	The electronic equipment will usually "select" the best of the three breathing tests.				
10. ★	Document patient compliance with and tolerance of the testing procedure. ***Sign the entry with your name and credentials.***				
11. ✦	Follow cleaning procedures to prepare the equipment and the area for the next patient.				
12. ✦	Wash your hands.				

Name: _____

Date: _____

Document: Enter the appropriate information in the chart below.

Grading

Points Earned	_____		
Points Possible	_____	81	81
Percent Grade (Points Earned/Points Possible)	_____		
PASS:	_____	❏ YES ❏ NO ❏ N/A	❏ YES ❏ NO ❏ N/A

Instructor Sign-Off

Instructor: _____   **Date:** _____

Name: _____

Date: _____

Procedure 36-2:

Measuring Oxygen Saturation Using a Pulse Oximeter

Objective: Correctly measure oxygen saturation using a pulse oximeter.

Supplies: Pulse oximeter, alcohol wipe, nail polish remover as needed, patient chart

Affective Behaviors: Affective behaviors provide a professional approach to a skill that enhances the patient encounter. These behaviors may also display sensitivity to a patient's rights and enhance communication. Pay close attention to these skills, which will be in **bold, italicized** font.

Notes to the Student

_____

_____

_____

_____

_____

_____

_____

Skills Assessment Requirements

Read and familiarize yourself with the procedure; complete the minimum practice requirements. Document each MPR using proper charting technique. Complete each procedure within a reasonable amount of time, with a minimum of 85 percent accuracy.

Name: _____

Date: _____

POINT VALUE ✦ = 3–6 points ⋆ = 7–9 points	PRACTICE TRIAL	GRADED TRIAL #1	GRADED TRIAL #2	NOTES
1. ✦ Wash your hands and gather equipment and supplies.				
2. ⋆ **Greet and identify the patient, introduce yourself and guide the patient to the treatment area.**				
3. ✦ **Explain the procedure to the patient.**				
4. ✦ Select the appropriate size sensor (pediatric, small or large).				
5. ✦ Instruct the patient to breathe normally.				
6. ⋆ Prepare the selected site (earlobe or finger). Remove nail polish or earring if necessary.				
7. ✦ Wipe the selected site with alcohol and allow to dry.				
8. ⋆ Attach the sensor to the site and connect to the pulse oximeter. Turn on the pulse oximeter and listen to the tone.				
9. ⋆ Read the saturation level and document in the patient's chart. **Sign the entry with your name and credentials.** Report to the physician readings that are less than 95%.				

Name: _____

Date: _____

Document: Enter the appropriate information in the chart below.

Grading

Points Earned	_____		
Points Possible	_____	66	66
Percent Grade (Points Earned/Points Possible)	_____		
PASS:	_____	❏ YES ❏ NO ❏ N/A	❏ YES ❏ NO ❏ N/A

Instructor Sign-Off

Instructor: _____ **Date:** _____

Procedure 36-3:

Demonstrate the Performance of Peak Flow Testing

Objective: The student, using the supplies and equipment listed below, will demonstrate how to assist the patient in the performance of peak flow testing.

Supplies: Peak flow meter, patient log or diary of peak flow readings, patient chart

Affective Behaviors: Affective behaviors provide a professional approach to a skill that enhances the patient encounter. These behaviors may also display sensitivity to a patient's rights and enhance communication. Pay close attention to these skills, which will be in ***bold, italicized*** font.

Notes to the Student

_____

_____

_____

_____

_____

_____

Skills Assessment Requirements

Read and familiarize yourself with the procedure; complete the minimum practice requirements. Document each MPR using proper charting technique. Complete each procedure within a reasonable amount of time, with a minimum of 85 percent accuracy.

POINT VALUE ✦ = 3–6 points ⋆ = 7–9 points	PRACTICE TRIAL	GRADED TRIAL # 1	GRADED TRIAL # 2	NOTES
1. ✦	Wash your hands. Gather equipment and supplies.			
2. ⋆	**Greet and identify the patient, introduce yourself and guide the patient to the treatment area.**			
3. ⋆	**Explain the procedure to the patient:** Instruct the patient to take as deep a breath as possible, place the mouthpiece just in front of the teeth, then use his or her lips to make a complete seal. Ask the patient to exhale as hard and as fast as possible.			
4. ✦	Have the patient repeat step 3 times.			
5. ✦	If test results also need to be taken after medication, allow the patient to rest. Administer the medication, then repeat the test.			
6. ✦	Clean the equipment and dispose of contaminated materials appropriately.			
7. ✦	Wash your hands.			
8. ⋆	Record the results. **Sign the entry with your name and credentials.** Compare the results with previous readings.			

Document: Enter the appropriate information in the chart below.

Grading

Points Earned	_____		
Points Possible	_____	57	57
Percent Grade (Points Earned/Points Possible)	_____		
PASS:	_____	❏ YES ❏ NO ❏ N/A	❏ YES ❏ NO ❏ N/A

Instructor Sign-Off

Instructor: _____ **Date:** _____

Name: _____

Date: _____

Procedure 36-4:

Demonstrate the Performance of the Mantoux Test by Intradermal Injection

Objective: The student, using the supplies and equipment listed below, will demonstrate how to perform the Mantoux test.

Supplies: Patient chart, disposable gloves, alcohol wipes, sharps container, tuberculin syringe with needle, vial of medication, bandage strips

Affective Behaviors: Affective behaviors provide a professional approach to a skill that enhances the patient encounter. These behaviors may also display sensitivity to a patient's rights and enhance communication. Pay close attention to these skills, which will be in **bold, *italicized*** font.

Notes to the Student

_____

_____

_____

_____

_____

_____

Skills Assessment Requirements

Read and familiarize yourself with the procedure; complete the minimum practice requirements. Document each MPR using proper charting technique. Complete each procedure within a reasonable amount of time, with a minimum of 85 percent accuracy.

Name: _____

Date: _____

POINT VALUE ✦ = 3–6 points ⋆ = 7–9 points		PRACTICE TRIAL	GRADED TRIAL # 1	GRADED TRIAL # 2	NOTES
1. ✦	Wash your hands and gather the equipment.				
2. ⋆	**Greet and identify the patient, introduce yourself and guide the patient to the treatment area.**				
3. ✦	Wash your hands again and put on disposable gloves. **Explain the procedure to the patient.**				
4. ✦	Ask the patient to reach out with one hand and turn the palm upward. Find a site without hair or blemishes on the forearm.				
5. ✦	Cleanse the skin with an alcohol wipe and allow it to thoroughly air dry.				
6. ✦	Cleanse the top of the PPD vial with an alcohol wipe and allow it to air dry. Withdraw 0.1 cc from the vial and hold it in your dominant hand.				
7. ✦	Place your nondominant hand under the patient's forearm and gently pull the skin tight. Ask the patient to keep the arm still. Insert the needle bevel just into and under the skin at a 10- to 15-degree angle.				
8. ⋆	Inject the medication slowly to create a raised blister, or wheal.				
9. ✦	Release the skin, then withdraw the needle and blot the area gently with an alcohol wipe. **Instruct the patient not to bandage the area.**				
10. ✦	Discard the syringe in the sharps container.				

Name: _____

Date: _____

		PRACTICE TRIAL	GRADED TRIAL # 1	GRADED TRIAL # 2	NOTES
11. ✦	Make an appointment for the patient to return and have the injection site checked after 48 to 72 hours.				
12. ⋆	Document the procedure, including a description of the Mantoux test site. **Sign the entry with your name and credentials.**				
13. ⋆	When the patient returns, measure only the induration, not the redness. For positive results, measure in millimeters (mm) and follow local public health guidelines for reporting.				

Name: _____

Date: _____

Document: Enter the appropriate information in the chart below.

Grading

Points Earned	_____		
Points Possible	_____	90	90
Percent Grade (Points Earned/Points Possible)	_____		
PASS:	_____	❏ YES ❏ NO ❏ N/A	❏ YES ❏ NO ❏ N/A

Instructor Sign-Off

Instructor: _____ **Date:** _____

Procedure 36-5:

Demonstrate Patient Instruction in the Use of an Inhaler

Objective: The student, using the supplies and equipment listed below, will demonstrate how to instruct and/or help the patient use an inhaler for the first time.

Supplies: Patient's prescription inhaler, patient's chart

Affective Behaviors: Affective behaviors provide a professional approach to a skill that enhances the patient encounter. These behaviors may also display sensitivity to a patient's rights and enhance communication. Pay close attention to these skills, which will be in **bold, *italicized*** font.

Notes to the Student

_____

_____

_____

_____

_____

_____

Skills Assessment Requirements

Read and familiarize yourself with the procedure; complete the minimum practice requirements. Document each MPR using proper charting technique. Complete each procedure within a reasonable amount of time, with a minimum of 85 percent accuracy.

Name: _____

Date: _____

POINT VALUE ✦ = 3–6 points ⋆ = 7–9 points	PRACTICE TRIAL	GRADED TRIAL # 1	GRADED TRIAL # 2	NOTES
1. ✦ Wash your hands and gather the equipment.				
2. ⋆ **Greet and identify the patient, introduce yourself and guide the patient to the treatment area.**				
3. ⋆ **Review the patient's prescription.** Give the patient the following instructions: • Shake the canister thoroughly. • Hold the canister upright within 2 inches of the mouth. Place the mouthpiece in your mouth, sealing the opening with your lips. • Activate the inhaler (usually by pressing the canister down) to spray. Breathe slowly but deeply after the medication is delivered. • Hold your breath for as long as possible, up to 10 seconds. • Begin breathing normally again.				
4. ✦ Follow the physician's instructions for immediate repeat use. **Ask the patient if he or she has any questions prior to leaving the examination room.**				
5. ⋆ Document the patient's ability to follow instructions. **Sign the entry with your name and credentials.** Inform the physician if the patient has any problems with self-administration. **Give the patient backup written instructions.**				

Name: _____

Date: _____

Document: Enter the appropriate information in the chart below.

Grading

Points Earned	_____		
Points Possible	_____	39	39
Percent Grade (Points Earned/Points Possible)	_____		
PASS:	_____	❏ YES ❏ NO ❏ N/A	❏ YES ❏ NO ❏ N/A

Instructor Sign-Off

Instructor: _____   **Date:** _____

Procedure 36-6:

Demonstrate Patient Assistance in the Use of a Nebulizer

Objective: The student, using the supplies and equipment listed below, will demonstrate how to assist the patient in the use of a nebulizer.

Supplies: Compressor, nebulizer with mask and tubing, medications, patient's chart

Affective Behaviors: Affective behaviors provide a professional approach to a skill that enhances the patient encounter. These behaviors may also display sensitivity to a patient's rights and enhance communication. Pay close attention to these skills, which will be in **bold, *italicized*** font.

Notes to the Student

_____

_____

_____

_____

_____

_____

Skills Assessment Requirements

Read and familiarize yourself with the procedure; complete the minimum practice requirements. Document each MPR using proper charting technique. Complete each procedure within a reasonable amount of time, with a minimum of 85 percent accuracy.

Name: _____

Date: _____

POINT VALUE ✦ = 3–6 points ⋆ = 7–9 points		PRACTICE TRIAL	GRADED TRIAL # 1	GRADED TRIAL # 2	NOTES
1. ✦	Wash your hands. Gather equipment and supplies.				
2. ⋆	**Greet and identify the patient, introduce yourself and guide the patient to the treatment area.**				
3. ✦	Obtain vital signs and **explain the procedure to the patient.**				
4. ✦	Wash your hands again.				
5. ✦	Prepare the nebulizer cup with medication(s) as ordered and/or prescribed.				
6. ✦	Turn on the compressor.				
7. ✦	Instruct, or help, the patient to hold the mask while the medication is being delivered.				
8. ⋆	Continue treatment until no medication remains in the nebulizer. Monitor the patient's pulse every 5 minutes throughout the treatment. If the pulse rises to 120 beats per minute or the patient's condition worsens, stop the treatment and tell the physician.				
9. ✦	Dispose of used materials in the appropriate containers.				
10. ✦	Wash your hands. **Ask the patient if he or she has any questions prior to leaving the examination room.**				
11. ⋆	Document the patient's vital signs at the beginning, middle, and end of the treatment. Also describe patient signs and symptoms at beginning and end of treatment. **Sign the entry with your name and credentials.**				

Document: Enter the appropriate information in the chart below.

Grading

Points Earned	_____		
Points Possible	_____	75	75
Percent Grade (Points Earned/Points Possible)	_____		
PASS:	_____	❏ YES ❏ NO ❏ N/A	❏ YES ❏ NO ❏ N/A

Instructor Sign-Off

Instructor: _____ **Date:** _____

Procedure 37-1:

Measure Distance Visual Acuity with a Snellen Chart

Objective: The student, using the supplies and equipment listed below, will demonstrate how to assist the patient in testing the visual acuity of both eyes.

Supplies: Snellen chart, occluder, spatula, or card, patient chart

Affective Behaviors: Affective behaviors provide a professional approach to a skill that enhances the patient encounter. These behaviors may also display sensitivity to a patient's rights and enhance communication. Pay close attention to these skills, which will be in **_bold, italicized_** font.

Notes to the Student

_____

_____

_____

_____

_____

_____

Skills Assessment Requirements

Read and familiarize yourself with the procedure; complete the minimum practice requirements. Document each MPR using proper charting technique. Complete each procedure within a reasonable amount of time, with a minimum of 85 percent accuracy.

Name: _____

Date: _____

POINT VALUE ✦ = 3–6 points ★ = 7–9 points		PRACTICE TRIAL	GRADED TRIAL # 1	GRADED TRIAL # 2	NOTES
1. ✦	Wash your hands. Gather equipment and supplies.				
2. ★	**Greet and identify the patient, introduce yourself and escort the patient to the examination room.**				
3. ✦	Record the patient's history and main complaint. **Explain the entire procedure to the patient.**				
4. ✦	Position the patient, standing or sitting, at the 20-foot line. Give the patient the occluder. Observe patient during the procedure for head tilting, squinting, and tearing.				
5. ✦	Ask the patient to cover the left eye, keeping it open, and to read aloud from the top line to the smallest line of readable letters.				
6. ★	Record the right-eye vision with the number of errors. For one or two errors, record the vision fraction and minus one or two. For more than two errors, record the vision fraction as noted one line above on the Snellen chart. **For example**, if the patient reads the 20/40 line with the right eye and two errors, the result is recorded as OD 20/40-2. If the patient reads the 20/40 line with the right eye and three errors, the result is OD 20/50, or one line above the 20/40 line.				

	PRACTICE TRIAL	GRADED TRIAL # 1	GRADED TRIAL # 2	NOTES
7. ✦ Next, ask the patient to repeat the procedure, covering the right eye and reading with the left.				
8. ⋆ **Record the left-eye vision with the number of errors. Sign the entry including your name and credentials.**				
9. ✦ Wash your hands and report the results to the physician.				

Document: Enter the appropriate information in the chart below.

Grading

Points Earned	_____		
Points Possible	_____	63	63
Percent Grade (Points Earned/Points Possible)	_____		
PASS:	_____	❏ YES ❏ NO ❏ N/A	❏ YES ❏ NO ❏ N/A

Instructor Sign-Off

Instructor: _____ **Date:** _____

Procedure 37-2:

Perform the Ishihara Color Vision Test

Objective: The student, using the supplies and equipment listed below, will demonstrate how to determine color vision acuity using Ishihara color plates.

Supplies: Ishihara color plates book, pen, patient chart

Affective Behaviors: Affective behaviors provide a professional approach to a skill that enhances the patient encounter. These behaviors may also display sensitivity to a patient's rights and enhance communication. Pay close attention to these skills, which will be in **_bold, italicized_** font.

Notes to the Student

_____

_____

_____

_____

_____

_____

Skills Assessment Requirements

Read and familiarize yourself with the procedure; complete the minimum practice requirements. Document each MPR using proper charting technique. Complete each procedure within a reasonable amount of time, with a minimum of 85 percent accuracy.

Name: _____

Date: _____

POINT VALUE ✦ = 3–6 points ⋆ = 7–9 points		PRACTICE TRIAL	GRADED TRIAL #1	GRADED TRIAL #2	NOTES
1. ✦	**Explain the procedure to the patient.**				
2. ⋆	Follow the physician's directions for administering the total book, or sections.				
3. ✦	Ask the patient to identify the number in each plate with both eyes.				
4. ✦	Have the patient cover the left eye and read the book again, then the right eye. Write down the page number of any plates the patient misses. (The correct answer is on the back of each page.)				
5. ✦	Follow the directions on the last page of the book to determine the level of color blindness, if any.				
6. ⋆	Document the procedure in the patient's chart. **Sign the entry with your name and credentials.**				

Name: _____

Date: _____

Document: Enter the appropriate information in the chart below.

Grading

Points Earned	_____		
Points Possible	_____	42	42
Percent Grade (Points Earned/Points Possible)	_____		
PASS:	_____	❑ YES ❑ NO ❑ N/A	❑ YES ❑ NO ❑ N/A

Instructor Sign-Off

Instructor: _____ **Date:** _____

Procedure 37-3:

Perform Eye Irrigation

Objective: The student, using the supplies and equipment listed below, will demonstrate how to irrigate the patient's eye.

Supplies: Irrigating solution, sterile basin, irrigating syringe, protective gear (gown, face shield, disposable gloves), towels, kidney-shaped basin, tissues, patient chart

Affective Behaviors: Affective behaviors provide a professional approach to a skill that enhances the patient encounter. These behaviors may also display sensitivity to a patient's rights and enhance communication. Pay close attention to these skills, which will be in **_bold, italicized_** font.

Notes to the Student

_____

_____

_____

_____

_____

_____

Skills Assessment Requirements

Read and familiarize yourself with the procedure; complete the minimum practice requirements. Document each MPR using proper charting technique. Complete each procedure within a reasonable amount of time, with a minimum of 85 percent accuracy.

Name: _____

Date: _____

POINT VALUE ✦ = 3–6 points ⋆ = 7–9 points		PRACTICE TRIAL	GRADED TRIAL # 1	GRADED TRIAL # 2	NOTES
1. ✦	Wash your hands. Gather equipment and supplies.				
2. ⋆	**Greet and identify the patient, introduce yourself and escort the patient to the examination room.**				
3. ✦	Record the patient's history and main complaint.				
4. ✦	Review the physician's order for the patient's name, the volume and name of the irrigating solution, and which eye to irrigate.				
5. ⋆	Ask the patient about medication allergies. **Explain the entire procedure.**				
6. ⋆	Check the label of the irrigating solution against the physician's order before pouring it into the sterile basin for irrigation.				
7. ✦	Wash your hands.				
8. ✦	Put on the gown, face shield, and gloves before proceeding with irrigation.				
9. ✦	Ask the patient to lie or sit down with the head tilted toward the eye to be irrigated. Place a towel and the kidney-shaped basin next to the patient's face to catch irrigating fluid.				
10. ✦	With your dominant hand, fill the irrigating syringe with the prescribed irrigating solution.				
11. ✦	With your nondominant hand, press with a tissue against the patient's cheekbone beneath the eye to expose more of the eye surface.				

		PRACTICE TRIAL	GRADED TRIAL #1	GRADED TRIAL #2	NOTES
12.★	While holding the syringe approximately 1/2 inch from the eye, gently direct the fluid toward the inside surface of the lower conjunctiva and from the inner to outer corner of the eye.				
13. ◆	Continue irrigating until the prescribed volume is used. Depending on the cause and symptoms, the physician may order further irrigation.				
14. ◆	When irrigation is complete, dry the area around the affected eye with tissues.				
15. ◆	Remove your protective clothing and place it in the proper laundry and waste containers.				
16. ◆	Wash your hands. **Prior to leaving the examination room, ask the patient if he or she has any questions.**				
17. ★	Document the patient's tolerance of the procedure, the amount and kind of irrigating solution, and the eye irrigated. **Sign the entry with your name and credentials.**				

Name: _____

Date: _____

Document: Enter the appropriate information in the chart below.

Grading

Points Earned	_____		
Points Possible	_____	117	117
Percent Grade (Points Earned/Points Possible)	_____		
PASS:	_____	❑ YES ❑ NO ❑ N/A	❑ YES ❑ NO ❑ N/A

Instructor Sign-Off

Instructor: _____ Date: _____

Name: _____

Date: _____

Procedure 37-4:

Perform Instillation of Eye Medication

Objective: The student, using the supplies and equipment listed below, will perform eye medication instillation.

Supplies: Prescription medication (drops or ointment), disposable gloves, tissues, patient chart

Affective Behaviors: Affective behaviors provide a professional approach to a skill that enhances the patient encounter. These behaviors may also display sensitivity to a patient's rights and enhance communication. Pay close attention to these skills, which will be in ***bold, italicized*** font.

Notes to the Student

_____

_____

_____

_____

_____

_____

Skills Assessment Requirements

Read and familiarize yourself with the procedure; complete the minimum practice requirements. Document each MPR using proper charting technique. Complete each procedure within a reasonable amount of time, with a minimum of 85 percent accuracy.

POINT VALUE ✦ = 3–6 points ⋆ = 7–9 points		PRACTICE TRIAL	GRADED TRIAL #1	GRADED TRIAL #2	NOTES
1. ✦	Wash your hands. Gather equipment and supplies.				
2. ✦	Take the medication from the storage shelf. Check the label against the physician's order.				
3. ⋆	*Identify the patient and guide him or her to the treatment area. Check the patient's identification against the physician's order and medication name.*				
4. ✦	Note the medication dosage to be administered.				
5. ⋆	*Ask the patient about allergies. Explain the entire procedure.*				
6. ✦	Wash your hands and put on disposable gloves.				
7. ✦	Ask the patient to lie down or sit with the head tilted back with both eyes open. (It may be necessary to ask the sitting patient to look at the ceiling.) If the patient is wearing an eye patch, remove it.				
8. ✦	Give the patient a tissue to hold in each hand until after the procedure. With your nondominant hand and a tissue, press on the lower cheekbone and gently pull the lower eyelid down to expose the cornea and conjunctival sac.				

		PRACTICE TRIAL	GRADED TRIAL # 1	GRADED TRIAL # 2	NOTES
9. ✱	*To administer eye drops:* Fill the eyedropper with your dominant hand. Hold the dropper approximately 1/2 inch away from the patient's eye, and administer the prescribed dose into the conjunctival sac. *To administer the ointment:* Rest your dominant hand on the patient's forehead, hold the tube, and lightly squeeze ointment into the conjunctival sac from the inner to outer corner of the patient's eye.				
10. ✦	Release the patient's lower eyelid and tell the patient to close the eye.				
11. ✦	Repeat the procedure in the other eye, if ordered by the physician.				
12. ✦	Instruct the patient to use a separate tissue for each eye to wipe away excess medication.				
13. ✦	Apply an eye patch, if ordered by the physician.				
14. ✦	Provide a waste container for the patient to discard the used tissue into. Dispose of the gloves and tissue.				
15. ✦	Wash your hands. **Prior to leaving the examination room, ask the patient if he or she has any questions.**				
16. ✱	Document the patient's tolerance of the procedure, the amount and kind of medication administered, and the eye(s) treated. **Sign the entry with your name and credentials.**				

Name: _____

Date: _____

Document: Enter the correct information in the chart below.

Grading

Points Earned	_____		
Points Possible	_____	108	108
Percent Grade (Points Earned/Points Possible)	_____		
PASS:	_____	❏ YES ❏ NO ❏ N/A	❏ YES ❏ NO ❏ N/A

Instructor Sign-Off

Instructor: _____   **Date:** _____

Name: _____

Date: _____

Procedure 37-5:

Perform Simple Audiometry

Objective: Correctly perform bilateral audiology testing.

Supplies: Audiometer, earphones, audiometric test report form, patient chart

Affective Behaviors: Affective behaviors provide a professional approach to a skill that enhances the patient encounter. These behaviors may also display sensitivity to patients' rights and enhance communication. Pay close attention to these skills which will be in **_bold, italicized_** font.

Notes to the Student

_____

_____

_____

_____

_____

_____

Skills Assessment Requirements

Read and familiarize yourself with the procedure; complete the minimum practice requirements. Document each MPR using proper charting technique. Complete each procedure within a reasonable amount of time, with a minimum of 85 percent accuracy.

Name: _____

Date: _____

POINT VALUE ✦ = 3–6 points ∗ = 7–9 points		PRACTICE TRIAL	GRADED TRIAL # 1	GRADED TRIAL # 2	NOTES
1. ✦	Wash your hands. Gather equipment and supplies.				
2. ∗	Prepare the testing area to ensure quiet during the procedure.				
3. ∗	**Warmly greet and identify the patient and introduce yourself.** Guide him or her to the testing area.				
4. ✦	Inform the patient that only one ear at a time will be tested. Instruct the patient to raise one finger or nod when he or she first hears the sound, no matter how soft. **Prior to beginning the test, ask the patient if he or she has any questions.**				
5. ✦	Place earphones on the patient.				
6. ✦	Administer low-frequency sounds to one ear to determine the patient's base-line hearing measurements and ability to follow test instructions.				
7. ∗	Plot the results from each tone on the graph immediately.				
8. ✦	Continue raising the tone frequency by 10 db (decibles) and recording the results until the patient can no longer hear in the first ear.				

Name: _____

Date: _____

	PRACTICE TRIAL	GRADED TRIAL # 1	GRADED TRIAL # 2	NOTES
9. ✦ Lower the tone by 5 db until the patient signals to confirm the lowest frequency the patient can hear in that ear.				
10. ✦ Repeat the procedure with the other ear.				
11. * **Document the results in the patient's chart, sign the entry and include your initials. Give the audiometric test results to the physician.**				
12. ✦ Prepare the audiometric equipment and room for the next patient.				

Name: _____

Date: _____

Document: Enter the appropriate information in the chart below.

Grading

Points Earned	_____		
Points Possible	_____	84	84
Percent Grade (Points Earned/Points Possible)	_____		
PASS:	_____	❏ YES ❏ NO ❏ N/A	❏ YES ❏ NO ❏ N/A

Instructor Sign-Off

Instructor: _____ **Date:** _____

Procedure 37-6:

Perform Ear Irrigation

Objective: The student, using the supplies and equipment listed below, will demonstrate how to irrigate the patient's ear.

Supplies: Irrigating solution, sterile basin, irrigating syringe, towels, cotton ball(s), patient chart

Affective Behaviors: Affective behaviors provide a professional approach to a skill that enhances the patient encounter. These behaviors may also display sensitivity to a patient's rights and enhance communication. Pay close attention to these skills, which will be in ***bold, italicized*** font.

Notes to the Student

_____

_____

_____

_____

_____

_____

Skills Assessment Requirements

Read and familiarize yourself with the procedure; complete the minimum practice requirements. Document each MPR using proper charting technique. Complete each procedure within a reasonable amount of time, with a minimum of 85 percent accuracy.

POINT VALUE ✦ = 3–6 points ⋆ = 7–9 points		PRACTICE TRIAL	GRADED TRIAL # 1	GRADED TRIAL # 2	NOTES
1. ✦	Wash your hands. Gather equipment and supplies.				
2. ⋆	**Greet and identify the patient, introduce yourself and escort the patient to the examination room.**				
3. ⋆	Check the label of the irrigating solution when you take it from the shelf and against the physician's order.				
4. ✦	Position the patient in a sitting position and instruct him or her to lean the head toward the side to be irrigated.				
5. ✦	Check the condition of the external auditory canal with the otoscope.				
6. ✦	Drape a towel across the patient's shoulder, under the ear.				
7. ✦	Fill the irrigating syringe with prescribed solution.				
8. ✦	Place the basin under the ear and against the skin. Instruct the patient or other office personnel to hold the basin in place.				
9. ⋆	For a child under 3 years, gently pull the auricle down and back. For a child over 3 years or an adult, gently pull the auricle ear up and back.				
10. ✦	Gently place the tip of the irrigating syringe into the external auditory canal and point to the side or top. Do not point directly toward the tympanic membrane.				

		PRACTICE TRIAL	GRADED TRIAL # 1	GRADED TRIAL # 2	NOTES
11. ★	Instill the irrigating solution with gentle pressure on the plunger of the syringe.				
12. ✦	Place the irrigation basin aside.				
13. ✦	Use the otoscope to determine if more irrigation is needed.				
14. ✦	Repeat the procedure until the desired results are obtained. If the patient experiences discomfort or other difficulties, report to the physician.				
15. ✦	After irrigation, instruct and/or assist the patient to lie down with the head tilted toward the irrigated ear.				
16. ✦	Place a towel under the head to catch the drainage.				
17. ✦	**Help the patient to a sitting, then standing position.** Assess the patient for light-headedness or dizziness. **Escort the patient to the waiting room.**				
18. ✦	Clean the treatment area and remove reusable equipment to the utility cleaning area.				
19. ✦	Wash your hands. **Prior to leaving the examination room, ask the patient if he or she has any questions.**				
20. ★	Document the patient's tolerance and the results of the procedure. **Sign the entry with your name and credentials.**				

Document: Enter the appropriate information in the chart below.

Grading

Points Earned	_____		
Points Possible	_____	135	135
Percent Grade (Points Earned/Points Possible)	_____		
PASS:	_____	❏ YES ❏ NO ❏ N/A	❏ YES ❏ NO ❏ N/A

Instructor Sign-Off

Instructor: _____ Date: _____

Name: _____

Date: _____

Procedure 37-7:

Perform Instillation of Ear Medication

Objective: The student, using the supplies and equipment listed below, will demonstrate how to instill medication into the patient's ear.

Supplies: Medication, disposable gloves, cotton balls, patient chart

Affective Behaviors: Affective behaviors provide a professional approach to a skill that enhances the patient encounter. These behaviors may also display sensitivity to a patient's rights and enhance communication. Pay close attention to these skills, which will be in **_bold, italicized_** font.

Notes to the Student

_____

_____

_____

_____

_____

_____

Skills Assessment Requirements

Read and familiarize yourself with the procedure; complete the minimum practice requirements. Document each MPR using proper charting technique. Complete each procedure within a reasonable amount of time, with a minimum of 85 percent accuracy.

Name: _____

Date: _____

POINT VALUE ✦ = 3–6 points ⋆ = 7–9 points		PRACTICE TRIAL	GRADED TRIAL # 1	GRADED TRIAL # 2	NOTES
1. ✦	Wash your hands. Gather equipment and supplies.				
2. ⋆	Check the label when removing the medication from the shelf and against the physician's order.				
3. ✦	Do not administer the medication unless it is at room temperature.				
4. ⋆	**Greet and identify the patient, introduce yourself and escort the patient to the examination room.** Check the patient name against the physician's order and against the medication.				
5. ✦	Explain the entire procedure to the patient. Ask about any allergies.				
6. ✦	Instruct the patient to lie on the side opposite the ear to be treated.				
7. ✦	Position the auricle as in procedure 19-6.				
8. ⋆	Hold the ear dropper or bottle tip about 1/2 inch above the external auditory canal and gently squeeze the bulb to administer the prescribed number of drops.				
9. ✦	Instruct the patient to lie still for 10 minutes.				
10. ✦	Loosely place a small cotton ball, if the physician orders it, at the opening to the canal.				

		PRACTICE TRIAL	GRADED TRIAL # 1	GRADED TRIAL # 2	NOTES
11. ✦	Repeat the procedure for the other ear, if ordered. Recap the medication bottle and dispose of waste materials.				
12. ✦	Remove and dispose of the gloves. Wash your hands.				
13. ✦	**Ensure that the patient does not have any questions and escort the patient back to the waiting room.**				
14. ⋆	Document the patient's tolerance of the procedure, the medication, the dosage administered, and which ear received treatment. **Sign the entry with your name and credentials.**				

Name: _____

Date: _____

Document: Enter the appropriate information in the chart below.

Grading

Points Earned	_____		
Points Possible	_____	96	96
Percent Grade (Points Earned/Points Possible)	_____		
PASS:	_____	❏ YES ❏ NO ❏ N/A	❏ YES ❏ NO ❏ N/A

Instructor Sign-Off

Instructor: _____ **Date:** _____

Name: _____

Date: _____

Procedure 37-8:

Assist with the Nasal Examination and Obtain a Nasopharyngeal Specimen

Objective: Correctly perform collection of a nasopharyngeal specimen and prepare it for transport.

Supplies: Penlight, tongue blade, sterile swab with transport device, specimen label, personal protective equipment, patient chart, waste container

Affective Behaviors: Affective behaviors provide a professional approach to a skill that enhances the patient encounter. These behaviors may also display sensitivity to a patient's rights and enhance communication. Pay close attention to these skills, which will be in **_bold, italicized_** font.

Notes to the Student

_____

_____

_____

_____

_____

_____

Skills Assessment Requirements

Read and familiarize yourself with the procedure; complete the minimum practice requirements. Document each MPR using proper charting technique. Complete each procedure within a reasonable amount of time, with a minimum of 85 percent accuracy.

POINT VALUE ✦ = 3–6 points ⋆ = 7–9 points		PRACTICE TRIAL	GRADED TRIAL # 1	GRADED TRIAL # 2	NOTES
1. ✦	Wash your hands.				
2. ✦	Gather equipment and supplies.				
3. ⋆	***Identify and greet the patient, then escort the patient to the examination room. Introduce yourself and explain the process of collection.***				
4. ✦	Wash your hands and put on your personal protective equipment.				
5. ⋆	Nasopharyngeal specimen collection: • Position the patient with head tilted back. • Using a tongue blade and penlight, examine the nasopharyngeal area and make note of any discharge, lesions, swelling, obstructions, or redness. • Gently pass the swab through the nostril and into the nasopharynx. Rotate the swab quickly, then remove it and place it in the transport container and medium, if used.				
6. ⋆	Label the container with the patient's name (first and last), date and time of collection, and source of specimens.				
7. ✦	Dispose of any waste materials in the appropriate container(s).				

Name: _____

Date: _____

		PRACTICE TRIAL	GRADED TRIAL # 1	GRADED TRIAL # 2	NOTES
8. ✦	Transport the specimen to the testing area.				
9. ✦	Wash hands and remove PPE. **Ensure that the patient is comfortable and does not have any questions.**				
10. ✶	Perform the required charting or laboratory documentation relating to specimen collection. **Sign the entry with your name and credentials.**				

Document: Enter the appropriate information in the chart below.

Grading

Points Earned	_____		
Points Possible	_____	72	72
Percent Grade (Points Earned/Points Possible)	_____		
PASS:	_____	❏ YES ❏ NO ❏ N/A	❏ YES ❏ NO ❏ N/A

Instructor Sign-Off

Instructor: _____ **Date:** _____

Name: _____

Date: _____

Procedure 41-1:

Perform Adult Rescue Breathing and One-Rescuer CPR

Objective: The student, using the supplies and equipment listed below, will demonstrate how to administer rescue breathing for an adult and one-rescuer CPR for an adult.

Supplies: Approved mannequin, gloves, ventilator mask, mouth guard

Affective Behaviors: Affective behaviors provide a professional approach to a skill that enhances the patient encounter. These behaviors may also display sensitivity to a patient's rights and enhance communication. Pay close attention to these skills, which will be in **_bold, italicized_** font.

Notes to the Student

_____

_____

_____

_____

_____

_____

Skills Assessment Requirements

Read and familiarize yourself with the procedure; complete the minimum practice requirements. Document each MPR using proper charting technique. Complete each procedure within a reasonable amount of time, with a minimum of 85 percent accuracy.

POINT VALUE ✦ = 3–6 points ⋆ = 7–9 points		PRACTICE TRIAL	GRADED TRIAL # 1	GRADED TRIAL # 2	NOTES
1. ✦	Assess the victim and determine if help is needed. Shout "Are you OK?" while gently shaking the victim's shoulders. **State your name and inform the victim that you are there to help.**				
2. ✦	If the adult victim is determined to be unresponsive, activate EMS immediately by calling 911 and get an AED if available. **Remain calm and collected during the next steps.**				
3. ⋆	Assess the ABCs. *Airway*: Perform a head-tilt chin lift, or, if a neck injury is suspected, a jaw thrust. Look and feel for breath and chest movements. Attempt to get another person to call 911. If you are alone, begin the rescue sequence for 1 minute and then attempt to call, yourself. If gloves are available, put them on. If you have a ventilator mask, place it on the victim.				
4. ✦	If breathing is absent, put on a mouth guard and administer two rescue breaths. If your breaths do not cause the chest to rise, look in the victim's mouth and remove the object if one is seen. If no object is seen, make a second attempt to administer a rescue breath. If the breath still does not enter the chest, proceed to abdominal thrusts for unconscious victims.				

		PRACTICE TRIAL	GRADED TRIAL # 1	GRADED TRIAL # 2	NOTES
5. ★	If the breaths cause the chest to rise, assess the patient's circulation by feeling for a pulse at the carotid artery. If you feel a pulse, begin rescue breathing. Administer 1 breath every 5 seconds, or 10–12 every minute. After 1 minute, reassess the victim for breathing and pulse.				
6. ★	If you do not feel a pulse, begin chest compressions. Kneel at the victim's side. Find the sternum and place the heel of one hand just below the nipple line.				
7. ✦	Place your other hand on top of the first hand, making sure to lift your fingers off the chest, using only the heels of your hands to administer compressions.				
8. ✦	Keeping your shoulders directly over your hands, compress the chest 1 1/2 to 2 inches, then allow the sternum to relax. Do not lift your hands off the chest.				
9. ✦	Continue to compress the chest a total of 30 times, then administer 2 breaths.				
10. ✦	Repeat this sequence for 4 total cycles. Reassess the victim.				
11. ✦	If necessary, continue CPR until pulse and breathing return or you are relieved by more advanced medical personnel.				

Name: _____

Date: _____

Document: Enter the appropriate information in the chart below.

Grading

Points Earned	_____		
Points Possible	_____	75	75
Percent Grade (Points Earned/Points Possible)	_____		
PASS:	_____	❏ YES ❏ NO ❏ N/A	❏ YES ❏ NO ❏ N/A

Instructor Sign-Off

Instructor: _____ **Date:** _____

Procedure 41-2:

Use of an Automated External Defibrillator (AED)

Objective: The student, using the supplies and equipment listed below, will demonstrate how to use an AED.

Supplies: AED machine, patient chart

Affective Behaviors: Affective behaviors provide a professional approach to a skill that enhances the patient encounter. These behaviors may also display sensitivity to a patient's rights and enhance communication. Pay close attention to these skills, which will be in **_bold, italicized_** font.

Notes to the Student

_____

_____

_____

_____

_____

Skills Assessment Requirements

Read and familiarize yourself with the procedure; complete the minimum practice requirements. Document each MPR using proper charting technique. Complete each procedure within a reasonable amount of time, with a minimum of 85 percent accuracy.

Name: _____

Date: _____

POINT VALUE ✦ = 3–6 points ⋆ = 7–9 points	PRACTICE TRIAL	GRADED TRIAL #1	GRADED TRIAL #2	NOTES
1. ✦ **State your name and inform the victim that you are there to help.** Place the AED next to the victim's left ear.				
2. ⋆ Turn the AED on and follow the voice prompts. **Remain calm and collected during the next steps.**				
3. ✦ You will be prompted to attach the electrode pads to the patient's chest, on the sternum and at the apex of the heart, following the diagram for correct placement.				
4. ✦ Next, you will be directed to allow the machine to analyze the heart rhythm to determine if it is a shockable rhythm. CPR should cease while the machine is analyzing.				
5. ✦ The machine will begin a charging sequence prior to shocking and warn rescuers to stand back. The voice prompt will then tell you to press the "shock" button to administer the electrical current to the patient.				
6. ⋆ If the machine indicates "No shock is advised," assess the patient for breathing and circulation. Continue CPR as needed until advanced medical personnel arrive. **Always act within your scope of practice.**				

Name: _____

Date: _____

Document: Enter the correct information in the chart below.

Grading

Points Earned	_____		
Points Possible	_____	81	81
Percent Grade (Points Earned/Points Possible)	_____		
PASS:	_____	❏ YES ❏ NO ❏ N/A	❏ YES ❏ NO ❏ N/A

Instructor Sign-Off

Instructor: _____ **Date:** _____

Procedure 41-3:

Respond to an Adult with an Obstructed Airway

Objective: The student, using the supplies and equipment listed below, will demonstrate how to administer the Heimlich maneuver to an adult.

Supplies: Approved mannequin, gloves, ventilation mask with one-way valve for an unconscious victim

Affective Behaviors: Affective behaviors provide a professional approach to a skill that enhances the patient encounter. These behaviors may also display sensitivity to a patient's rights and enhance communication. Pay close attention to these skills, which will be in **_bold, italicized_** font.

Notes to the Student

_____

_____

_____

_____

_____

_____

Skills Assessment Requirements

Read and familiarize yourself with the procedure; complete the minimum practice requirements. Document each MPR using proper charting technique. Complete each procedure within a reasonable amount of time, with a minimum of 85 percent accuracy.

Name: _____

Date: _____

POINT VALUE ✦ = 3–6 points ⋆ = 7–9 points		PRACTICE TRIAL	GRADED TRIAL # 1	GRADED TRIAL # 2	NOTES
1. ⋆	Once it has been established that the victim is choking, with no air exchange, direct someone to call 911 and shout, "Are you choking?" or "Can you speak?" If the answer is no—as indicated by a head shake—**state your name and tell the victim you are going to begin emergency treatment.**				
2. ✦	Stand behind the victim with your feet slightly apart, placing one foot between the victim's feet and one to the outside. This stance will give you greater stability, and if the victim should pass out, you can safely guide them to the ground by sliding them down your thigh.				
3. ✦	Place the index finger of one hand at the person's navel or belt buckle. If the victim is a pregnant woman, place your finger above the enlarged uterus.				
4. ✦	Make a fist with your other hand and place it, thumb side to victim, above your other hand. If the person is very pregnant, the uterus is pushing the stomach and other internal organs under the rib cage and you may have to do chest compressions.				
5. ✦	Place your marking hand over your curled fist and begin to give quick inward and upward thrusts.				

Name: _____

Date: _____

		PRACTICE TRIAL	GRADED TRIAL # 1	GRADED TRIAL # 2	NOTES
6. ✦	There is no set number of thrusts to give to an adult who remains conscious. Continue to give thrusts until the object is removed or the victim becomes unconscious.				
7. ✦	If the victim becomes unconscious, gently lower them to the ground.				
8. ✦	Activate EMS and put on gloves.				
9. ★	Immediately begin CPR with 30 chest compressions and two rescue breaths.				
10. ★	Before administering rescue breaths, open the airway with the head-tilt chin lift and look for a foreign body in the victim's mouth and remove if visible. **Blind finger sweeps are no longer recommended and should not be performed.**				
11. ✦	Continue with cycles of 30 compressions and two rescue breaths until the foreign body is expelled or advance medical personnel arrive to relieve you.				

Name: _____

Date: _____

Document: Enter the correct information in the chart below.

Grading

Points Earned	_____		
Points Possible	_____	75	75
Percent Grade (Points Earned/Points Possible)	_____		
PASS:	_____	❏ YES ❏ NO ❏ N/A	❏ YES ❏ NO ❏ N/A

Instructor Sign-Off

Instructor: _____ **Date:** _____

Name: _____

Date: _____

Procedure 41-4:

Administer Oxygen

Objective: The student, using the supplies and equipment listed below, will demonstrate how to administer oxygen therapy to an adult.

Supplies: Portable oxygen tank, pressure regulator, oxygen flow meter, sterile, prepackaged, disposable nasal cannula with tubing, gloves, oximeter, patient chart

Affective Behaviors: Affective behaviors provide a professional approach to a skill that enhances the patient encounter. These behaviors may also display sensitivity to a patient's rights and enhance communication. Pay close attention to these skills, which will be in **_bold, italicized_** font.

Notes to the Student

_____

_____

_____

_____

_____

_____

Skills Assessment Requirements

Read and familiarize yourself with the procedure; complete the minimum practice requirements. Document each MPR using proper charting technique. Complete each procedure within a reasonable amount of time, with a minimum of 85 percent accuracy.

Name: _____

Date: _____

POINT VALUE ✦ = 3–6 points ⋆ = 7–9 points		PRACTICE TRIAL	GRADED TRIAL # 1	GRADED TRIAL # 2	NOTES
1. ✦	Gather all needed equipment.				
2. ✦	Wash your hands.				
3. ⋆	***Warmly greet and identify the patient, state your name and confirm the physician's order for oxygen therapy.***				
4. ✦	Check the pressure reading on the oxygen tank to make sure it has enough oxygen in it.				
5. ✦	Start the flow of oxygen by opening the cylinder.				
6. ✦	Attach the cannula tubing to the flow meter. Adjust the oxygen flow to the physician's order.				
7. ✦	Hold the cannula tips over the inside of your wrist, without touching the skin, to determine if the oxygen is flowing.				
8. ✦	Don gloves, if necessary. You may prefer to wear gloves with patients who demonstrate a chronic cough, nasal drip, or other situation of potential exposure.				
9. ✦	Place the tips of the nasal cannula into the patient's nostrils. Wrap the tubing behind the patient's ears.				
10. ✦	Instruct the patient to breathe normally through the mouth and nose. Some patients instinctively hold their breath or avoid breathing through the nose when an object is placed in the nostrils.				

Name: _____

Date: _____

		PRACTICE TRIAL	GRADED TRIAL # 1	GRADED TRIAL # 2	NOTES
11. ✦	Check the patient's oxygen level with an oximeter. Place the probe over the index finger and record the reading. If necessary, have the patient take a short walk to verify that the oxygen flow rate is sufficient for activity.				
12. ⋆	**Ask the patient if he or she has any questions, thank the patient and bid him or her a good day,** and document the procedure in the patient's chart.				

Document: Enter the correct information in the chart below.

Grading

Points Earned	_____		
Points Possible	_____	78	78
Percent Grade (Points Earned/Points Possible)	_____		
PASS:	_____	❏ YES ❏ NO ❏ N/A	❏ YES ❏ NO ❏ N/A

Instructor Sign-Off

Instructor: _____ Date: _____

Procedure 41-5:

Respond to a Patient Who Has Fainted

Objective: Care correctly for a patient who has fainted within the time limit set by the instructor.

Supplies: Blanket, footstool, or box

Affective Behaviors: Affective behaviors provide a professional approach to a skill that enhances the patient encounter. These behaviors may also display sensitivity to a patient's rights and enhance communication. Pay close attention to these skills, which will be in **_bold, italicized_** font.

Notes to the Student

_____
_____
_____
_____
_____
_____

Skills Assessment Requirements

Read and familiarize yourself with the procedure; complete the minimum practice requirements. Document each MPR using proper charting technique. Complete each procedure within a reasonable amount of time, with a minimum of 85 percent accuracy.

POINT VALUE ✦ = 3–6 points ⋆ = 7–9 points		PRACTICE TRIAL	GRADED TRIAL # 1	GRADED TRIAL # 2	NOTES
1. ✦	If the patient communicates a faint feeling, help the patient sit, bend forward, and place the head on the knees. If the patient collapses with no warning, do not move the patient. The patient may have sustained a neck or back injury.				
2. ✦	**Remain calm, notify the physician, and always act within your scope of practice.**				
3. ✦	Loosen any tight clothing, and cover the patient with a blanket for warmth.				
4. ✦	If the physician directs, use the footstool to support the patient's legs in a raised position.				
5. ✦	Check the patient's carotid artery. If the physician directs, call for emergency services.				
6. ⋆	Once the emergency passes, document all activities in the patient's medical record.				

Name: _____

Date: _____

Document: Enter the appropriate information in the chart below.

Grading

Points Earned	_____		
Points Possible	_____	39	39
Percent Grade (Points Earned/Points Possible)	_____		
PASS:	_____	❏ YES ❏ NO ❏ N/A	❏ YES ❏ NO ❏ N/A

Instructor Sign-Off

Instructor: _____   **Date:** _____

Procedure 41-6:

Demonstrate the Application of a Pressure Bandage

Objective: The student, using the supplies and equipment listed below, will demonstrate the application of a pressure dressing.

Supplies: Dressing supplies or makeshift materials, gloves and/or other PPE available

Affective Behaviors: Affective behaviors provide a professional approach to a skill that enhances the patient encounter. These behaviors may also display sensitivity to a patient's rights and enhance communication. Pay close attention to these skills, which will be in **_bold, italicized_** font.

Notes to the Student

_____

_____

_____

_____

_____

_____

Skills Assessment Requirements

Read and familiarize yourself with the procedure; complete the minimum practice requirements. Document each MPR using proper charting technique. Complete each procedure within a reasonable amount of time, with a minimum of 85 percent accuracy.

Name: _____

Date: _____

POINT VALUE ✦ = 3–6 points ⋆ = 7–9 points		PRACTICE TRIAL	GRADED TRIAL # 1	GRADED TRIAL # 2	NOTES
1. ✦	***Identify the patient and escort the patient immediately to an examination room. Introduce yourself and try to calm the patient.***				
2. ✦	Wash your hands. Put on disposable gloves.				
3. ⋆	***Under physician's supervision,*** apply direct pressure with a dressing placed on the open wound. If possible, elevate the affected part.				
4. ✦	After assessment, the physician will decide if EMS should be activated.				
5. ✦	Apply additional dressings as needed. Do not remove the original dressing.				
6. ⋆	Apply pressure to pressure points as necessary and ***with the physician's supervision.***				
7. ✦	If bleeding is controlled, anchor the dressing to maintain pressure.				
8. ✦	Prepare the patient for transport to an emergency care facility.				
9. ✦	Dispose of waste in a biohazard container.				
10. ✦	Remove your gloves and discard. Wash your hands.				
11. ⋆	Document the procedure. ***Sign the entry with your name and credentials.***				

Competency Check-Offs **1183**

Name: _____

Date: _____

Document: Enter the correct information in the chart below.

Grading

Points Earned	_____		
Points Possible	_____	75	75
Percent Grade (Points Earned/Points Possible)	_____		
PASS:	_____	❏ YES ❏ NO ❏ N/A	❏ YES ❏ NO ❏ N/A

Instructor Sign-Off

Instructor: _____ **Date:** _____

Procedure 41-7:

Demonstrate the Application of Triangular, Figure 8, and Tubular Bandages

Objective: The student, using the supplies and equipment listed below, will demonstrate how to apply triangular, figure 8, and tubular bandaging.

Supplies: Elastic bandage, roller bandage, Kling™ bandage, tubular gauze and applicator, triangular bandage, tape, scissors

Affective Behaviors: Affective behaviors provide a professional approach to a skill that enhances the patient encounter. These behaviors may also display sensitivity to a patient's rights and enhance communication. Pay close attention to these skills, which will be in **bold, *italicized*** font.

Notes to the Student

_____

_____

_____

_____

_____

_____

Skills Assessment Requirements

Read and familiarize yourself with the procedure; complete the minimum practice requirements. Document each MPR using proper charting technique. Complete each procedure within a reasonable amount of time, with a minimum of 85 percent accuracy.

POINT VALUE ✦ = 3–6 points ⋆ = 7–9 points		PRACTICE TRIAL	GRADED TRIAL # 1	GRADED TRIAL # 2	NOTES
1. ✦	**Escort the patient immediately to an examination room. Identify youself to the patient.** You may need to assist the patient, depending on the severity, location, and type of injury.				
2. ✦	**Explain the procedure to the patient.**				
3. ✦	Wash your hands.				
4. ✦	Gather necessary supplies.				
5. ⋆	**Triangular bandage:** • Keep the injured arm as immobile as possible. • Carefully slide the triangular bandage under the area to be held. The two shorter sides of the triangle should be pointing toward the elbow, and the remaining longer edge should be parallel to the opposite body side. • Bring the lowest side of the triangle up and over the arm. • Tie the ends of the bandage behind and slightly to the side of the neck. • Tuck the peak of the bandage in toward the elbow point of the bandage. • The triangular bandage may also be wrapped around the head as a turban to anchor dressings onto the head.				

		PRACTICE TRIAL	GRADED TRIAL # 1	GRADED TRIAL # 2	NOTES
6. ★	**Figure 8 bandage:** • Place the thumb of one hand on one end of the bandage to hold it in place. • Anchor the bandage with your other hand, then complete one circle around the extremity or body part. • Continue to alternate wrapping above and below the body joint or dressing and circling behind the joint or dressing area until the injured area is covered adequately.				
7. ★	**Tubular bandage:** • Choose an applicator that is larger than the extremity to be bandaged. • Cut an approximate amount of tubular gauze bandage and slide the gathered bandage onto the applicator. • Slide the applicator over the extremity. • Hold the bandage against the proximal end of the extremity and pull the applicator approximately 1 inch past the distal end. • Twist the bandage gauze one complete turn. • Next, slide the applicator toward the proximal end of the injury. • Hold the proximal end of the tubular bandage gauze in place, and pull the applicator toward the distal end. • After pulling past the distal end, complete one twist.				

		PRACTICE TRIAL	**GRADED TRIAL # 1**	**GRADED TRIAL # 2**	**NOTES**
	• Slide back and forth and twist the distal end of the dressing until the injured area is adequately covered. Cut excess dressing, but remember to anchor the bandage at the proximal end. • Instruct the patient to watch for signs of circulation impairment.				
8. ✦	Wash your hands.				
9. ⋆	Document the procedure and patient teaching. **Sign the entry with your name and credentials.**				

Name: _____

Date: _____

Document: Enter the correct information in the chart below.

Grading

Points Earned	_____		
Points Possible	_____	66	66
Percent Grade (Points Earned/Points Possible)	_____		
PASS:	_____	❏ YES ❏ NO ❏ N/A	❏ YES ❏ NO ❏ N/A

Instructor Sign-Off

Instructor: _____ Date: _____

Procedure 41-8:

Demonstrate the Application of a Splint

Objective: The student, using the supplies and equipment listed below, will demonstrate how to apply a splint.

Supplies: Makeshift or sterile dressing supplies, stiff or solid materials to immobilize the extremity, bandages or strips of material to secure splint materials

Affective Behaviors: Affective behaviors provide a professional approach to a skill that enhances the patient encounter. These behaviors may also display sensitivity to a patient's rights and enhance communication. Pay close attention to these skills, which will be in **_bold, italicized_** font.

Notes to the Student

_____

_____

_____

_____

_____

_____

Skills Assessment Requirements

Read and familiarize yourself with the procedure; complete the minimum practice requirements. Document each MPR using proper charting technique. Complete each procedure within a reasonable amount of time, with a minimum of 85 percent accuracy.

Name: _____

Date: _____

POINT VALUE ✦ = 3–6 points ⋆ = 7–9 points	PRACTICE TRIAL	GRADED TRIAL #1	GRADED TRIAL #2	NOTES
1. ✦ **Greet and identify yourself to the patient.**				
2. ✦ Obtain vital signs.				
3. ✦ **Ask the patient, if conscious, to speak his or her name.**				
4. ⋆ Ask about medical allergies and medications and whether or not the patient has a medical history.				
5. ✦ Assess the area of suspected fracture for bruising, bleeding, and open areas or protruding bones.				
6. ⋆ Moving the limb as little as possible and with gentle traction on the distal side, place the splint with padding under the limb or alongside the limb. You may have to ask other clinical staff for help to ensure the least amount of discomfort for the least amount of time.				
7. ✦ Place sterile dressings or clean makeshift dressings gently over open areas.				
8. ⋆ Secure the splint by wrapping bandages or strips of material around the splint and the limb. The ties must be above and below the joints on both sides of the suspected fracture.				
9. ✦ Add additional ties as necessary along the length of the splint.				
10. ✦ If possible, leave an exposed area, such as toes or fingers, so that circulation can be monitored.				

		PRACTICE TRIAL	GRADED TRIAL # 1	GRADED TRIAL # 2	NOTES
11. ★	The splint should be snug enough to immobilize the limb, but not tight.				
12. ★	**Document the procedure in the patient's chart. Sign the entry with your name and credentials.**				

Name: _____

Date: _____

Document: Enter the correct information in the chart below.

Grading

Points Earned	_____		
Points Possible	_____	78	78
Percent Grade (Points Earned/Points Possible)	_____		
PASS:	_____	❏ YES ❏ NO ❏ N/A	❏ YES ❏ NO ❏ N/A

Instructor Sign-Off

Instructor: _____ **Date:** _____

Name: _____

Date: _____

Procedure 42-1:

Assist with a Colon Endoscopic/Colonoscopy Exam

Objective: Correctly set up an exam room and assist the physician with a colon endoscopic procedure.

Supplies: Two pairs of nonsterile gloves, instrument for viewing depending on procedure being performed, water-soluble lubricant, patient drapes and gown, sterile cotton-tipped applicators for collection of fecal samples, suction device, sterile biopsy forceps, disposable or sterile rectal speculum, specimen containers with lab requisition form, as needed, disposable tissue, biohazard container, patient chart

Affective Behaviors: Affective behaviors provide a professional approach to a skill that enhances the patient encounter. These behaviors may also display sensitivity to a patient's rights and enhance communication. Pay close attention to these skills, which will be in ***bold, italicized*** font.

Notes to the Student

_____

_____

_____

_____

_____

_____

Skills Assessment Requirements

Read and familiarize yourself with the procedure; complete the minimum practice requirements. Document each MPR using proper charting technique. Complete each procedure within a reasonable amount of time, with a minimum of 85 percent accuracy.

POINT VALUE ✦ = 3–6 points ⋆ = 7–9 points	PRACTICE TRIAL	GRADED TRIAL # 1	GRADED TRIAL # 2	NOTES
1. ✦ Gather all needed supplies.				
2. ⋆ **Identify the patient and explain the procedure. Introduce yourself and verify that the patient has followed pre-exam instructions regarding medications, foods, and activities to avoid, such as enemas.** The patient should be asked to empty the bladder prior to the exam.				
3. ✦ Give the patient drapes and a gown and instructions on proper gown opening placement.				
4. ✦ Take the patient's vital signs.				
5. ✦ **Assist the patient to the table and position him or her for the exam. Consider the patient's feelings, as this examination may cause the patient to be nervous.**				
6. ✦ Wash your hands and put on gloves.				
7. ⋆ Assist the physician by handing him or her supplies as requested. To ease equipment entry into the anal canal, the physician will use an anal speculum. A suction device may be required to remove any fecal matter that obstructs the physician's view. If polyp tissue samples are needed, the physician will use sterile biopsy forceps.				
8. ✦ **To ease any discomfort, instruct the patient to breathe slowly and deeply. Observe the patient for any change in vitals, increased pain level, or other undue reactions.**				

		PRACTICE TRIAL	GRADED TRIAL # 1	GRADED TRIAL # 2	NOTES
9. ✦	After the physician has collected any necessary samples, you will place them in sterile specimen containers.				
10. ✦	When the physician has completed the examination, cleanse the patient's anal area with tissues.				
11. ✦	Remove the gloves, wash your hands, and assist the patient into a recovery position.				
12. ✦	While the patient is resting, recheck vital signs. Invasive procedures often cause a drop in blood pressure.				
13. ✦	Once the blood pressure is stable, allow the patient to get off the exam table and get dressed. **Ensure that the patient is comfortable and ask if he or she has any questions.**				
14. ⋆	Complete laboratory forms. Seal the specimen containers in an appropriate biohazard transport bag.				
15. ⋆	When the patient has been released from the room, wash your hands, put on new gloves, and disinfect the area. A disposable speculum should be discarded into a biohazard container; a stainless steel speculum should be prepared for autoclaving.				
16. ⋆	Document the procedure in the patient's chart. **Sign the entry with your name and credentials.**				

Name: _____

Date: _____

Document: Enter the appropriate information in the chart below.

Grading

Points Earned	_____		
Points Possible	_____	111	111
Percent Grade (Points Earned/Points Possible)	_____		
PASS:	_____	❑ YES ❑ NO ❑ N/A	❑ YES ❑ NO ❑ N/A

Instructor Sign-Off

Instructor: _____   **Date:** _____

Procedure 42-2:

Assist with a Sigmoidoscopy

Objective: The student, using the supplies and equipment listed below, will demonstrate how to set up an exam room and assist the physician with a sigmoidoscopy procedure.

Supplies: Sigmoidoscope, insufflator, water-soluble lubricant, patient drapes and gown, sterile cotton-tipped applicators, suction device, sterile biopsy forceps as directed by physician, disposable or sterile rectal speculum, specimen containers with lab requisition form, as needed, disposable tissue, chucks pads, water basin, 500 ml of warmed water, gloves, biohazard container, patient chart

Affective Behaviors: Affective behaviors provide a professional approach to a skill that enhances the patient encounter. These behaviors may also display sensitivity to a patient's rights and enhance communication. Pay close attention to these skills, which will be in **bold, *italicized*** font.

Notes to the Student

_____

_____

_____

_____

_____

_____

Skills Assessment Requirements

Read and familiarize yourself with the procedure; complete the minimum practice requirements. Document each MPR using proper charting technique. Complete each procedure within a reasonable amount of time, with a minimum of 85 percent accuracy.

Name: _____

Date: _____

POINT VALUE ✦ = 3–6 points ⋆ = 7–9 points		PRACTICE TRIAL	GRADED TRIAL # 1	GRADED TRIAL # 2	NOTES
1. ✦	Gather all needed supplies.				
2. ⋆	**Identify the patient and explain the procedure. Introduce yourself** and verify that the patient has followed pre-exam instructions regarding medications, foods, and activities and performed an enema. The patient should be asked to empty the bladder prior to the exam for greater comfort.				
3. ✦	**Give the patient drapes and a gown and instructions on proper gown opening placement.**				
4. ✦	Take the patient's vital signs.				
5. ✦	Assist the patient to the table and position for the exam. **Consider the patient's feelings, as this examination may cause the patient to be nervous.**				
6. ✦	Place a chucks pad, examination pad, or other absorbent material under the patient's perineal area.				
7. ✦	Wash your hands and put on gloves.				
8. ⋆	Assist the physician as needed.				
9. ⋆	Attach the light source and insufflator to the sigmoidoscope, but do not turn on the light until the physician is ready to use it. The light generates heat the longer it is on and can potentially burn the patient.				

		PRACTICE TRIAL	GRADED TRIAL # 1	GRADED TRIAL # 2	NOTES
10. ✦	**To ease the patient's discomfort, instruct him or her to breathe slowly and deeply. Observe the patient for any change in vitals, increased pain level, or other undue reactions.**				
11. ✦	When the physician has completed the examination, cleanse the patient's anal area with tissues.				
12. ✦	Remove the gloves, wash your hands, and assist the patient into a recovery position.				
13. ✦	While the patient is resting, recheck vital signs. Invasive procedures often cause a drop in blood pressure.				
14. ✦	Once the blood pressure is stable, allow the patient to get off the exam table and get dressed. **Ensure that the patient is comfortable and ask if he or she has any questions.**				
15. ✦	Complete the laboratory forms and send samples to be examined.				
16. ✦	When the patient has been released from the room, wash your hands, put on new gloves, and disinfect the area.				
17. ⋆	Document the procedure in the patient chart. **Sign the entry with your name and credentials.**				

Document: Enter the correct information in the chart below.

Grading

Points Earned	_____		
Points Possible	_____	114	114
Percent Grade (Points Earned/Points Possible)	_____		
PASS:	_____	❏ YES ❏ NO ❏ N/A	❏ YES ❏ NO ❏ N/A

Instructor Sign-Off

Instructor: _____   **Date:** _____

Procedure 42-3:

Inserting a Rectal Suppository

Objective: The student, using the supplies and equipment listed below, will demonstrate how to administer a rectal suppository.

Supplies: Physician-prescribed rectal suppository, water-soluble lubricant, tissues, biohazard container, disposable gloves, patient instructions, patient chart

Affective Behaviors: Affective behaviors provide a professional approach to a skill that enhances the patient encounter. These behaviors may also display sensitivity to a patient's rights and enhance communication. Pay close attention to these skills, which will be in **_bold, italicized_** font.

Notes to the Student

_____

_____

_____

_____

_____

_____

Skills Assessment Requirements

Read and familiarize yourself with the procedure; complete the minimum practice requirements. Document each MPR using proper charting technique. Complete each procedure within a reasonable amount of time, with a minimum of 85 percent accuracy.

POINT VALUE ✦ = 3–6 points ⋆ = 7–9 points		PRACTICE TRIAL	GRADED TRIAL # 1	GRADED TRIAL # 2	NOTES
1. ✦	**Greet and identify the patient, introduce yourself and escort the patient to the examination room.** Check for any allergies.				
2. ⋆	Verify the physician's medication order.				
3. ✦	Collect all necessary supplies.				
4. ✦	**Explain the procedure to the patient.**				
5. ✦	Wash your hands and put on gloves.				
6. ✦	Ask the patient to remove all clothing from the waist area down.				
7. ✦	Assist the patient into a Sims position and provide proper drapes. **This will make the patient feel more comfortable.**				
8. ✦	Take the protective foil wrap from the suppository and carefully smooth any rough or jagged edges. Lubricate the suppository with the water-soluble lubricant.				
9. ✦	Expose the patient's buttocks.				
10. ⋆	Holding the suppository in one hand, lift the upper buttock with your other hand, exposing the anus.				
11. ⋆	Firmly guide the suppository into the anus with your index finger, past any fecal masses and the internal sphincter. This will prevent it from being expelled.				

		PRACTICE TRIAL	GRADED TRIAL # 1	GRADED TRIAL # 2	NOTES
12. ✦	With a tissue, apply firm pressure on the anus for 1–2 minutes to allow the medication to be retained. Discard the tissue into the biohazard container.				
13. ✦	With another tissue, wipe away any excess lubricant or fecal matter from the anus and discard the tissue into the biohazard container.				
14. ✦	Instruct the patient to get into a comfortable position and rest for 30 minutes as the medication is absorbed.				
15. ✦	**Clean the area, providing a new drape if necessary,** and dispose of all materials in the biohazard container.				
16. ✦	Remove the gloves and wash your hands. **Ensure that the patient does not have any questions prior to leaving the examination room.**				
17. ✶	Document the procedure in the patient chart. **Sign the entry with your name and credentials.**				

Name: _____

Date: _____

Document: Enter the correct information in the chart below.

Grading

Points Earned	_____		
Points Possible	_____	114	114
Percent Grade (Points Earned/Points Possible)	_____		
PASS:	_____	❏ YES ❏ NO ❏ N/A	❏ YES ❏ NO ❏ N/A

Instructor Sign-Off

Instructor: _____   **Date:** _____

Name: _____

Date: _____

Procedure 43-1:

Assist with Fiberglass Cast Application

Objective: The student, using the supplies and equipment listed below, will demonstrate how to assist with the application of a fiberglass cast.

Supplies: Rolls of fiberglass casting material, stockinette, padding, tape, blunt/sharp nose scissors (for cutting material), warm tap water, basin (2–4 liter), bandage, gloves, stool or low chair for support (if casting a foot or lower leg), patient drapes

Affective Behaviors: Affective behaviors provide a professional approach to a skill that enhances the patient encounter. These behaviors may also display sensitivity to a patient's rights and enhance communication. Pay close attention to these skills, which will be in **_bold, italicized_** font.

Notes to the Student

_____

_____

_____

_____

_____

_____

Skills Assessment Requirements

Read and familiarize yourself with the procedure; complete the minimum practice requirements. Document each MPR using proper charting technique. Complete each procedure within a reasonable amount of time, with a minimum of 85 percent accuracy.

Name: _____

Date: _____

		PRACTICE TRIAL	GRADED TRIAL # 1	GRADED TRIAL # 2	NOTES
1. ✦	Assist the patient to the exam room and into a comfortable position. **Explain that the patient should be comfortable to avoid having to shift the body weight during the lengthy casting process.**				
2. ★	**Identify the patient and verify the physician's orders. Introduce yourself to the patient.**				
3. ✦	**Explain the procedure.**				
4. ✦	Wash your hands and put on gloves.				
5. ★	Cleanse and inspect the area to which the cast will be applied. Note any open wounds, bruising, or excessive swelling and report these to the physician.				
6. ✦	**Drape the patient to protect clothing.**				
7. ✦	Open one package of fiberglass material. Do not open the other packages until they are needed, to prevent waste.				
8. ✦	Hand the physician the materials requested. If your clinic allows medical assistants to perform casting, cut the stockinette to fit the area.				
9. ★	Cover the affected body part with the stockinette, making sure it is smooth against the patient's skin and extends 1–2 inches beyond where the cast will end. If the stockinette is allowed to wrinkle or become bulky, it may cause a pressure sore on the patient's skin.				

Name: _____

Date: _____

		PRACTICE TRIAL	GRADED TRIAL # 1	GRADED TRIAL # 2	NOTES
10. ✦	If you are casting the ankle, cut away excess wrinkled stockinette from the bend in the front of the ankle.				
11. *	Use a spiral bandage turn to cover the casting area with padding. Apply extra padding to any bony areas.				
12. ✦	Soak the inner layer of fiberglass tape in the basin of warm water. The tape material will be activated on contact with the water, so only wet as much as you need at a time.				
13. ✦	The physician will roll and form the cast to the patient.				
14. ✦	Roll the excess stockinette over the edges of the casting material to form a smooth edge.				
15. ✦	Open the package of outer fiberglass tape for the physician.				
16. ✦	The physician will shape and smooth the cast or may direct you to do so.				
17. ✦	Clean up the work station. Remove the gloves and wash your hands. Ensure the patient does not have any questions prior to leaving the examination room.				
18. *	Document the procedure in the patient chart. **Sign the entry with your name and credentials.**				

Document: Enter the correct information in the chart below.

Grading

Points Earned	_____		
Points Possible	_____	123	123
Percent Grade (Points Earned/Points Possible)	_____		
PASS:	_____	❏ YES ❏ NO ❏ N/A	❏ YES ❏ NO ❏ N/A

Instructor Sign-Off

Instructor: _____ **Date:** _____

Procedure 43-2:

Assist with Cast Removal

Objective: The student, using the supplies and equipment listed below, will demonstrate how to assist in the removal of a cast.

Supplies: Cast-cutting device, cast spreader, bandage scissors, heavy-duty bag in which to discard cast materials, patient drape, 500 ml basin, 500 ml of warm water, hypoallergenic soap, towel, hypoallergenic lotion

Affective Behaviors: Affective behaviors provide a professional approach to a skill that enhances the patient encounter. These behaviors may also display sensitivity to a patient's rights and enhance communication. Pay close attention to these skills, which will be in **bold, italicized** font.

Notes to the Student

_____

_____

_____

_____

_____

_____

Skills Assessment Requirements

Read and familiarize yourself with the procedure; complete the minimum practice requirements. Document each MPR using proper charting technique. Complete each procedure within a reasonable amount of time, with a minimum of 85 percent accuracy.

POINT VALUE ✦ = 3–6 points ⋆ = 7–9 points	PRACTICE TRIAL	GRADED TRIAL # 1	GRADED TRIAL # 2	NOTES
1. ✦ Gather equipment and supplies.				
2. ⋆ **Greet and identify the patient. Introduce yourself and explain the procedure.**				
3. ⋆ Making certain that the limb is properly supported, make two cuts along the medial and lateral side of the long axis of the cast.				
4. ✦ Pry the cast apart with a cast spreader.				
5. ✦ Carefully remove the two halves of the cast.				
6. ✦ Cut away the stockinette and padding with the large bandage scissors.				
7. ✦ Wash the previously casted area with hypoallergenic soap.				
8. ✦ Dry the skin and apply a gentle skin lotion.				
9. ⋆ Provide the patient with written and verbal instructions for care of the limb. **Prior to leaving the examination room, ask the patient if he or she has any questions.**				
10. ⋆ Document the procedure in the patient chart. **Sign the entry with your name and credentials.**				

Name: _____

Date: _____

Document: Enter the correct information in the chart below.

Grading

Points Earned	_____		
Points Possible	_____	72	72
Percent Grade (Points Earned/Points Possible)	_____		
PASS:	_____	❏ YES ❏ NO ❏ N/A	❏ YES ❏ NO ❏ N/A

Instructor Sign-Off

Instructor: _____ Date: _____

Name: _____

Date: _____

Procedure 43-3:

Assist the Patient with Cold Application/Cold Compress

Objective: The student, using the supplies and equipment listed below, will demonstrate how to apply a cold compress.

Supplies: Water, 4 × 4 gauze pads or other absorbent material or water, 4 × 4 gauze pads or other absorbent material or washcloths, waterproof pad, waterproof wrap (plastic bag or plastic wrap), basin, ice cubes

Affective Behaviors: Affective behaviors provide a professional approach to a skill that enhances the patient encounter. These behaviors may also display sensitivity to a patient's rights and enhance communication. Pay close attention to these skills, which will be in **bold, italicized** font.

Notes to the Student

_____

_____

_____

_____

_____

_____

Skills Assessment Requirements

Read and familiarize yourself with the procedure; complete the minimum practice requirements. Document each MPR using proper charting technique. Complete each procedure within a reasonable amount of time, with a minimum of 85 percent accuracy.

Name: _____

Date: _____

POINT VALUE ✦ = 3–6 points ⋆ = 7–9 points		PRACTICE TRIAL	GRADED TRIAL # 1	GRADED TRIAL # 2	NOTES
1. ✦	Wash your hands.				
2. ⋆	**Identify the patient and verify the physician's order. Introduce yourself to the patient.**				
3. ✦	**Explain the procedure to the patient.**				
4. ✦	Fill the basin with ice and water and soak the gauze pads or washcloths.				
5. ✦	Wring out the compress so it is damp, but not dripping.				
6. ✦	Place the compress on the patient's injured body part and wrap it with plastic wrap to protect the patient's clothing.				
7. ⋆	Check the compress every 3–5 minutes, replacing it with a colder compress as needed. Remove water as necessary from the basin and add more ice to keep the water cold.				

		PRACTICE TRIAL	GRADED TRIAL # 1	GRADED TRIAL # 2	NOTES
8. ✦	After applying compresses for the time specified by the physician, remove them and dry the affected area. Call the physician if you notice increased swelling and red-ness, or if the pain intensifies. ***Ensure patient comfort and answer questions as necessary.***				
9. ✦	Launder the linens or place them in the appropriate laundry hamper, according to office protocol, and clean the room.				
10. *	Wash your hands and docu-ment the procedure. ***Sign the entry with your name and credentials.***				

Name: _____

Date: _____

Document: Enter the correct information in the chart below.

Grading

Points Earned	_____		
Points Possible	_____	69	69
Percent Grade (Points Earned/Points Possible)	_____		
PASS:	_____	❏ YES ❏ NO ❏ N/A	❏ YES ❏ NO ❏ N/A

Instructor Sign-Off

Instructor: _____ Date: _____

Procedure 43-4:

Assist the Patient with Hot Moist Application/Hot Compress

Objective: The student, using the supplies and equipment listed below, will demonstrate how to apply a cold compress.

Supplies: Water, digital or disposable strip thermometer, 4 × 4 gauze pads or other absorbent material or washcloths, waterproof pad, waterproof wrap (plastic bag or plastic wrap can be used), basin

Affective Behaviors: Affective behaviors provide a professional approach to a skill that enhances the patient encounter. These behaviors may also display sensitivity to a patient's rights and enhance communication. Pay close attention to these skills, which will be in **bold, italicized** font.

Notes to the Student

_____

_____

_____

_____

_____

_____

Skills Assessment Requirements

Read and familiarize yourself with the procedure; complete the minimum practice requirements. Document each MPR using proper charting technique. Complete each procedure within a reasonable amount of time, with a minimum of 85 percent accuracy.

Name: _____

Date: _____

POINT VALUE ✦ = 3–6 points ⋆ = 7–9 points		PRACTICE TRIAL	GRADED TRIAL # 1	GRADED TRIAL # 2	NOTES
1. ✦	Wash your hands.				
2. ⋆	**Identify the patient and verify the physician's order. Introduce yourself to the patient.**				
3. ✦	**Explain the procedure to the patient.**				
4. ✦	Fill the basin with water heated to 105–110° F, as verified with the thermometer, and soak the gauze pads.				
5. ✦	Wring out the compress so it is damp, but not dripping.				
6. ✦	Place the waterproof pad under the injured body part. Apply the compress to the patient's injured body part and wrap with plastic wrap to protect clothing. **Ask the patient to confirm that the temperature is comfortable, but not burning.**				
7. ⋆	Check the compress every 3–5 minutes, replacing it with a warmer compress as needed. Call the physician if you notice increased swelling and redness, or if pain increases.				

		PRACTICE TRIAL	GRADED TRIAL # 1	GRADED TRIAL # 2	NOTES
8. ✦	After applying the compress for the time specified by the physician, remove it and dry the affected area.				
9. ✦	Launder the linens or place them in the appropriate laundry hamper, according to office protocol, and clean the room.				
10. *	Wash your hands and document the procedure. **Sign the entry with your name and credentials.**				

Name: _____

Date: _____

Document: Enter the correct information in the chart below.

Grading

Points Earned	_____		
Points Possible	_____	69	69
Percent Grade (Points Earned/Points Possible)	_____		
PASS:	_____	❏ YES ❏ NO ❏ N/A	❏ YES ❏ NO ❏ N/A

Instructor Sign-Off

Instructor: _____ Date: _____

Procedure 43-5:

Assisting with Therapeutic Ultrasonography

Objective: The student, using the supplies and equipment listed below, will demonstrate how to assist with therapeutic ultrasonography.

Supplies: Ultrasound gel (coupling agent), ultrasound machine, tissue, patient chart

Affective Behaviors: Affective behaviors provide a professional approach to a skill that enhances the patient encounter. These behaviors may also display sensitivity to a patient's rights and enhance communication. Pay close attention to these skills, which will be in **_bold, italicized_** font.

Notes to the Student

_____

_____

_____

_____

_____

_____

Skills Assessment Requirements

Read and familiarize yourself with the procedure; complete the minimum practice requirements. Document each MPR using proper charting technique. Complete each procedure within a reasonable amount of time, with a minimum of 85 percent accuracy.

Name: _____

Date: _____

POINT VALUE ✦ = 3–6 points ★ = 7–9 points		PRACTICE TRIAL	GRADED TRIAL # 1	GRADED TRIAL # 2	NOTES
1. ★	Prepare the equipment and *identify the patient. Introduce yourself to the patient.*				
2. ★	Verify the physician's orders for duration and frequency of treatment.				
3. ✦	*Explain the procedure and encourage the patient to inform you of any pain or discomfort.*				
4. ✦	Have the patient remove clothing from the area to be treated.				
5. ✦	Apply warmed ultrasonic gel to the area to be treated and to the applicator head.				
6. ✦	Set the machine at the lowest treatment setting and increase gradually as needed. Set the timer to the specified treatment time.				
7. ★	Place the applicator head firmly against the patient's skin and move the applicator in a circular motion at a speed of 2 inches per second. Keep the applicator head in contact with the patient's skin and moving at all times when the machine is running.				
8. ✦	When the set time has expired, the machine will shut off automatically.				

		PRACTICE TRIAL	GRADED TRIAL # 1	GRADED TRIAL # 2	NOTES
9. ✦	Return the intensity control back to zero.				
10. ✦	Wipe the ultrasonic gel from the patient's skin and **assist with dressing if necessary. Ask the patient if he or she has any questions.**				
11. *	Wash your hands and document the procedure in the patient's chart. **Sign the entry with your name and credentials.**				

Name: _____

Date: _____

Document: Enter the correct information in the chart below.

Grading

Points Earned	_____		
Points Possible	_____	78	78
Percent Grade (Points Earned/Points Possible)	_____		
PASS:	_____	❏ YES ❏ NO ❏ N/A	❏ YES ❏ NO ❏ N/A

Instructor Sign-Off

Instructor: _____ Date: _____

Procedure 43-6:

Demonstrate Measuring for Axillary Crutches

Objective: The student, using the supplies and equipment listed below, will demonstrate how to measure for axillary crutches.

Supplies: Patient chart, order for axillary crutches, adjustable axillary crutches

Affective Behaviors: Affective behaviors provide a professional approach to a skill that enhances the patient encounter. These behaviors may also display sensitivity to a patient's rights and enhance communication. Pay close attention to these skills, which will be in **_bold, italicized_** font.

Notes to the Student

_____

_____

_____

_____

_____

_____

Skills Assessment Requirements

Read and familiarize yourself with the procedure; complete the minimum practice requirements. Document each MPR using proper charting technique. Complete each procedure within a reasonable amount of time, with a minimum of 85 percent accuracy.

Name: _____

Date: _____

POINT VALUE ✦ = 3–6 points ∗ = 7–9 points		PRACTICE TRIAL	GRADED TRIAL #1	GRADED TRIAL #2	NOTES
1. ✦	Wash your hands and gather the necessary materials.				
2. ∗	Greet and identify the patient, introduce yourself and escort the patient to the treatment area.				
3. ∗	**Assist the patient,** with shoes on, to a standing position. With the crutch armrests under the patient's axillae, adjust the crutches first for height and then for hand position, using the following criteria: (a) A space of two finger widths between the axilla and the crutch armrest (b) Body weight supported by the hands on the hand grips (c) Crutch tip placement approximately 2 inches in front of the foot and 4 to 6 inches from the lateral aspect				
4. ✦	After the crutches have been correctly measured and fitted to the patient, **provide verbal and written instruction about general guidelines, crutch gait, and symptoms of improper fit. Ask the patient if he or she has any questions prior to leaving the examination room.**				
5. ✦	Document the procedure and prepare the treatment area for the next patient. **Sign the entry with your name and credentials.**				

Document: Enter the correct information in the chart below.

Grading

Points Earned	_____		
Points Possible	_____	36	36
Percent Grade (Points Earned/Points Possible)	_____		
PASS:	_____	❏ YES ❏ NO ❏ N/A	❏ YES ❏ NO ❏ N/A

Instructor Sign-Off

Instructor: _____ **Date:** _____

Procedure 43-7:

Assist a Patient with Crutch Walking

Objective: The student, using the supplies and equipment listed below, will demonstrate how to assist a patient with crutch walking.

Supplies: Crutches correctly fitted to the patient

Affective Behaviors: Affective behaviors provide a professional approach to a skill that enhances the patient encounter. These behaviors may also display sensitivity to a patient's rights and enhance communication. Pay close attention to these skills, which will be in **_bold, italicized_** font.

Notes to the Student

_____

_____

_____

_____

_____

_____

Skills Assessment Requirements

Read and familiarize yourself with the procedure; complete the minimum practice requirements. Document each MPR using proper charting technique. Complete each procedure within a reasonable amount of time, with a minimum of 85 percent accuracy.

Name: _____

Date: _____

POINT VALUE ✦ = 3–6 points ⋆ = 7–9 points		PRACTICE TRIAL	GRADED TRIAL #1	GRADED TRIAL #2	NOTES
1. ✦	Wash your hands and gather the necessary materials.				
2. ⋆	**Greet the patient, identify yourself and escort the patient to the treatment area.**				
3. ✦	Inspect the crutches for correctly fitted arm pads, tight wingnuts, and comfortable handgrips.				
4. ✦	Instruct the patient to relax the injured knee and keep it slightly bent to avoid touching the foot to the ground.				
5. ✦	Instruct the patient in the crutch-walking gait ordered by the physician.				
6. ⋆	**Have the patient practice taking several steps to ensure correct technique. Ask the patient if he or she has any questions prior to leaving the examination room.**				
7. ⋆	Document patient education in the patient's chart. **Sign the entry with your name and credentials.**				

Document: Enter the correct information in the chart below.

Grading

Points Earned	_____		
Points Possible	_____	51	51
Percent Grade (Points Earned/Points Possible)	_____		
PASS:	_____	❏ YES ❏ NO ❏ N/A	❏ YES ❏ NO ❏ N/A

Instructor Sign-Off

Instructor: _____ **Date:** _____

Procedure 43-8:

Assist a Patient Using a Cane

Objective: The student, using the supplies and equipment listed below, will demonstrate how to instruct a patient on correct cane use.

Supplies: Single-tipped cane as ordered by physician, gait belt

Affective Behaviors: Affective behaviors provide a professional approach to a skill that enhances the patient encounter. These behaviors may also display sensitivity to a patient's rights and enhance communication. Pay close attention to these skills, which will be in ***bold, italicized*** font.

Notes to the Student

_____

_____

_____

_____

_____

_____

Skills Assessment Requirements

Read and familiarize yourself with the procedure; complete the minimum practice requirements. Document each MPR using proper charting technique. Complete each procedure within a reasonable amount of time, with a minimum of 85 percent accuracy.

Name: _____

Date: _____

POINT VALUE ✦ = 3–6 points ∗ = 7–9 points		PRACTICE TRIAL	GRADED TRIAL # 1	GRADED TRIAL # 2	NOTES
1. ∗	**Greet and identify the patient, introduce yourself to the patient and explain why instruction in cane use is necessary.**				
2. ✦	Wash your hands.				
3. ✦	Verify the type of cane the patient and physician have agreed on and assemble equipment.				
4. ✦	**For patient safety: Make sure the suction tip on the cane is in good condition.**				
5. ✦	Place the gait belt snugly around the patient's waist, tucking any excess length into the belt.				
6. ∗	Place the cane tip 4–6 inches to the side of the patient's foot, on the patient's stronger, unaffected side. Adjust the cane so that the handle grip is level with the patient's hip and the patient's elbow is flexed at a 20- to 30-degree angle.				
7. ✦	Stand on the patient's weaker side with a firm underhand grip on the gait belt.				
8. ✦	Instruct the patient to move the injured leg and cane forward simultaneously.				
9. ✦	The patient should then advance the stronger leg and rest it slightly in front of the injured leg. Repeat this process.				

1232 APPENDIX

		PRACTICE TRIAL	GRADED TRIAL # 1	GRADED TRIAL # 2	NOTES
10. ✦	*Going up stairs:* Instruct the patient to use hand rails whenever possible.				
11. ✦	The patient moves the stronger leg forward to the next step while the injured leg and cane rest on the lower step.				
12. ✦	With a firm grip on the cane and the handrail, the patient moves the injured leg up to the same step as the uninjured leg. Repeat as needed.				
13. ✦	*Going down stairs:* The patient steps down with the uninjured leg and the cane. The injured leg follows to the same step. **Ask the patient if he or she has any questions prior to leaving the examination room.**				
14. ★	Document patient education in the patient's chart. **Sign the entry with your name and credentials.**				

Name: _____

Date: _____

Document: Enter the correct information in the chart below.

Grading

Points Earned	_____		
Points Possible	_____	93	93
Percent Grade (Points Earned/Points Possible)	_____		
PASS:	_____	❏ YES ❏ NO ❏ N/A	❏ YES ❏ NO ❏ N/A

Instructor Sign-Off

Instructor: _____ Date: _____

Procedure 43-9:

Assist a Patient Using a Walker

Objective: The student, using the supplies and equipment listed below, will demonstrate how to teach a patient how to use a walker.

Supplies: Walker, gait belt

Affective Behaviors: Affective behaviors provide a professional approach to a skill that enhances the patient encounter. These behaviors may also display sensitivity to a patient's rights and enhance communication. Pay close attention to these skills, which will be in **_bold, italicized_** font.

Notes to the Student

_____

_____

_____

_____

_____

_____

Skills Assessment Requirements

Read and familiarize yourself with the procedure; complete the minimum practice requirements. Document each MPR using proper charting technique. Complete each procedure within a reasonable amount of time, with a minimum of 85 percent accuracy.

Name: _____

Date: _____

POINT VALUE ✦ = 3–6 points ⋆ = 7–9 points		PRACTICE TRIAL	GRADED TRIAL #1	GRADED TRIAL #2	NOTES
1. ⋆	**Greet and identify the patient. Introduce yourself and explain why instruction in walker use is necessary.**				
2. ✦	Wash your hands.				
3. ✦	Place a gait belt snugly around the patient's waist. Tuck any excess belt length under the belt near the hip.				
4. ✦	Position the patient inside the walker. Adjust the height of the walker as needed. The patient's arms should be flexed at a 30-degree angle when resting on the hand grips.				
5. ✦	Stand behind and slightly to the side of the patient, with an under-hand grip on the gait belt. **Remain aware of the patient's likelihood of falling.**				
6. ✦	Instruct the patient to move the walker directly ahead until the back supports of the walker are even with the patient's toes.				
7. ✦	Instruct the patient to grip the handles firmly and step toward the walker with the stronger leg first, then the other leg.				
8. ✦	Repeat: The patient moves the walker first, then moves toward the walker.				
9. ✦	**Watch the patient for signs of fatigue.** Some walkers are equipped with platforms on which the patient can sit to rest. **Ask the patient if he or she has any questions prior to leaving the examination room.**				
10. ⋆	Document patient education in patient's chart. **Sign the entry with your name and credentials.**				

Name: _____

Date: _____

Document: Enter the correct information in the chart below.

Grading

Points Earned	_____		
Points Possible	_____	66	66
Percent Grade (Points Earned/Points Possible)	_____		
PASS:	_____	❏ YES ❏ NO ❏ N/A	❏ YES ❏ NO ❏ N/A

Instructor Sign-Off

Instructor: _____ Date: _____

Procedure 43-10:

Assist a Patient in a Wheelchair to and from an Exam Table

Objective: The student, using the supplies and equipment listed below, will demonstrate how to transfer a patient from a wheelchair to an examination table and from an examination table to a wheelchair.

Supplies: Gait belt, long-handled stool (if exam table is not equipped with pull-out step)

Affective Behaviors: Affective behaviors provide a professional approach to a skill that enhances the patient encounter. These behaviors may also display sensitivity to a patient's rights and enhance communication. Pay close attention to these skills, which will be in **bold, *italicized*** font.

Notes to the Student

_____

_____

_____

_____

_____

_____

Skills Assessment Requirements

Read and familiarize yourself with the procedure; complete the minimum practice requirements. Document each MPR using proper charting technique. Complete each procedure within a reasonable amount of time, with a minimum of 85 percent accuracy.

Name: _____

Date: _____

POINT VALUE ✦ = 3–6 points ⋆ = 7–9 points		PRACTICE TRIAL	GRADED TRIAL # 1	GRADED TRIAL # 2	NOTES
1. ⋆	**Greet and identify the patient, introduce yourself and explain what you are going to do.**				
2. ✦	Wash your hands.				
3. ✦	Position the wheelchair so that the patient is sitting with his or her strongest side next to the examination table.				
4. ⋆	Lock the wheelchair brakes.				
5. ✦	Place the gait belt snugly around the patient's waist, making certain the belt is tight enough that it will not slip and put unnecessary pressure on the ribs. Tuck any excess belt length under the belt.				
6. ✦	If the wheelchair allows, remove the foot rests. If not, move them as far out as possible to avoid hitting your shins against them during the transfer. **Ensure that the patient is ready prior to beginning the transfer.**				
7. ⋆	Standing directly in front of and as close to the patient as possible, grip the gait belt with both hands in an underhand grip. Bend at the knees and hips to avoid back strain.				
8. ✦	If the patient is able, have him or her grip the arm rests and push off at the same time that you lift, for added leverage. If possible, the patient can also assist by pushing upward with his or her legs. **Instill confidence by encouraging the patient.**				

Name: _____

Date: _____

		PRACTICE TRIAL	GRADED TRIAL # 1	GRADED TRIAL # 2	NOTES
9. ★	With the patient now standing, have him or her place the stronger leg on the stool or exam table step, and together you will lift as the patient steps up.				
10. ✦	Have the patient place one hand on the table and guide him or her to a sitting position.				
11. ✦	Move the wheelchair out of the way.				
12. ★	*To transfer the patient back to the wheelchair:* After identifying the patient, explaining the procedure, and washing your hands, place the stool (if the exam table does not have a step) next to the exam table.				
13. ✦	Place the wheelchair next to the exam table with the brakes locked.				
14. ★	With a firm underhand grip on the gait belt, assist the patient to a standing position. If the patient is able, have him or her push off with the legs and arms. Once the patient is steady on the step or stool, have him or her step to the floor with the stronger leg.				
15. ✦	Have the patient take small steps backward until the backs of the knees touch the wheelchair.				

		PRACTICE TRIAL	GRADED TRIAL # 1	GRADED TRIAL # 2	NOTES
16. ✦	Ask the patient to reach back and place the hands on the wheelchair armrests for support. Bending at the hips and knees, slowly lower the patient to the chair.				
17. ✦	Help the patient adjust to a comfortable position in the wheelchair. **Ask the patient if he or she has any questions prior to leaving the examination room.**				
18. ✦	Replace the foot rests.				

Name: _____

Date: _____

Document: Enter the correct information in the chart below.

Grading

Points Earned	_____		
Points Possible	_____	126	126
Percent Grade (Points Earned/Points Possible)	_____		
PASS:	_____	❑ YES ❑ NO ❑ N/A	❑ YES ❑ NO ❑ N/A

Instructor Sign-Off

Instructor: _____ **Date:** _____

Procedure 44-1:

Assist with a Prenatal Exam

Objective: The student, using the supplies and equipment listed below, will demonstrate how to assist with a prenatal exam.

Supplies: EDD calculator, full pap and pelvic exam setup, gloves, patient's chart

Affective Behaviors: Affective behaviors provide a professional approach to a skill that enhances the patient encounter. These behaviors may also display sensitivity to a patient's rights and enhance communication. Pay close attention to these skills, which will be in **bold, italicized** font.

Notes to the Student

_____

_____

_____

_____

_____

_____

Skills Assessment Requirements

Read and familiarize yourself with the procedure; complete the minimum practice requirements. Document each MPR using proper charting technique. Complete each procedure within a reasonable amount of time, with a minimum of 85 percent accuracy.

POINT VALUE ✦ = 3–6 points ⋆ = 7–9 points		PRACTICE TRIAL	GRADED TRIAL # 1	GRADED TRIAL # 2	NOTES
1. ⋆	**Greet the patient and introduce yourself. Verify the patient's identification.**				
2. ✦	**Explain the tests that will be done as a baseline to compare to in the later stages of pregnancy.**				
3. ✦	Measure the patient's height and weight. **Relay this information privately to the patient. Return the scale bars to zero.**				
4. ⋆	Depending on your office requirements, you may be asked to take a complete physical history of the patient. Obtain her menstrual history (age of onset, duration, flow rate, and intervals) and pregnancy history (number of pregnancies, number of live births, number of miscarriages, number of abortions).				
5. ✦	Obtain a urine sample to run a UA.				
6. ✦	Assist the physician with the Pap and pelvic examination as required by office protocol.				
7. ⋆	Document required information in the patient's chart. **Sign the entry with your name and credentials.**				

Document: Enter the correct information in the chart below.

Grading

Points Earned	_____		
Points Possible	_____	51	51
Percent Grade (Points Earned/Points Possible)	_____		
PASS:	_____	❏ YES ❏ NO ❏ N/A	❏ YES ❏ NO ❏ N/A

Instructor Sign-Off

Instructor: _____ **Date:** _____

Procedure 44-2:

Instruct the Patient in Breast Self-Examination

Objective: The student, using the supplies and equipment listed below, will demonstrate how to instruct the patient in the performance of breast self-examination.

Supplies: Patient chart, educational materials such as patient brochures or breast models

Affective Behaviors: Affective behaviors provide a professional approach to a skill that enhances the patient encounter. These behaviors may also display sensitivity to a patient's rights and enhance communication. Pay close attention to these skills, which will be in **_bold, italicized_** font.

Notes to the Student

_____

_____

_____

_____

_____

_____

Skills Assessment Requirements

Read and familiarize yourself with the procedure; complete the minimum practice requirements. Document each MPR using proper charting technique. Complete each procedure within a reasonable amount of time, with a minimum of 85 percent accuracy.

POINT VALUE ✦ = 3–6 points ★ = 7–9 points		PRACTICE TRIAL	GRADED TRIAL # 1	GRADED TRIAL # 2	NOTES
1. ✦	Wash your hands and gather the necessary supplies.				
2. ✦	Escort the patient to the patient education area. **Introduce yourself to the patient if you haven't already done so.**				
3. ★	Emphasize the following habits for the monthly self-exam: a. Premenopausal women should perform the examination about one week after the menstrual period, when the breasts are not swollen. Postmenopausal women should select a specific date of the month. b. Perform a visual inspection while standing in front of a mirror. With the arms hanging at the sides, above the head, or forward, away from the body, or with the hands positioned on the hips, observe for bilateral similarities or differences, for color or texture changes in the skin and nipples, and for nipple discharge. c. Examine each breast in side-lying and flat positions, starting with the same breast each time. For the flat position, place a pillow under the shoulder on each side. d. Palpate each breast with the fingertip pads of the opposite hand, using a dime-sized, circular motion. Use the same search pattern of vertical strip, wedge, or circle search for both breasts.				

		PRACTICE TRIAL	GRADED TRIAL # 1	GRADED TRIAL # 2	NOTES
	e. Finish the breast examination by squeezing for nipple discharge and palpating the breast into the axillary area. f. Report any abnormalities or changes to the physician. ***Recognize that this may be embarrassing for some patients and remain sensitive to their feelings and needs. Prior to leaving the examination room, ask the patient if she has any questions.***				
4. ★	Document your patient instruction in breast self-examination. Note the patient's level of understanding. ***Sign the entry with your name and credentials.***				
5. ✦	Perform any necessary cleaning of teaching models and store for the next patient use.				

Document: Enter the correct information in the chart below.

Grading

Points Earned	_____		
Points Possible	_____	36	36
Percent Grade (Points Earned/Points Possible)	_____		
PASS:	_____	❏ YES ❏ NO ❏ N/A	❏ YES ❏ NO ❏ N/A

Instructor Sign-Off

Instructor: _____   **Date:** _____

Name: _____

Date: _____

Procedure 44-3:

Assist the Physician in the Performance of a Pelvic Examination and Pap Test

Objective: The student, using the supplies and equipment listed below, will demonstrate how to assist the physician during the performance of a pelvic examination and pap test.

Supplies: Patient chart; examination gloves; water-soluble lubricant; physician's gown and eye protection; vaginal speculum; gooseneck or other light source; slide container, glass slides, marker to label slides, and slide fixative for pap smear; cervical/spatula scraper, cotton-tipped applicators, lab requisition form

Affective Behaviors: Affective behaviors provide a professional approach to a skill that enhances the patient encounter. These behaviors may also display sensitivity to a patient's rights and enhance communication. Pay close attention to these skills, which will be in ***bold, italicized*** font.

Notes to the Student

_____

_____

_____

_____

_____

_____

Skills Assessment Requirements

Read and familiarize yourself with the procedure; complete the minimum practice requirements. Document each MPR using proper charting technique. Complete each procedure within a reasonable amount of time, with a minimum of 85 percent accuracy.

POINT VALUE ✦ = 3–6 points ★ = 7–9 points		PRACTICE TRIAL	GRADED TRIAL # 1	GRADED TRIAL # 2	NOTES
1. ✦	Wash your hands and assemble the equipment. Label the slide containers with patient information. Label the frosted edge of each slide with patient information and the location from which the specimen was taken.				
2. ★	**Greet and identify the patient and escort her to the examination room. Introduce yourself to the patient.** Obtain the mensuration required by the physician (usually weight, temperature, blood pressure, pulse, and respirations).				
3. ✦	Interview the patient for the following information: • Chief complaint (reason for visit) • Medications and known allergies • Start date of last menstrual period • Date of most recent pap smear				
4. ✦	**Explain the procedure to the patient.**				
5. ✦	Before the procedure, assist the patient to the bathroom to void.				
6. ★	When the patient returns to the examination room, instruct her to remove clothing from the waist down. Assist as necessary. Provide a drape for the body from the waist down. If a breast examination is also to be performed, the patient will need to completely disrobe. Provide a gown cover for the chest area as well. The patient may sit on the examination table or lie comfortably until the physician arrives.				

		PRACTICE TRIAL	GRADED TRIAL # 1	GRADED TRIAL # 2	NOTES
7. ✦	When the physician is present, assist the patient into a supine/dorsal recumbent position if a breast exam is to be performed. Slide the patient toward the stirrups and into the lithotomy position for the remainder of the pelvic examination and the pap test.				
8. ⋆	*This is often an uncomfortable procedure for women; be sensitive to their needs. Observe the patient's tolerance of the procedure* and hand the slides, cervical/spatula scraper, and cotton-tipped applicators to the physician for the pap smear. After the physician has placed the specimen on the slides, immediately spray or apply ethyl alcohol liquid fixative. Give the physician water-soluble lubricant for the pelvic examination.				
9. ✦	When the procedure has been completed, assist the patient to a sitting position. *Leave the room to allow her to dress in private, or assist if necessary. Prior to leaving the examination room, ask the patient if she has any questions.*				
10. ✦	Remove the used implements to the cleaning area. Dispose of disposable and biohazardous materials in the appropriate containers. Wash your hands				

		PRACTICE TRIAL	GRADED TRIAL # 1	GRADED TRIAL # 2	NOTES
11. ✦	Transport the labeled specimen to the laboratory, or arrange for transport, with the appropriate lab requisitions. Assist the patient with the scheduling of additional procedures, if necessary.				
12. ★	Document the patient's response to the procedure, any future appointments, and other patient information, including prescriptions or patient instruction. **Sign the entry with your name and credentials.**				

Name: _____

Date: _____

Document: Enter the correct information in the chart below.

Grading

Points Earned	_____		
Points Possible	_____	84	84
Percent Grade (Points Earned/Points Possible)	_____		
PASS:	_____	❏ YES ❏ NO ❏ N/A	❏ YES ❏ NO ❏ N/A

Instructor Sign-Off

Instructor: _____ Date: _____

Procedure 44-4:

Perform a Urine Pregnancy Test

Objective: The student, using the supplies and equipment listed below, will demonstrate how to test a patient's urine for the presence of hCG.

Supplies: Gloves, urine sample, hCG test, hCG positive urine control, hCG negative urine control, timer, disinfectant, patient chart

Affective Behaviors: Affective behaviors provide a professional approach to a skill that enhances the patient encounter. These behaviors may also display sensitivity to a patient's rights and enhance communication. Pay close attention to these skills, which will be in **_bold, italicized_** font.

Notes to the Student

_____

_____

_____

_____

_____

_____

Skills Assessment Requirements

Read and familiarize yourself with the procedure; complete the minimum practice requirements. Document each MPR using proper charting technique. Complete each procedure within a reasonable amount of time, with a minimum of 85 percent accuracy.

Name: _____

Date: _____

POINT VALUE ✦ = 3–6 points ⋆ = 7–9 points		PRACTICE TRIAL	GRADED TRIAL # 1	GRADED TRIAL # 2	NOTES
1. ✦	Assemble all necessary equipment.				
2. ✦	Wash your hands and put on gloves.				
3. ⋆	Follow the manufacturer's directions for using the negative control serum.				
4. ✦	When you are satisfied that the tests are reliable, test the patient's urine sample.				
5. ✦	Report the results to the physician.				
6. ✦	Disinfect the work area.				
7. ⋆	Document the test and results in the patient's chart. ***Sign the entry with your name and credentials.***				

Name: _____

Date: _____

Document: Enter the correct information in the chart below.

Grading

Points Earned	_____		
Points Possible	_____	48	48
Percent Grade (Points Earned/Points Possible)	_____		
PASS:	_____	❏ YES ❏ NO ❏ N/A	❏ YES ❏ NO ❏ N/A

Instructor Sign-Off

Instructor: _____   Date: _____

Name: _____

Date: _____

Procedure 44-5:

Assist with Cryosurgery

Objective: The student, using the supplies and equipment listed below, will demonstrate how to assist with a cryosurgery.

Supplies: Gloves, patient drapes, light source, liquid nitrogen, vaginal speculum, sterile specimen container (if needed), patient chart

Affective Behaviors: Affective behaviors provide a professional approach to a skill that enhances the patient encounter. These behaviors may also display sensitivity to a patient's rights and enhance communication. Pay close attention to these skills, which will be in **_bold, italicized_** font.

Notes to the Student

_____

_____

_____

_____

_____

_____

Skills Assessment Requirements

Read and familiarize yourself with the procedure; complete the minimum practice requirements. Document each MPR using proper charting technique. Complete each procedure within a reasonable amount of time, with a minimum of 85 percent accuracy.

Name: _____

Date: _____

POINT VALUE ✦ = 3–6 points ⋆ = 7–9 points		PRACTICE TRIAL	GRADED TRIAL #1	GRADED TRIAL #2	NOTES
1. ⋆	**Greet the patient, introduce yourself and verify the patient's identification.**				
2. ✦	**Explain the procedure to the patient.**				
3. ✦	If necessary, assist the patient in undressing from the waist down. **Provide proper patient drapes.**				
4. ✦	When the patient is undressed and draped, assist her into the lithotomy position. **Reassure the patient, as this can be an uncomfortable procedure for a woman.**				
5. ⋆	Assist the physician as needed.				
6. ✦	**Reassure the patient that as the probe moves over the affected tissue and the liquid nitrogen freezes and kills the tissue, she will feel some discomfort, similar to menstrual cramping. The discomfort should not be unbearable, however.**				
7. ✦	After the procedure, assist the patient to a seated position and help her dress as needed. **Prior to leaving the examination room, ask the patient if she has any questions.**				
8. ✦	Clean and disinfect the room.				

Name: _____

Date: _____

Document: Enter the correct information in the chart below.

Grading

Points Earned	_____		
Points Possible	_____	54	54
Percent Grade (Points Earned/Points Possible)	_____		
PASS:	_____	❏ YES ❏ NO ❏ N/A	❏ YES ❏ NO ❏ N/A

Instructor Sign-Off

Instructor: _____ Date: _____

Procedure 45-1:

Perform and Record Measurements of Height or Length, Weight, and Head or Chest Circumference

Objective: The student, using the supplies and equipment listed below, will demonstrate how to measure the child's length (height), weight, and head and/or chest circumference.

Supplies: Plastic or paper tape measure, infant or platform scale, stadiometer, growth charts, patient chart

Affective Behaviors: Affective behaviors provide a professional approach to a skill that enhances the patient encounter. These behaviors may also display sensitivity to a patient's rights and enhance communication. Pay close attention to these skills, which will be in **bold, italicized** font

Notes to the Student

_____

_____

_____

_____

_____

_____

Skills Assessment Requirements

Read and familiarize yourself with the procedure; complete the minimum practice requirements. Document each MPR using proper charting technique. Complete each procedure within a reasonable amount of time, with a minimum of 85 percent accuracy.

Name: _____

Date: _____

POINT VALUE ✦ = 3–6 points ⋆ = 7–9 points		PRACTICE TRIAL	GRADED TRIAL #1	GRADED TRIAL #2	NOTES
1. ✦	Wash your hands and gather equipment and supplies.				
2. ⋆	**Greet and identify the parent or guardian with the child and guide them to the treatment area. Introduce yourself to the parent or guardian.**				
3. ✦	Remove all clothing except the diaper before weighing. **Recognize the necessity to remain calm and attentive to the patient and parent/guardian.**				
4. ✦	Weigh the child on the platform scale.				
5. ⋆	Record the weight on the growth charts and/or progress notes within the child's chart.				
6. ✦	Wash your hands.				
7. ✦	Move or ask the parent or guardian to move the child to the exam table.				
8. ✦	Measure the length of the child.				
9. ⋆	Record the height on the growth charts and/or progress notes within the child's chart.				
10. ✦	Measure the child's head circumference.				
11. ⋆	Record the head circumference on the growth charts and/or progress notes within the child's chart.				
12. ✦	Measure the child's chest circumference, if necessary.				

		PRACTICE TRIAL	GRADED TRIAL # 1	GRADED TRIAL # 2	NOTES
13. ★	Record the chest circumference on the growth charts and/or progress notes within the child's chart.				
14. ✦	Tell the physician that the child is ready.				
15. ✦	After the physician has examined the child, tell the parent or guardian to redress the child. **Prior to leaving the examination room, ask the parent/guardian if he or she has any questions.**				
16. ✦	Dispose of disposables.				
17. ✦	Clean the room. Wash your hands.				

Name: _____

Date: _____

Document: Enter the correct information in the chart below.

Grading

Points Earned	_____		
Points Possible	_____	117	117
Percent Grade (Points Earned/Points Possible)	_____		
PASS:	_____	❏ YES ❏ NO ❏ N/A	❏ YES ❏ NO ❏ N/A

Instructor Sign-Off

Instructor: _____ **Date:** _____

Name: _____

Date: _____

Procedure 45-2:

Perform and Record Pediatric Vital Signs and Vision Screening

Objective: The student, using the supplies and equipment listed below, will demonstrate how to measure a child's temperature, pulse, respirations, and blood pressure and perform a vision screening test.

Supplies: Pediatric blood pressure cuff, Snellen E chart, watch with a sweeping second hand, digital thermometer, patient chart

Affective Behaviors: Affective behaviors provide a professional approach to a skill that enhances the patient encounter. These behaviors may also display sensitivity to a patient's rights and enhance communication. Pay close attention to these skills, which will be in **bold, *italicized*** font.

Notes to the Student

_____

_____

_____

_____

_____

_____

Skills Assessment Requirements

Read and familiarize yourself with the procedure; complete the minimum practice requirements. Document each MPR using proper charting technique. Complete each procedure within a reasonable amount of time, with a minimum of 85 percent accuracy.

Name: _____

Date: _____

POINT VALUE ✦ = 3–6 points ★ = 7–9 points		PRACTICE TRIAL	GRADED TRIAL # 1	GRADED TRIAL # 2	NOTES
	Pulse, respirations, axillary temperature, and blood pressure:				
1. ✦	Gather equipment and supplies. Wash your hands.				
2. ★	***Greet and identify the patient, introduce yourself and explain the procedure to the parent or guardian.***				
3. ✦	Have the parent disrobe the child down to the diaper. ***Recognize and communicate with the patient at his or her own level of understanding.***				
4. ✦	Place the child in the supine position or allow him or her to remain in the parent's lap for greater compliance.				
5. ★	Locate the apex of the heart by feeling for the fifth intercostal space to the left of the sternum on the midclavicular line.				
6. ✦	Make sure the stethoscope head is warmed and place it on the space, listening for the "lub-dub" of the heart. Count for 1 minute (each lub-dub equals one beat).				
7. ✦	Record the results.				
8. ✦	Place your hand on the child's chest and count inspirations and expirations for 1 minute. The rise and fall of the chest is counted as one breath.				
9. ★	Record the results.				

		PRACTICE TRIAL	GRADED TRIAL # 1	GRADED TRIAL # 2	NOTES
10. ✦	Take the temperature probe and apply a disposable sheath.				
11. *	Place the probe in the infant's axillary space, holding the child's arm down close to his or her side.				
12. ✦	Wait for the beep to indicate the reading has been completed, then dispose of the probe cover.				
13. *	Record the results.				
14. ✦	If the physician orders that blood pressure be taken, follow the directions for taking an adult BP reading.				
15. ✦	Palpate the blood pressure first to avoid over-inflating the cuff. Make sure the cuff size is correct for the patient size.				
16. *	Record the results.				
	Vision screening:				
17. ✦	Take the child to the vision screening area, accompanied by the parent. Explain the chart and ask the child to stand at the correct distance from the chart. (Each chart indicates the recommended distance.)				

		PRACTICE TRIAL	GRADED TRIAL # 1	GRADED TRIAL # 2	NOTES
18. *	Have the child cover one eye and read as many lines as possible. If the child misses two objects, directions, or letters in a single line, stop the test and record the line number. For example, if the child reads line 20/20 correctly with the left eye but misses multiple letters on line 20/15, the vision would be 20/20 in the left eye.				
19. ✦	Repeat the procedure for the other eye, then both eyes reading together. *Escort the patient back to the examination room if necessary. Ask the parent/guardian if he or she has any questions prior to leaving the examination room.*				
20. *	Record the results in the patient's chart. *Sign the completed entry with your name and credentials.*				

Name: _____

Date: _____

Document: Enter the correct information in the chart below.

● Grading

Points Earned	_____		
Points Possible	_____	144	144
Percent Grade (Points Earned/Points Possible)	_____		
PASS:	_____	❏ YES ❏ NO ❏ N/A	❏ YES ❏ NO ❏ N/A

Instructor Sign-Off

Instructor: _____ **Date:** _____

Name: _____

Date: _____

Procedure 45-3:

Perform Documentation of Immunization, Both Stored and Administered

Objective: The student, using the supplies and equipment listed below, will demonstrate how to provide the parent or guardian instruction and give childhood immunizations.

Supplies: Vaccine information sheets (VIS), vaccination dosage, sterile gloves, patient chart

Affective Behaviors: Affective behaviors provide a professional approach to a skill that enhances the patient encounter. These behaviors may also display sensitivity to a patient's rights and enhance communication. Pay close attention to these skills, which will be in ***bold, italicized*** font

Notes to the Student

_____

_____

_____

_____

_____

_____

Skills Assessment Requirements

Read and familiarize yourself with the procedure; complete the minimum practice requirements. Document each MPR using proper charting technique. Complete each procedure within a reasonable amount of time, with a minimum of 85 percent accuracy.

Name: _____

Date: _____

POINT VALUE ✦ = 3–6 points ✱ = 7–9 points		PRACTICE TRIAL	GRADED TRIAL #1	GRADED TRIAL #2	NOTES
1. ✦	Wash your hands. Gather the equipment and supplies.				
2. ✱	**Greet and identify the parent or guardian with the child, introduce yourself and guide them to the treatment area.**				
3. ✦	Ask the parent or guardian about the child's recent health and if there is medical history that would exclude the child temporarily or permanently from any of the immunizations.				
4. ✱	Provide vaccine information sheets for each immunization to be given. **Ask the parent/ guardian if he or she has any questions prior to administering the vaccines.**				
5. ✦	Take and record the child's vital signs.				
6. ✦	After the physician has seen the patient, wash your hands and put on gloves.				
7. ✦	Administer the immunizations.				
8. ✦	Dispose of sharp or biohazardous materials in the appropriate containers.				
9. ✦	Wash your hands. **Ensure that the parent/guardian does not have any more questions prior to leaving the examination room.**				
10. ✱	Document on the child's immunization record for the parent or guardian and on the child's chart. **Sign the entry with your name and credentials.**				

Name: _____

Date: _____

Document: Enter the correct information in the chart below.

Grading

Points Earned	_____		
Points Possible	_____	69	69
Percent Grade (Points Earned/Points Possible)	_____		
PASS:	_____	❏ YES ❏ NO ❏ N/A	❏ YES ❏ NO ❏ N/A

Instructor Sign-Off

Instructor: _____   **Date:** _____

Name: _____

Date: _____

Procedure 45-4:

Perform Urine Collection with a Pediatric Urine Collection Bag

Objective: The student, using the supplies and equipment listed below, will demonstrate how to collect a urine specimen in a urine collection bag.

Supplies: Urine collection bag for newborn or pediatric patient, sterile gloves, sterile container with label, cotton balls, prepackaged sterile cleansing swabs or towelettes, laboratory requisition form, patient chart

Affective Behaviors: Affective behaviors provide a professional approach to a skill that enhances the patient encounter. These behaviors may also display sensitivity to a patient's rights and enhance communication. Pay close attention to these skills, which will be in **bold, *italicized*** font.

Notes to the Student

_____

_____

_____

_____

_____

_____

Skills Assessment Requirements

Read and familiarize yourself with the procedure; complete the minimum practice requirements. Document each MPR using proper charting technique. Complete each procedure within a reasonable amount of time, with a minimum of 85 percent accuracy.

POINT VALUE ✦ = 3–6 points ✭ = 7–9 points		PRACTICE TRIAL	GRADED TRIAL # 1	GRADED TRIAL # 2	NOTES
1. ✦	Wash your hands. Gather the equipment and supplies.				
2. ✭	**Identify the parent or guardian with the child and guide them to the treatment area. Introduce yourself and explain the procedure to the parent or guardian.**				
3. ✦	Put on sterile gloves.				
4. ✦	Remove the diaper and dispose of it in the appropriate container. **Demonstrate sensitivity by trying to maintain the patient's modesty during this procedure.**				
5. ✭	Wipe the child's genital area with sterile towelettes or cleansing swabs. For boy infants, wipe around and away from the urinary meatus. For girl infants, wipe from the clitoris toward the rectal area. Repeat the wipe with a separate towelette or cleansing swab a second and third time to cleanse the area immediately surrounding the urinary meatus, then cleanse the wider surrounding area.				
6. ✦	Dry the cleansed area with dry cotton balls.				
7. ✦	Remove the adhesive tabs of the urine collection bag and apply the bag to the genital area securely, without gaps between the tabs and the skin.				
8. ✦	Diaper the child.				
9. ✦	Wash your hands.				

		PRACTICE TRIAL	GRADED TRIAL # 1	GRADED TRIAL # 2	NOTES
10. ✦	Instruct the parent or guardian to encourage the infant or toddler to drink or nurse.				
11. ✦	Recheck the diaper every 20 minutes until a specimen is obtained in the bag.				
12. *	Wash your hands and put on sterile gloves.				
13. ✦	Remove the urine collection bag. Place the bagged urine specimen in the sterile cup and cover the container tightly.				
14. ✦	Diaper the child. *Prior to leaving the examination room, ask the parent/guardian if he or she has any questions.*				
15. ✦	Remove the gloves and wash your hands.				
16. *	Prepare the container label and laboratory requisition. Transport or arrange for transport of the specimen to the laboratory.				
17. *	Document the procedure in the child's chart. *Sign the entry with your name and credentials.*				
18. ✦	Dispose of biohazardous materials in the proper containers.				
19. ✦	Clean the area. Wash your hands.				

Name: _____

Date: _____

Document: Enter the correct information in the chart below.

Grading

Points Earned	_____		
Points Possible	_____	129	129
Percent Grade (Points Earned/Points Possible)	_____		
PASS:	_____	❏ YES ❏ NO ❏ N/A	❏ YES ❏ NO ❏ N/A

Instructor Sign-Off

Instructor: _____ **Date:** _____

Procedure 46-1:

Assisting in a Neurological Exam

Objective: The student, using the supplies and equipment listed below, will demonstrate how to assist with a neurological exam.

Supplies: Reflex hammers; penlight; pinwheel; tongue blade; tuning fork; ophthalmoscope; cold object, as determined by physician; warm object, as determined by physician; scent object (coffee grounds, for example), as determined by physician; patient drapes as determined by office protocol; patient chart

Affective Behaviors: Affective behaviors provide a professional approach to a skill that enhances the patient encounter. These behaviors may also display sensitivity to a patient's rights and enhance communication. Pay close attention to these skills, which will be in ***bold, italicized*** font

Notes to the Student

_____

_____

_____

_____

_____

_____

Skills Assessment Requirements

Read and familiarize yourself with the procedure; complete the minimum practice requirements. Document each MPR using proper charting technique. Complete each procedure within a reasonable amount of time, with a minimum of 85 percent accuracy.

Name: _____

Date: _____

POINT VALUE ✦ = 3–6 points ⋆ = 7–9 points		PRACTICE TRIAL	GRADED TRIAL # 1	GRADED TRIAL # 2	NOTES
1. ✦	Wash your hands and gather equipment and supplies.				
2. ⋆	**Greet and identify patient. Introduce yourself and escort patient to examination room.**				
3. ✦	Interview the patient according to office protocol. Ask standard questions such as: • What is your full name? • Who is the current president of the United States? • What is the date, including the month and year?				
4. ✦	If your office protocol requires patients to change into cotton shorts and a tank top, assist the patient as necessary.				
5. ✦	Provide patient drapes as needed. **Recognize the importance of being sensitive to the patient's feelings regarding modesty.**				
6. ⋆	Follow office protocol for assisting the patient into the required positions. If the physician tests reflexes with a hammer first, assist the patient into a seated position on the exam table. Have the patient remove socks and shoes in preparation for testing the Babinski reflex.				
7. ✦	After the physician has finished reflex testing, assist the patient to dress, as needed. Escort the patient to the gait-and-movement testing area.				
8. ⋆	Document any changes in the patient chart. **Sign the entry with your name and credentials.**				

Name: _____

Date: _____

Document: Enter the correct information in the chart below.

Grading

Points Earned	_____		
Points Possible	_____	57	57
Percent Grade (Points Earned/Points Possible)	_____		
PASS:	_____	❏ YES ❏ NO ❏ N/A	❏ YES ❏ NO ❏ N/A

Instructor Sign-Off

Instructor: _____ **Date:** _____

Procedure 46-2:

Assisting with a Lumbar Puncture

Objective: The student, using the supplies and equipment listed below, will demonstrate how to assist the physician with a lumbar puncture to obtain CSF.

Supplies: Lumbar puncture kit: iodine antiseptic, iodine applicator, adhesive bandages, spinal puncture needle, four testing tubes, patient drape, BP cuff, manometer, xylocaine 1–2%, syringe and needle for anesthetic, sterile gloves, gauze sponges, fenestrated drape

Affective Behaviors: Affective behaviors provide a professional approach to a skill that enhances the patient encounter. These behaviors may also display sensitivity to a patient's rights and enhance communication. Pay close attention to these skills, which will be in **_bold, italicized_** font

Notes to the Student

_____

_____

_____

_____

_____

_____

Skills Assessment Requirements

Read and familiarize yourself with the procedure; complete the minimum practice requirements. Document each MPR using proper charting technique. Complete each procedure within a reasonable amount of time, with a minimum of 85 percent accuracy.

POINT VALUE ✦ = 3–6 points ⋆ = 7–9 points	PRACTICE TRIAL	GRADED TRIAL #1	GRADED TRIAL #2	NOTES
1. ✦ Wash your hands and gather equipment and supplies.				
2. ⋆ **Greet and identify patient. Introduce yourself and escort patient to examination room.**				
3. ✦ Interview the patient according to office protocol. Ask standard questions such as: • What is your full name? • Who is the current president of the United States? • What is the date, including the month and year?				
4. ✦ If your office protocol requires patients to change into cotton shorts and a tank top, assist the patient as necessary.				
5. ✦ Provide patient drapes as needed. **Recognize the importance of being sensitive to the patient's feelings regarding modesty.**				
6. ⋆ Follow office protocol for assisting the patient into the required positions. If the physician tests reflexes with a hammer first, assist the patient into a seated position on the exam table. Have the patient remove socks and shoes in preparation for testing the Babinski reflex.				
7. ✦ After the physician has finished reflex testing, assist the patient to dress, as needed. Escort the patient to the gait-and-movement testing area.				
8. ⋆ Document any changes in the patient chart. **Sign the entry with your name and credentials.**				

Name: _____

Date: _____

Document: Enter the correct information in the chart below.

Grading

Points Earned	_____		
Points Possible	_____	57	57
Percent Grade (Points Earned/Points Possible)	_____		
PASS:	_____	❏ YES ❏ NO ❏ N/A	❏ YES ❏ NO ❏ N/A

Instructor Sign-Off

Instructor: _____   **Date:** _____

Procedure 46-3:

Prepare a Patient for an Electroencephalogram

Objective: The student, using the supplies and equipment listed below, will demonstrate how to assist the physician with an EEG.

Supplies: EEG machine, electrodes, approved EEG electrode adhesive

Affective Behaviors: Affective behaviors provide a professional approach to a skill that enhances the patient encounter. These behaviors may also display sensitivity to a patient's rights and enhance communication. Pay close attention to these skills, which will be in **bold, italicized** font.

Notes to the Student

_____

_____

_____

_____

_____

Skills Assessment Requirements

Read and familiarize yourself with the procedure; complete the minimum practice requirements. Document each MPR using proper charting technique. Complete each procedure within a reasonable amount of time, with a minimum of 85 percent accuracy.

POINT VALUE ✦ = 3–6 points ★ = 7–9 points		PRACTICE TRIAL	GRADED TRIAL # 1	GRADED TRIAL # 2	NOTES
1. ★	*Identify the patient. Introduce yourself and explain the procedure and why the physician has ordered it. Try to allay any anxiety the patient might be feeling.*				
2. ✦	Verify that the patient has followed pretesting procedures—avoiding caffeine and other stimulants and eating a well balanced diet to avoid hypoglycemia.				
3. ✦	Instruct the patient to remain absolutely motionless during the baseline reading. Even tongue or eyelid movements will alter the baseline.				
4. ★	Connect the electrodes to the patient's scalp with the appropriate adhesive.				
5. ✦	If a sleep EEG has been ordered, the patient should not alter his or her sleeping patterns and avoid using sleep aids.				
6. ✦	The patient will be shown flickering lights to stimulate the brain. This activity will be recorded by the technician.				
7. ✦	Remove the electrodes from the patient's scalp. *If the patient has been lying supine for the exam, help him or her to a sitting position.* The patient should remain seated for a minimum of 1 minute to avoid dizziness caused by orthostatic hypotension. *Ask the patient if he or she has any questions prior to leaving the examination room.*				
8. ★	Document the procedure in the patient's chart. *Sign the entry with your name and credentials.*				

Document: Enter the correct information in the chart below.

Grading

Points Earned	_____		
Points Possible	_____	57	57
Percent Grade (Points Earned/Points Possible)	_____		
PASS:	_____	❏ YES ❏ NO ❏ N/A	❏ YES ❏ NO ❏ N/A

Instructor Sign-Off

Instructor: _____ **Date:** _____

Procedure 49-1:

Role-Play Sensorimotor Changes of the Elderly

Objective: The student, using the supplies and equipment listed below, will demonstrate how to understand the changes that aging patients undergo.

Supplies: Two pairs of laboratory goggles, yellow tissue paper (such as gift wrap), pastel-colored candy, Vaseline, earmuffs, black construction paper, swimming goggles with one lens blacked out, heavy dishwashing gloves, long (50″ or more) belt, walker, tongue depressors, ace bandages, regular print newspaper, coins (pennies and dimes), button-front shirts, textbook, tape, gallon jug of water

Notes to the Student

_____

_____

_____

_____

_____

_____

Skills Assessment Requirements

Read and familiarize yourself with the procedure; complete the minimum practice requirements. Document each MPR using proper charting technique. Complete each procedure within a reasonable amount of time, with a minimum of 85 percent accuracy.

POINT VALUE ✦ = 3–6 points ⋆ = 7–9 points		PRACTICE TRIAL	GRADED TRIAL # 1	GRADED TRIAL # 2	NOTES
1. ✦	**Vision loss:** a. Put on the swimming goggles and wait for your partner's directions. b. Have your partner stand out of the line of vision and give directions to cross the room and pick up a specific textbook.				
2. ✦	**Vision loss accompanied by hearing loss:** a. Continue to wear the swimming goggles and put on the earmuffs. b. Have your partner stand out of the line of sight and tell you to retrieve a different textbook.				
3. ✦	**Difficulty distinguishing colors:** a. Remove the goggles and earmuffs. Put on the laboratory goggles, which should be covered with yellow paper to simulate yellowing of the lens. b. Have your partner spread the pastel candy on a table and give you directions to pick up specific colors and quantities of each color.				
4. ✦	**Difficulty focusing:** a. Put on a set of lab goggles that have been smeared with Vaseline. b. Without speaking, your partner must get you to walk a specific distance using hand signals.				

Name: _____

Date: _____

		PRACTICE TRIAL	GRADED TRIAL # 1	GRADED TRIAL # 2	NOTES
5. ✦	**Loss of peripheral vision:** a. While wearing goggles with black construction paper taped to the sides, have your partner stand out of your line of vision and give you directions to follow. b. Have your partner lead you through several turns and doors if possible.				
6. ✦	**Aphasia and partial paralysis:** a. Bend one arm at the elbow, with your fingertips touching your shoulder. Have another student wrap the ace bandage around your arm, securing it in this position. Bend one leg at the knee with your foot near your buttocks. Have another student secure your leg in place with the belt. Finally, have someone tape your mouth shut. b. Your partner should stand several feet away. Communicate to your partner that you need to go to the bathroom.				
7. ✦	**Loss of dexterity:** a. Put on the dishwashing gloves and try to button a shirt, tie your shoes, and pick up the coins off a flat surface.				
8. ✦	**Problems with mobility:** a. Use a walker to move across the room. b. When you have traveled 2 feet, have your partner hand you a gallon of water to carry.				

1288 APPENDIX

Name: ______________________________

Date: ______________________________

Document: Enter the correct information in the chart below.

Grading

Points Earned	______		
Points Possible	______	48	48
Percent Grade (Points Earned/Points Possible)	______		
PASS:	______	❑ YES ❑ NO ❑ N/A	❑ YES ❑ NO ❑ N/A

Instructor Sign-Off

Instructor: ______________________________ **Date:** ______________

Procedure 51-1:

Write an Effective Resume

Objective: Compose your resume correctly within the time limit set by the instructor.

Supplies: Computer with word processing software

Affective Behaviors: Affective behaviors provide a professional approach to a skill that enhances the patient encounter. These behaviors may also display sensitivity to a patient's rights and enhance communication. Pay close attention to these skills, which will be in **_bold, italicized_** font.

Notes to the Student

_____

_____

_____ ●

_____

_____

_____

Skills Assessment Requirements

Read and familiarize yourself with the procedure; complete the minimum practice requirements. Document each MPR using proper charting technique. Complete each procedure within a reasonable amount of time, with a minimum of 85 percent accuracy.

Name: _____

Date: _____

POINT VALUE ✦ = 3–6 points ★ = 7–9 points		PRACTICE TRIAL	GRADED TRIAL # 1	GRADED TRIAL # 2	NOTES
1. ✦	Choose a resume template in the word processing program.				
2. ✦	Enter your name, address, telephone number, and e-mail address.				
3. ✦	Enter an objective (e.g., "To obtain a position as a certified medical assistant in a medical practice where my skills can be used to their full potential.")				
4. ✦	Enter your educational background, including degrees. **Never exaggerate or falsify this information.**				
5. ✦	Enter your employment history, including dates. **Never exaggerate or falsify this information.**				
6. ✦	List references or a phrase like, "References available upon request."				
7. ★	**Review the document for typographical and grammatical errors.**				
8. ✦	Print the resume on quality paper.				
9. ★	**Review the resume again for typographical and grammatical errors.**				

Name: _____

Date: _____

Document: Enter the correct information in the chart below.

Grading

Points Earned	_____		
Points Possible	_____	60	60
Percent Grade (Points Earned/Points Possible)	_____		
PASS:	_____	❏ YES ❏ NO ❏ N/A	❏ YES ❏ NO ❏ N/A

Instructor Sign-Off

Instructor: _____ Date: _____

Procedure 51-2:

Composing a Cover Letter

Objective: Compose a cover letter correctly within the time limit set by the instructor.

Supplies: Computer with word processing software

Affective Behaviors: Affective behaviors provide a professional approach to a skill that enhances the patient encounter. These behaviors may also display sensitivity to a patient's rights and enhance communication. Pay close attention to these skills, which will be in **_bold, italicized_** font.

Notes to the Student

_____

_____

_____

_____

_____

_____

Skills Assessment Requirements

Read and familiarize yourself with the procedure; complete the minimum practice requirements. Document each MPR using proper charting technique. Complete each procedure within a reasonable amount of time, with a minimum of 85 percent accuracy.

Name: _____

Date: _____

POINT VALUE ✦ = 3–6 points ★ = 7–9 points		PRACTICE TRIAL	GRADED TRIAL # 1	GRADED TRIAL # 2	NOTES
1. ✦	Using the word processing software, enter the date and name, company, and address of the letter recipient.				
2. ★	Compose a letter that addresses the desired job and the reasons the employer should consider you for the position.				
3. ✦	List any information that directly relates to your ability to perform the desired job. ***Never exaggerate or be untruthful about your experience.***				
4. ★	Request an interview.				
5. ✦	State that you will call the employer to follow up in a few days.				

Name: _____

Date: _____

Document: Enter the correct information in the chart below. _____

Grading

Points Earned	_____		
Points Possible	_____	36	36
Percent Grade (Points Earned/Points Possible)	_____		
PASS:	_____	❑ YES ❑ NO ❑ N/A	❑ YES ❑ NO ❑ N/A

Instructor Sign-Off

Instructor: _____ **Date:** _____

Procedure 51-3:

Following Up After an Interview

Objective: Follow up after an interview with a thank-you note to the potential employer correctly within the time limit set by the instructor.

Supplies: Note card, blue or black ink pen

Affective Behaviors: Affective behaviors provide a professional approach to a skill that enhances the patient encounter. These behaviors may also display sensitivity to a patient's rights and enhance communication. Pay close attention to these skills, which will be in **_bold, italicized_** font.

Notes to the Student

_____

_____

_____

_____

_____

_____

Skills Assessment Requirements

Read and familiarize yourself with the procedure; complete the minimum practice requirements. Document each MPR using proper charting technique. Complete each procedure within a reasonable amount of time, with a minimum of 85 percent accuracy.

Name: _____

Date: _____

		PRACTICE TRIAL	GRADED TRIAL # 1	GRADED TRIAL # 2	NOTES
POINT VALUE ✦ = 3–6 points ★ = 7–9 points					
1. ✦	**Handwrite or type a note to the interviewer.**				
2. ✦	Thank the person for the interview time.				
3. ★	List something about the position or office that inspires excitement.				
4. ✦	Express a desire to meet again.				
5. ★	**Send the note 3 to 5 days after the interview.**				

Name: _____

Date: _____

Document: Enter the correct information in the chart below. _____

Grading

Points Earned	_____		
Points Possible	_____	36	36
Percent Grade (Points Earned/Points Possible)	_____		
PASS:	_____	❏ YES ❏ NO ❏ N/A	❏ YES ❏ NO ❏ N/A

Instructor Sign-Off

Instructor: _____ **Date:** _____